AF526852

A COLOUR ATLAS OF WILDLIFE DISEASES AND DISORDERS

B.M. Arora

MVSc, PhD, PGD (J & MC)
Principal Scientist (Wildlife) & Head (Retd.)
Division of Epidemiology & Wildlife Centre
IVRI, Izatnagar, U.P.
Former Director, National Zoological Park, New Delhi

Co-author

A. Chakraborty

MVSc, PhD
Professor of Pathology
College of Veterinary Science
Khanapara, Guwahati, Assam

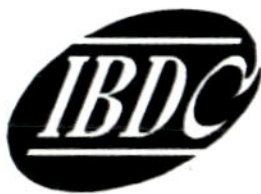

International Book Distributing Co.
(Publishing Division)

Published by

INTERNATIONAL BOOK DISTRIBUTING CO.
(Publishing Division)
Khushnuma Complex Basement
7, Meerabai Marg (Behind Jawahar Bhawan),
Lucknow 226 001 U.P. (INDIA)
Tel. : 91-522-2209542, 2209543, 2209544, 2209545
Fax : 0522-4045308
E-Mail : ibdco@airtelmail.in

First Edition 2009

Price : [illegible]

ISBN 81-8189-244-5

Composed & Designed at :

Panacea Computers
3rd Floor, Agarwal Sabha Bhawan, Subhash Mohal
Sadar Cantt. Lucknow-226 002
Tel. : 0522-2483312, 9335927082, 9452295008
E-mail : prasgupt@rediffmail.com

Printed at:

Salasar Imaging Systems
C-7/5, Lawrence Road Industrial Area
Delhi - 110 035
Tel. : 011-27185653, 9810064311

KARNATAKA
VETERINARY, ANIMAL & FISHERIES SCIENCES
UNIVERSITY
Nandinagar, P.B. No. 6, BIDAR-585 401

Prof. R.N.Sreenivas Gowda
Vice- Chancellor

Office : 08482-245264/9341478770
Fax : 08482-245107
E-mail : vckvafsu@yahoo.co.in
www.kvafsu.kar.nic.in

Foreword

Though disease diagnosis and investigation facilities have become well established in veterinary domestic livestock management science and it is only during the past 3 decades its scientific importance in, in-situ & ex-situ wildlife conservation has been seriously realized. This has been brought by knowledge body which has been built recently by Dr B.M. Arora, Ex Director National Zoological Park, and Principal Scientist (Wildlife) and Head, Div. Epidemiology (IVRI), who has contributed so much to understand wildlife management and their health problems. This is evident from his earlier publications: Rehabilitation in Free living Animals (2007), Indian Wildlife Diseases and Disorders (2003), Reproduction in Wild Mammalia & Conservation (2002), Dietary Husbandry in Wild Mammalia (2001), Restraint & Translocation of Wild Mammalia (2000) and Wildlife Diseases in India (1994). Besides he is editor of Indian Wildlife Yearbook being published by AIZ&WV since, 2002 .His expertise in wildlife has put to good use for professionals and forest officials with the background of wildlife health working in the Zoos, National Parks, and Sanctuaries.

Recognizing his services in wildlife, Ministry of Environment & Forests has encouraged him to help in establishing the Wildlife Health and Disease diagnosis Centers in certain Veterinary Institutes in the country in 2001. He has also been instrumental for strengthening wildlife health and disease monitoring surveillance programmes in India. Thus trend of involvement of professionals in health and husbandry management in-situ and ex-situ wildlife conservation has increased in the country. His contributions in wildlife have also helped in conservation of endangered native wild animal species. It is heartening to see that Dr B.M. Arora has compiled "A Colour Atlas of Wildlife Diseases and Disorders " with full of information having interdisciplinary approach. It is truly compliment since it covers Clinico-pathological illustrations of mammals, birds, reptiles and amphibians. The value of Atlas has increased by macroscopic, microscopic and clinico-pathological studies contributed by many veterinary professionals, who worked on wildlife disease investigation and health management.

I greatly appreciate the co-author Dr Apurba Chakraborty, Professor of Pathology, College of Veterinary science, Guwahati (Assam) for his contribution to this Atlas of Wildlife Diseases and Disorders. I know him personally working him on wildlife pathologist since last two decades and the Indian Association of Veterinary pathologoists had recognized his work with Varsha award in 2002.

. I am sure this Atlas will provide valuable information to professionals engaged in wildlife health, management and conservation. It appears that no body have made any attempts so far in bring out such practical guide for the professionals working in the field of wildlife health, management and conservation. I am confident that this Atlas will serve as useful guide for the all those professionals engaged in disease investigation and diagnosis (including veterolegal aspects), research and academic persuits of in-situ and ex-situ wildlife conservation.

Prof. R.N.Sreenivas Gowda
Vice- Chancellor, KVAFSU

Preface

Presently country has a vast in-situ wildlife network (501 wildlife Sanctuaries, 90 National Parks, 28 tiger reserves (10 more are propsed), 11 elephant reserves) where veterinary science professionals to monitor wildlife health, to evaluate disease carrier status (for example, avian flu, kayasanur disease, plague) in migratory as well as in resident fauna, management and conservation implications to endangered flagship species due to extrinsic and intrinsic factors, care of orphans and destitute, to investigate medico-legal cases, and undertake necropsy investigations etc are woefully inadequate. Once the disease out break occurs in closed species population in a reserve, where survival of species is already at risk and its extinction for forever cannot be ruled out. This compilation will be an eye opener to the conservationists who happen to believe that deaths of wild animals in wildlife habitats are natural and under the misconception that disease has hardly any role in dwindling of their population. For example, death of 73 rhinoceros (*Rhinoceros unicornis*) in Kaziranga National Park, between 2001-2005 due to old age is not convincing. Even they have not learned from loss of 50 percent of tiger (*P.tigris tigris*) in a decade and recently experiencing of heavy mortality in Asiatic lions (*P. leo persica*), gharials (*Gavialis gangeticus*), and vultures (three *Gyps* species), which have been seriously viewed with concern at national and international welfare organizations. Despite woefully inadequate veterinary professionals in ex-situ wildlife management to some extent wildlife healthcare has recently gained momentum after my persistent persuasion to bureaucrats. But still there is lot to be done particularly to provide services to in-situ wildlife network. Indian Veterinary Research Institute (ICAR), Izatnagar, Institute of Animal health, Bangalore and recently established disease insvestigation centres in veterinary Colleges are regularly conducting training, teaching and organizing scientific workshops, symposia and conferences in colloboration with Association of Indian Zoo & Wildlife Veterinarians and Dept of Forests and Animal Husbandry and updating the reference works, documenting and publishing research works have been great steps towards conservation of wildlife diversity by the veterinary professionals. Using advanced methods of diagnoses we may not only eliminate scope of any biased opinion about causative factors of mortality and morbidity but also take timely measures to improve their health and husbandry standards and help in medico-legal cases too. A need to write an Atlas depicting in detail the recorded cases of diseases and disorders encountered in mammalian, avian, and reptilian and amphibian species and to be at the desk of every concerned professional was felt by me. Fortunately, department of science and technology, Govt. of India came forward for financial help in this venture. After tiresome efforts of about 22 months it was possible for me to develop and write "A Colour Atlas of Wildlife Diseases and Disorders " to provide an exhaustive pictorial scientific information to take precedence over the books written on the subject. The Atlas is planned to give an account of clinico-pathological anomalies and diseases attributed for morbidity and mortality captive and free-living vertebrate wildlife but excluding marine species. In general presentation in each chapter proceeds in the following order; development disorders, eco-husbandry related health hazards (physical trauma and chemical poisoning, nutritional and metabolic disorders) health hazards, systemic infectious and parasitic diseases and neoplasms in four different groups of wild fauna namely, mammals, birds, reptiles and amphibians. Practically there appears to been no records of diseases in rodent and insectivore species and bat species except a trifle information in respect of squirrels, porcupines, pangolins. Each chapter per se Animal Orderwise presents a prologue related to species morbidity and mortality conditions illustrated. The photographs received from the contributors are listed with captions and indexed separately with their addresses. References to published works are cited at the end of each chapter.

The Atlas is unique, not only in illustrating and expressing in detail clinical, gross necropsy and laboratory findings of diseases and disorders pictorially in diverse species but entailing their magnitude in two different, in-situ and ex-situ management environments. This would facilitate the research scientist, scholars and academicians in understanding impact of health problem in two different situations and encourage looking further into nutritional, metabolic and genetic disorders in zoological collections particularly in species representing poor gene pools. Thus, Atlas is perspective treasure, likely to aid and guide for the workers of discipline of wildlife health management and those engaged in disease investigation and diagnoses, which are difficult and always involves cumbersome laboratory procedures coupled with field studies. Over all eventually it will be baneful to the field professionals engaged in wildlife health and eco-husbandry management practices. Both the contributors as well as readers are welcome to draw the author's attention to any errors or scope for improvement of this Atlas.

15 August, 2008

B.M.Arora

Acknowledgements

"A Colour Atlas of Wildlife Diseases & Disorders" has been prepared with the financial support to the principal author from Department of Science and Technology, Ministry of Science and Technology, Govt. of India which was processed with kind sanction of the Director CARI (ICAR) - Izatnagar (U.P.) through his account section. I am thankful to Shri J.B.V. Reddy Scientist –B, SERC, Division of the Ministry of Science & Technology, New Delhi, who has been instrument in completion of the formalities with his benevolence and help in preparation of the Atlas.

The Atlas is compilation of contributions of clinico-pathological conditions of wild mammalian, avian, and reptilian and amphibian species belonged to ex-situ and in-situ facilities from many disease investigation and diagnosis scientists, and Zoo & Wildlife Veterinarians who have been duly acknowledged in the publication. I am grateful for their help to enrich the contents of the Atlas.

The author acknowledges with humility and respects the help and cooperation received from IVRI, Izatnagar, State Veterinary Colleges and Wildlife Veterinary Science professionals. Certain case reports appeared in context to wildlife health problems in various Indian journals and periodicals with consent of authors and from print media have been adopted too.

My special thanks are due to Dr. N. S. Parihar, Ex Principal Scientist & Head, Division of Pathology, I.V.R.I. for extending his indispensable and valuable suggestions in preparation of scientific interpretation of pathological illustrations in the Atlas. The inspiration and constant encouragement received from Prof. R.N.Sreenivas Gowda, Vice-Chancellor, KVAFSU has been guiding source in my endurance. I appreciate the help extended by Dr Apurba Chakraborty, Co-author of this Atlas. Last but not the least I am thankful to Dr Sanjay Arora, Assistant Professor, SKUAS& T, Jammu who facilitated the author throughout the period in processing E-mail correspondence with different sources.

Dr. B.M. Arora

CONTENTS

ARTIODACTYLIDS

Introduction

The genera of families of the order- artiodactylida include representative native common and endangered species and subspecies (Table 1). The endangered species such as musk deer, sangai deer, hungul, barasingha, chousingha, Tibetan antelope, mouse deer, Himalayan, nilgiri tahr, ibex, wild buffalo, takin, pigmy hog are listed in schedule 1 of Indian Wildlife Protection Act (IWPA). The common native species are chital, sambar, hog and barking deer, nilgai, and blackbuck, wild boar, which breed prolifically to surplus in captivity. This chapter gives clinco-pathological illustrations of developmental congenital and acquired anomalies, eco-husbandry associated health hazards and infectious and parasitic diseases and neoplasms, attributed for captive and free living artiodactylid species.

Table 1: Common and endangered wild artiodactylid species and subspecies.

SN	Family & Subfamily	Genus	Species/ subspecies
	(A)Ruminants		
1.0	**Family: *Cervidae*** Subfamily: *Cervinae*	*Cervus*	Sambar (*Cervus unicolor*); Sangai (*Cervus eldi eldi*); Barasingha (*Cervus duvauceli duvauceli*); Hangul/Kashmir stag (*Cervus elaphus*)
		Axis	Chital (*Axis axis*); Hog- deer (*Axis porcinus*)
	Subfamily *Muntiacinae*	*Muntiacus*	Barking deer (*Muntiacus muntjak*)
2.0	**Family :*Moschidae***	*Moschus*	Musk deer (*Moschus chrysogaster*)
3.0	**Family :*Tragulidae***	*Tragulus*	Indian chevrotain (*Tragulus meminna*)
4.0	**Family : *Bovidae*** Subfamily: :*Bovinae*	*Bos*	Gaur (*Bos gaurus gaurus*)
		Bubalus	Wild buffalo (*Bubalus bubalis*)
		Anoa	Anoa (*Anoa depressicornis)*
	Subfamily: *Boselaphilnae/ Tragelaphinae*	*Boselaphus*	Blue bull/Nilgai (*Boselaphus tragocamelus)*
		Tetraceros	Chousingha *(Tetraceros quardricornis)*
	Subfamily:*Antilopinae*	*Antilope*	Blackbuck (*Antilope cervicapra*)
		Gazella	Chinkara (*Gazella gazella*)
	Subfamily: *Caprinae* (also includes goat antelopes)	*Capra*	Wild goat (*Capra hircus blythi*); Ibex (*Capra ibex*); Markhor (*Capra falconeri*)
		Hemitragus	Himalayan tahr (*Hemitragus jamlahicus*); Nilgiri tahr (*Hemitragus hylocrius*)
		Nemorhaedus	Goral (*Nemorhaedus goral*)
		Capricornis	Serow (*Capricornis sumatraensis*)
		Budorcas	Takin/Musk oxen (*Budorcas taxicolor*)
		Pantholops	Tibetan antelope/Chiru (*Pantholops. hodgsoni*)
		Ovis	Shapu (*Ovis orientalis*); Nagan (*Ovis ammon hodgsoni*); Bharal (*Pseudois nayaur nayaur*)
4.0	**Family : *Camelidae***	*Camelus*	Bacterian/Two humped camel (*Camelus bacterianus*)
	(B) Non –Ruminants		
6.0	**Family :*Suidae***	*Sus*	Wild pig/boar (*Sus scrofa cristatus*); Pigmy hog(*P.salvania*)

Developmental anomalies : Birth of white (albino) deer and antelopes **(Figures,169a-d)** are recorded more frequently in Zoological Garden, Ahmedabad as compared to other zoos but rarely in natural reserves. Development of antlers or horns in female of the species not possessing them is an abnormal condition related to hormonal imbalance **(Figure 170)**. Deformed antlers and antlers with persisting velvet are recorded in deer and those conditions are due to one of the reasons, like hormonal imbalance, congenital defective testis or castration/ orcheectomy **(Figures 174-178)**. Necropsy of a hog deer (*A. porcinus*) fawn that died after a couple of hours of its birth showed occluded ends of arterial trunks **(Figure 1).** Growths in the nostrils were observed in a stillborn sangai deer (*C. eldi eldi*) fawn **(Figure 23).** Necropsy of a young adult blackbuck (*A. cervicapra*) died in captivity showed presence of a distinct accessory diaphragmatic lobe -a congenital anatomical anomaly **(Figure 24).** No such cases ever recorded in any other artiodactylid species. Morpho – anatomical difference in the form, shape, size and number difference in teeth are recorded frequently in deer and antelope species. Supernumerary teeth **(Figures 56- 58)**, one or two ridges instead of three ridges of equal height but less in diameter, presence of a spur shaped small tooth embedded between the roots of molars with curved roots **(Figure 59)** are the dental anomalies found in deer and antelope species. In case of adult blackbuck (*A. cervicapra*) mandibles, very often contain five cheek teeth **(Figure 62).**

Eco-husbandry associated health hazards : In the early 2008 nearly 5,500 Tibetan gazelles have died during Snow disaster **(Figure 269)** in Ganzi Tibetan Autonomous Prefacture in South Western China (The Tianfu Morning Post, March 15, 2008- Source e-mail ERN of WTI, 4th April, 2008). Tibetan antelope/ Chiru (*Panthelops hodgsoni*) is listed in IWPA. Floods are the major perennial threats in certain in-situ wildlife reserves such as Kaziranga National Park (Assam), Dudwa National Park (Uttar Pradesh) and in certain unplanned captive facilities. To make zoo look natural, water moat barriers in front of animal enclosures/ cages were constructed on the pattern imbibed from the foreign experts, however, it has been observed that enclosures of bovine and cervine species having water moats proved to be death traps for their offsprings, as after couple of hours of birth due to their frolic activities they often accidentally fell in to the water moats and are drowned **(Figure 25).** During a period of 5 years Biological Park, Bhubneshwar had experienced 4.3 per cent mortality in its deer collections due to drowning (Rao and Acharjyo, 1992). Such deaths are due to asphyxiation and fibrillation of heart. Accidental forest fires may cause losses in terrestrial wildlife.

Skin and muscular lacerations, and bone fractures in cervid and bovid species are exceedingly common due to infighting particularly during mating season, and various threat or stress such as capture and restraint **(Figures 54,55,159,194).** Traumatic wounds of skin on different areas **(Figure 195, 212)** and hoofs often aggravate because of crow pecking, and getting invaded by pathogen **(Figures 262 to 265)**. At times rupture of internal vital organ due to goring of horn /antlers may occur in infighting **(Figures 2, 28)**. On any disturbances in the animal cage such as capture operation some traumatic insult is likely to inflict upon the cage denizens. Stealthily entering of stray dog causes commotion to animals' tranquility and as a result group is fragmented into individuals running helter-skelter and several met head-on collision against hard object of the cage/ enclosure or fall in the water moat and get severely injured or die instantaneously due to traumatic shock **(Figures 270 to 273).** Poaching of deer/ antelope for venison with bullet shot directly into the animal heart, lungs, pleura or traumatizing head/ vertebra column **(Figures 214, 215),** although rare, may occurs.

The other management related problems of artiodactylid of zoo, mentioned include asphyxiation due to strangulation of neck in the enclosure fence **(Figure 26),** rumenal impaction due to ingestion of foreign objects and due to formation enteroliths **(Figures 78 to 83)**. Animals that ingested foreign objects always manifest sign of recurrent tympani and also aspiration pneumonia due to regurgitation of ingesta and the condition usually proves fatal particularly when such animal is tranquilized. An environment pollution hazard is recognized in the form of pneumoconiosis **(Figure 27)** in Zoo animals. Histological findings include occurrence of pigmentation as sparse to moderate deposits of brownish black amorphous matter diffusely or aggregates in the alveolar walls and perivascular and peribronchial tissues. In most of the cases these carbon particles were present within the macrophages but massive accumulation may incite fibrosis.Contamination of enclosure substarte with infected animals discharges can not be ruled out.

Nutritional & Metabolic disorders : Massive irregular wears of M_2 and M_3 is more common than in other cheek teeth **(Figures,63 to 73)**, which is mainly due to harsh grinding pressure on them for mastication and chewing of the roughage foods. Heavy wear forms a cavity between the teeth and food is packed therein as debris, which in due course may decay and facilitate anaerobic bacteria to multiply and infect the injured mucosa around. Ingestion of foreign matters from the enclosures and causing gastric trouble in animals is not uncommon in zoological captive facilities **(Figures 78-81)**. Information on food poisoning is scarce. In captivity, excess feeding of shoo babul fodder (*Leucaena leucocephala*) and Soy bean chunks (*Gycine max*) alleged for death in antelopes and deer **(Figure 84)**. Hand reared animals often suffers with some kind of nutritional deficiency **(Figures, 132 a,b)** and are prone to diseases. Lesions of dry deep cracks in the skin mainly from thigh region to stifle joint of blackbuck (*A. cervicapra*) were associated to zinc deficiency as result of feeding mainly on Lucerne **(Figure 197)**. In all 13 animals in a herd of 50 individuals had died in a period of three months in a captive facility located. This appears to be first report of its kind made by College of Veterinary Science, Mumbai. Ingestion of plants, high in oxalate, or diets high in phosphates, is attributed for calculus formation in the kidney. Infections in the urinary tract by urea- splitting organisms may lead to increase ammonia levels and the formation of magnesium-ammonium phosphate stones. Thus, the shape of the calculus also varies however; no such case is presented here.

Lesions of fatty streaks, fibrous plaque/ nodule, intimal thickening, metaplastic change in the large blood vessels **(Figures 6 to 7)** could be of arteriosclerosis/ atheroma related to senility. Pulmonary ossification and mineralization due to metabolic disorders **(Figure 29)** are often-accidental histopathological findings.

Nutritional and senility cataracts have not been specifically identified in zoo artiodactylid species. However, corneal opacity, usually visible grossly, is found in free living and captive antelopes (**Figures 165-166**). Severe traumatic injury due to rubbing against the broken fence of the exhibit may lead to complete damage of the eye **(Figure 167).**

Debility **(Figure 130)** in deer and antelopes in captivity is often either due to intimidation to sub-ordinates by the herd stronger companions and the victims are mostly females as they lack horns for defenseor due to some chronic disease like fasciolasis, tuberculosis, etc. Congenital myopathies or muscle weakness due to vitamin E and selenium deficiencies etc. are likely to occur which generally are identified in the form of abnormal anatomical structures and physiological functions in postnatal life.

Diseases. (A) Infectious & Parasitic : Clinical and gross lesion based diagnoses are made in most of animals barring a few diseases such as tuberculosis, paratuberculosis, foot and mouth disease, rinderpest, rabies, stephanofilirial dermatitis in which they are showing / causing pathogonomic manifestations. The gross and histopathological findings of certain systemic infectious and parasitic diseases are pictorially presented in the chapter and are briefly recounted and interpreted here under.

(a) Cardio-vascular system: There are many septicaemic infectious diseases in which haemorrhage (petechiae) lesions are seen. Such lesions are seen when endothelium is destroyed by bacterial toxins and in viral infections where pathogens replicate in vascular endothelium. Haemorrhagic lesions subcutaneously and in internal organ are also due to damage caused by impact of infighting. Tuberculous pericarditis and endocarditis **(Figures 10 to 12)** concomitant to lung lesions are not uncommon.

Anaplasma infection is demonstrated in the blood smear **(Figure 13)** of captive nilgai (*B. tragocamelus*). It has also been reported from a chital (*A. axis*) died in wild having ectoparasitic dermatitis (Arora, 2003). Trypanosomosis (*Trypanosoma evansi*) is related to impaired vision in a blackbuck **(Figure 14)**. Outbreaks of trypanosomosis in captive and wild deer have been encountered (Arora, 2003). Sarcocystic infection in the cardiac muscle of deer is usually an incidental finding in histopathological examinations **(Figure 15)**.

(b) Respiratory system: Acute to subacute form of pasteurellosis in deer and antelope is caused by *Pasteurella haemolytica* as well as *P. multocida*. The lesions recorded are presented in **Figures 33-36.** A case of pseudotuberculosis (*Corynebacterium ovis*) is recorded in blackbucks (*A. cervicapra*) died in captivity **(Figure 37).** Suppurative bronchopneumonia in deer and bovide species are mainly caused due to tuberculosis. Pulmonary tuberculous lesions in deer and antelopes vary from milliary, caseated bronchopneumonia to granulomatous form **(Figures 39 to 42).** The only pulmonary mycosis recorded is zygomycotic infection in pigmy hog (*Porcula salvania*) and of nasal cavity of hog-deer (*A. porcinus*) died in captivity **(Figures 43 to 44)**. *Balantdium coli* in the lung **(Figure 45)** of giraffe (*Giraffe camelopardus*, an exotic sp.) might have the sequelae of aspiratory pneumonia. Verminous pneumonia due to *Dcityocaulus* sp. infection in a hangul deer (*Cervus elaphus hanglu*) and *Muellerius capillaris* infection in musk deer (*M. crysogaster*), chinkara (*G. gazella*) and blackbuck (*A. cervicapra*) and Strongyloides in barking deer (*Muntiacus muntjack*) were diagnosed histopathologically **(Figures 48 to 51)**. A high occurrence of subclincal mulleriasis in chitals (*A.axis*) inhabiting in tropical environment has already been reported (Arora, 2003).

(c) Digestive system: Periodontitis and dental caries **(Figure 77)** are not uncommon in deer and antelopes in captivity **(Figures 74-75).** Staphylococcous parotiditis was recorded in eland (*Taurotragus oryx*,an exotic sp.) Focal tuberculous lesion in the rumen **(Figure 89)** and generalized lesions involving intestine and mesentery lymph glands in addition to pulmonary lesions in chitals (*A. axis*) and blackbucks (*A. cervicapra*) were due to *Mycobacterium avium* (**Figures 88 to 89**). Paratuberculosis (Johne's disease) is recorded in gaur (*Bos gaurus*) in captivity **(Figure 90)** and in free ranging artiodactylid species (Arora, 2003). Gingivitis with stomatitis **(Figure 91)** in FMD was recorded in antelope. Occurrence of rinderpest (RP) in wild gaurs **(Figure 92)** and in deer in captivity **(Figure 93)** has been known since long. Presently the disease appears to be contained but Peste Des Petitis Ruminants (PPR) and blue tongue species are emerging viral diseases. The latter one has been diagnosed histopathologically in deer **(Figure 94)**. Classical swine fever claimed death of nine (9) wild pigs (*S. scrofa cristatus*) in Gorumara National Park (WB). The lesions included Catarrhal enteritis, haemorrhages and raised circular encrusted lesions like button ulcers mostly on the colon and ceacal **(Figure 95)**. Petechial haemorrhages over the surface of kidneys and enlargement and haemorrhages of the thymus and mesenteric lymph nodes and enlargement of spleen with focal infarcts were also marked.

Intestinal ulcerative lesions related to candidiasis in a blackbuck (*Antelope cervicapra*) and in a sambar (*Cervus unicolor*) and zygomycosis in the latter has been documented. Salmonellosis (*Salmonella enteritidis*) claimed 7 deaths in captive population of pigmy hog (*P. salvania*). Zygomycotic infection was demonstrated concurrently from lesions of necrotic gastritis **(Figure 96).** *Candida albicans* was isolated from ulceration and perforation lesions **(Figure 97)** of duodenum and caseated lymph node of blackbuck (*A. cervicapra*).A variety of hepatitis encountered in artiodactylids dying in captivity were attributed for *E. coli* **(Figures 120-122)** and *Spherophorous necrophorus* **(Figures 123, 124).** Incidence of *Fasciola gigantica* **(Figures 125-127)** in cheetal (*A.axis*)belonged to certain zoos has been found to be high.

Immature *Amphistom sp.* **(Figures 100 to 103),** adult tapeworms in the intestine and single to multiple cysticerci (*Cysticercus tenuicollis*) attached to mesentery **(Figure 104 to 106) a**nd *Oesophagostomum* sp**. (Figure 107)** in intestine were recorded atgross necropsy examinations in certain artiodactylid species. An abomasum specimen of nilgai (*B.tragocamelus*) showed *Ashworthius mertinagliae* **(Figure 109)**. *Gongylonema* sp. in oral cavity **(Figure 110)** of giraffe (*G. camelopardus,* an exotic sp.) and in oesophagus **(Figure111)** of chital (A. axis) were identified in histparasitological studies.

(d) Urinary system: Wild artiodactylids are also susceptible to bacterial pathogens like *Corynebacterium renale, Actinomyces pyogenes, Streptococcus sp, Leptospira sp., Mycobacterium sp.,* may cause nephritis and cystitis Focal tuberculous abscess in the medulla of kidney was noticed in a chital (*Axis axis*) died of generalized form of disease **(Figure 137).**

Renal amyloidosis has been described in certain mammalian species (deer, large cats). It has been found in histopathological examinations as concomitant finding, in case of deer and antelope **(Figure 113).**

(e) Reproductive system: Endometritis, metritis, vaginitis have been recorded at necropsy **(Figures 156-157)** and cases of abortion, still birth and other reproductive disorders though encountered in captive cervids and bovids, however could not be investigated for the causative infectious agents.

(f) Nervous system: In a serow (*C. sumataraensus*) died in captivity lesion of encephalomalacia with congestion and demyelination **(Figure 160)** was recorded, but without relating to its cause. Tuberculous lesions in the brain were found in a chital (*A. axis*) died of generalized form of the disease **(Figure 161)**. Severe meningeal congestion in wild boar (*S. scrofa*) died of swine fever was recorded **(Figure 162).** Specimen collected from cerebrum of a Beisa oryx (*Beisa oryx,* an exotic sp.) died at National Zoological Park after a prolonged illness marked for loss of vision and circling movement (Gid) was identified as *Cysticercus tenuicollis* **(Figure 164)**.

(g) Sense organs: Ophthalmic problems in Indian wild artiodactylid species are poorly studied. Two cases of corneal opacity diagnosed in antelope species are only gross observations **(Figures 165 - 166).** *Trypanosoma evansi* in blood smear of a blackbuck (*A. cervicapra*) suffering from corneal opacity was found **(Figure 14).** Conjunctivitis / severe congestion **(Figure 168)** was also observed in addition to other clinical signs in a gaur (*B. gaurus*) suffering from pasteurellosis.

(h) Integumentary: Foot lesions due to foot and mouth disease (FMD) appear to be more severe in gaur, deer, antelopes and wild boars **(Figures 188 to 192)** as compared to oral lesions. Deformity of hooves as sequel to FMD occurred in wild hog-deer (*A. porcinus*). Foot rot **(Figure 187)** outbreak has been recorded in deer inhibiting Bandipur Reserve. Suppurative lesions of hoofs in deer species are encountered as a result of supervening of traumatic injury of skin and hoofs **(Figures 253,263-265).** *Stephanofilaria* outbreak in captive stock of barking deer (*Muntiacus muntjak*) has been documented. The lesions in six deer caused were formation of small nodules on the face and groin region mainly **(Figure 200).** In wild sambar (C. *unicolour*) and nilgai (*Bos tragocamelus*) ear sore lesions **(Figure 201)** were related to *Stephanofilaria* infection. Nodular swellings often seen are suppurative lesion due to secondary Infection. Not many external dermal mycotic infections have been diagnosed. *Hypoderma dianna* **(Figure 203)** infestation of dermis is recorded in hog-deer (*A. porcinus*). In the species lesions of dermatitis and folliculitis with calcified mite (scabies) have also been demonstrated histologically **(Figure 202)**. Severe infestation of ticks **(Figure 204)** was recorded in wild boar (*Sus scrofa cristatus*).

(i) Musculo-Skeletal system: *Staphylococcus aureus* infection causing alveolar bone recession and mandibular (suppurative) osteitis **(Figure 228)** are recorded in deer. The bones and the joints of chitals (*A. axis*) in captivity died of generalized tuberculosis have been recorded **(Figures 268 to 269)**.

(B) Neoplasms : Illustrations of respiratory tract neoplasms of includeded are, cystadenocarcinoma **(Figure 52)** of nasal chamber of frontonasal region of sangi deer (*C. eldi eldi*) and squamous cell carcinoma **(Figure 53)** of ethmoid region in sika deer (*Cervus nippon*, an exotic sp.). One case each of hepatocellular carcinoma **(Figure 128)** and adenocarcinoma of liver **(Figure 129)** were diagnosed in wild chitals *(A. axis*), which appear to be first reports in wild deer. Gross appearance of adenocarcinomatous growth in the uterus of an adult female hog- deer (*A.porcinus*) died in captivity is presented **(Figure 158)**.

There is hardly any report on the bone neoplasms in Indian wild artiodactylid species. Based on radiological examination a specimen of fused radius and ulna of chital (*A. axis*) showing irregular spongy mass suggestive of tumourous growth **(Figure 267)** was observed. Similarly based on radiological findings of periosteal thickening of radius bone of wild blackbuck (*A. cervicapra*) was diagnosed for bone tumour **(Figure 268)**.

Figure 1: Photograph of heart of a stillborn hog-deer (*A. porcinus*) showing arterial trunk incompletely developed. Note occluded ends.

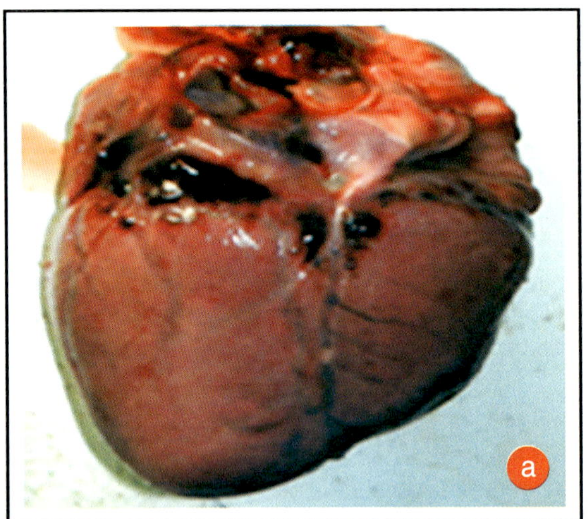

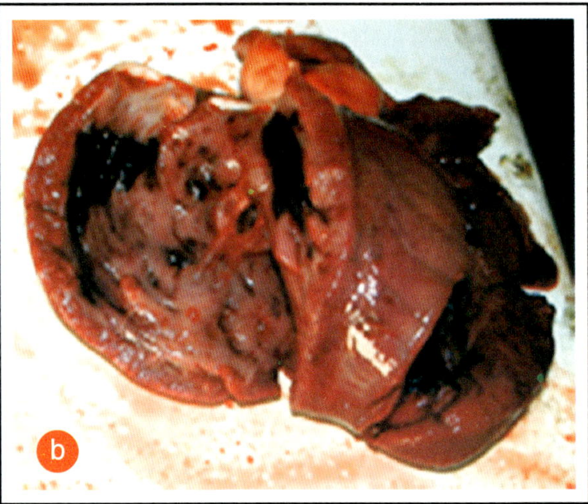

Figure 2: Photograph of heart of blackbuck (*A. cervicapra*) showing haemorrhagic lesion of (a) epicardium and (b) endocardium caused due to horns gored by a stronger male.

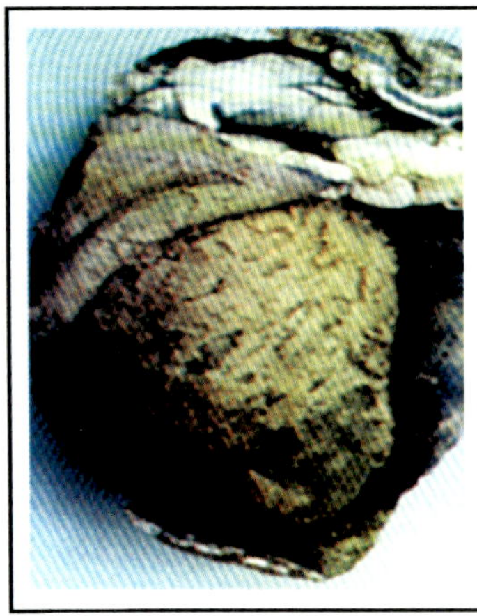

Figure 3: Photograph showing truamatic pericarditis in sika deer (*Cervus nippon*, an exotic sp.). (Rao & Acharjyo, 2003)

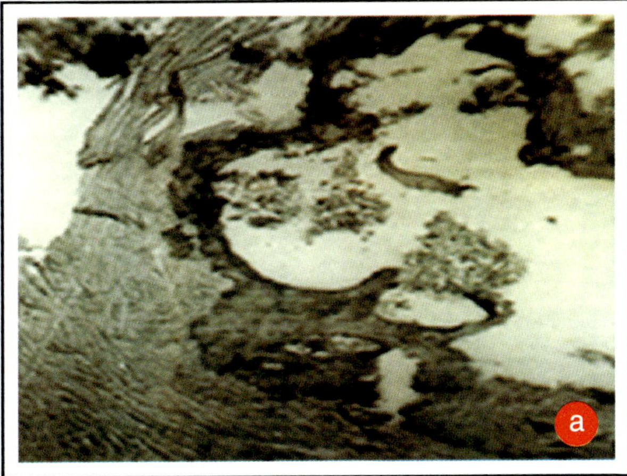

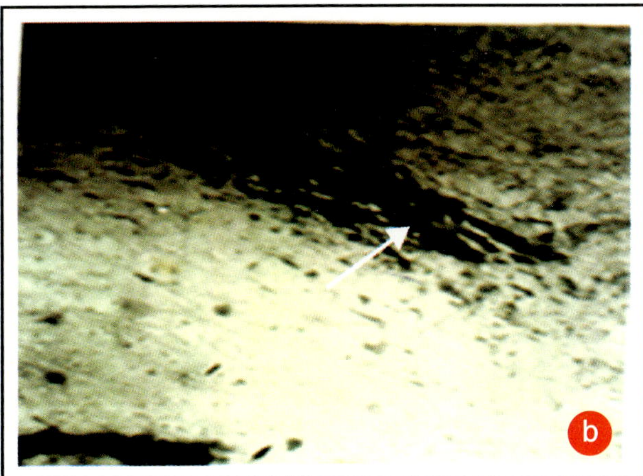

Figure 4: (a) Photomicrograph showing metaplastic changes in the artioventricular septa of heart of sambar (*C. unicolor*). H&E,x140. (b) Photomicrograph showing calcified lesion in the aorta of blackbuck (*A. cervicapra*). H & E, x 140.

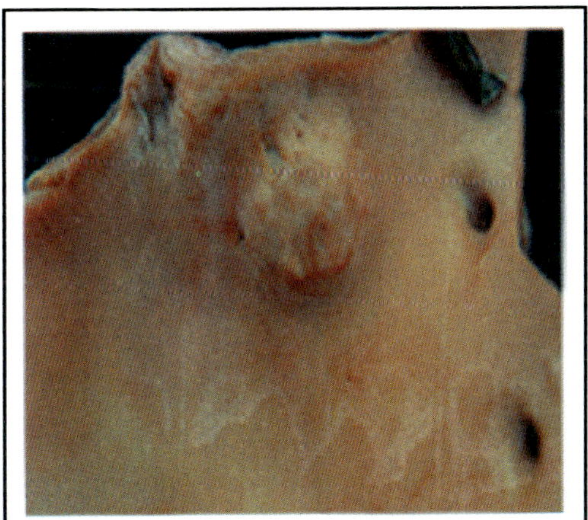

Figure 5: Photograph showing sudanophilic fibrous plaque in the aorta arch of a giraffe (*Giraffe camelopardus*, an exotic sp.)died at Zoological Garden,Guwahati, Assam.

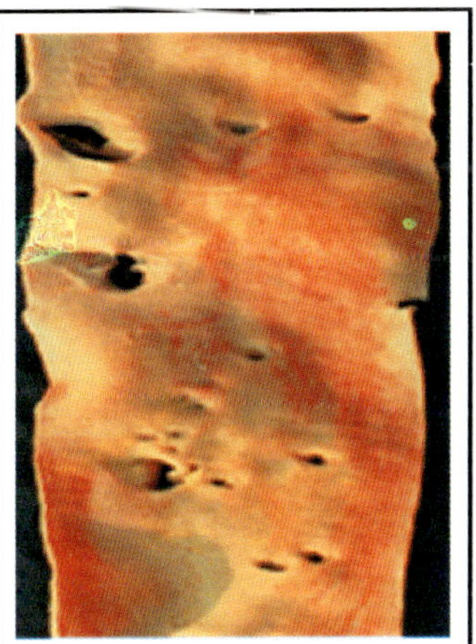

Figure 6: Photograph of abdominal aorta of chital (*A. axis*) showing sudanophilic fatty streaks .

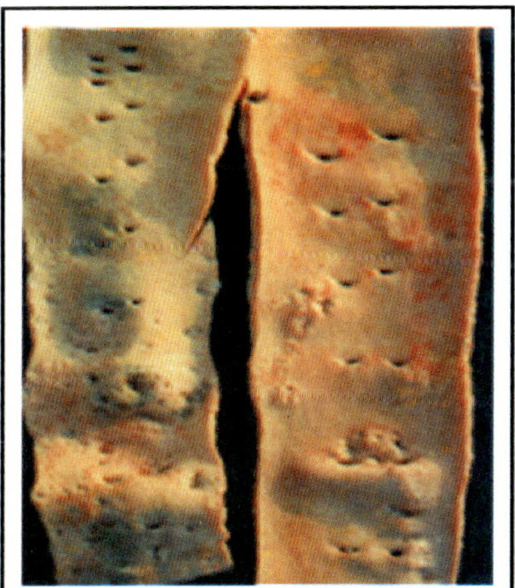

Figure 7 : Photograph showing uneven masses in aorta of blackbuck (*A. cervicapra)* and Nilgai *(B. tragocamelus)* died in captivity.

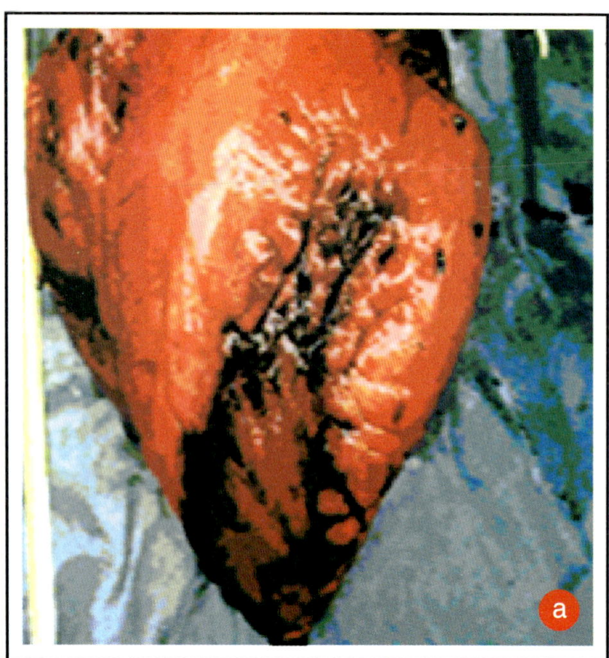

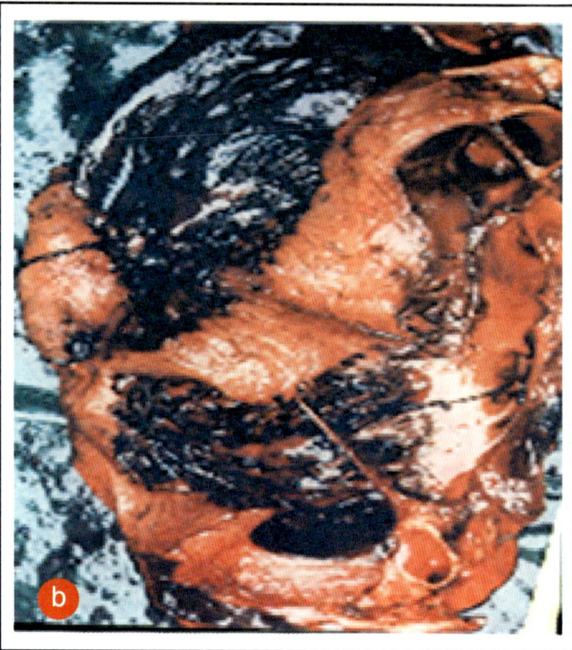

Figure 8: Photographs showing epicardial (a) and endocardial (b) haemorrhagic lesions in Hippopotamus (*H. amphibius*, an exotic species) that died of acute salmonellosis at Zoological Garden, Guwahati, Assam. The case is also referred under digestive system.

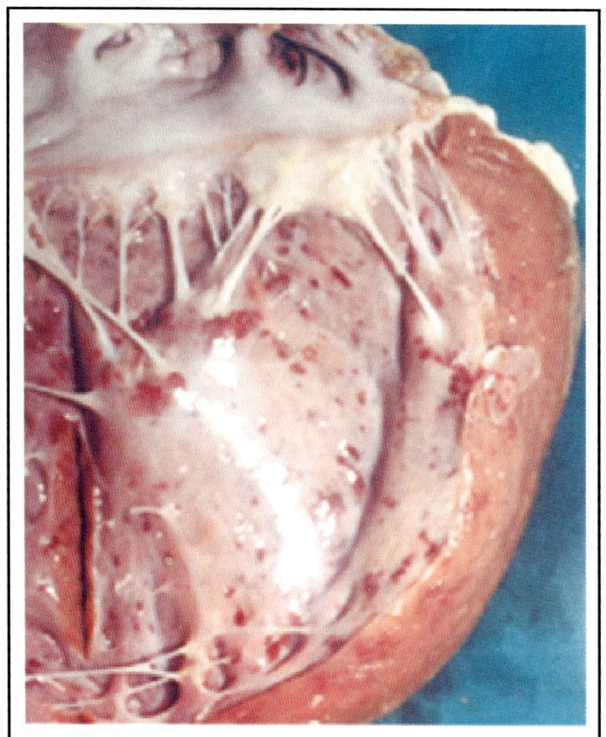

Figure 9: Pinpoint haemorrhages on endocardium of deer died due to Clostradial infection.(Courtesy: Suryawanshi, D.S.).

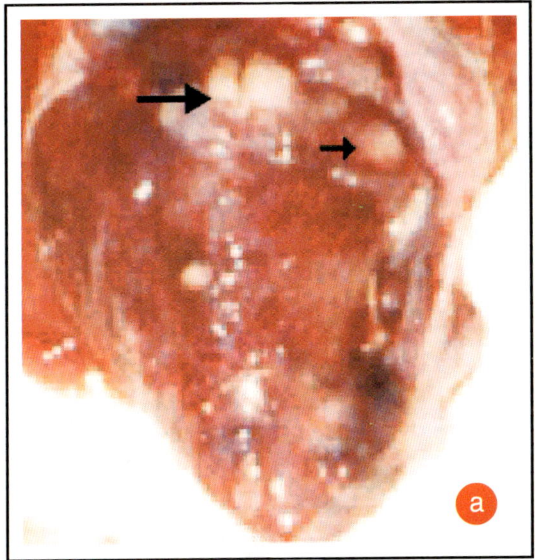

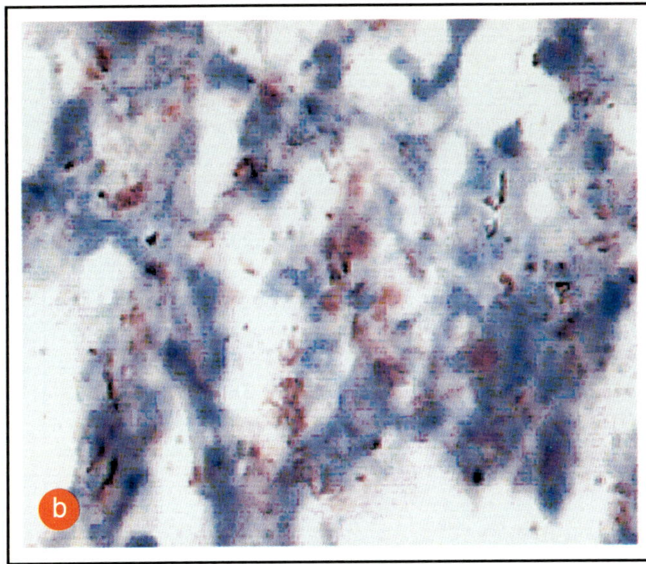

Figure 10: (a) Photograph showing tuberculous nodules on the epicardium concurrent with extensive pulmonary lesions of the disease in chital (*A. axis*).(b) Acid-fast bacilli in lung tissue of (a). x 1000.(Courtesy:Singh,K.P.).

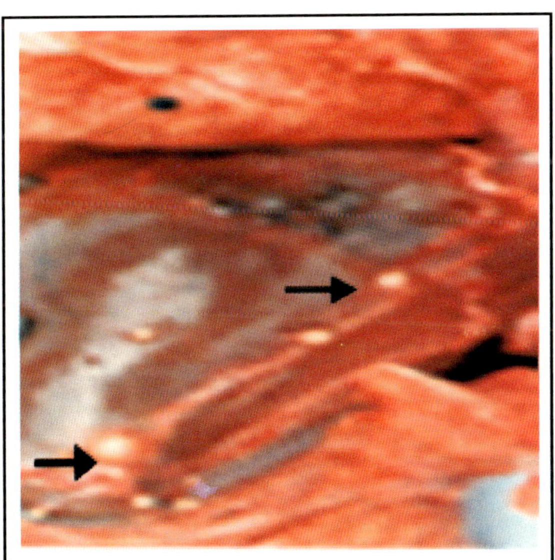

Figure 11: Photograph showing pericardium with small tuberculous nodules in adult blackbuck (*A.cervicapra*).

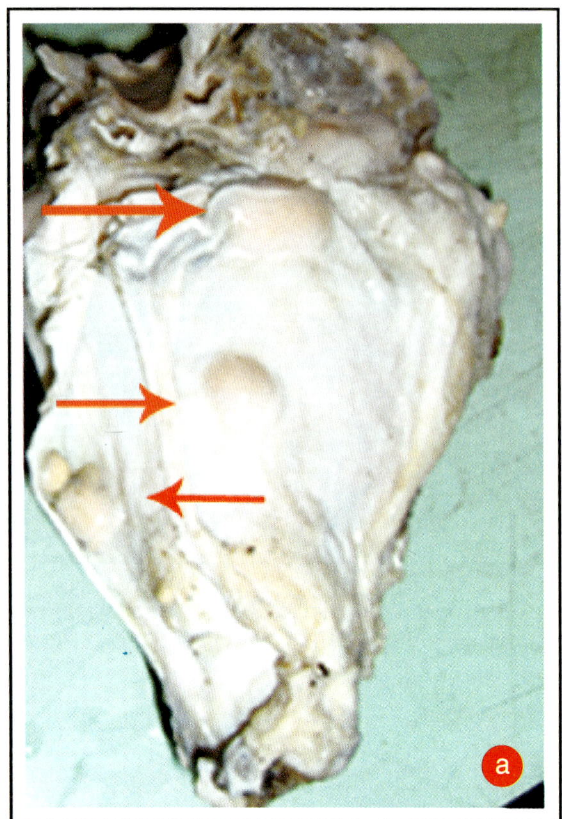

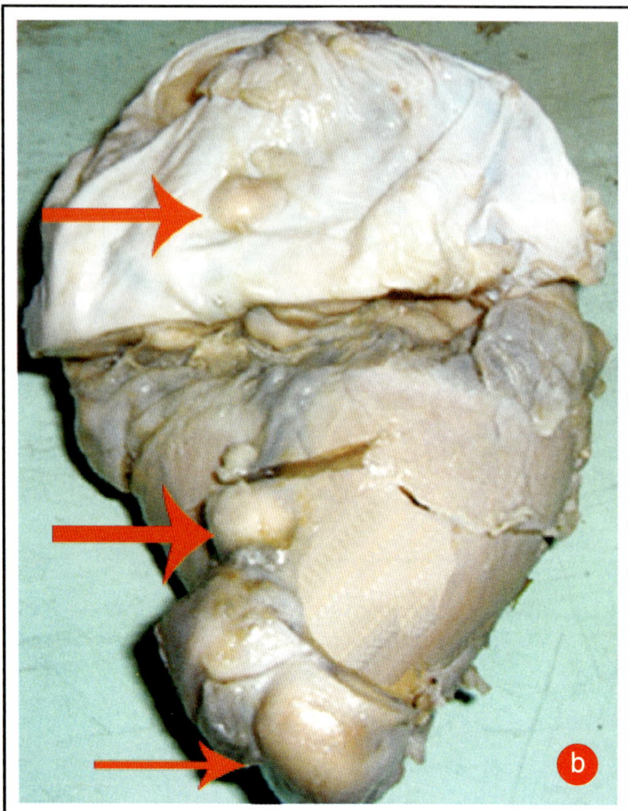

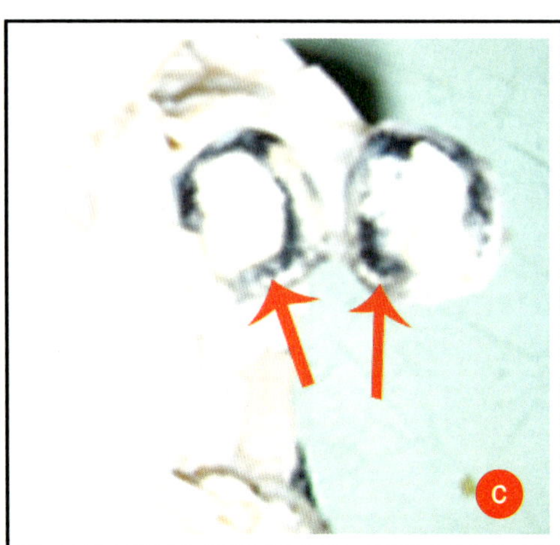

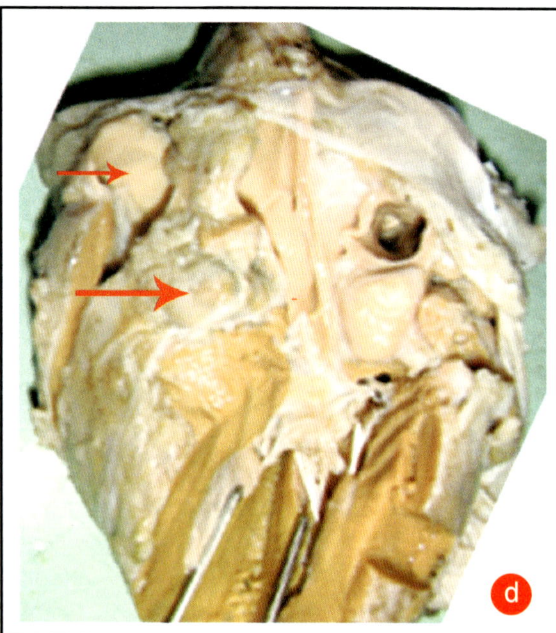

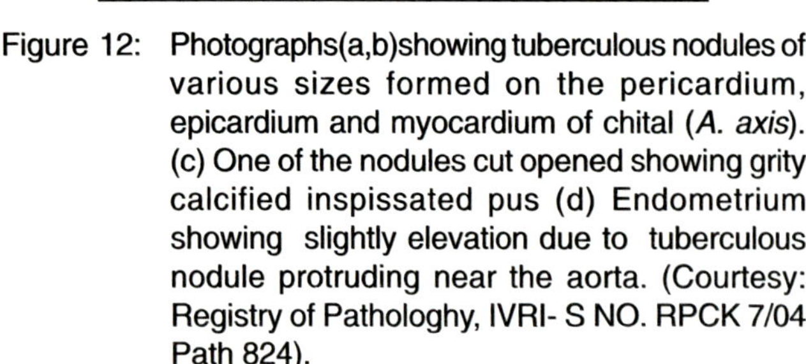

Figure 12: Photographs(a,b)showing tuberculous nodules of various sizes formed on the pericardium, epicardium and myocardium of chital (*A. axis*). (c) One of the nodules cut opened showing grity calcified inspissated pus (d) Endometrium showing slightly elevation due to tuberculous nodule protruding near the aorta. (Courtesy: Registry of Pathologhy, IVRI- S NO. RPCK 7/04 Path 824).

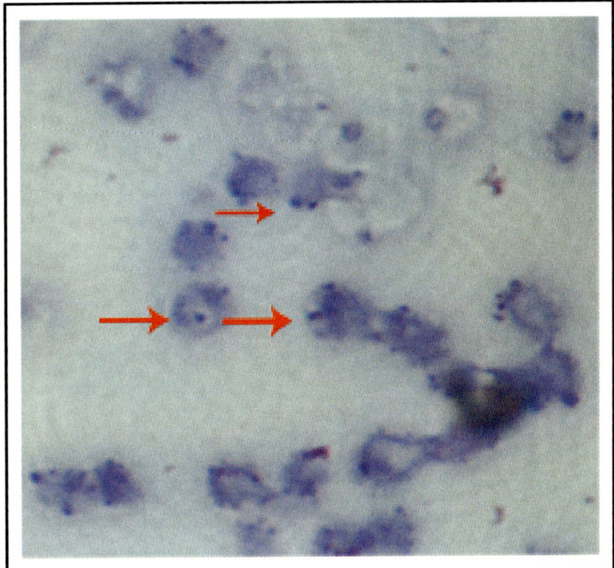

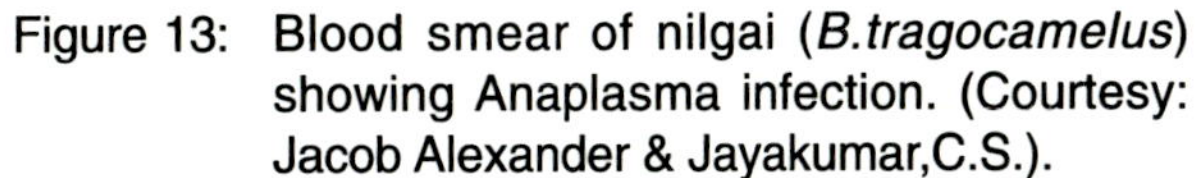

Figure 13: Blood smear of nilgai (*B.tragocamelus*) showing Anaplasma infection. (Courtesy: Jacob Alexander & Jayakumar,C.S.).

Figure 14: *Trypanosoma evansi* in the blood smear of white mouse experimentally infected with trypanosoma positive blood of blackbuck (*A.cervicapra*) suffering with corneal opacity.(Courtesy: Gupta,M.P.).

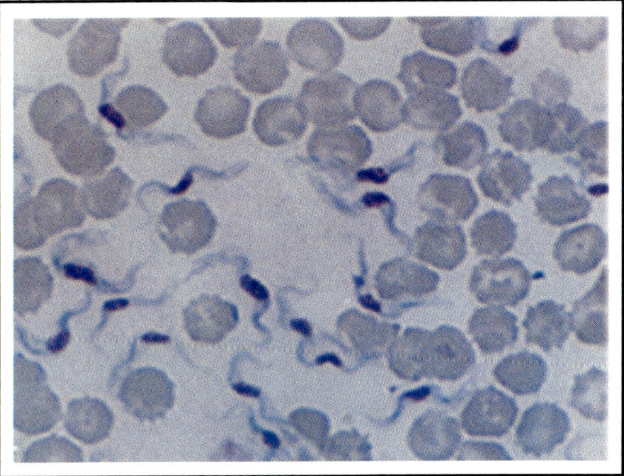

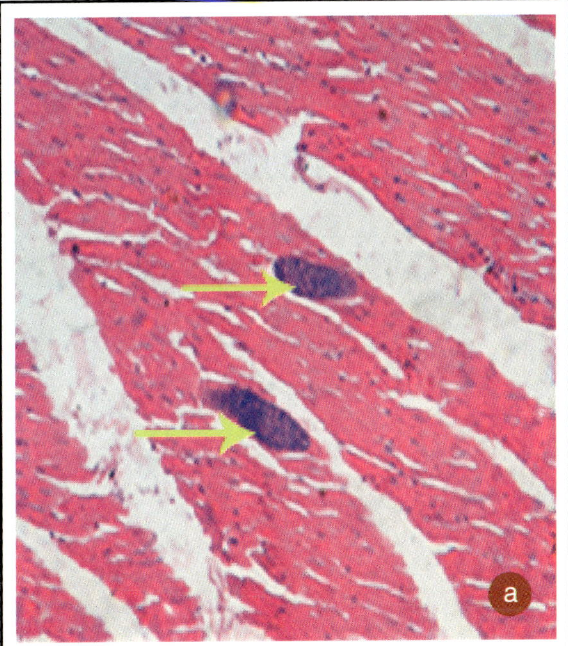

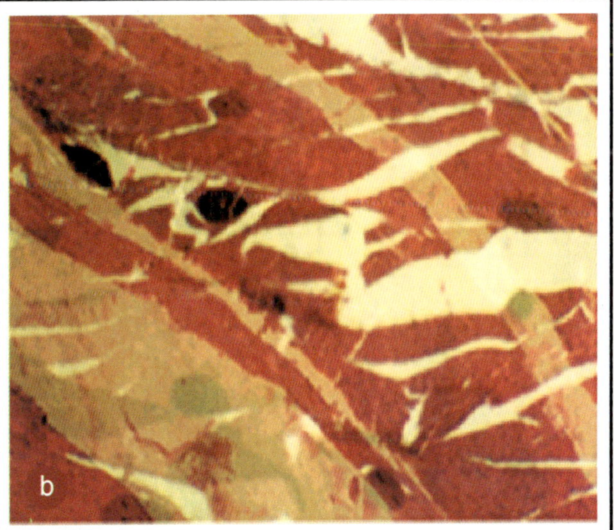

Figure 15: Photomicrographs showing sarcocyst in the cardiac muscle of (a) Chital (*A.axis*) H & E, x 100 (Courtesy: Dept.of Pathology, CVSc,Nagpur, M.S.). (b) Barasingha (*C. d. branderi*) H & E, x 100 (*C. d. branderi*). (Courtesy: Srivastava, A.B.).

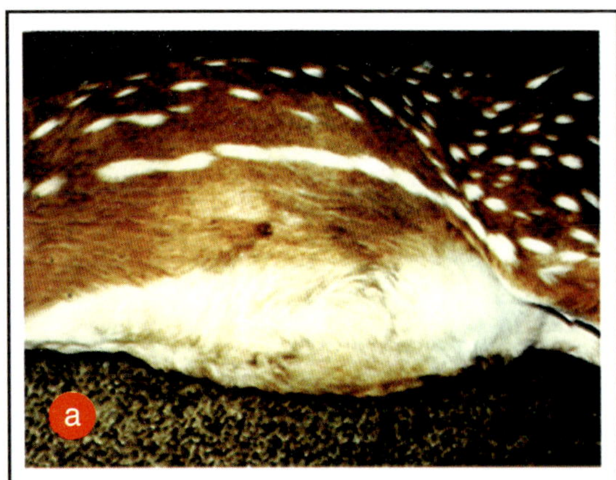

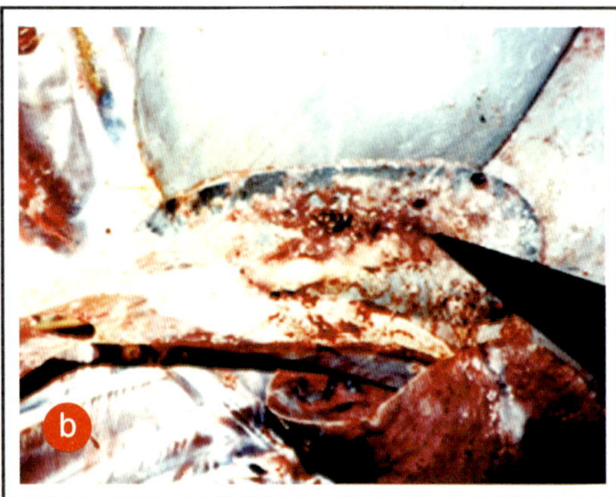

Figure 16: (a) Chital (*A. axis*)carcass marked for enlarged abdomen.(b)Dissected abdomen of (a) showing suppurative lesion on the left side with enlarged spleen adhering abdominal wall.This might be result of some external traumatic impact.

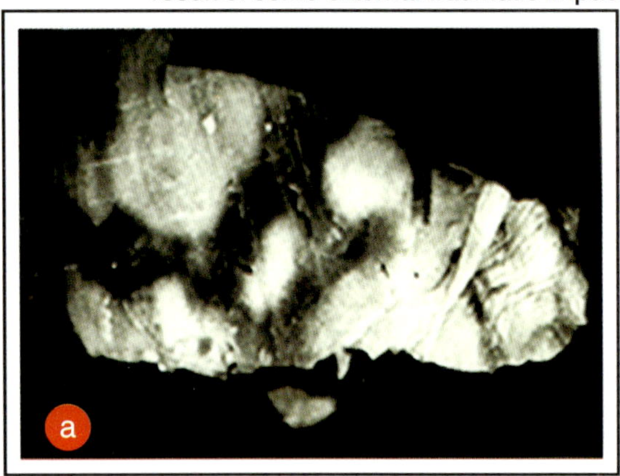

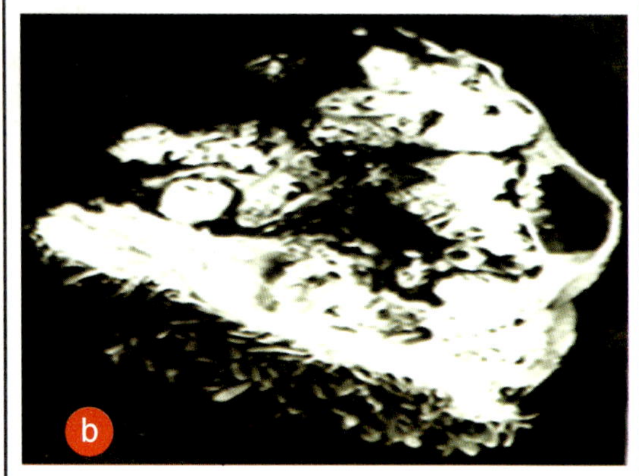

Figure 17: (a) Photograph of spleen of nilgai (*B. tragocamelus*) died in Zoological Park, Hyderabad (A.P.) showing: (a) Multiple abscesses (b) Incised abscess showing pockets of pus. The condition was related to traumatic reticulo splenitis.

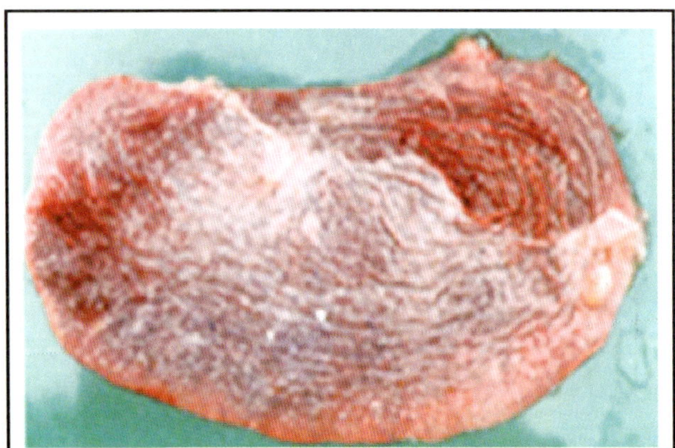

Figure 18: Photograph of spleen of hog-deer (*A. porcinus*) showing tuberculous nodules. Animal had died of disseminated form of disease.

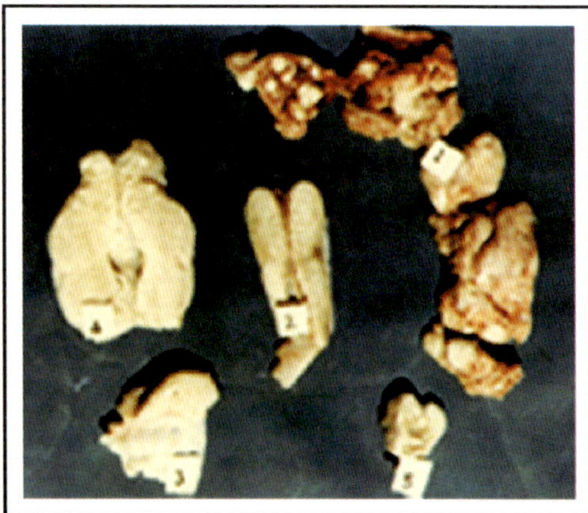

Figure 19: Photograph showing tuberculous lesion in lymph nodes of blackbuck (*A.cervicapra*).

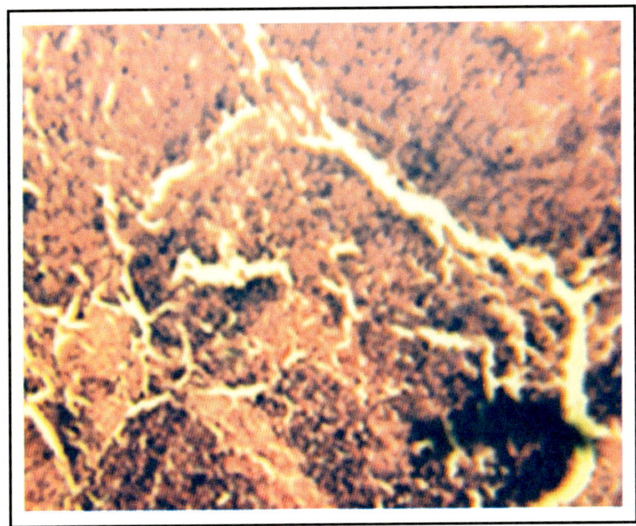

Figure 20: Photograph showing tuberculous necrotic lesion in lymph node of hog-deer (*A. porcinus*).

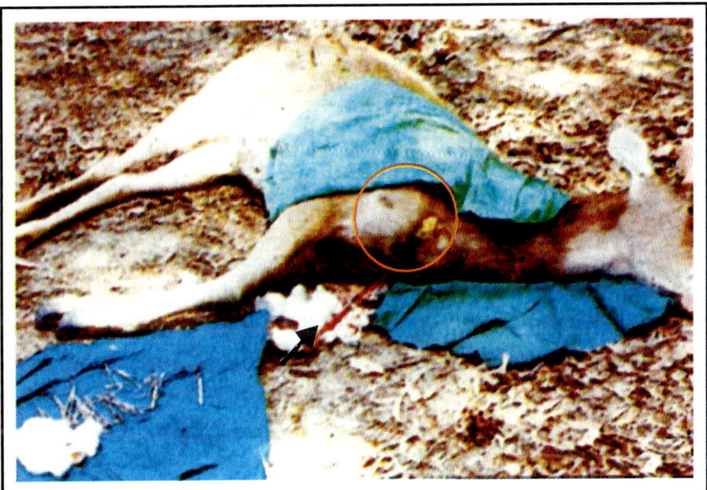

Figure 21 : Photograph showing enlarged prescapluar lymph gland in Barasingha (*Cervus d. duvauceli*) due to tuberculosis. (Note Caseated mass (arrow) from the enlarged gland)

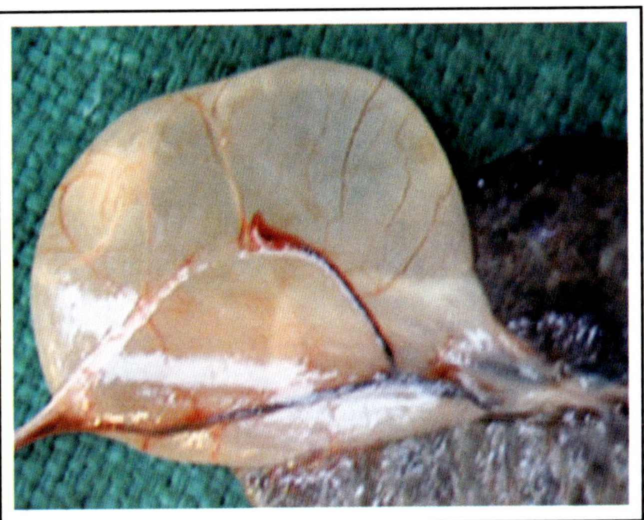

Figure 22: Photograph showing *Taenia hydatigena* cyst attached to the serosal surface of the spleen of a pigmy hog (*Porcula salvania*).

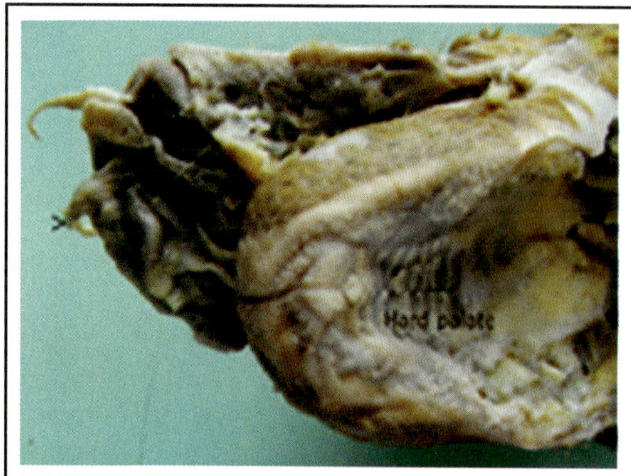

Figure 23 : Photograph showing wartlike growths in the nostrils of a just born sangai (*C. eldi eldi*) fawn. The case is also referred under skeletal anomalies.

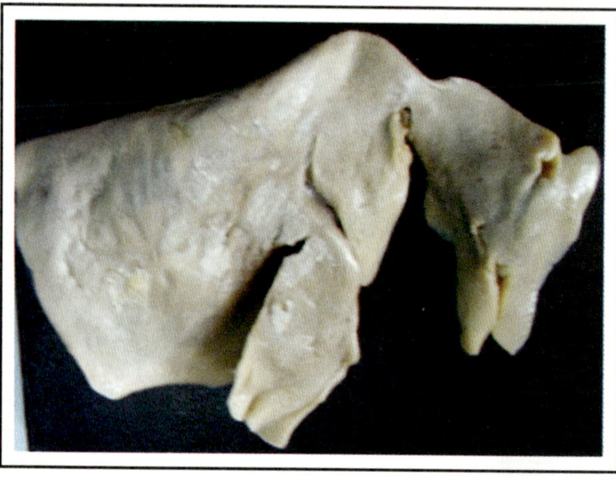

Figure 24 : Photograph of right diaphragmatic lobe of lung of an adult blackbuck (*A.cervicapra*) having an accessory lobe (anatomical anomaly).

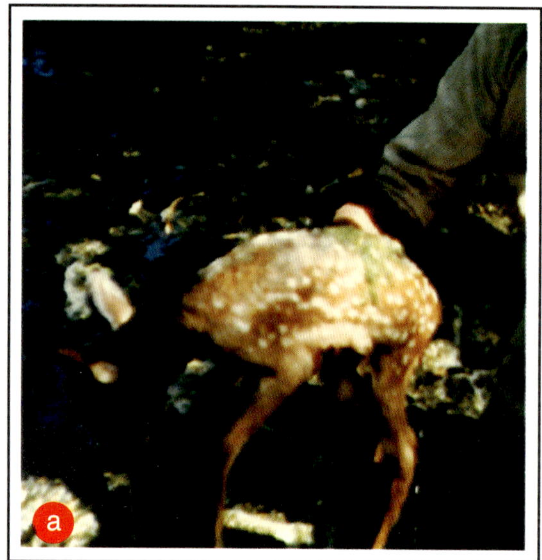

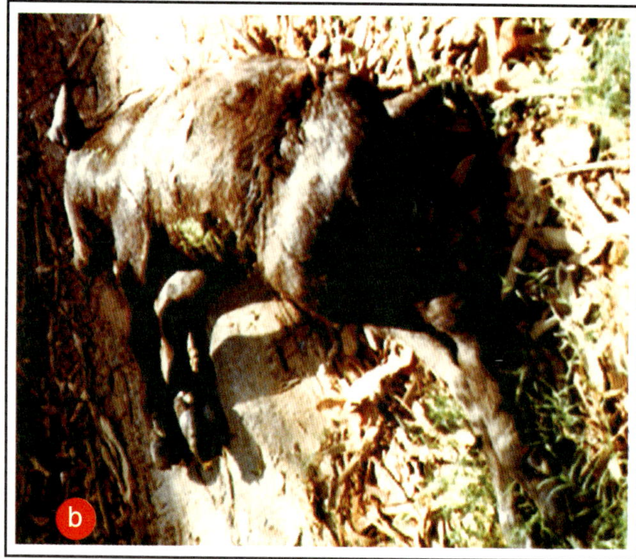

Figures 25 : Neonatal deaths due to drowning in the water moats of the enclosure encountered at National Zoological Park, New Delhi:(a) Sika deer (*Cervus nippon*, an exotic sp.) fawn. (b) Cape buffalo (*Syncerus caffer*, an exotic sp.) calf .

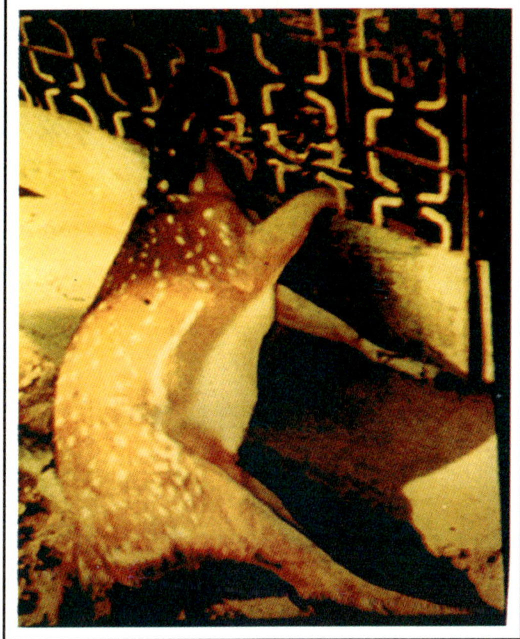

Figure 26 : Photograph showing chital (*A. axis*) neck strangulated in the enclosure fence at Zoological Garden, Mysore (Courtesy: Nagaraju, S.).

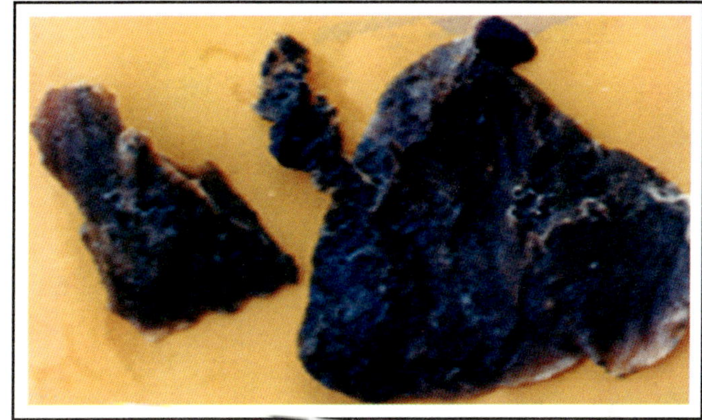

Figure 27 : Photograph of lung of blackbuck (*A. cervicapra*) showing Pneumonoconiosis.

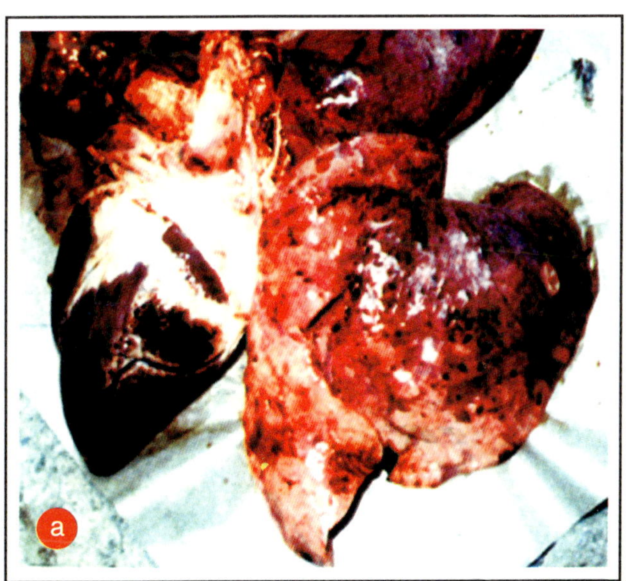

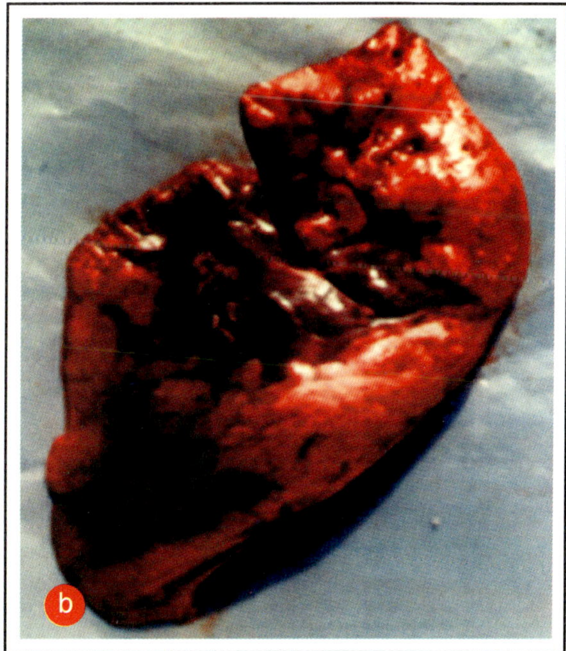

Figure 28 : (a) An estrus female barasingha (*C. d. duvauceli*) was hit by its male partner and died due to fracture of cervical vertebrae. Necropsy showed haemorrhages on pericardium and lung. The lungs also showed *Echinococcus granulosus* cysts. (b) Photograph showing rupture of lung of sub-adult blackbuck (*A. cervicapra*) caused due to goring by companion male.

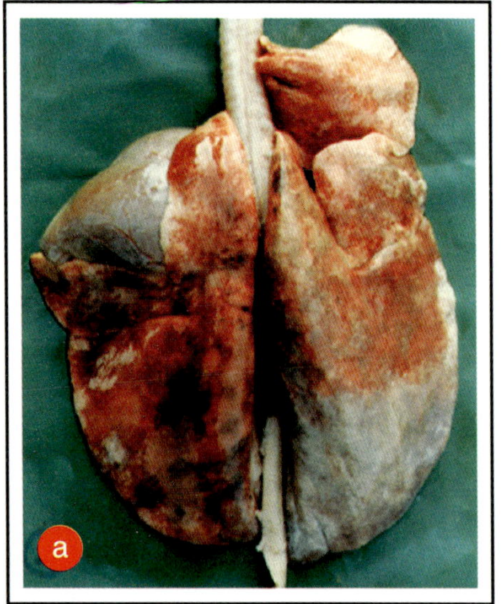

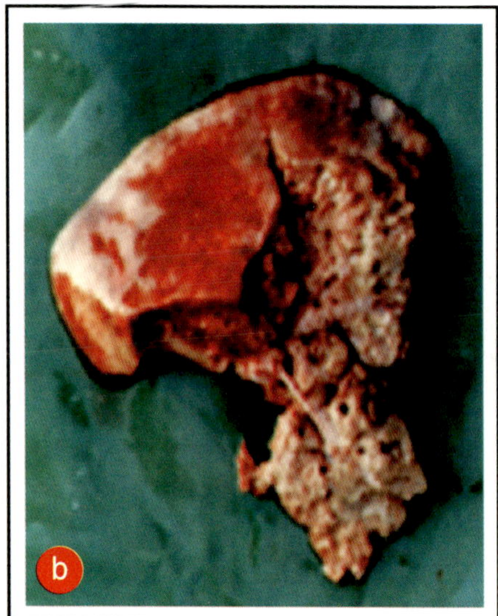

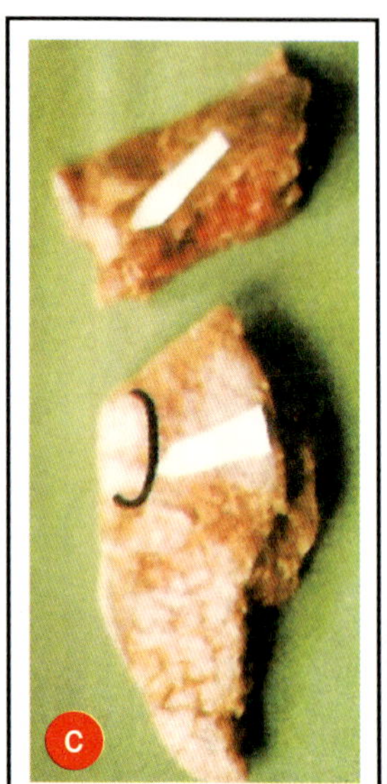

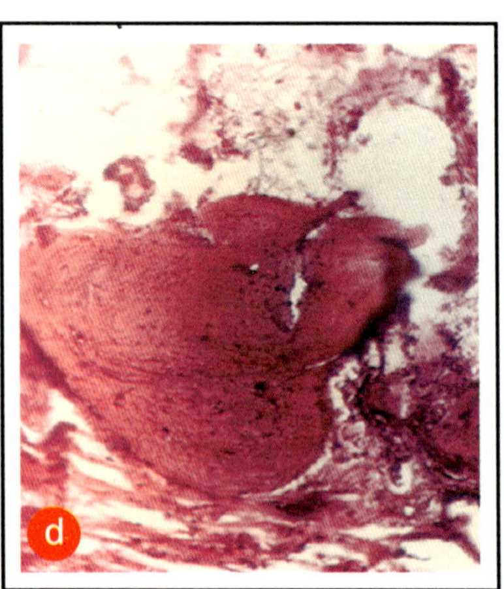

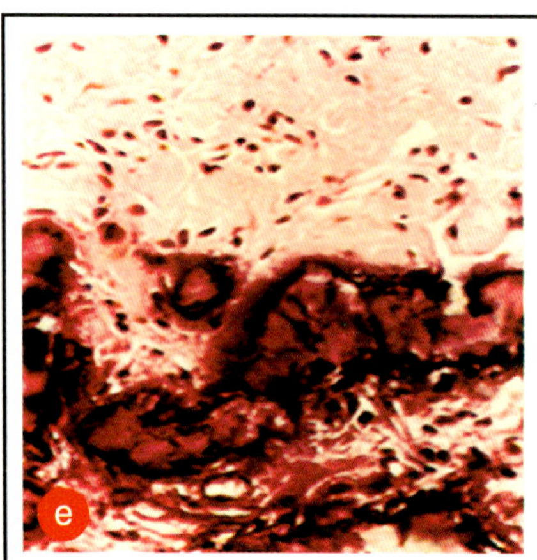

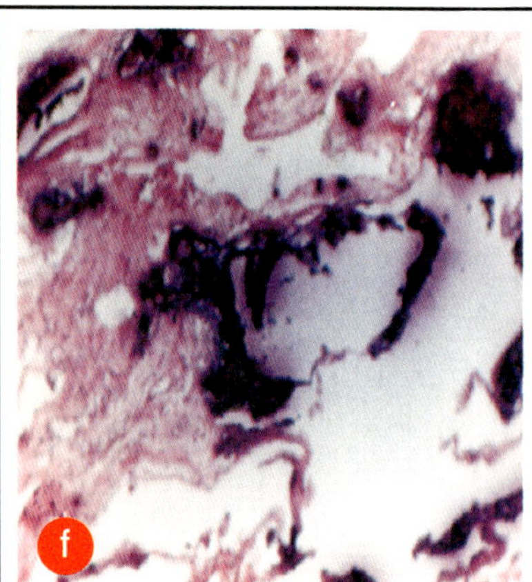

Figure 29 : Photographs (a-c) showing: (a) Grayish white foci in lung of blackbuck (*A. cervicapra*). (b) Cut piece of (a) having grayish white granular mass. (c) Ossified areas in the lung parenchyma. Photomicrographs of (a) showing: (d) A large ossicle in the lung tissue. H & E, x 100 (e, f)Lung tissue undergoing metaplastic transformation into fibrous and osseous tissue. H & E, x 128.

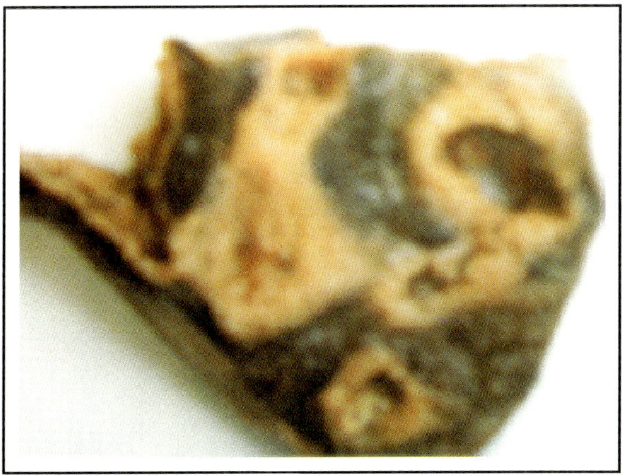

Figure 30 : Photograph of lung section of sangai deer (*C. eldi eldi*) died in National Zoological Park,showing fibrinonecrotic pneumonia.

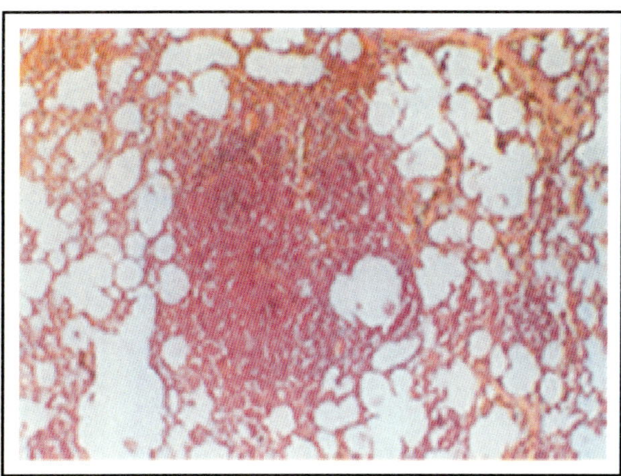

Figure 31 : Photomicrograph of lung of blackbuck (*A. cervicapra*) showing suppurative pneumonia. (Courtesy: Dept of Wildlife Science, C.V. Sc, Chennai).

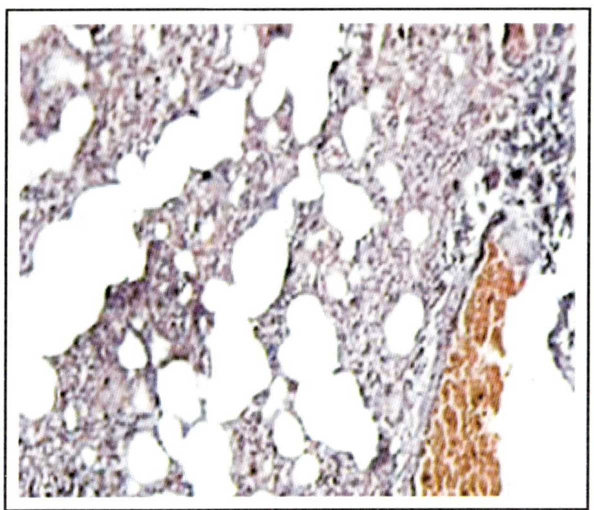

Figure 32 : Photomicrograph showing the areas of haemorrhages and congestion in lungs related to hypovolemic shock in nilgai (*B. tragocarnelus*) H & E, x 400 (Courtesy: Somesh Singh).

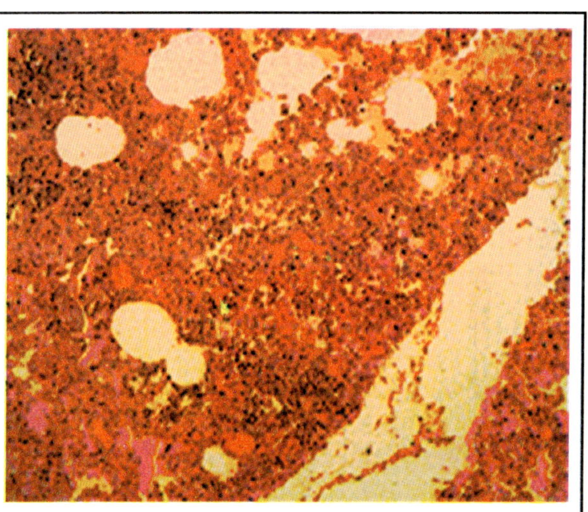

Figure 33: Photomicrograph of lung of sangai deer (*C. eldi eldi*) showing severe haemorrhages and congestion in the parenchyma.Interstitial spaces filled with oedematous fluid and infiltrated with inflammatory cells due to Pasteurella infection.(Courtesy : Harish, B. R. & Shivashankar).

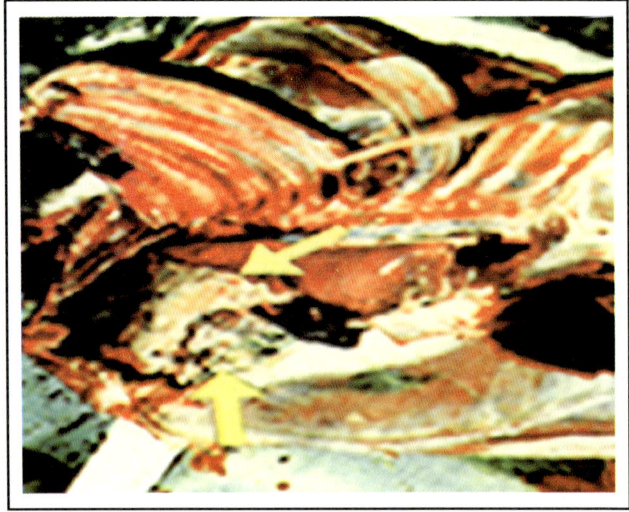

Figure 34: Photograph showing pneumonic lesions due to *Pasteurella haemolytica* infection in blackbuck (*A.cervicapra*) died at V. P.U. IVRI Izatnagar, Bareilly. (U.P)

Figure 35: Photomicrograph of lung from hog-deer (*A. porcinus*) showing bronchopneumonia due to Pasteurella infection.H&E x100 (Courtesy:Bhowmik,M.K.).

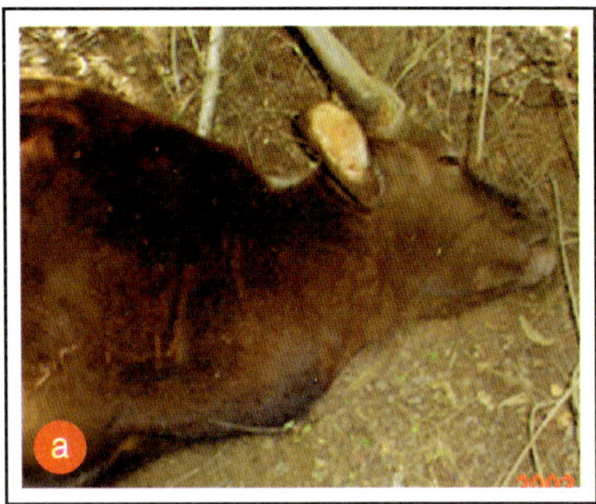

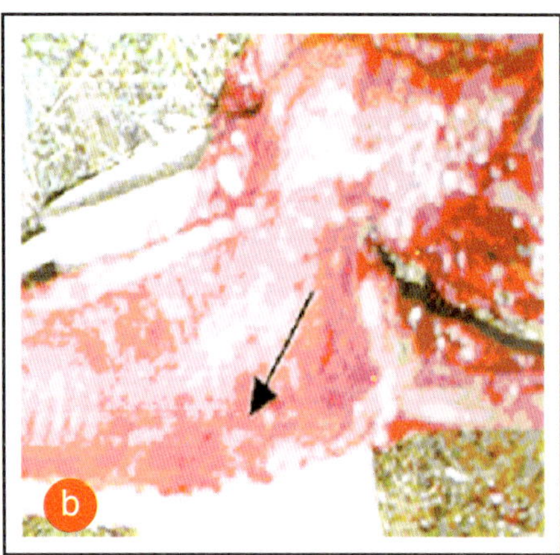

Figure 36 : (a) Carcass of gaur (*B. gaurus*) died of pasteurellosis at Zoological Park, Chennai (T.N). Note swelling of the throat region due to accumulation of serous/sero-fibrinous fluid.Necropsy of (a) showed.(b) Haemorrhages in the upper respiratory tract. (c) Pneumonic lesion. The case is also referred under sense organs. (Courtesy: Dept. of Wildlife Science, C.V. Sc, & Z.P. Chennai,TN).

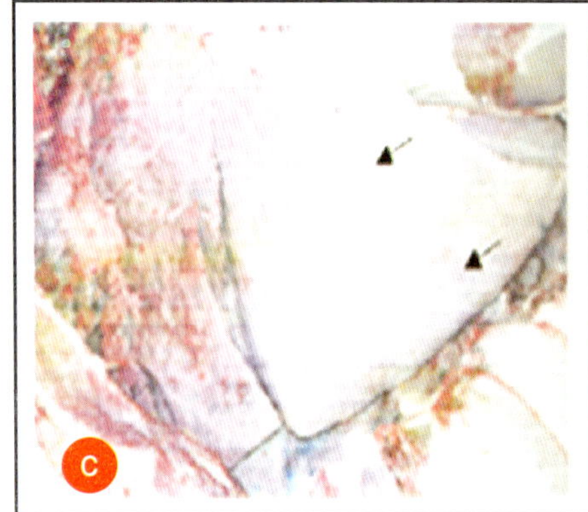

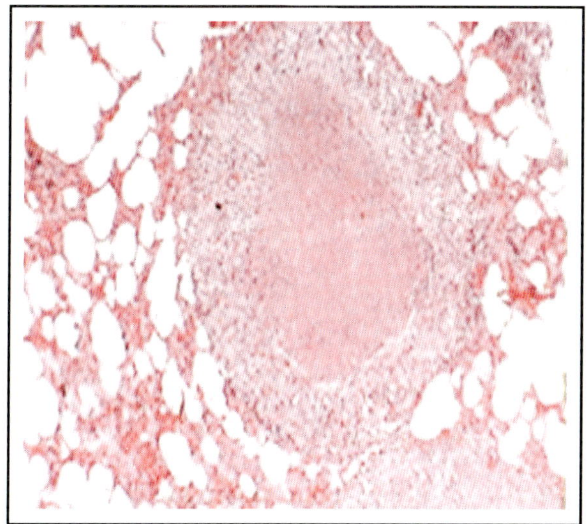

Figure 37 : Photomicrograph showing caseated nodules in lung of blackbuck (*A.cervicapra*) caused due to *Corynebactrium ovis*. The case is also referred under reproductive system.

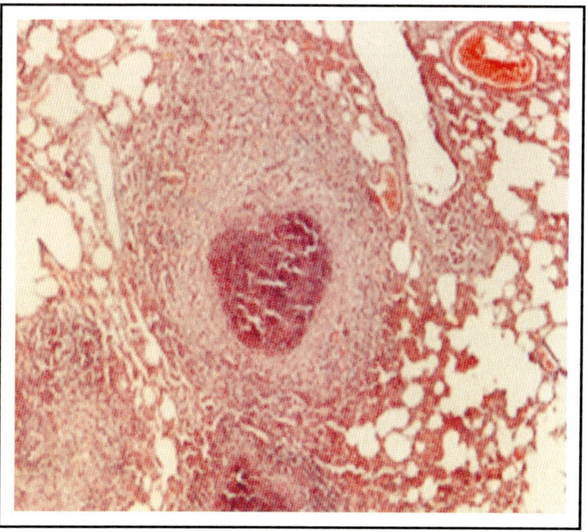

Figure 38 : Photomicrograph of lung of nilgai (*B.tragocamelus*) showing central necrosis surrounded by leucocytes and thin layer of connective tissues. N & E, x 100. The condition was diagnosed as *E. coli* granuloma (Courtesy: Suryawanshi, D.S.).

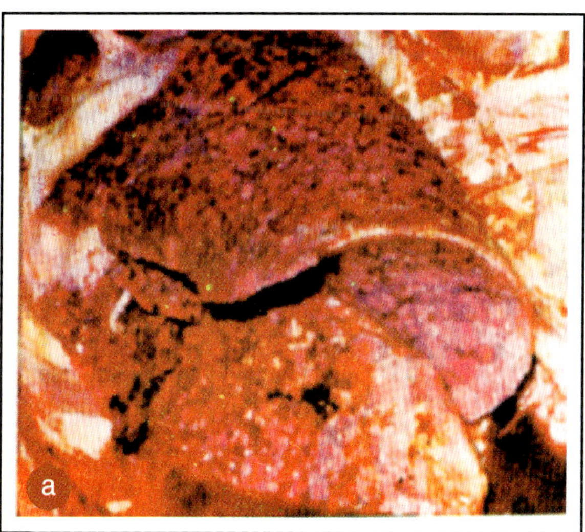

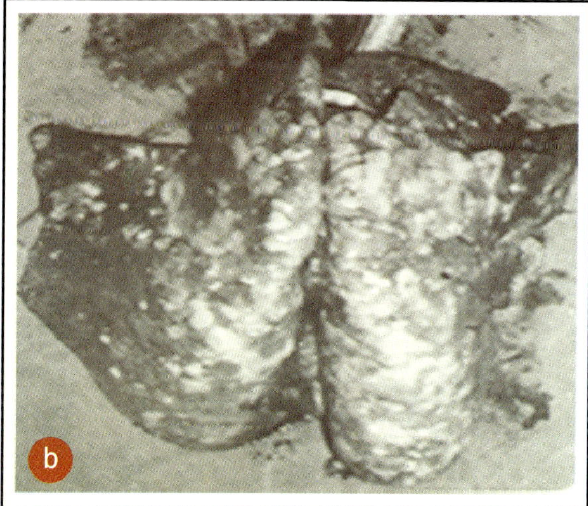

Figure 39 : Photograph showing pulmonary tuberculous lesions in:(a) Chital (*A. axis*).(b) Barking deer (*M. muntjak*).

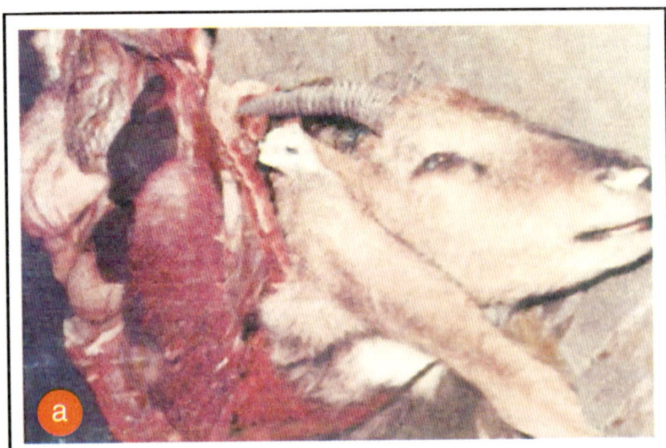

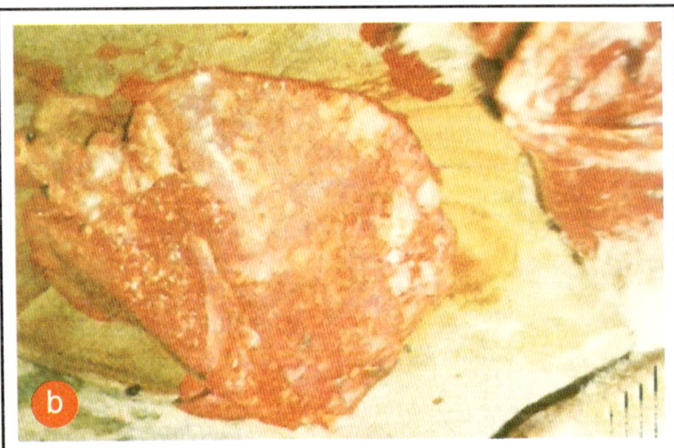

Figure 40: (a) Photoghaph showing pus with frothy discharge from nostrils of goral (*N.goral*) died in National Zoological Park. (b)Lungs of (a) showing caseated tuberculous lesion.

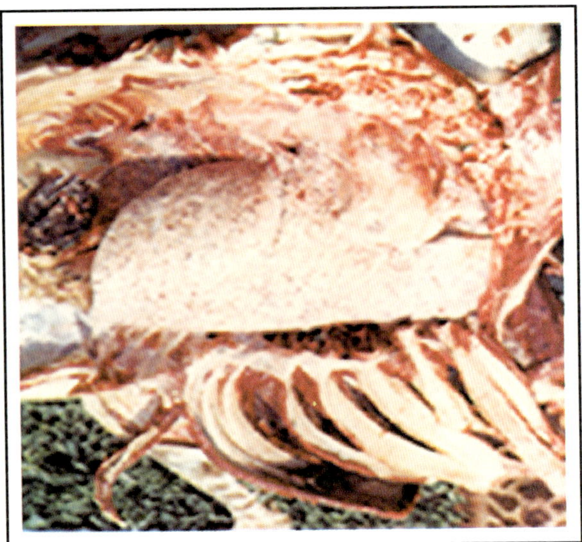

Figure 41 : Photograph showing pulmonary tuberculosis lesions in giraffe (*G. camelopardus*, an exotic sp.)

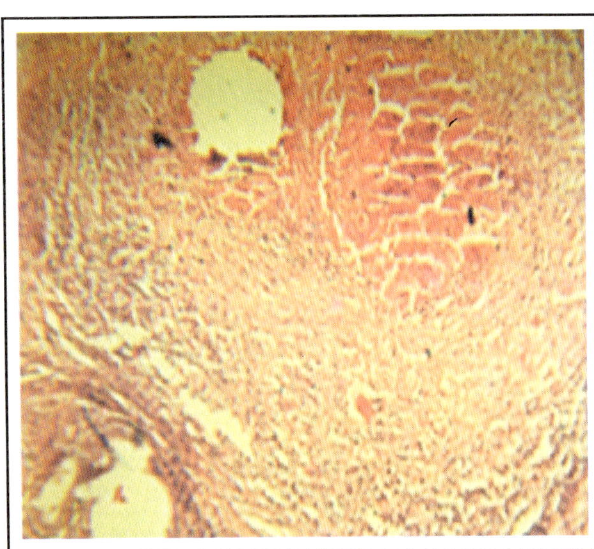

Figure 42 : Photomicrograph showing tuberculous granuloma in lung of hog-deer (*A.porcinus*). H&E, x 100 (Courtesy: Bhowmik,M.K).

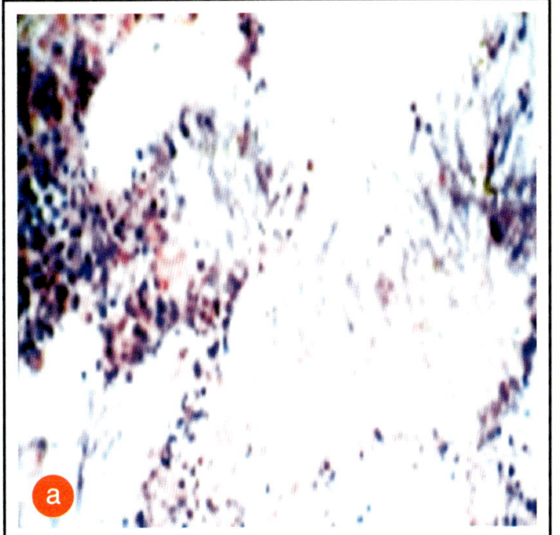

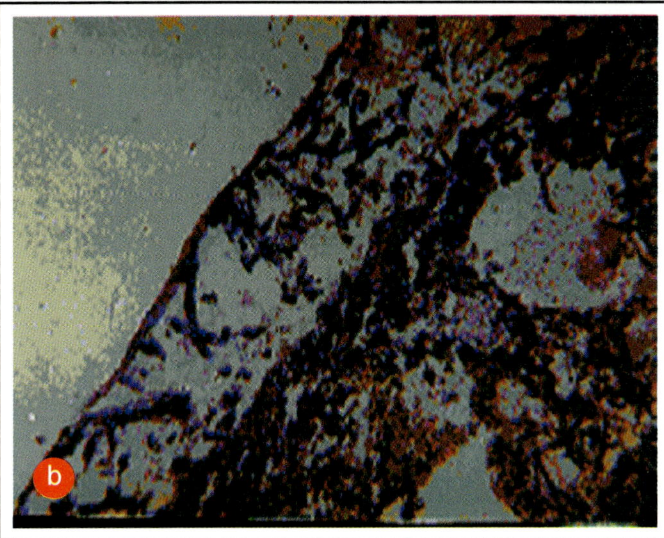

Figure 43 : (a) Pulmonary zygomycosis in pigmy hog (*P. salvania*) affected with Salmonella infection. (a) Photomicrograph showing fungal elements within the alveoli and infiltration of polymorph nuclear cells. H&E, x 100 (b) Lesion showing zygomycotic fungus in pleura.H & E, x 100.

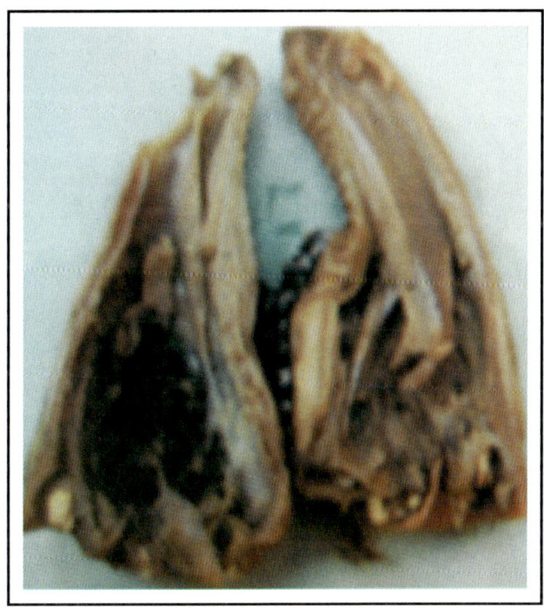

Figure 44 : Zygomycosis in hog-deer (*A. porcinus*). Photograph showing nasal chamber filled with caseo-necrotic mass mixed with blood clot. Dissolution of turbinate bones is also discerned (Rao & Acharjyo,2003).

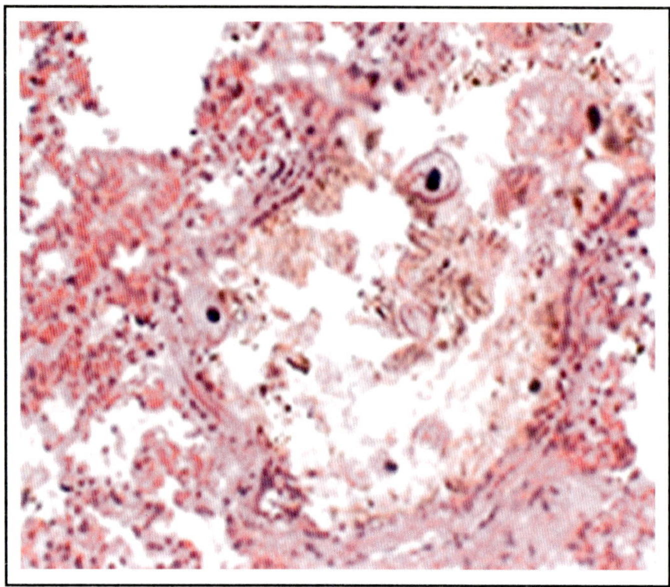

Figure 45 : Photomicrograph of lung of giraffe (*Giraffe camelopardus*,an exotic sp.) showing protozoa indistinguishable from *Blantidium coli* in the bronchioles along with massive haemorrhages in the alveoli. H&E,x400. The condition was related to aspiratory pneumonia.

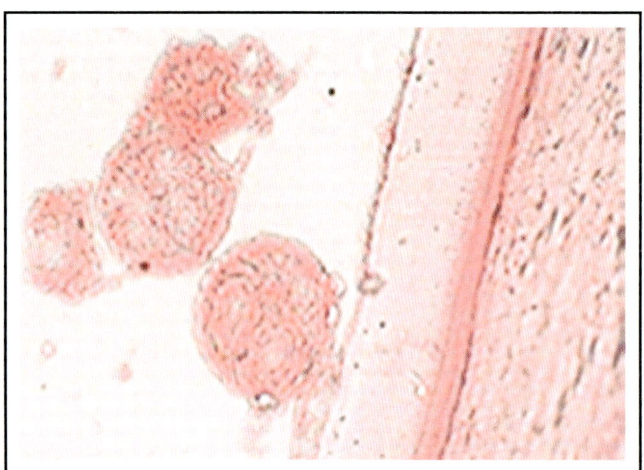

Figure 46 : Photomicrograph of lung of blackbuck (*A.cervicapra*) showing cysticercus with daughter cysts H&E,x400.

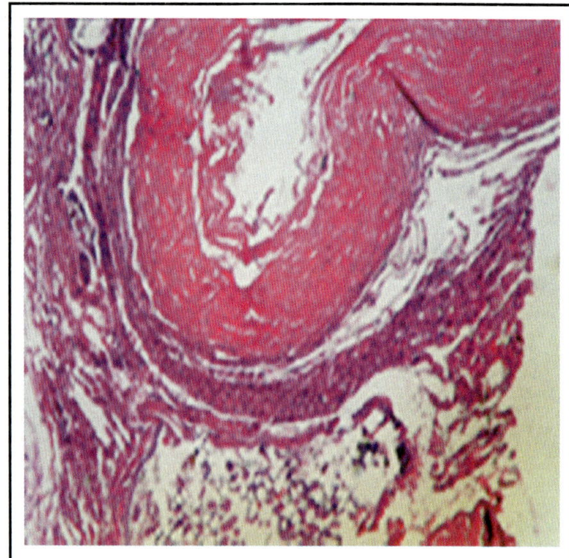

Figure 47 : Photomicrograph of lung of chital (*A. axis*) showing cyst H&E, x100 (Courtesy:Dept of Pathology, C.V.Sc, Nagpur, M.S.).

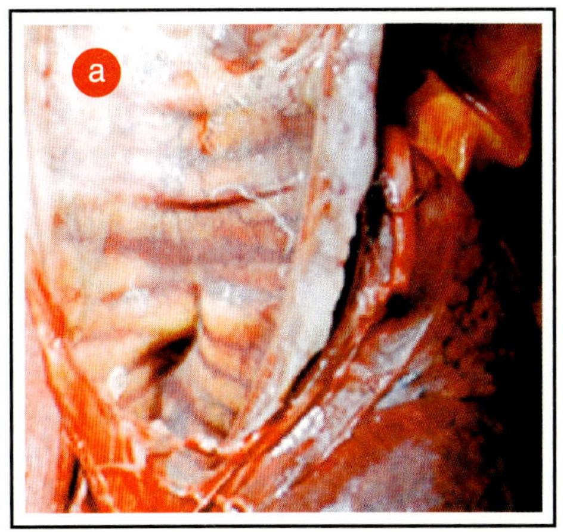

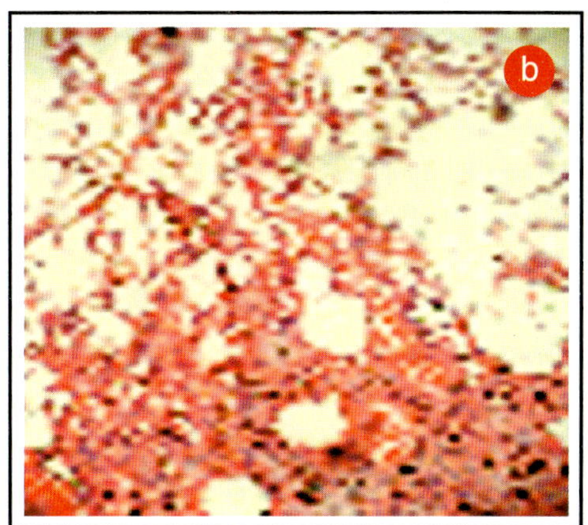

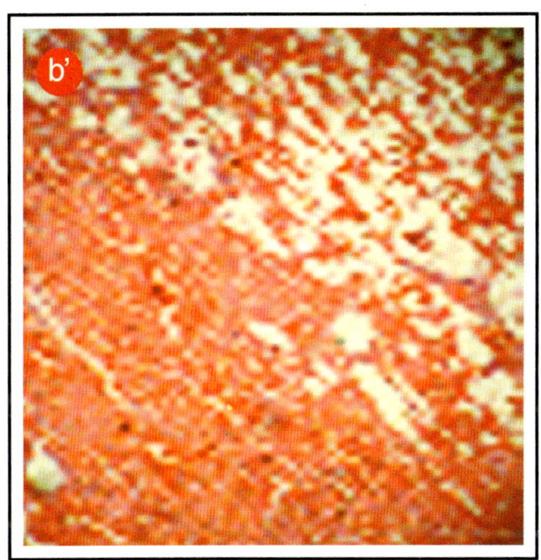

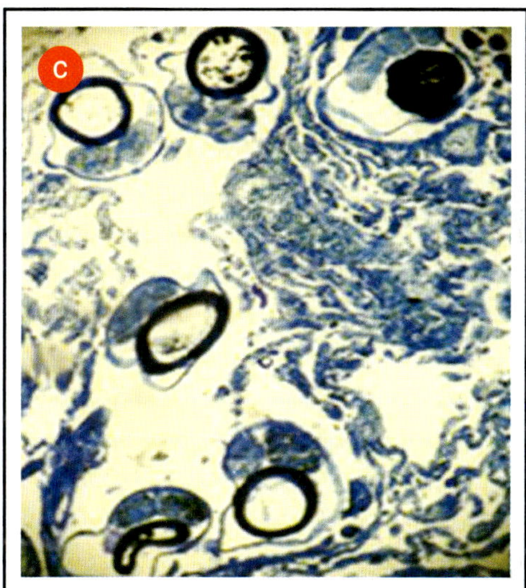

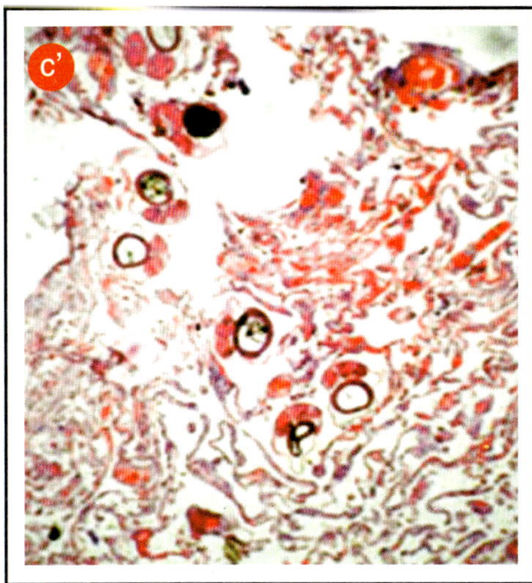

Figure 48 : (a) Photograph of trachea of hangul (*Cervus elaphus hanglu*) showing congestion and mucinous froth and *Dictyocaulus* sp. worms. Photomicrographs showing: (b,b') Patchy areas of pneumonia, congestion, atelectasis and emphysema. (c,c') Variable cellular reaction around parasites and larvae H & E, x 100

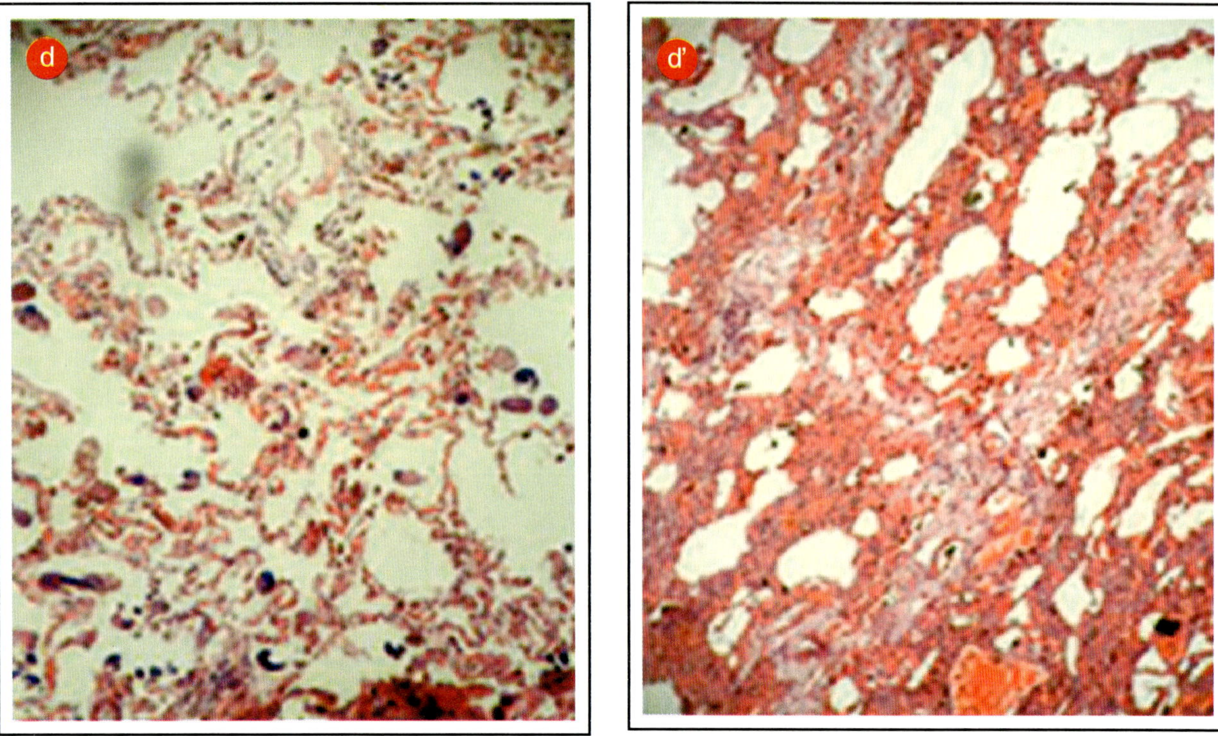

Figure 48 : (d,d') Larvae and their migratory tract along the lung parenchyma H & E, x 100.

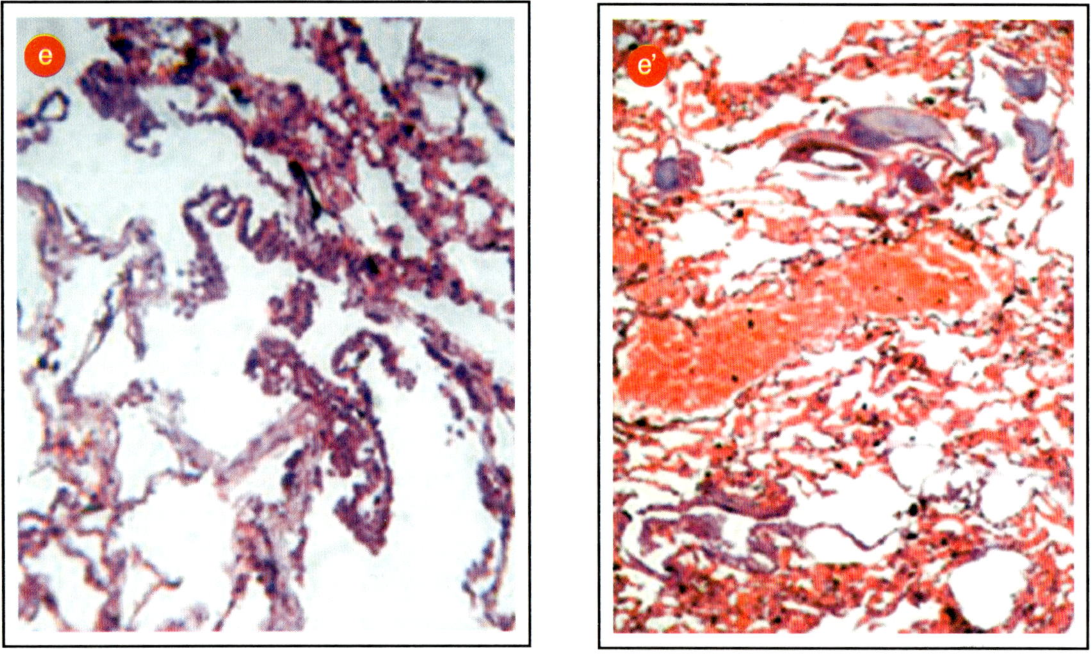

Figure 48 : (e, e') Epithelial hyperplasia with epithelialisation in alveoli and airways, H & E, x 100

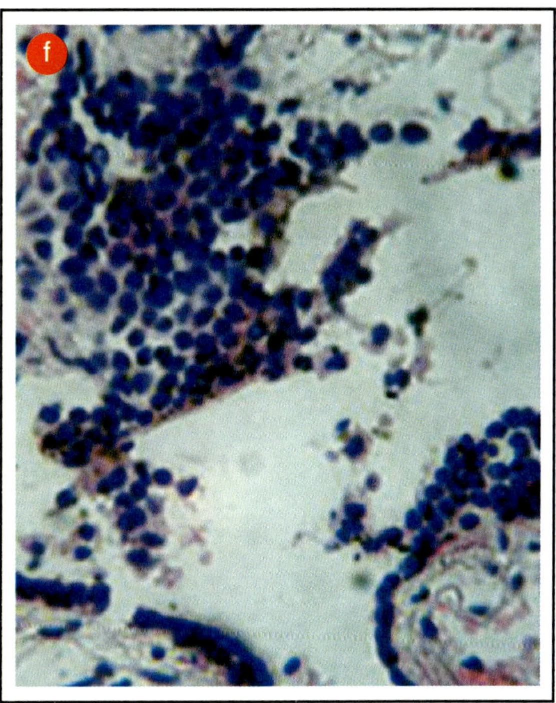

Figure 48 : (f) Nodular epithelial hyperplasia. (Nashiruddullah *et al.*, 2007).

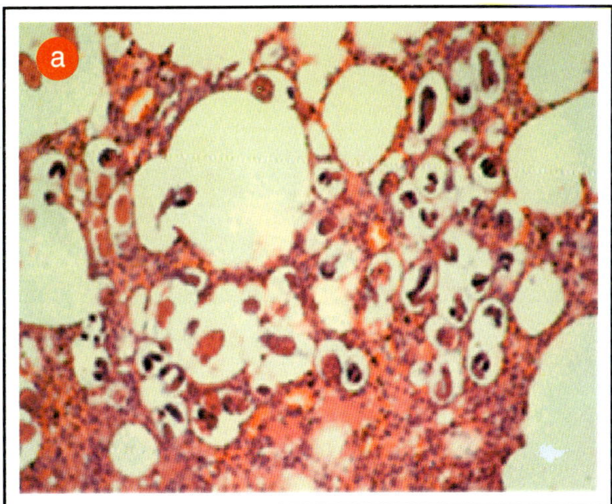

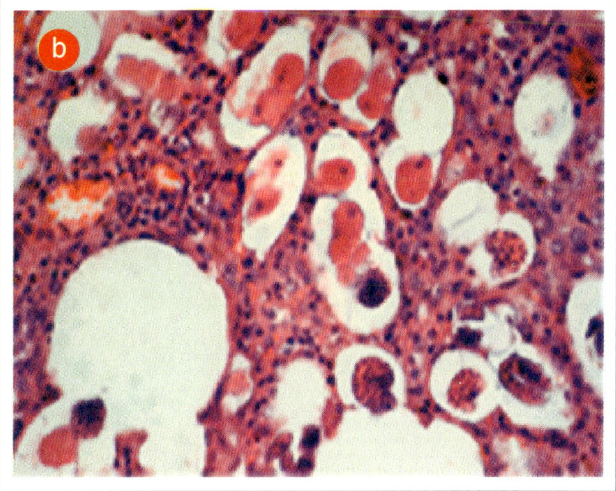

Figure 49: (a) Photomicrograph of lung of musk deer (*Moschus chrysogaster*) showing ova and larve of lung worm (verminous pneumonia). Magnification (a) x 200 and (b) x 400 (Courtesy: Singh, K.P.).

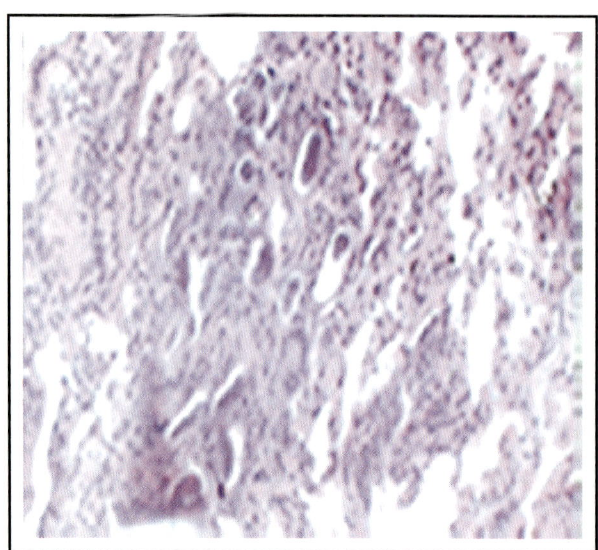

Figure 50 : Histopathologic section of lung from barking deer (*M. muntjak*) showing parasite and eggs (verminous pneumonia). H&E, x100.

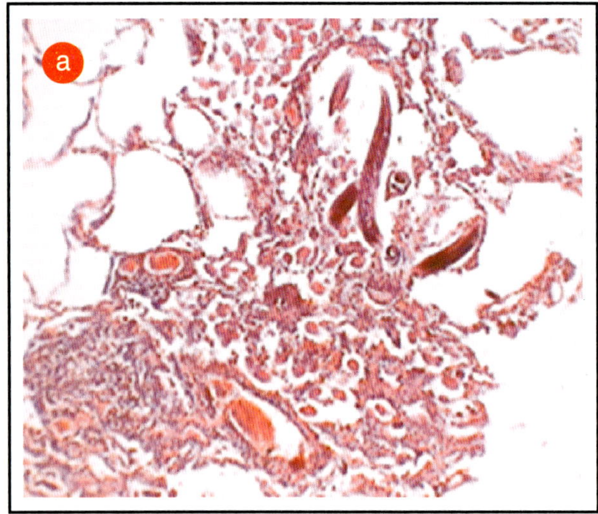

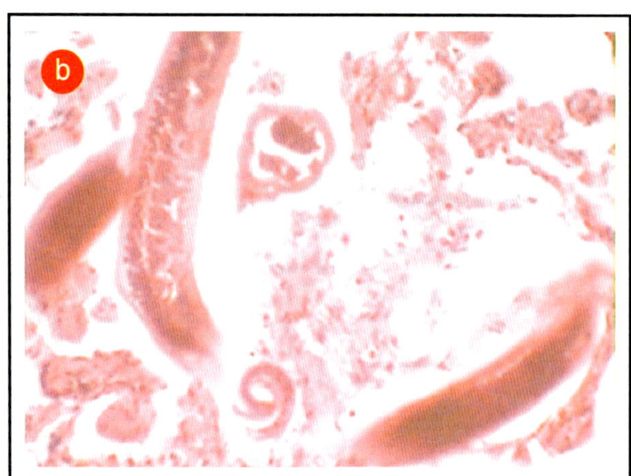

Figure 51 : (a) Photomircrograph of lung of barking deer (*Muntiacus muntjak*) showing Strongyloides H&E, x100. (b) Another view of (a) H&E, x 400.

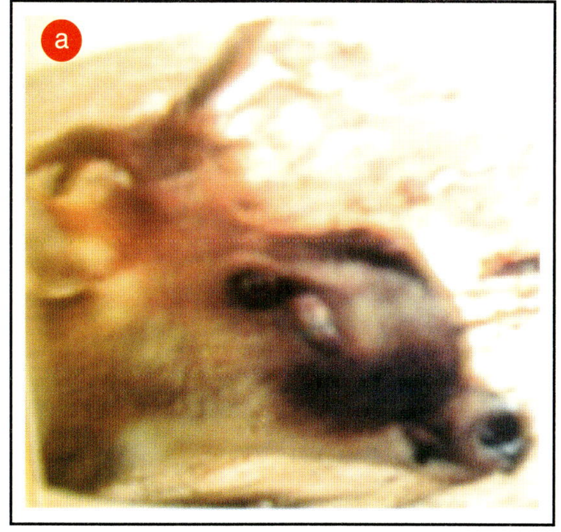

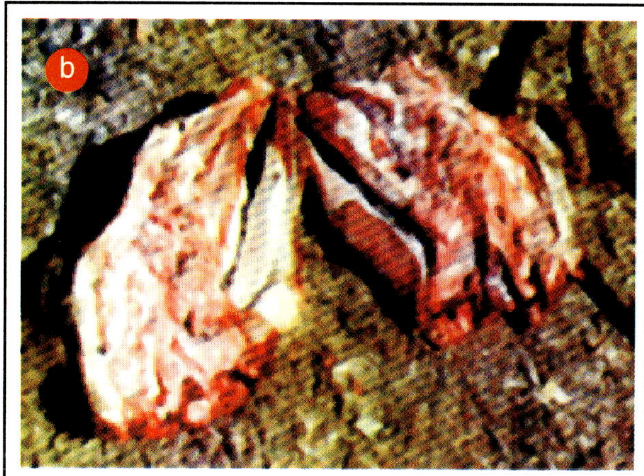

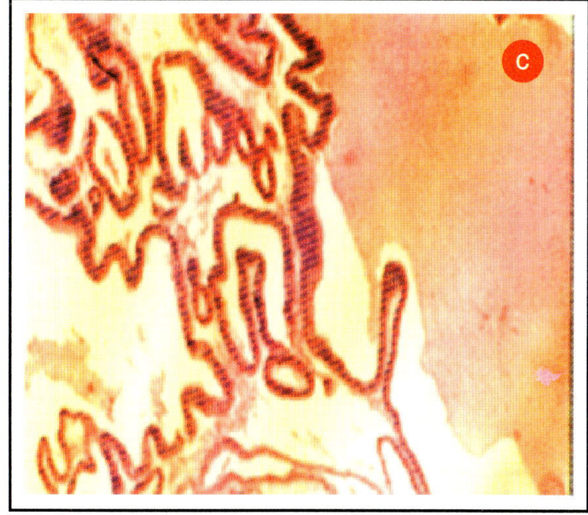

Figure 52 : Cystadenocarcinoma in sangai deer (*C. eldi eldi*).Photographs showing: (a) Swelling of frontonasal region. (b) Extirpated cancerous growth from the nasal chamber of (a). Photomicrograph(c) of (b) (Rao and Acharjyo, 2003.).

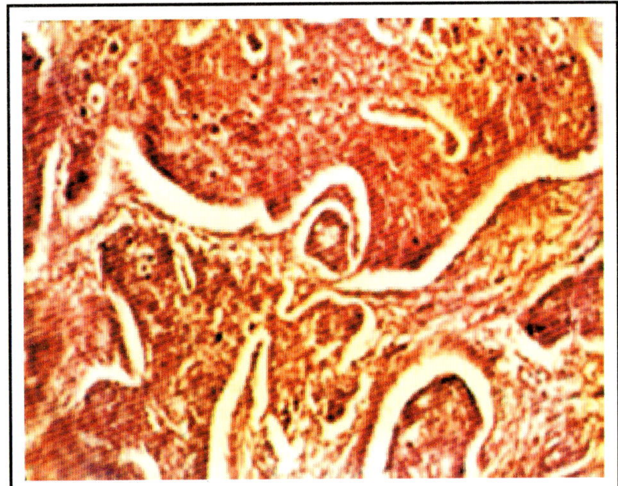

Figure 53 : Photomicrograph showing squamous cell carcinoma from ethmoid region of sika deer (*Cervus nippon*, an exotic sp.). (Rao and Acharjyo, 2003)

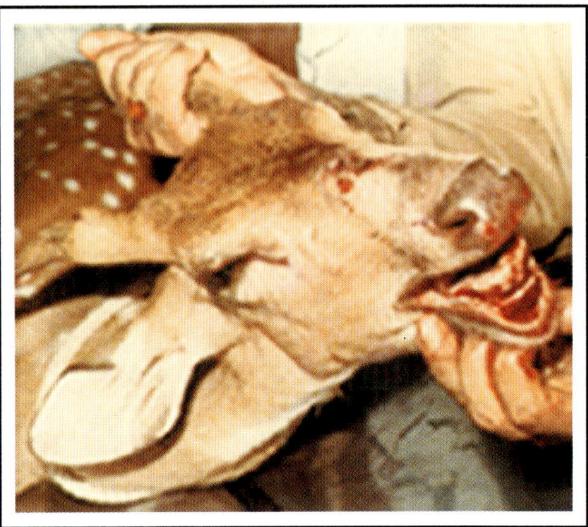

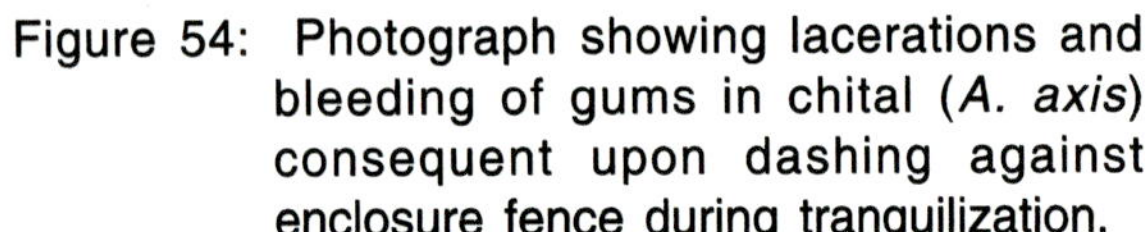

Figure 54: Photograph showing lacerations and bleeding of gums in chital (*A. axis*) consequent upon dashing against enclosure fence during tranquilization.

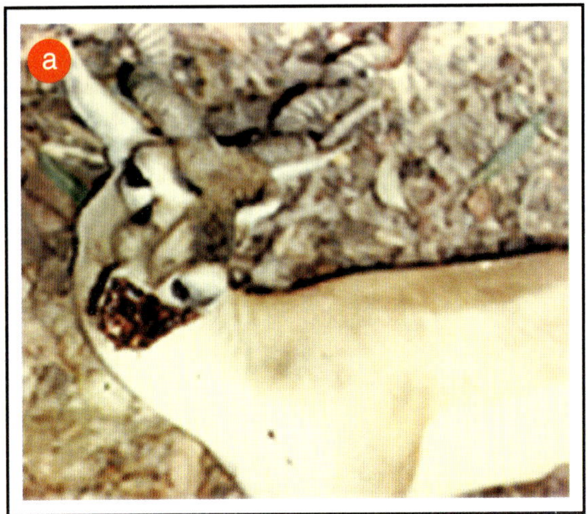

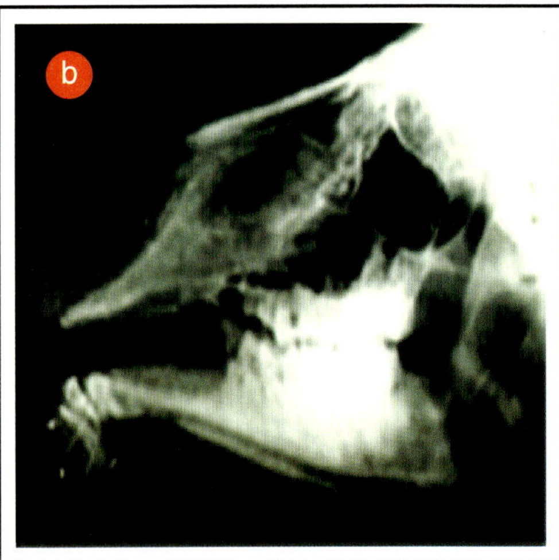

Figure 55 : Photograph showing: (a) Severe lacerations of lower gums of male blackbuck (*A. cervicapra*) caused due to dashing repeatedly against the enclosure fence in efforts to get mixed with a herd in the adjacent enclosure. (b) Radiograph of (a) showing severity of the damaged gums and shattered incisors.

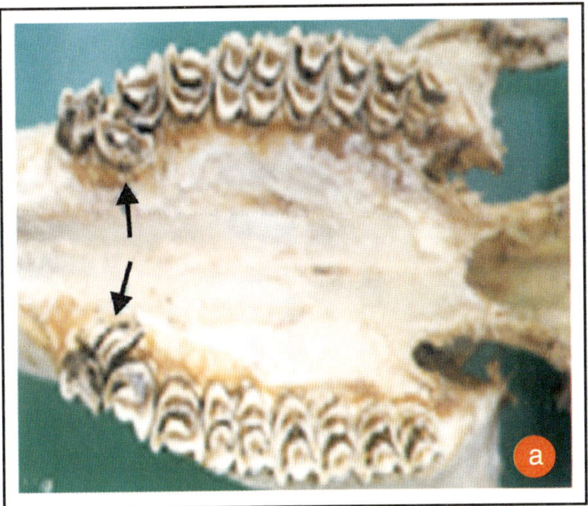

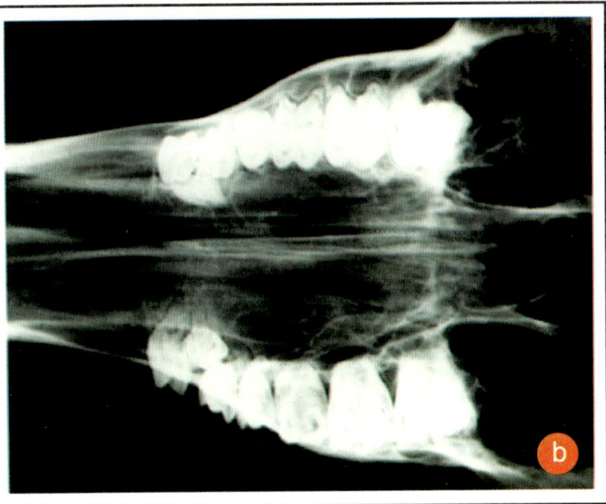

Figure 56: (a) Photograph showing a supernumerary tooth on either side of maxillary jaw of nilgai (*B. tragocamelus*). (b) Radiograph of (a) showing location of supernumerary tooth.

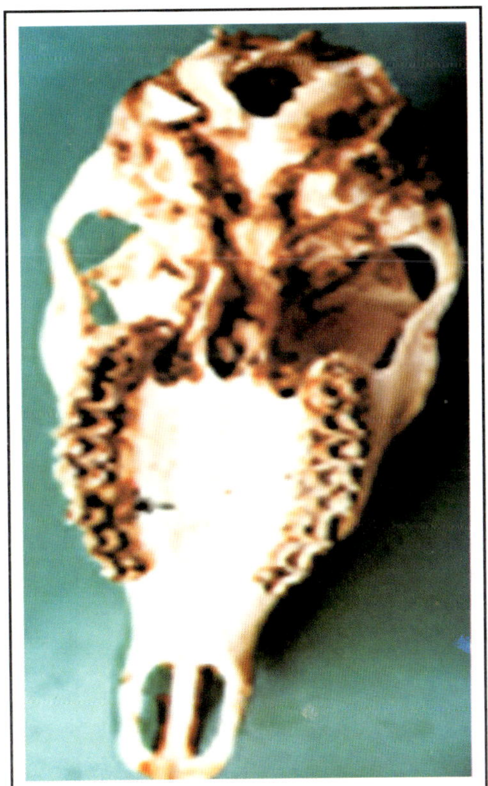

Figure 57: Photograph showing a growth on lingual aspect of left upper 3rd maxillary premolar in chital (*A. axis*).

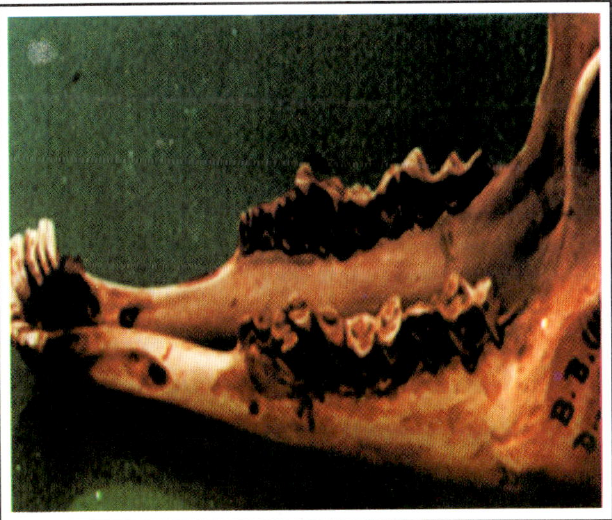

Figure 58: Photograph of blackbuck (*A. cervicapra*) mandible showing varying degree of wear in its cheek teeth. Note left ramus also showing a supernumerary premolar.

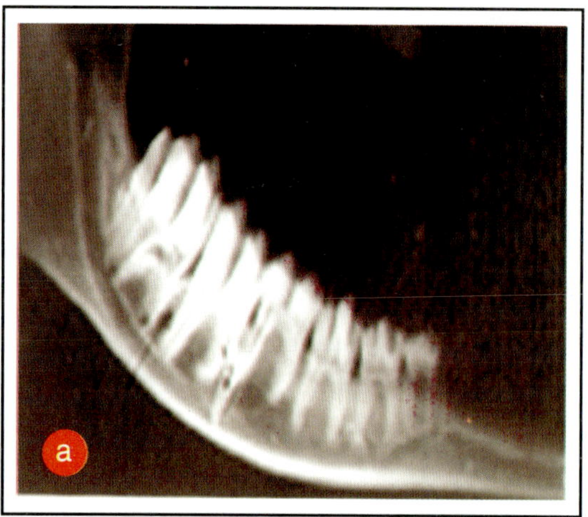
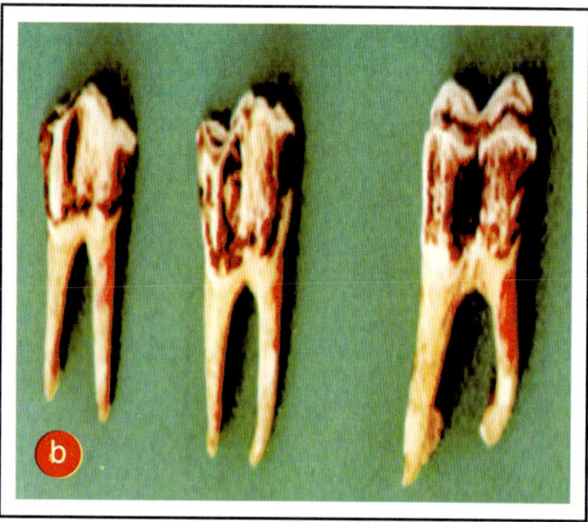

Figure 59: (a) Radiograph of sambar (*C. unicolor*) mandible showing formation of a spur between roots of first and 2nd molar teeth and its root extending beyond the mandibular canal. (b) 2nd molar showing bent root.

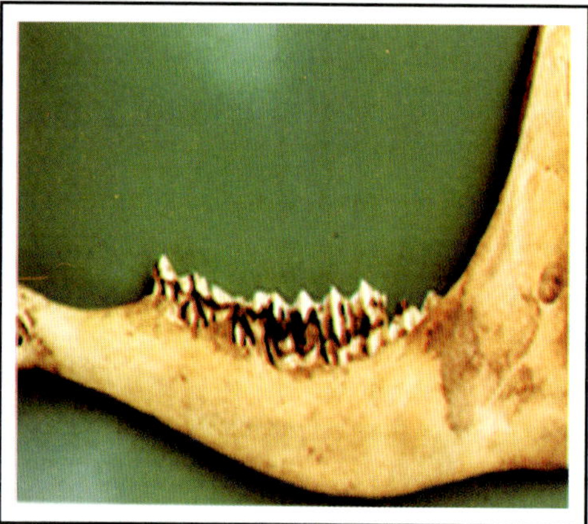

Figure 60: Photograph of an adult hog-deer (*A. porcinus*) mandible showing existing 2nd and 3rd premolars being replaced by the new ones.

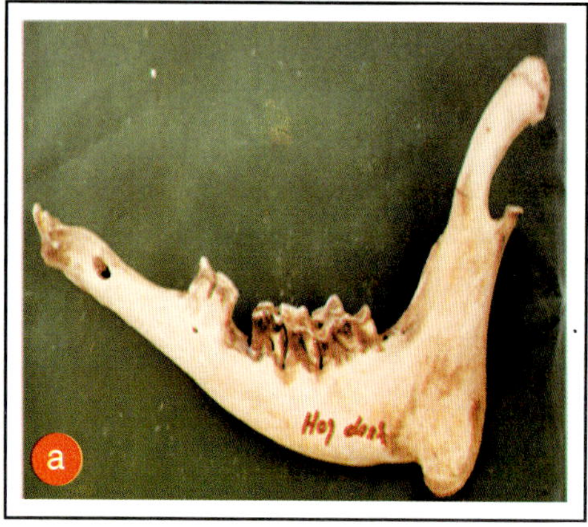

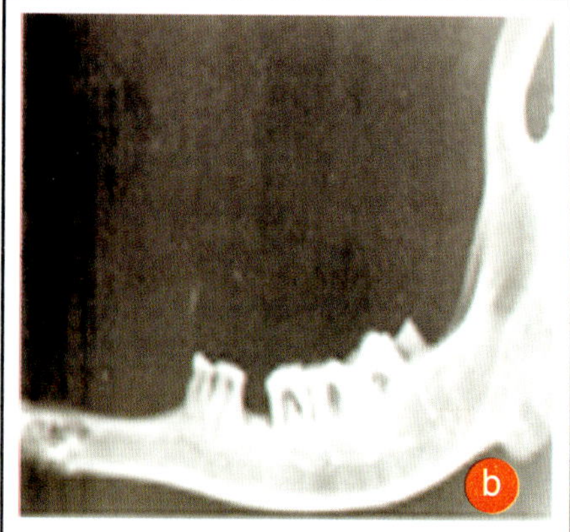

Figure 61: (a) Photograph of hog-deer (*A. porcinus*) mandible showing: (a) Loss of 3rd premolar (b) Radiograph of (a) showing obliterated alveolus. Note wearing of occlusal surfaces of cheek teeth.

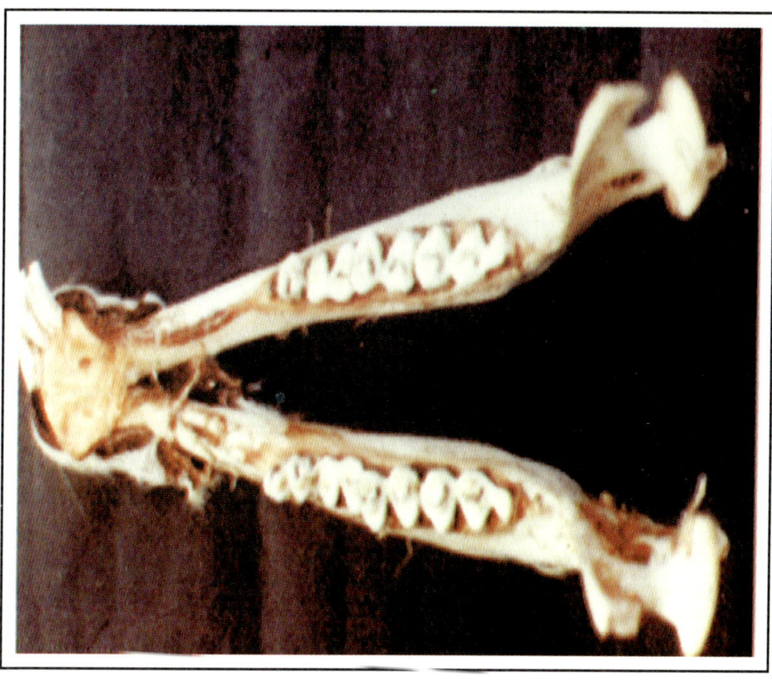

Figure 62: Photograph showing absence of left side incisors in blackbuck (*A. cervicapra*). Note their alveoli obliterated, which could be due to impact of some traumatic blow, the animal had experienced in its early life.

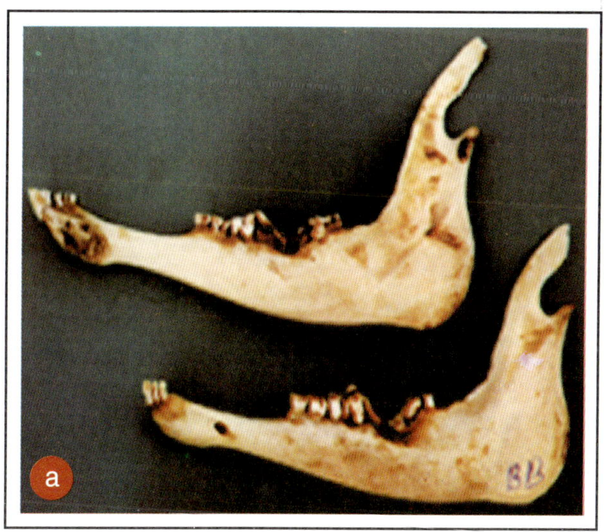

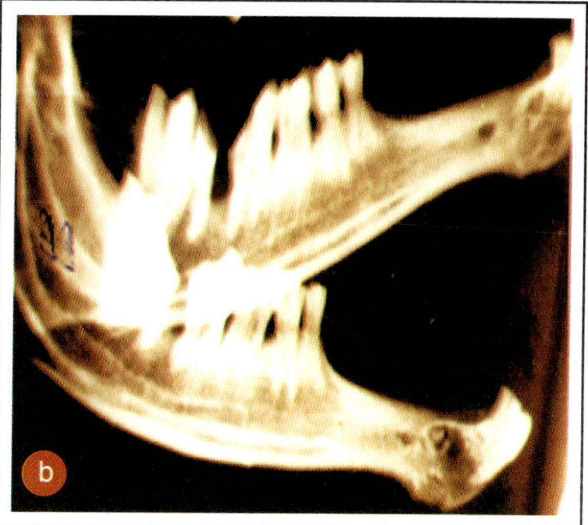

Figure 63: (a) Photograph of blackbucks (*A. cervicapra*) mandible showing rare half of M_3 of either side damaged. (b) Radiograph of (a) discerening the same.

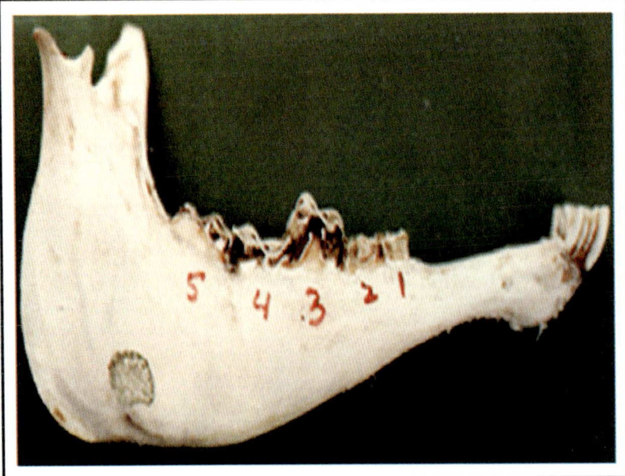

Figure 64: Photograph showing uneven wears of lower cheek teeth in blackbuck (*A. cervicapra*).

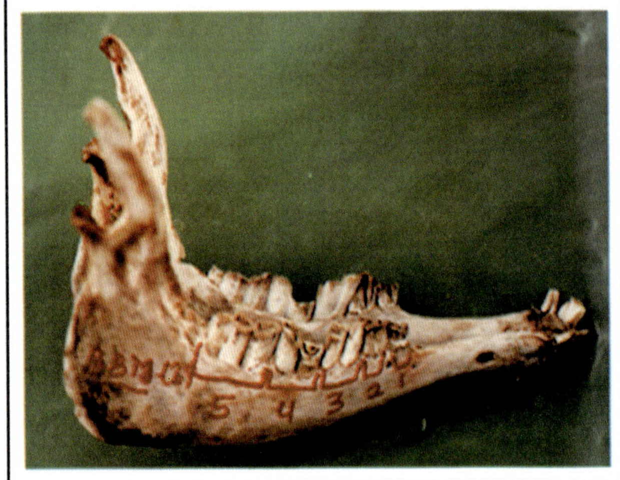

Figure 65: Photograph showing uneven wears of mandible premolars in blackbuck (*A. cervicapra*).

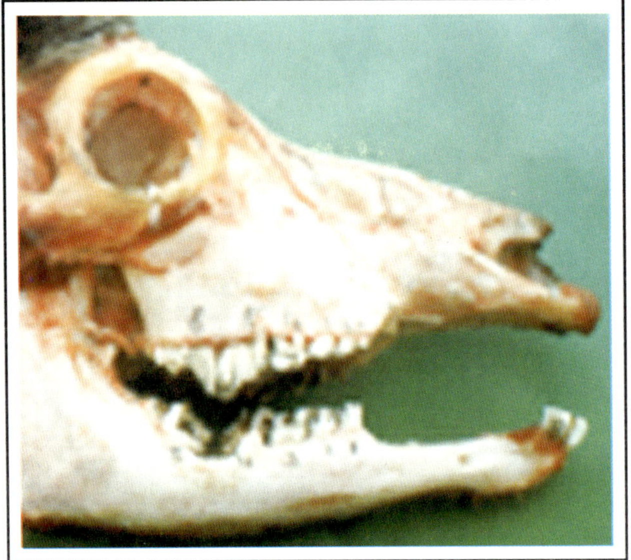

Figure 66: Photograph showing uneven wears of upper cheek teeth and also 1st and 2nd molars of lower jaw in blackbuck (*A. cervicapra*)

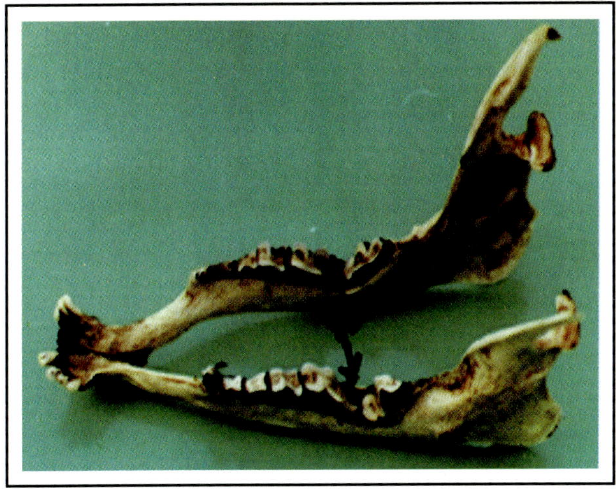

Figure 67: Photograph of chinkara (*G. gazella*) mandible showing severe wear of cheek teeth.

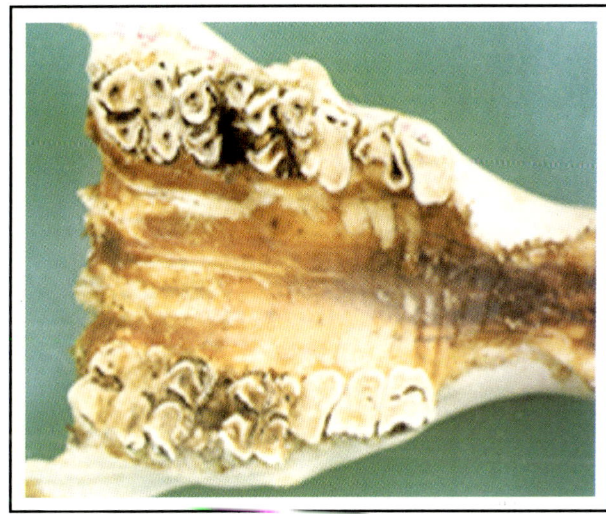

Figure 68: Photograph showing wear and loss of maxillary teeth in chital (*A. axis*). Note signs of caries.

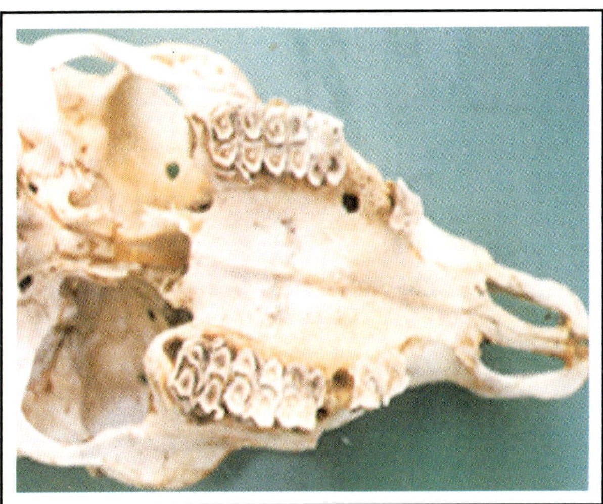

Figure 69: Photograph showing wear and loss of maxillary teeth in chital (*A. axis*).

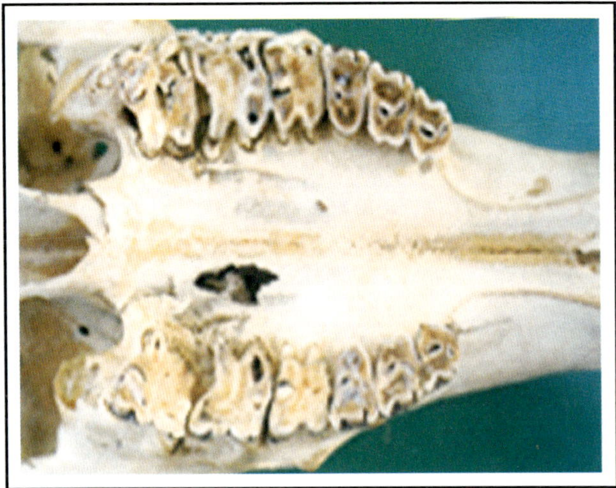

Figure 70: Photograph showing wear as well as caries in maxillary teeth of barasingha (*C.d. duvauceli*).

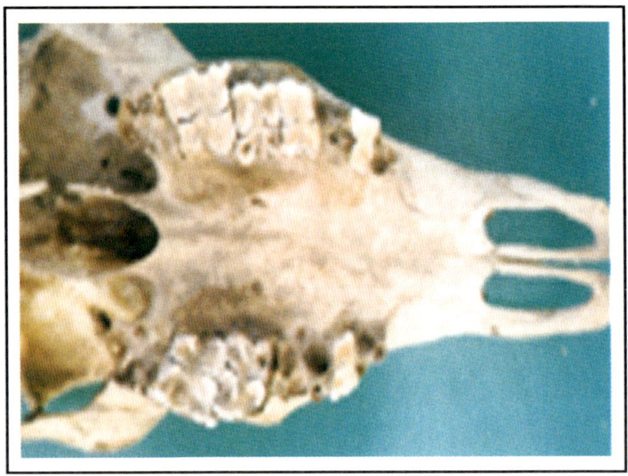

Figure 71: Photograph showing wear and caries in upper premolars of hog-deer (*A. porcinus*).

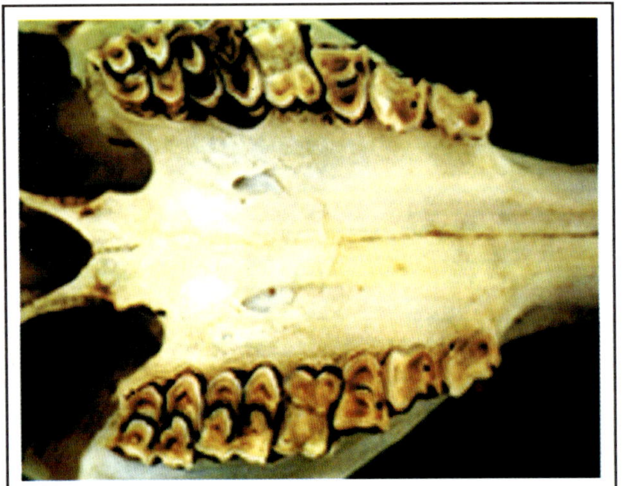

Figure 72: Photograph showing wear (also caries in 2nd right molar) in maxillary teeth of barking deer (*M. muntjak*).

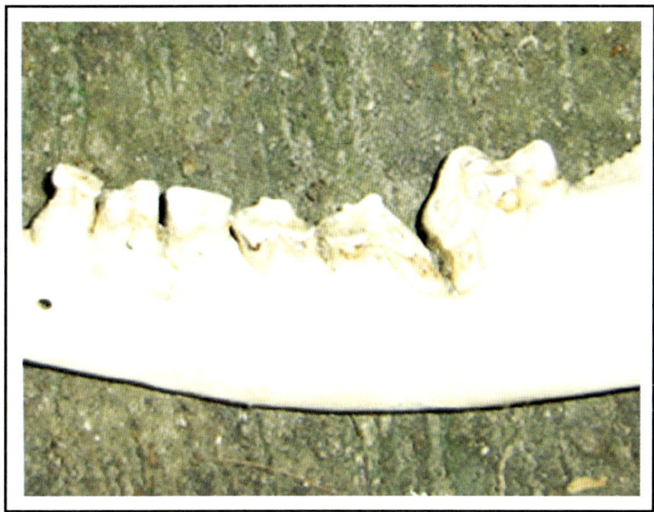

Figure 73: Photograph showing uneven wears in mandibular cheek teeth of chital (*A. axis*). Note recession of alveolar border between the last two cheek teeth.

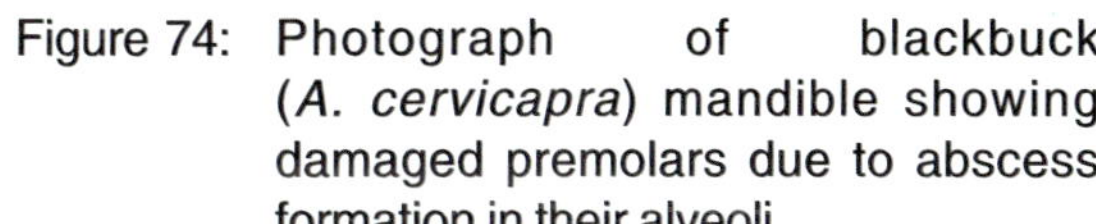

Figure 74: Photograph of blackbuck (*A. cervicapra*) mandible showing damaged premolars due to abscess formation in their alveoli.

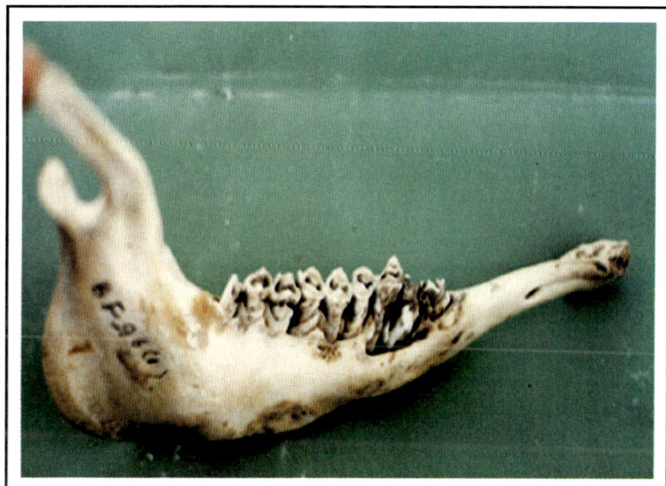

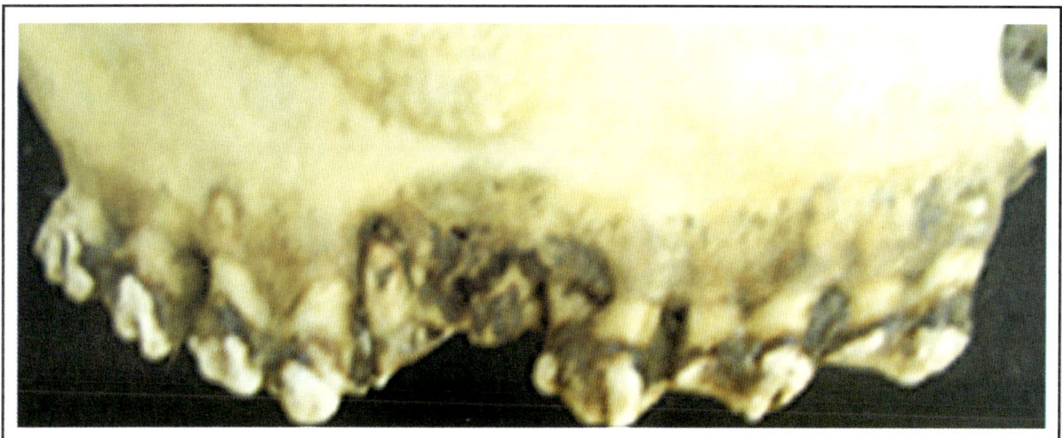

Figure 75: Photograph of maxillary jaw of sambar (*C. unicolor*) showing decaying of last premolar and 1st molar teeth.

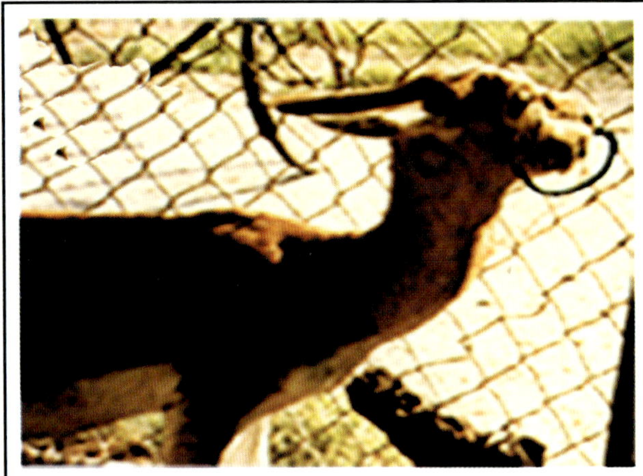

Figure 76: Photograph showing swollen right cheek of the blackbuck (*A. cervicapra*) due to chewing of broken fence wire piece.

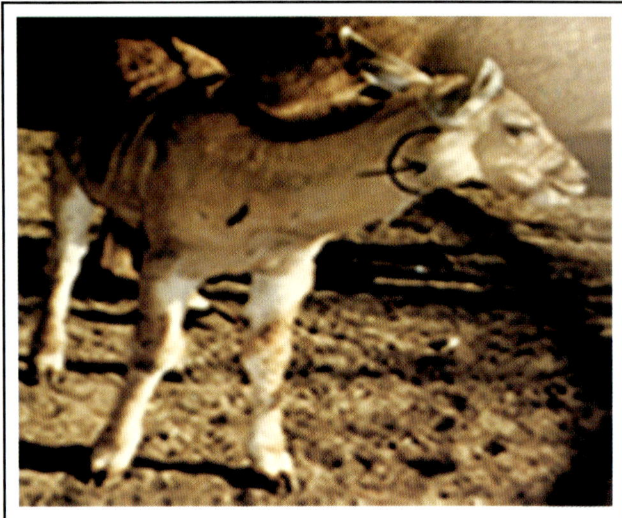

Figure77 : Photograph showing parotiditis in eland (*Taurotragus oryx*, an exotic sp.) calf due to Staphylococcus infection.

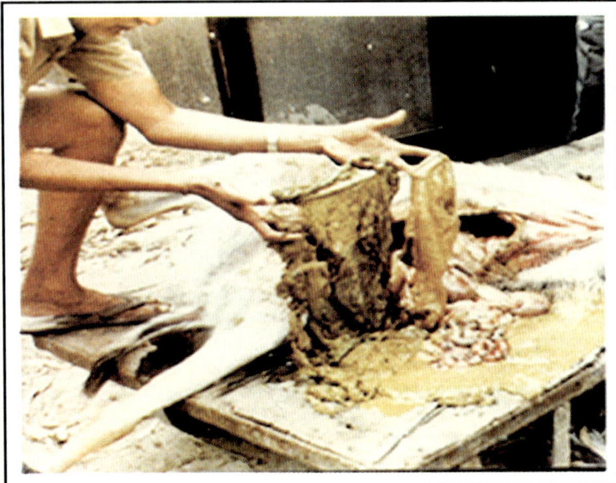

Figure 78: Photograph showing mass of polythene bags causing impaction of rumen of red lechwe (*Kobus lechee*,an exotic antelope).

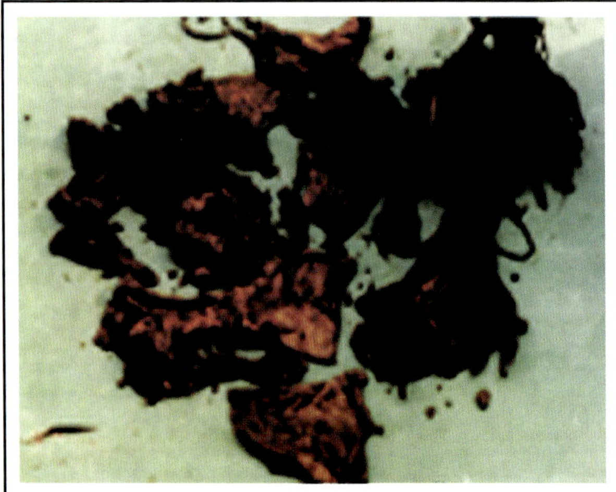

Figure 79: Photograph showing mass of 3.5 kg of polythene bags recovered from the rumen of an adult blackbuck (*A. cervicapra*).

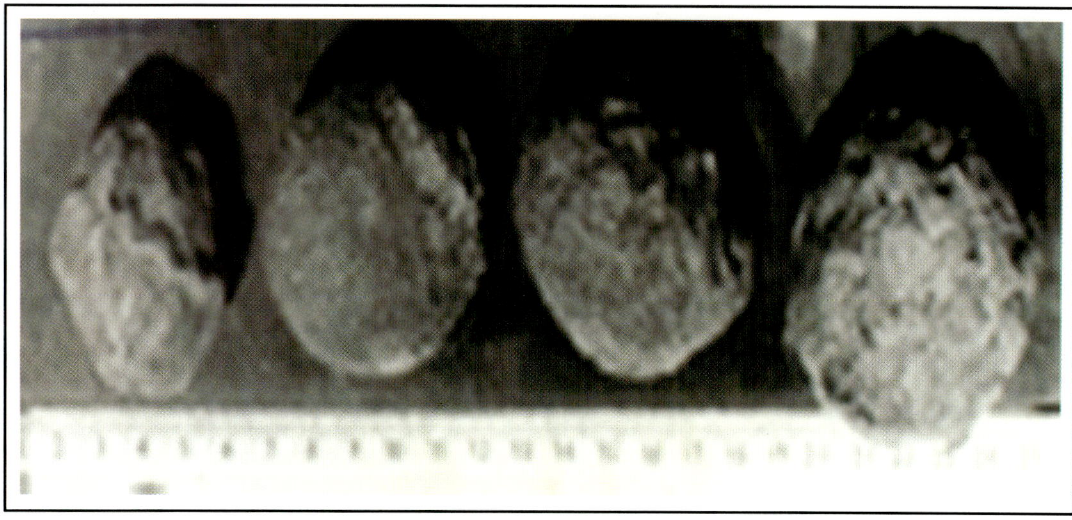

Figure 80: Photograph of phytobezoars recovered from the rumen during necropsy of a giraffe (*G. camelopardus*, an exotic sp.). One such phytobezoar caused obstruction at the oesophageal end of rumen.

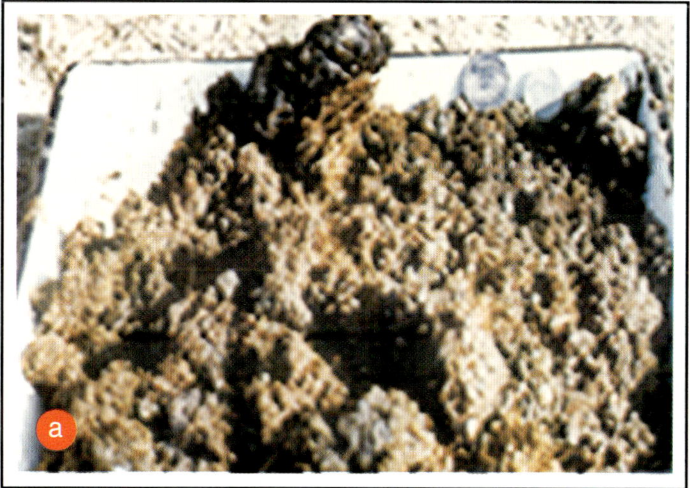

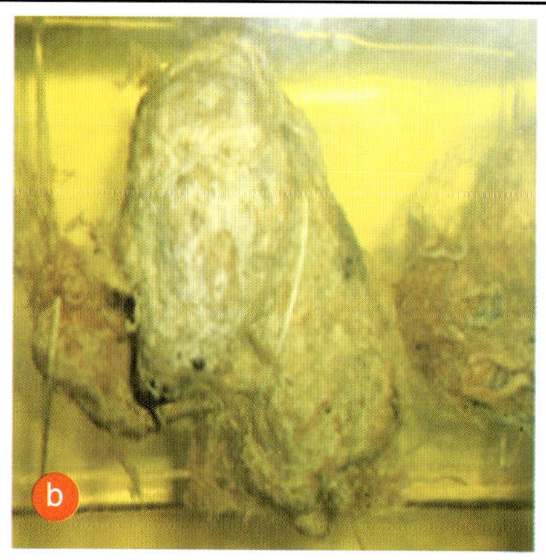

Figure 81: Photograph of gastroliths recovered from the stomach of hippopotamus (*H. amphibius*, an exotic sp.) died in Zoological Garden, Lucknow (U.P.). (b) Photograph showing hair balls recovered from the stomach of Llama (*Lama glama*, an exotic sp.) died in the Zoological Garden, Chennai, TN (Courtesy: Dept. of Wildlife Sci,C.V.Sc. Chennai, TN).

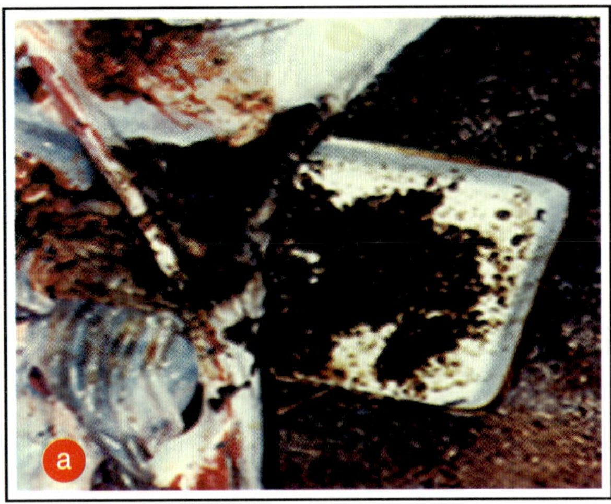

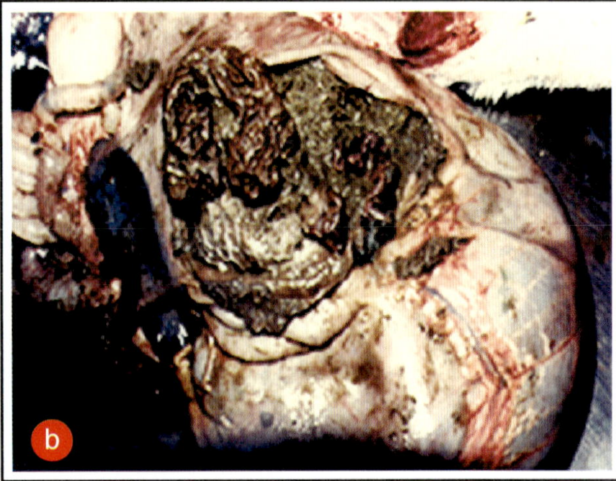

Figure 82: (a) Photograph showing sand collected from rumen of an adult chital (*A.axis*) which died of tuberculosis (b) Photograph showing leather pieces in the rumen of blackbuck (*A. cervicapra*).Due to which animal used to suffer from episodes of recurrent tympany.

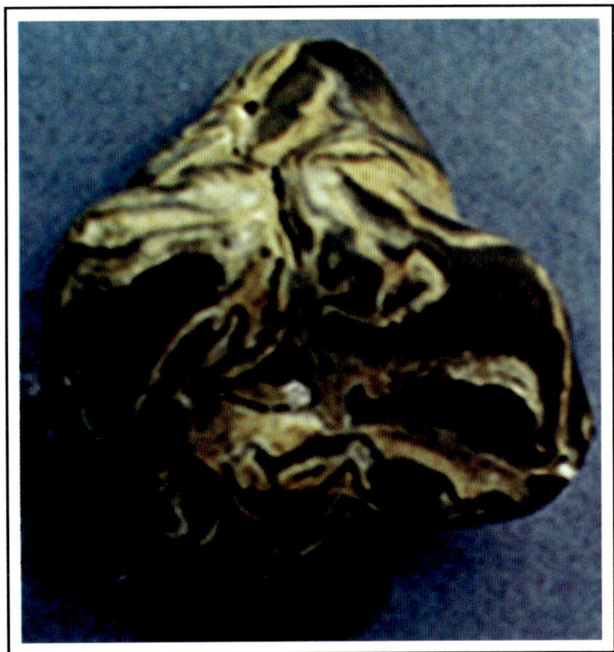

Figure 83: Photograph of a prism shaped hard fibrous matter recovered from rumen during necropsy of barking deer (*M.muntjak*).

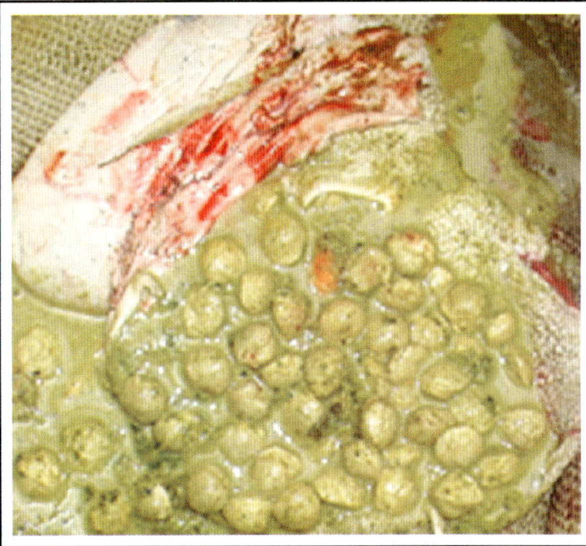

Figure 84: Photograph showing soybean chunks (*Glycine max*) in rumen of barking deer (*M. muntjak*), died due to bloat after consuming a large quantity of these chunks (Courtesy: Thirumurugan, R.).

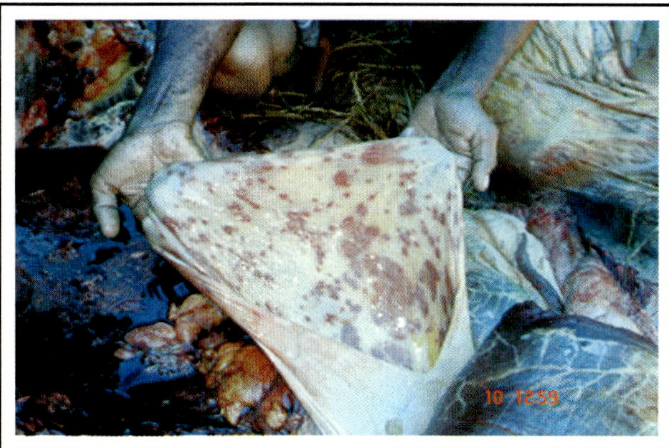

Figure 85: Photograph of abomasum of gaur (*B. gaurus*) showing haemorrhagic lesions related to Haemorrhagic septicaemia (Courtesy: Nanjappa, K.A.).

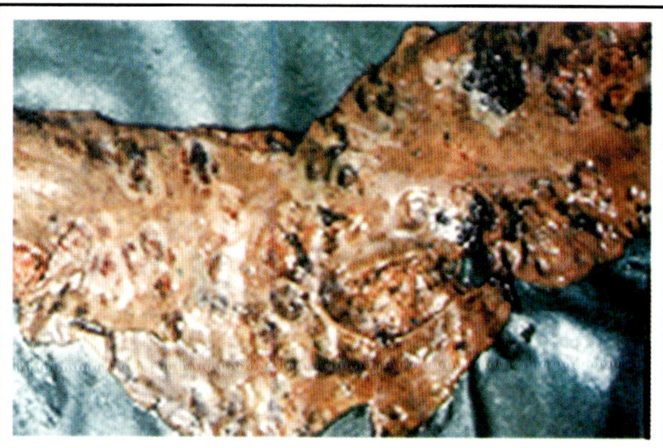

Figure 86: Photograph showing haemorrhagic and necrotic ulceration in the intestine of hippopotamus (*H. amphibius*, an exotic sp.) related to salmonellosis.

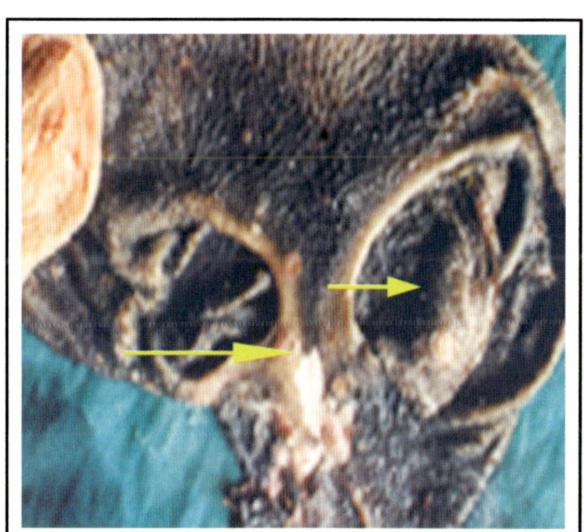

Figure 87: Photograph showing tuberculous abscess in the rumen of chousingha (*T. quadricornis*) died in captivity. (Courtesy: Suryawanshi, D.S.).

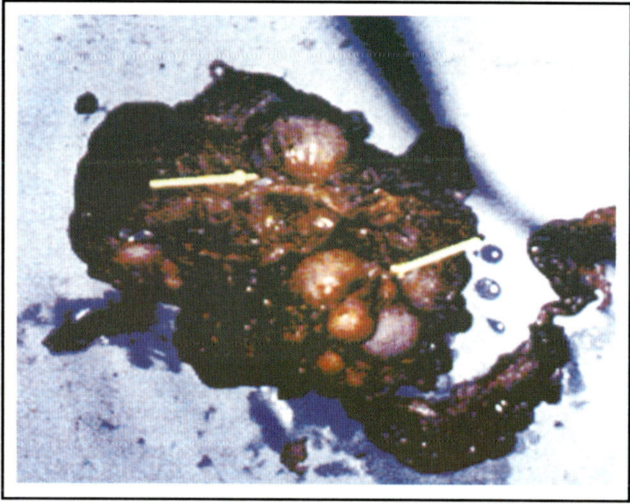

Figure 88: Photograph showing tuberculous nodules in the small intestine and mesentery of an adult female chital (*A. axis*) died in captivity.

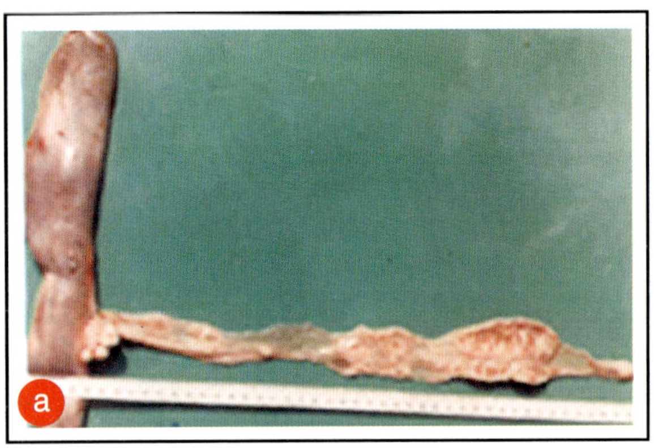

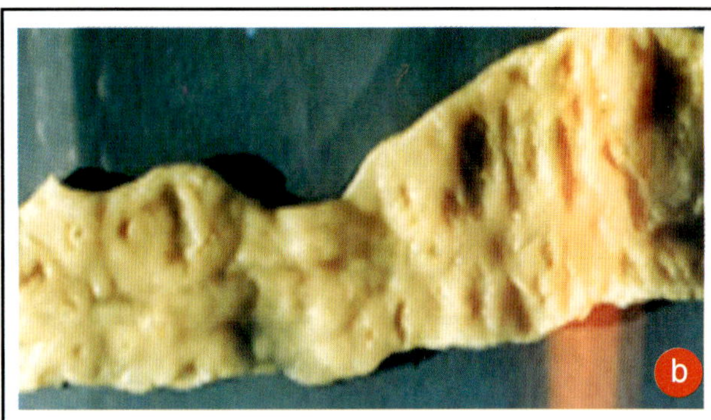

Figure 89: (a) Photograph showing tuberculous nodules at the ileo-caecal junction and (b) crateous tuberculous lesions in the small intestine of blackbuck (*A. cervicapra*).

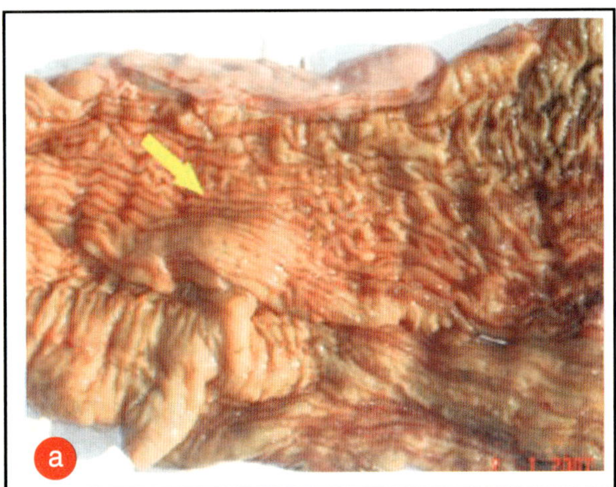

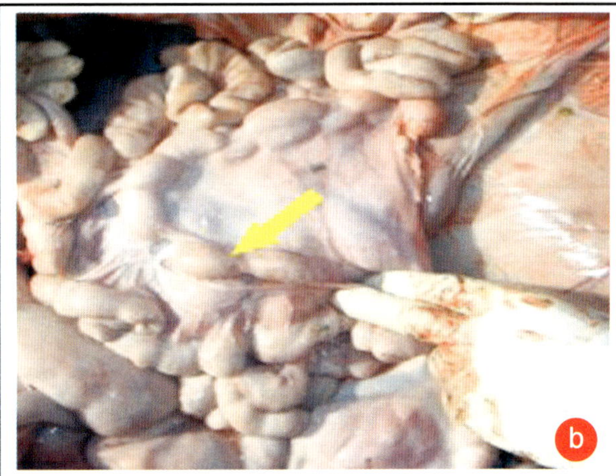

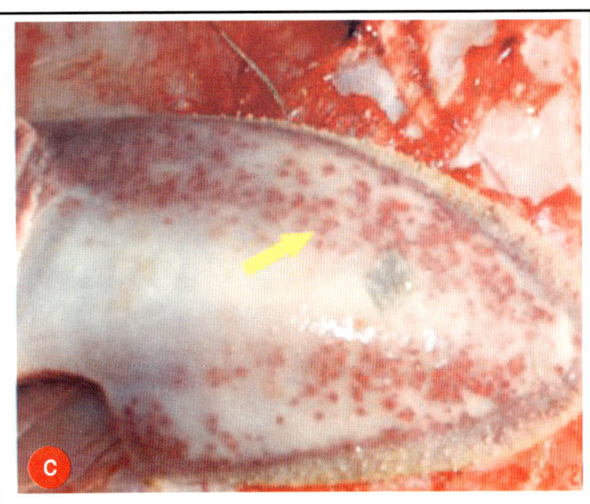

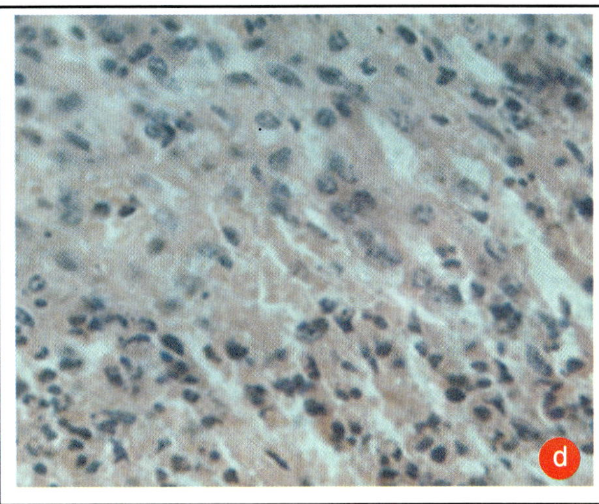

Figure 90: (a) Photograph of intestine from gaur (*B. gaurus*) showing corrugated and thickened folds of paratuberculosis. (b) Enlarged mesenteric lymph nodes. (c) Haemorrhagic and necrotic lesions on the ventral surface of tongue. (d) Photomicrograph of (a) showing mononuclear cell infiltration. H&E,x200 (Courtesy: Gupta, M.P.).

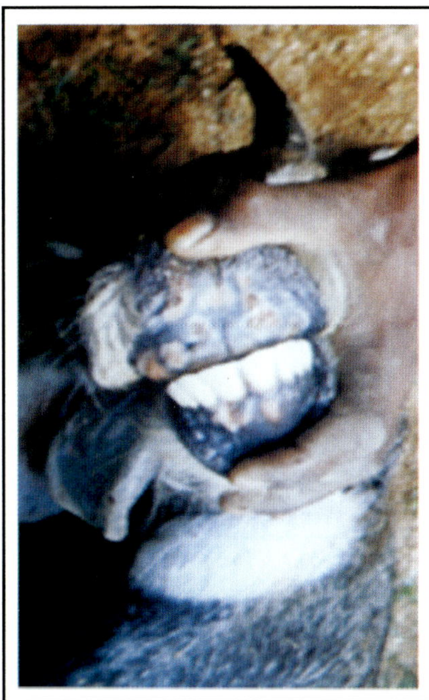

Figure 91: Photograph showing foot and mouth (FMD) lesions - Burst vesicles on the muzzle and gums of nilgai (*B. tragocamelus*). Courtesy:(Dept. of Pathology, C.V.Sc, Tirupati, A.P).

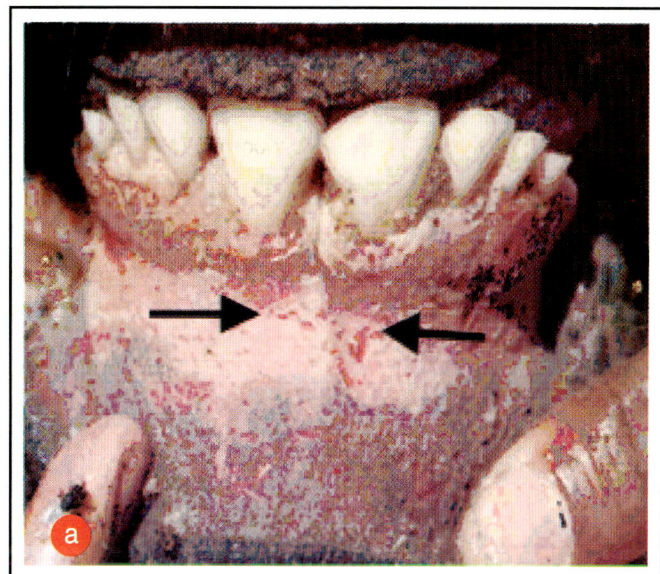

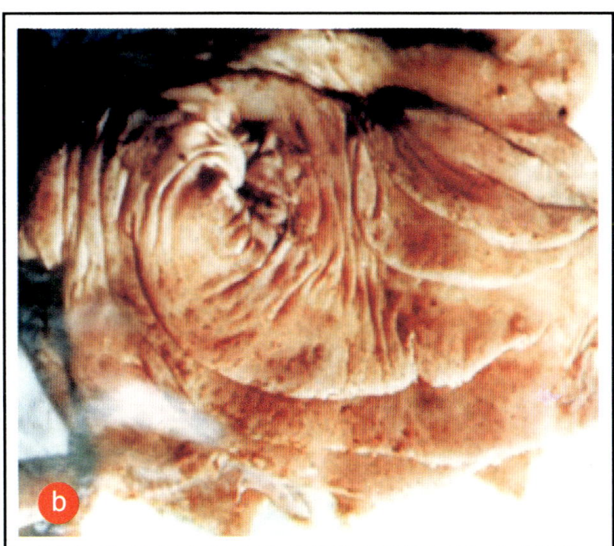

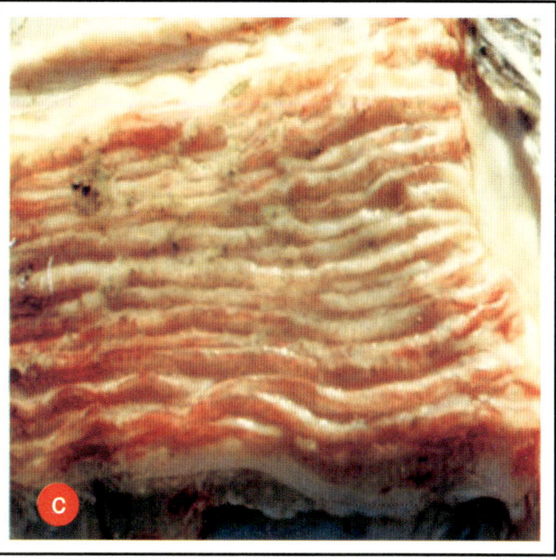

Figure 92: Rinderpest in gaur (*B. gaurus*) died in Bhadra Wildlife Sanctuary, Karnataka (Courtesy: Ranuka prasad, C. and Babu, M. M.).Photographs showing : (a) Rinderpest lesions on dental pad. (b,c) Corrugations of mucosal folds in abomasum and rectum.

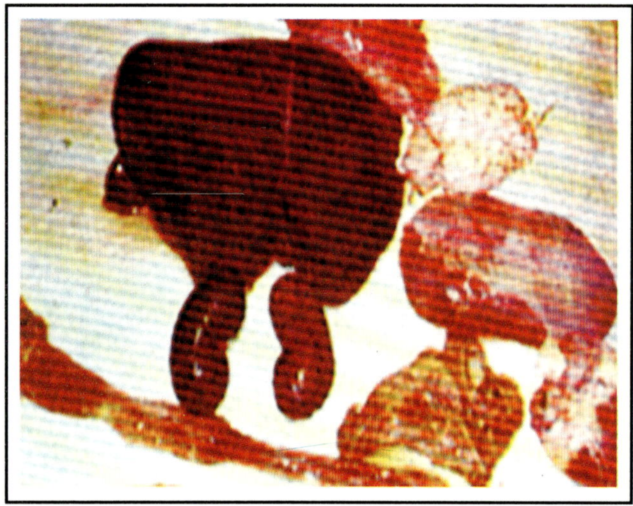

Figure 93: Rinderpest in chital (*A. axis*). Photograph showing haemorrhagic lesion in the abomasum and small intestine and severe congestion in other organs.

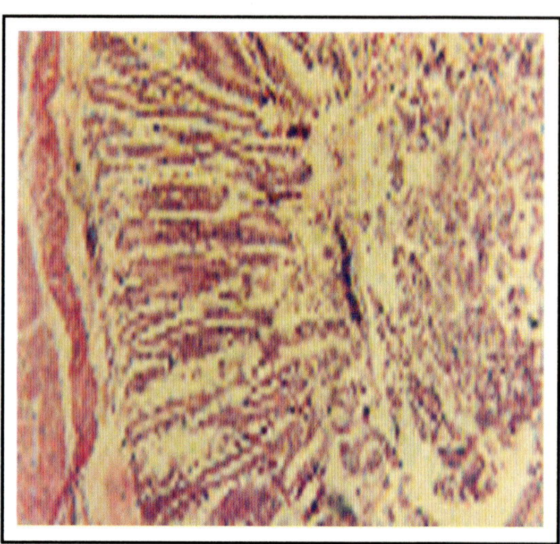

Figure 94: Photomicrograph showing necrotic gastritis indistinguishable from blue tongue in hog-deer (*A. porcinus*). H & E, x100. (Courtesy: Bhowmik, M.K.).

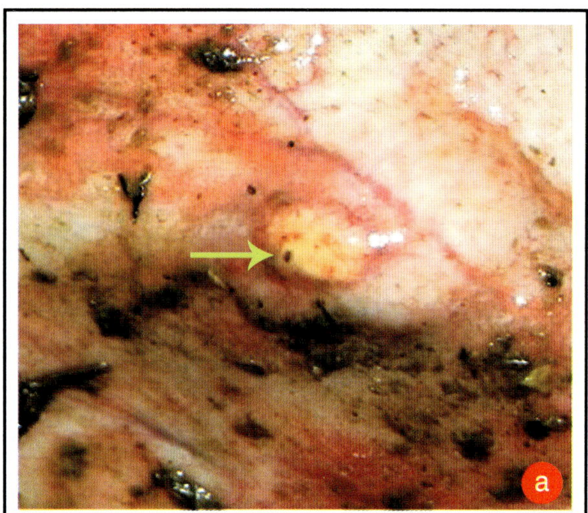

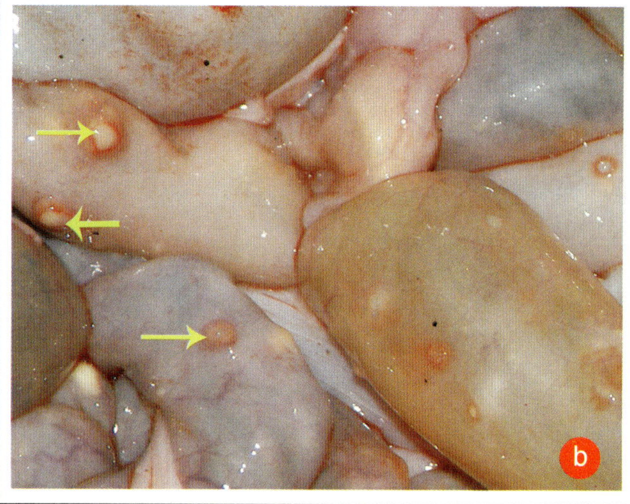

Figure 95: Swine fever encountered in wild boars (*S.scrofa cristatus*) died in the Garumara National Park (WB) Photographs showing:(a) Button like ulcers on the mucosa of intestine (b) Nodular lesion on the serosal surface of intestine. (Courtesy : Anupam Rakshit)

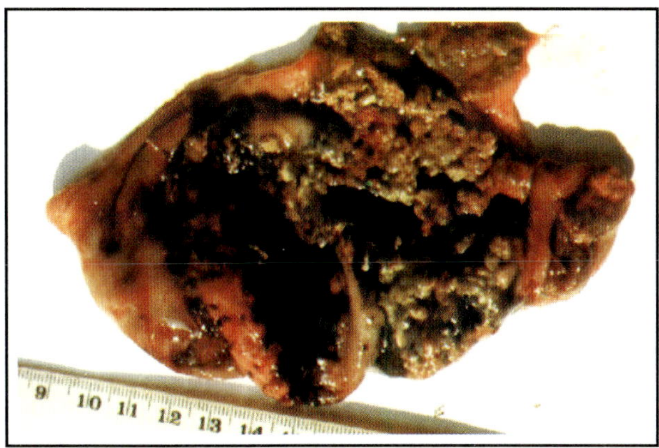

Figure 96: Photograph of pigmy hog (*P. salvania*) showing caseo-necrotic gastritis related to zygomycosis and *Salmonella enteritidis* infection.

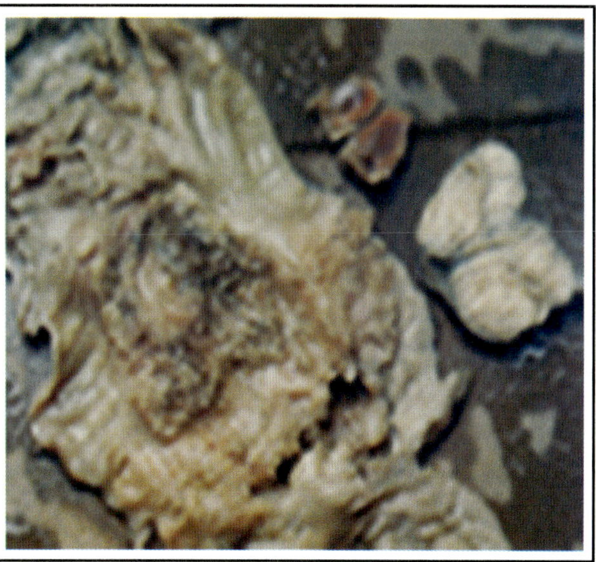

Figure 97: Photograph showing *Candida albicans* infection with ulceration and perforation in the duodenum of blackbuck (*A. cervicapra*). Note a caseated and enlarged lymph node and a normal mesenteric lymph node placed nearby.

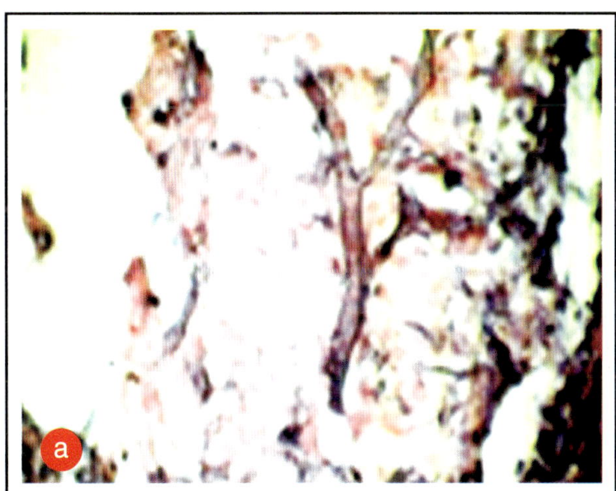

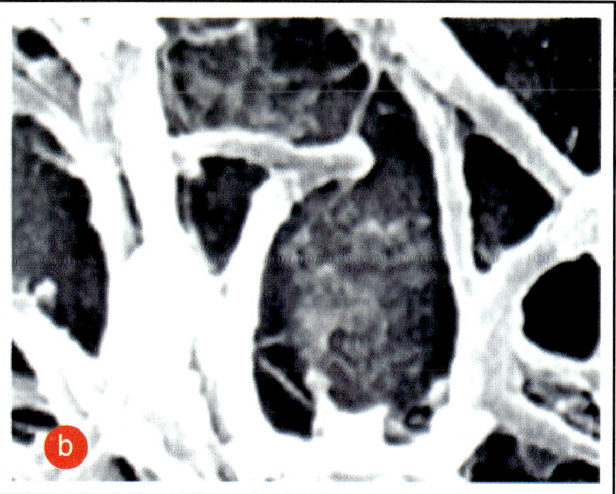

Figure 98: (a) Photomicrograph of stomach of pigmy hog (*P. salvania*) showing broad aseptated thin walled fungal hyphae in the necrotic mucosa. H&E,x400. (b) Scan EM photograph of the section (a) showing necrosis and different sizes of fungal hyphae x 8600.

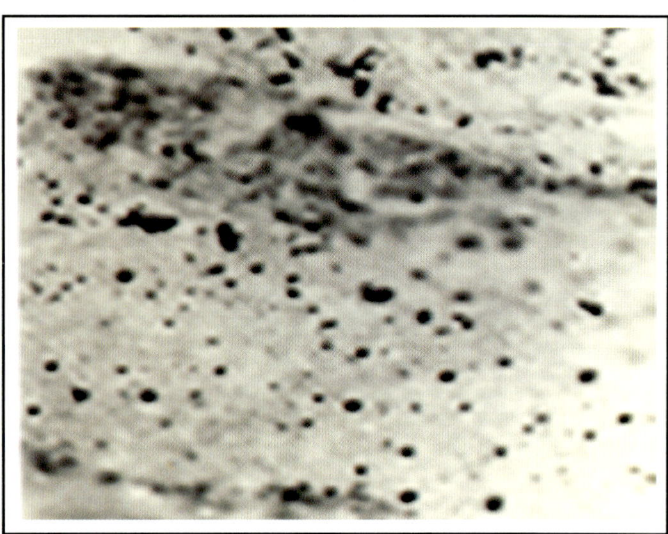

Figure 99: Photomicrograph showing spores and pseudohyphaes of *Candida* sp. causing ulcer in the duodenum of sambar (*C. unicolor*). H&E, x 280

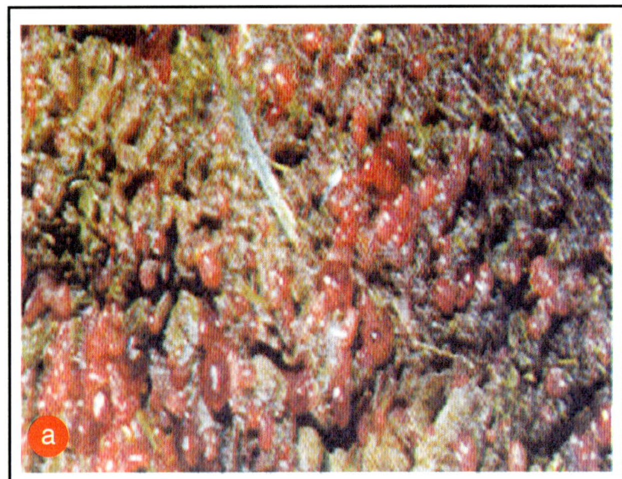

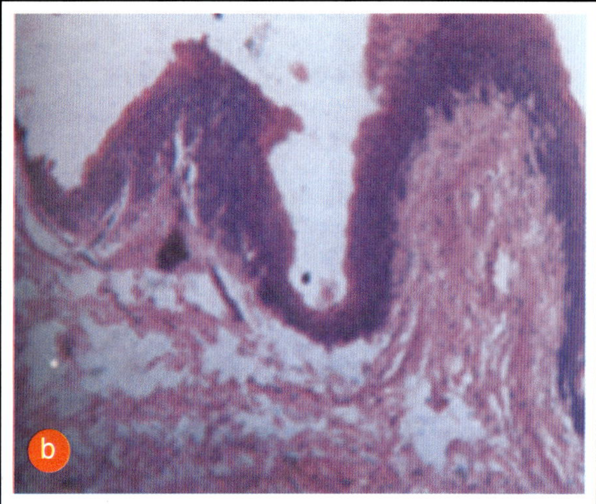

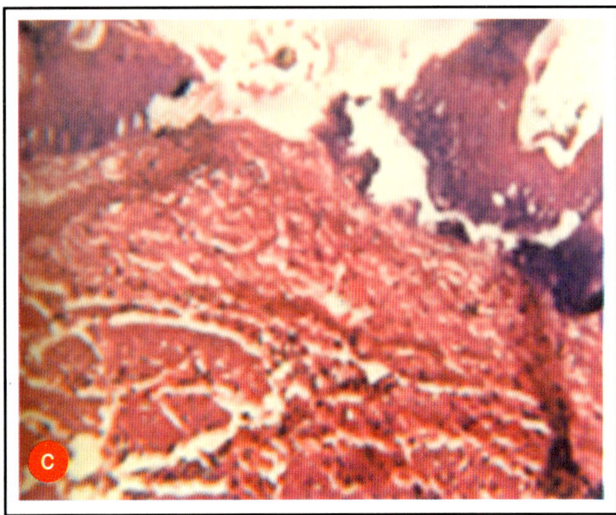

Figure 100: (a) Photograph of rumen of chital (*A. axis*) showing immature amphistomes. (b) Photomicrographs of (a) showing hyperplastic changes in different layers and (c) destruction /denudation of papillae layer. H&E, x100 (Courtesy: Mukhopadhayay, S.K.).

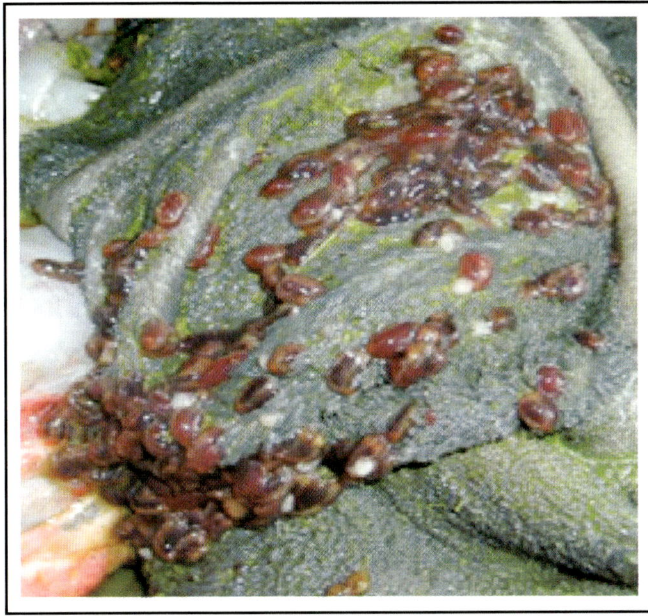

Figure 101: Photograph of rumen of blackbuck (*A. cervicapra*) showing immature amphistomes.

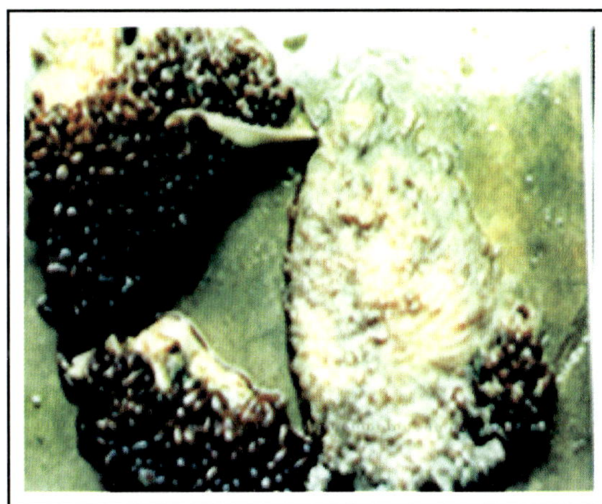

Figure 102: Pieces of rumen and reticulum from chital (*A. axis*) showing massive infection with *Paramphistomum*, *Gastrothalax* and *Fischederius* flukes.

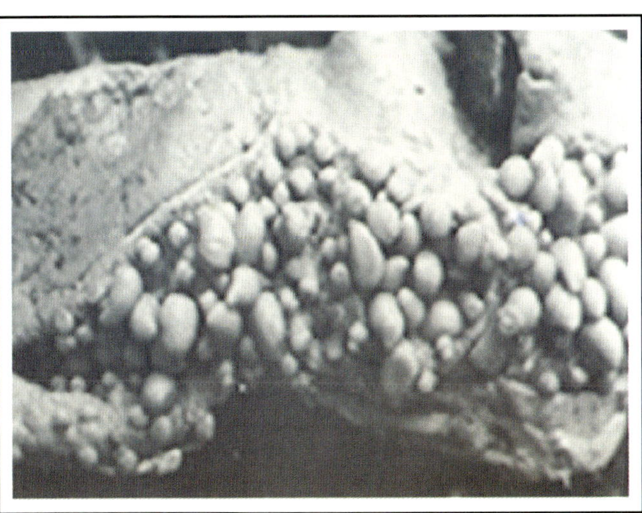

Figure 103: Photograph showing *Gigantocotyle explanatum* in the bile duct of water buffalo (*B. bubalis*) died in Kaziranga National Park, Assam.

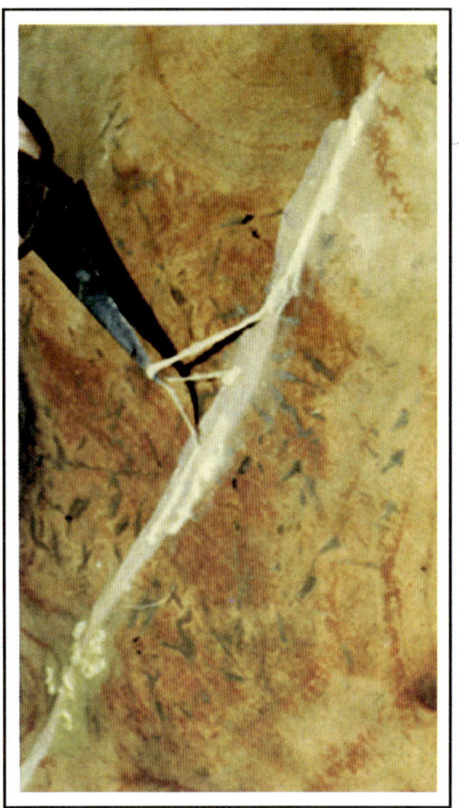

Figure 104:Tapeworms in the intestine of 79-day- old female blackbuck (*A. cervicapra*).

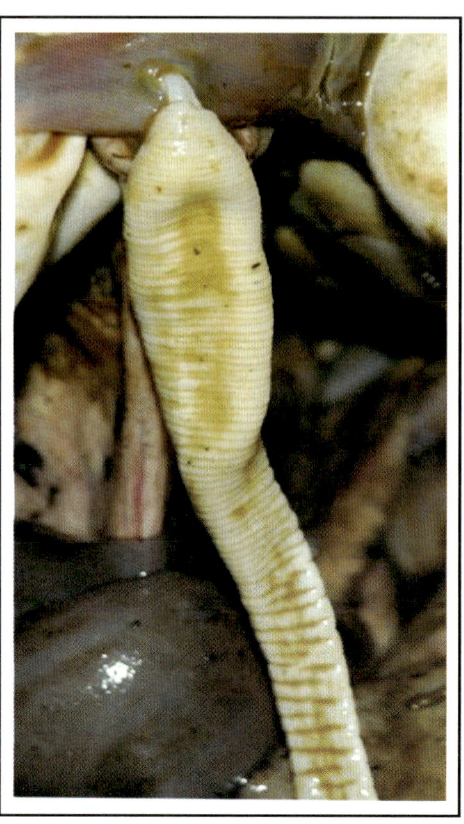

Figure 105: Tapeworm in the intestine of wild boar (*S. scrofa*). Courtesy : Anupam Rakshit.

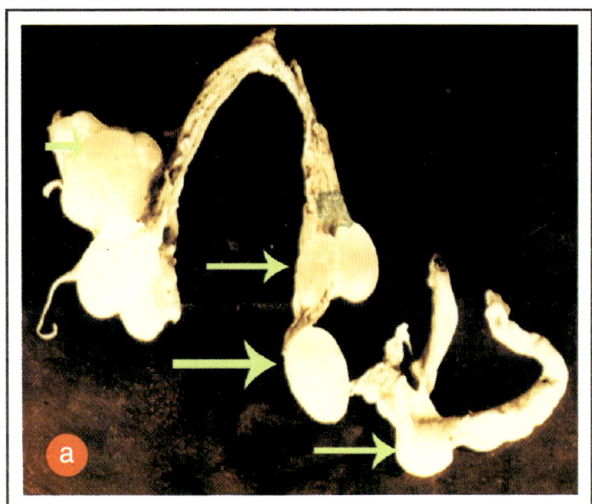

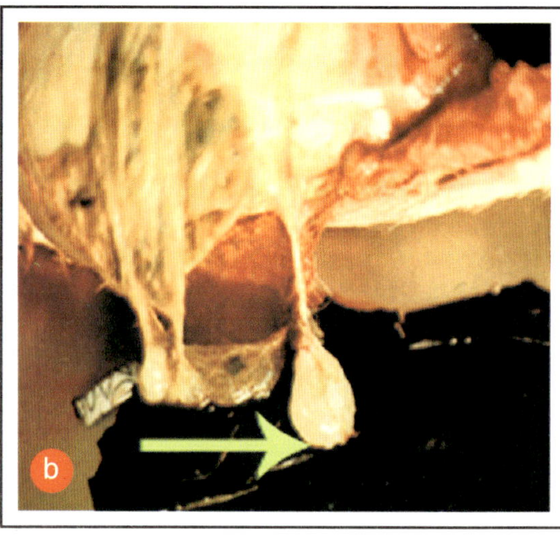

Figure 106: Photographs showing: (a) Cysticerci (*Cysticercus tenuicollis*) ranging from 2.25 to 3.85 cm in diameter attached with mesentery encountered during necropsy of 3- month old blackbuck (*A. cericapra*). (b) A large *C. tenuicollis* cyst attached to mesentery of chital (*A.axis*).

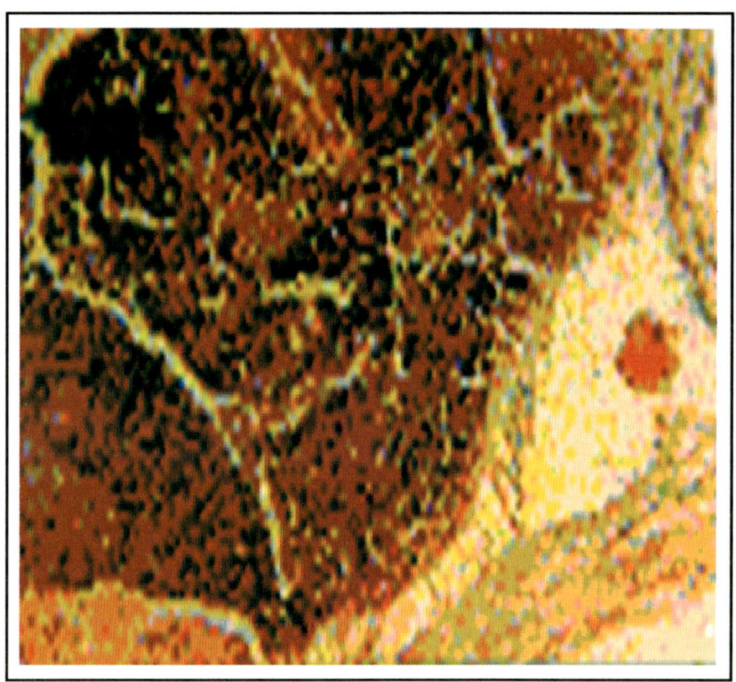

Figure 107: Photomicrograph showing granuloma caused by *Oesophagostomum* sp. infection in the intestine of hog-deer (*A. porcinus*). H&E, x 100 (Courtesy: Bhowmik, M.K.).

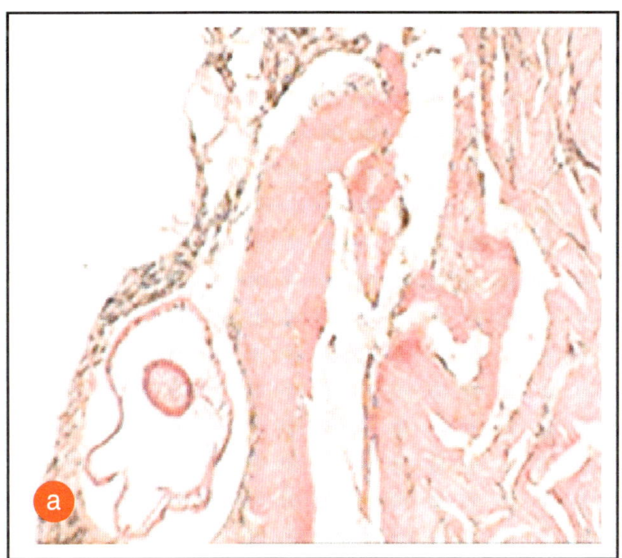

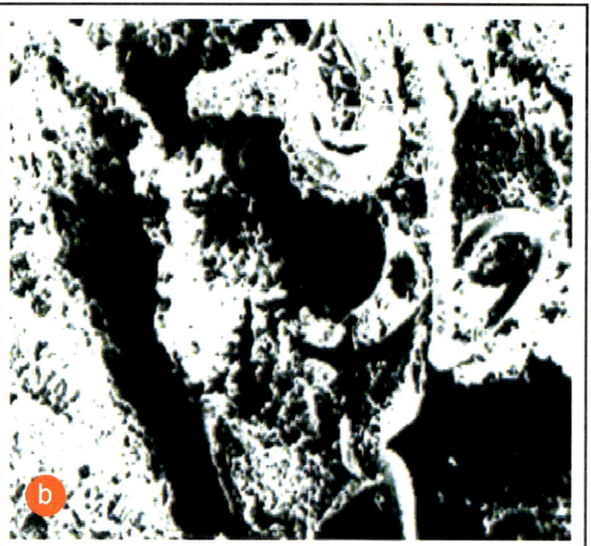

Figure 108: (a) Photomicrograph showing *Trichuris* sp. in the colon of giraffe (*G. camelopardus*, an exotic sp.). H&E x 100. (b) SEM of (a)showing distortion and disruption of mucosa and "tunnel" formation in the affected part. x 28.

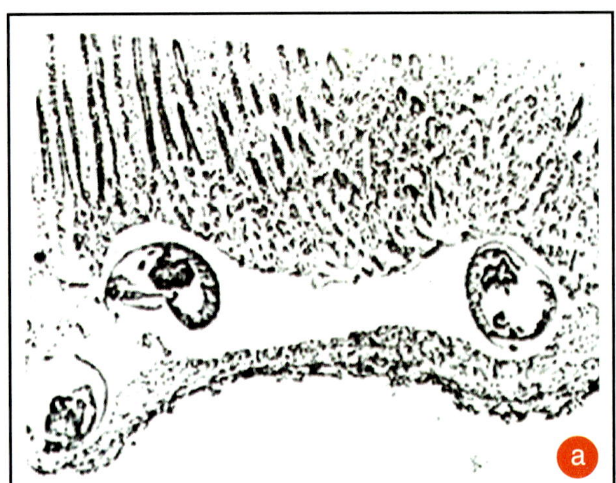

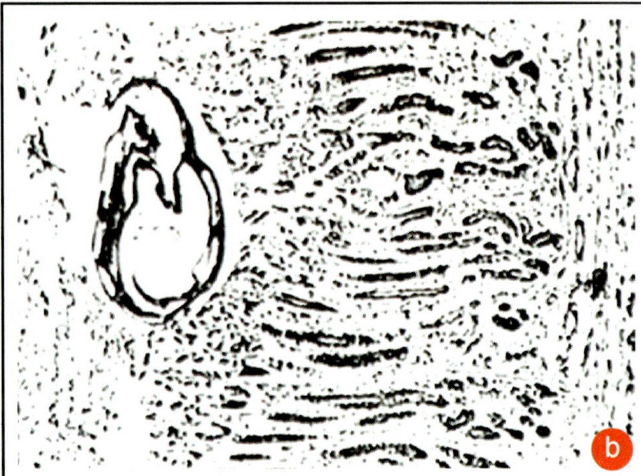

Figure 109: Photomicrographs of sections of abomasum of nilgai (*B. tragocameus*) showing:(a) transversely cut nematode-*Ashworthius mertinagliae* in a tunnel superficially x700 (b) Desquamation of the superficial lining with a part of male worm cut through the bursal region x750 (Chauhan *et al.*, 1972).

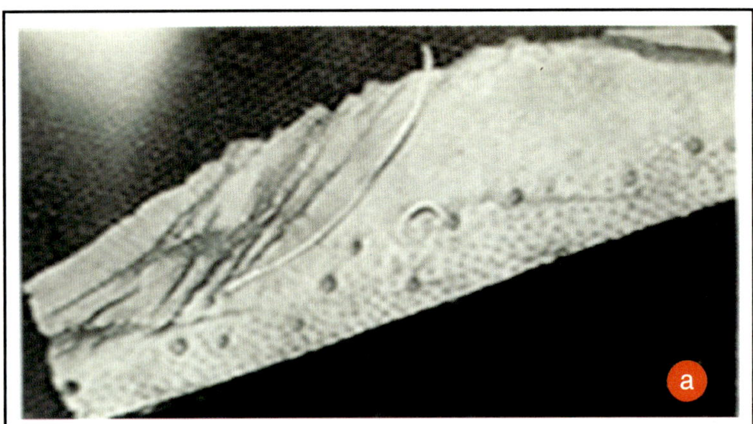

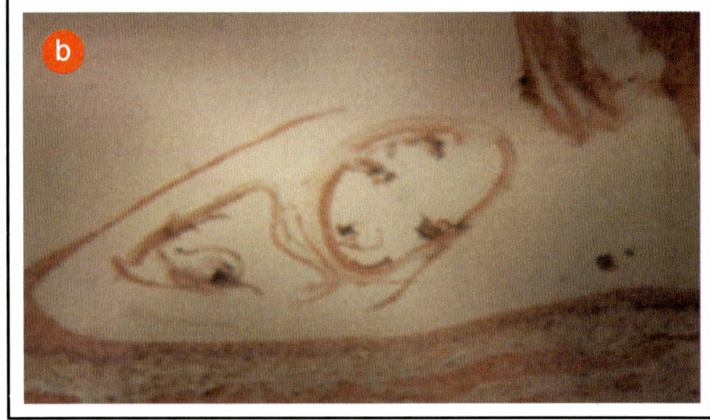

Figure 110: Cut portion of tongue of giraffe (*G. camelopardus*, an exotic sp.):(a)Showing *Gongylonema pulchrum* of which both ends were embedded in tongue substance (b) Histologic section of (a) showing parasite embedded in the tongue without inciting pathogenic alterations H&E,x70.

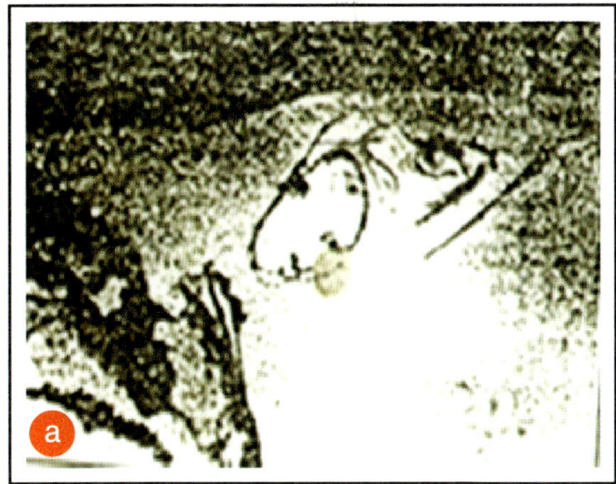

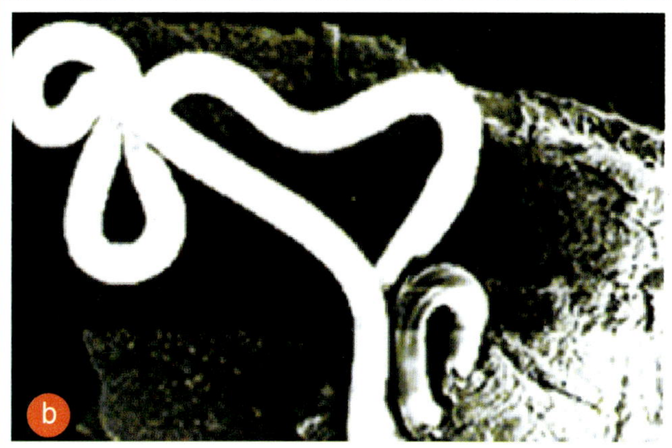

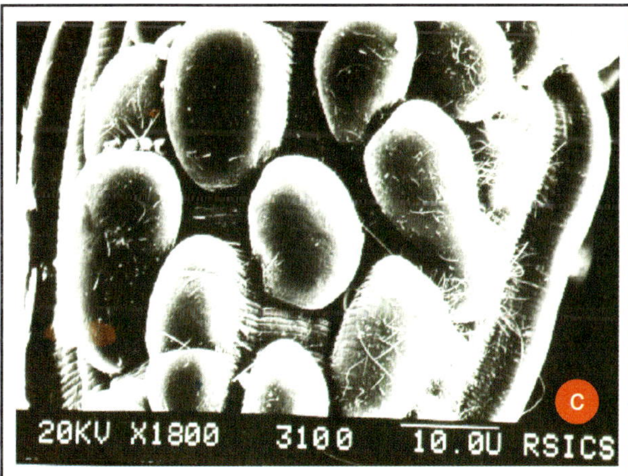

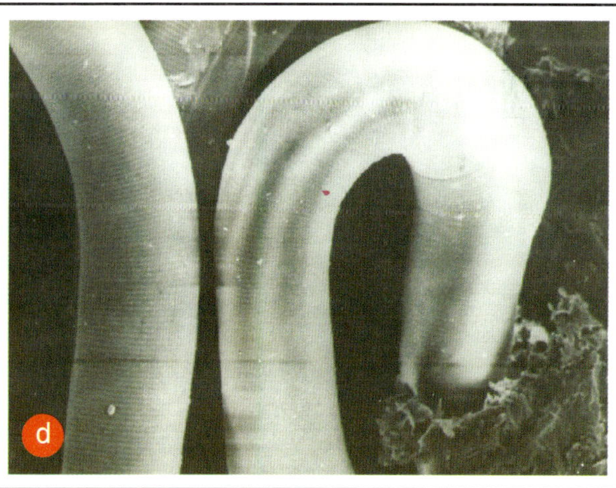

Figure 111: (a) Photomicrograph of oesophagus of chital (*A. axis*) showing *Gongylonema* sp.with hypertrophy and cornification of epithelium H & E.x70 (b) SEM Photo showing both the ends of the parasite embedded in epithelial tissue (sloughing also marked) of the oesophagus (c) Higher magnification of anterior part of *Gongylonema* sp. showing cuticular plates. x 1800. (d) Scanning electron micrograph of *Gongylonema* sp., showing cuticular transverse striation throughout the body x 3600

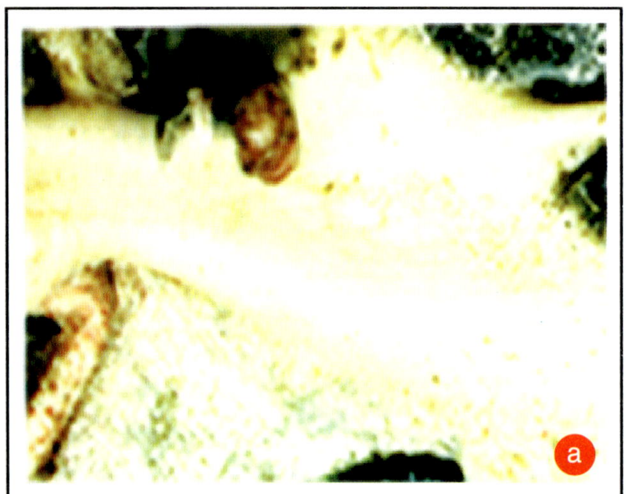

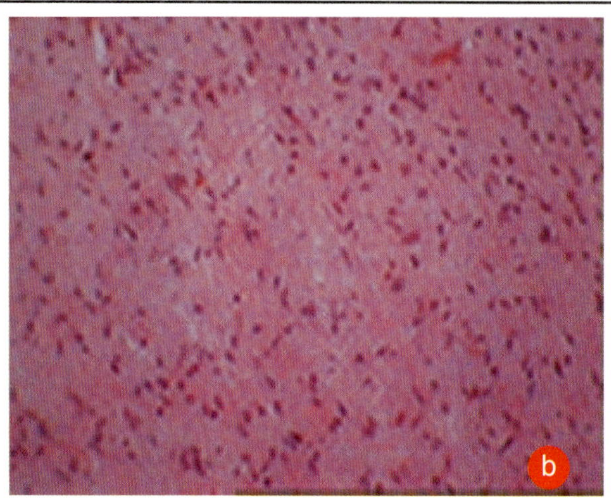

Figure 112: Photograph showing soft fibroma in the raphae of rumen of sambar (*C. unicolor*). (b) Histopathological section of (a) showing whorl forming arrangements of fibrous connective tissue. H&E, x 400.

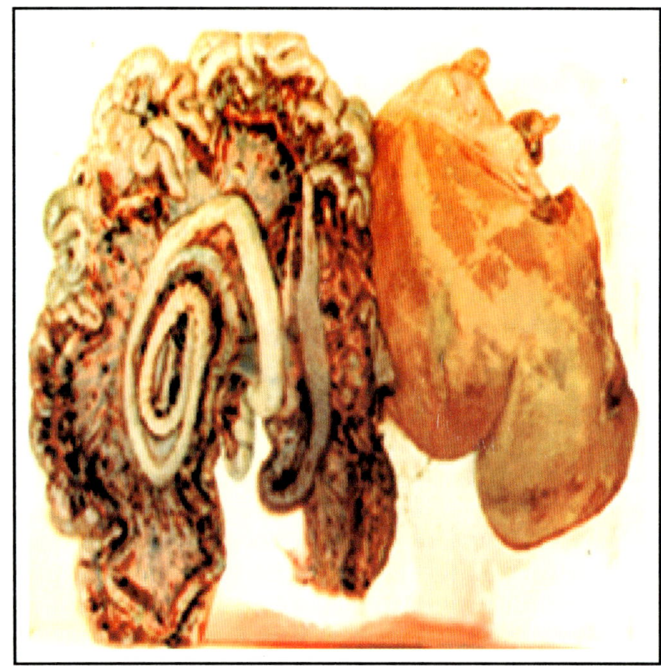

Figure 113: Photograph showing fatty liver in blackbuck (*A. cervicapra*) died in captivity.

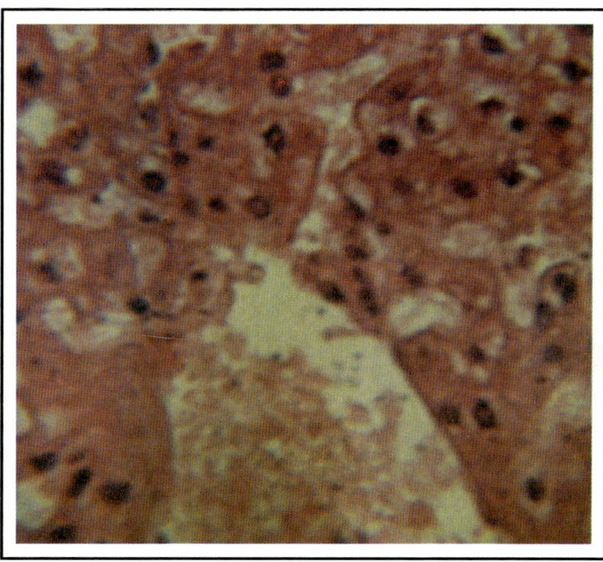

Figure 114: Acute toxic hepatitis in hog-deer (*A. porcinus*). Photomicrograph showing centrilobular necrosis and degeneration with haemorrhagc, sorofibrinous exudation and cellular infiltration. H&E, x 400 (Courtesy: Bhowmik, M.K.)

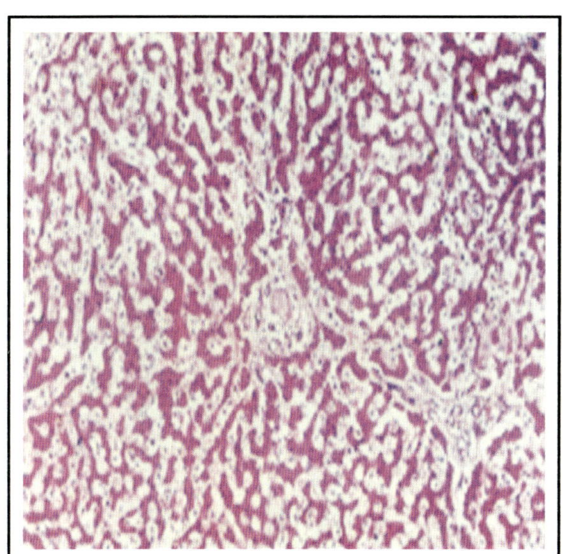

Figure 115: Histopathological section of liver of nilgai (*B. tragocamelus*) died of traumatic injury showing chronic venous congestion. Note dilatation of sinusoidal spaces and atrophy of few hepatocytes. H&E, x 100. (Courtesy: Suryawanshi, D.S.).

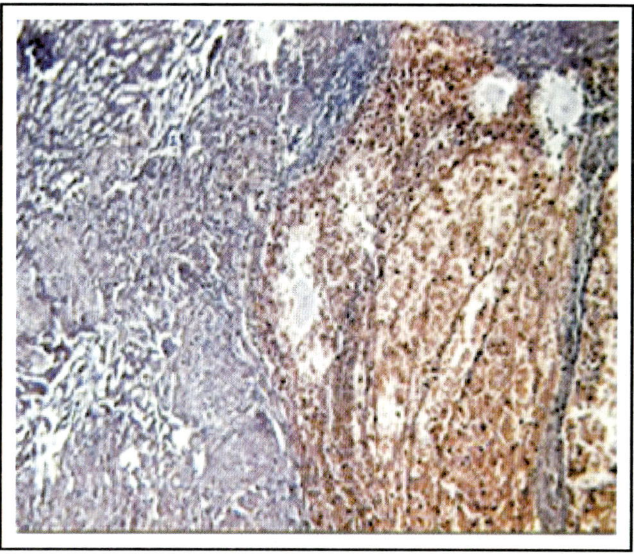

Figure 116: Photomicrograph showing the haemorrhages and congestion in nilgai (*B. tragocamelus*) liver related to hypovolemic shock. H & E, x 100 (Courtesy: Somesh Singh)

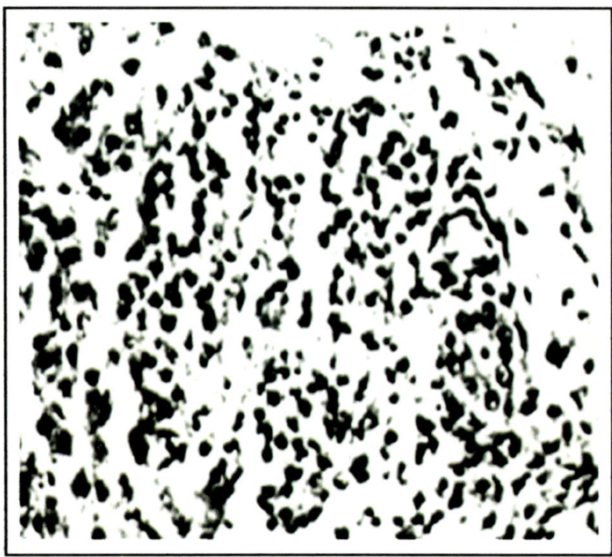

Figure 117: Photomicrograph of liver of blackbuck (*A. cervicapra*) showing a granuloma consisting of mononuclear cells aggregate replacing the liver parenchyma. H&E, x 400 (Singh *et al.*, 1981).

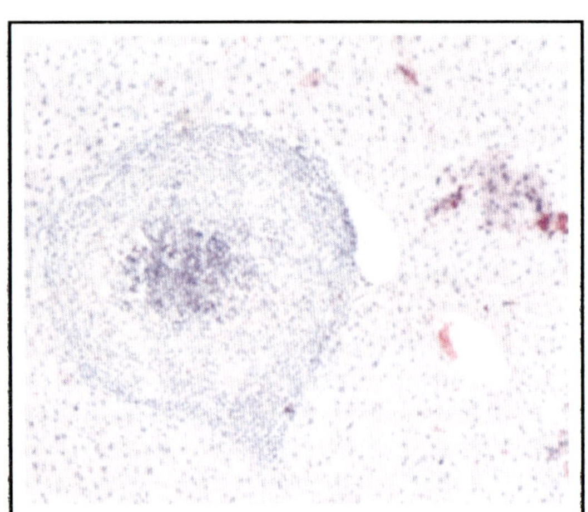

Figure 118 : Photomicrograph of liver of deer showing tuberculous granuloma with central caseous mass surrounded by mononuclear cells and connective tissues. H & E, x 100 (Courtesy: Suryawanshi, D.S.).

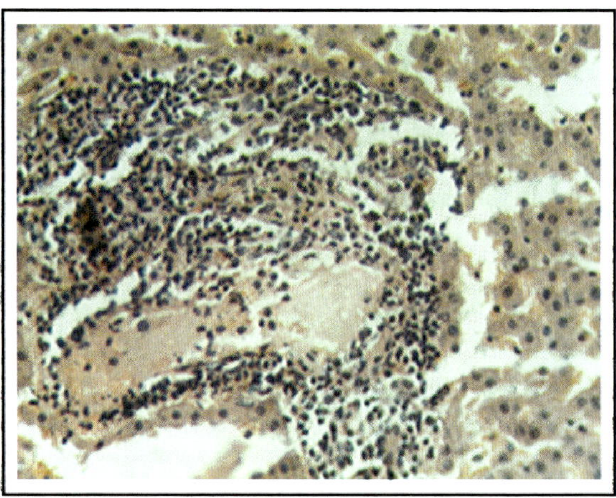

Figure 119 : Photomicrograph of liver of gaur (*B. gaurus*) showing hepatitis, periportal infiltration and vasculitis in case of paratuberculosis H&E,x200 (Courtesy: Gupta,M.P.)

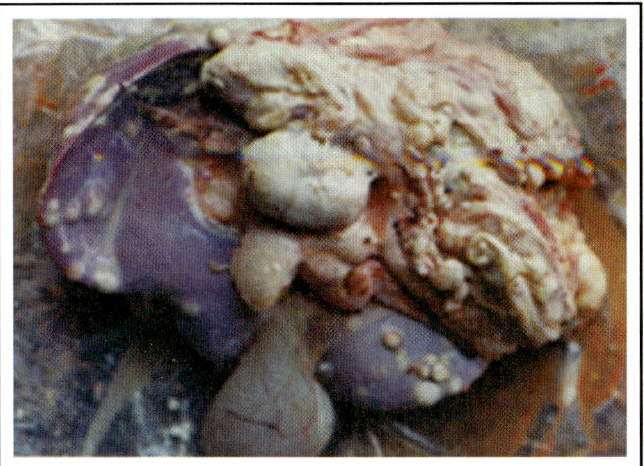

Figure 120 : Photograph showing various sized abscesses in liver and enlarged lymph nodes in sambar (*C. unicolor*) fawn. Adhesions between intestinal loops and mesentery also marked. Lesions were related to *E. coli* infection (Navel ill).

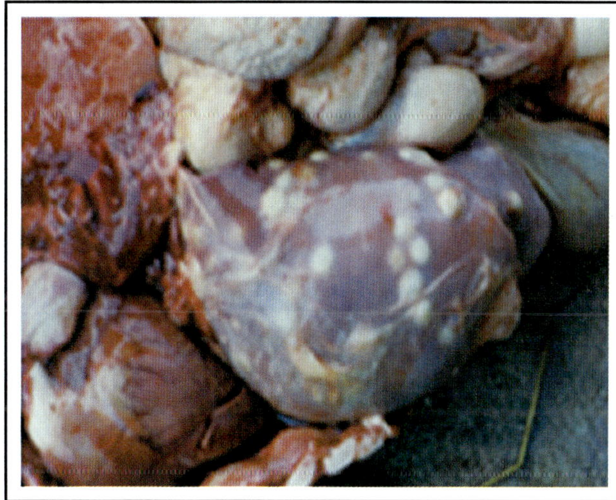

Figure 121 : Photograph showing *E. coli* abscess in the liver of hog-deer (*A. porcinus*)

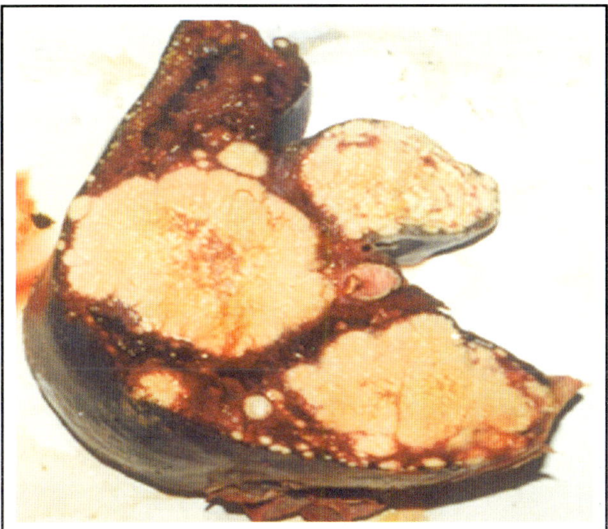

Figure 122 : Photograph of liver of nilgai (*B.tragocamelus*) showing granulomatous lesion due to *E. coli* infection (Courtesy: Suryawanshi, D.S.).

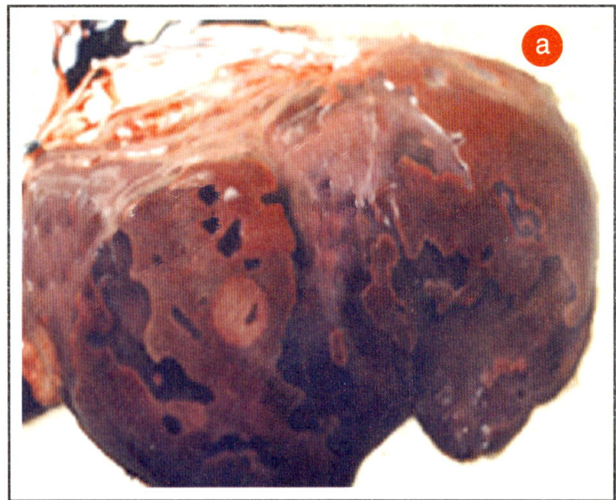

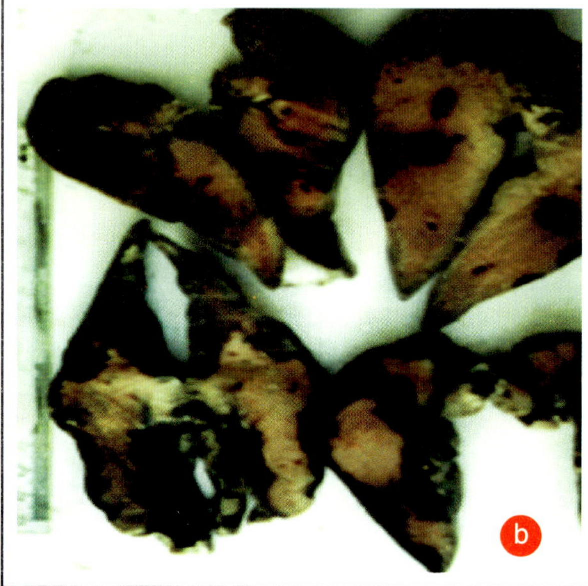

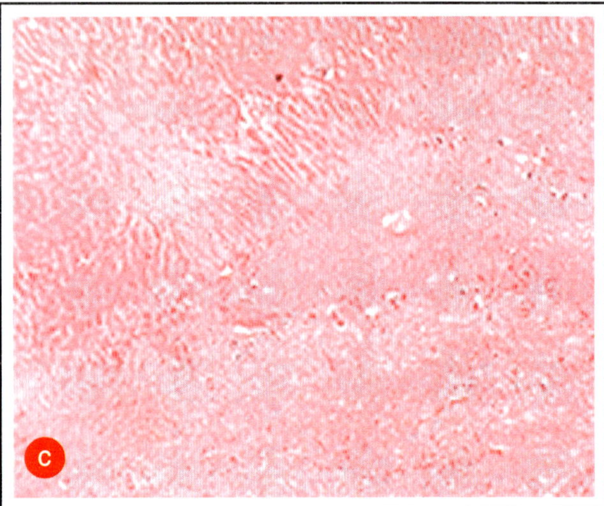

Figure 123: Photograph of liver of sambar (*C. unicolor*) showing: (a) Well- defined necrotic lesion on the dorsal surface. (b) Irregular necrotic areas on cut surface. (c) Photomicrograph showing coagulative necrosis of hepatocytes caused by *Fusobacterium necrophorum*. H&E,x100

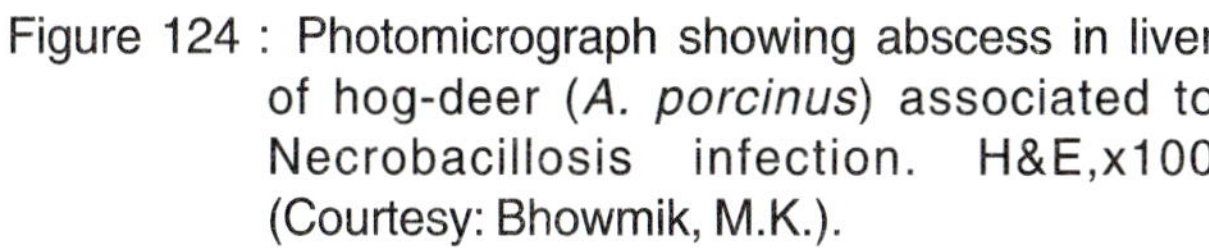

Figure 124 : Photomicrograph showing abscess in liver of hog-deer (*A. porcinus*) associated to Necrobacillosis infection. H&E,x100 (Courtesy: Bhowmik, M.K.).

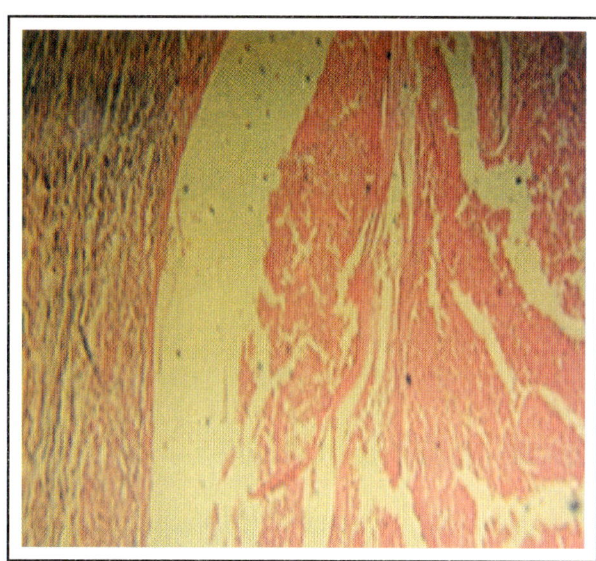

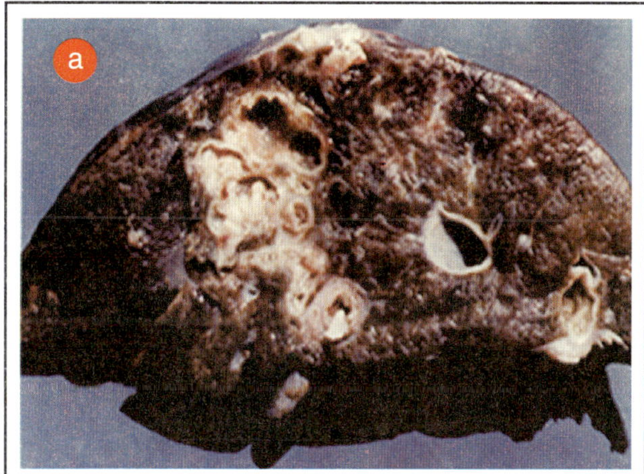

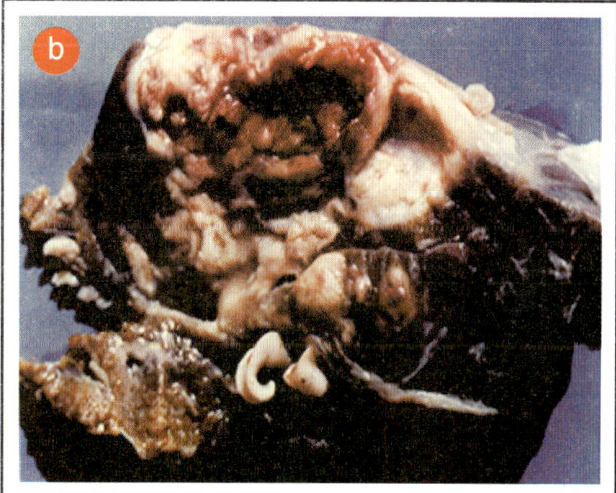

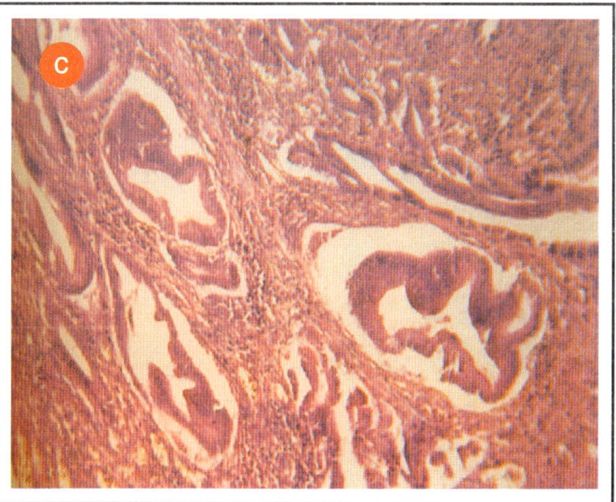

Figure 125: Photographs (a, b) of cut section of liver from chital (*A. axis*) died in captivity showing damage to the parenchyma by *Fasciola gigantica*. (c) Photomicrograph of bile duct of chital (*A. axis*) showing *Fasciola* sp. (Courtesy: Mukhopadhayay, S.K.).

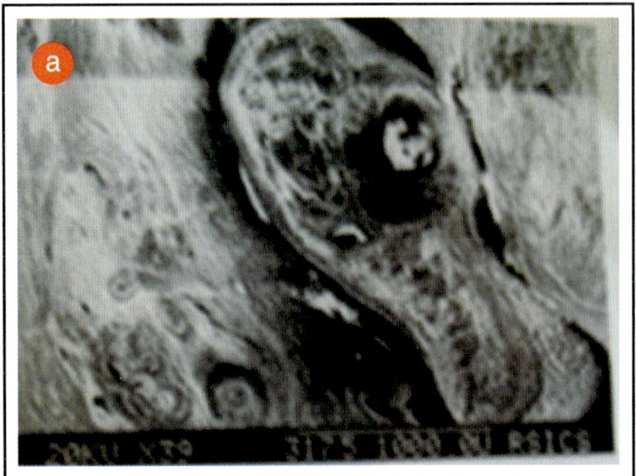

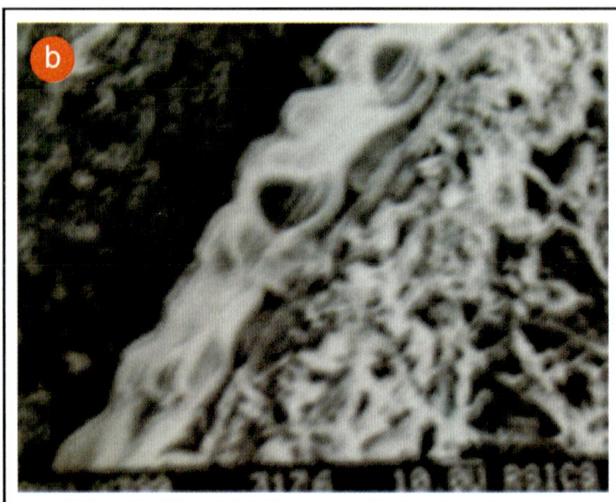

Figure 126: SEM photograph showing cross section of *Fasciola gigantica* in the bile duct of chital (*A. axis*) (a) low magnification x 39. (b) Note extensive damage caused by the cuticular spine of the parasite x 780.

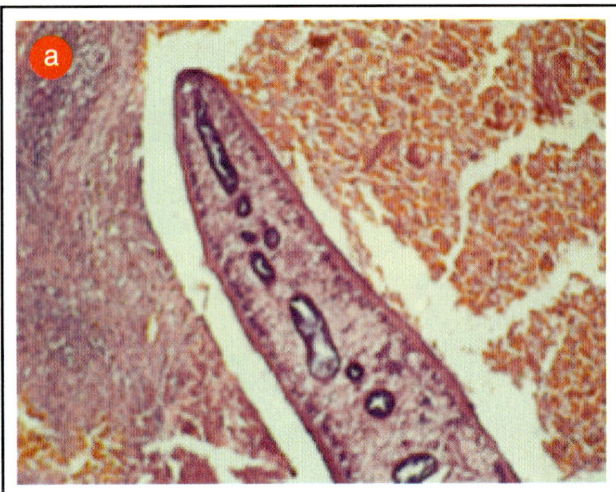

Figure 127: Photomicrographs of Chital (*A. axis*) liver showing:(a) Fasciola migrated tracts. H&E, x 100. (b) Same as (a) in higher magnification, x 200 (Courtesy: Singh, K.P.).

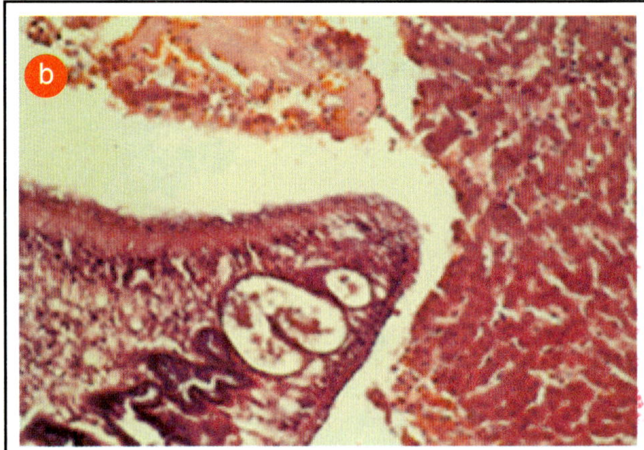

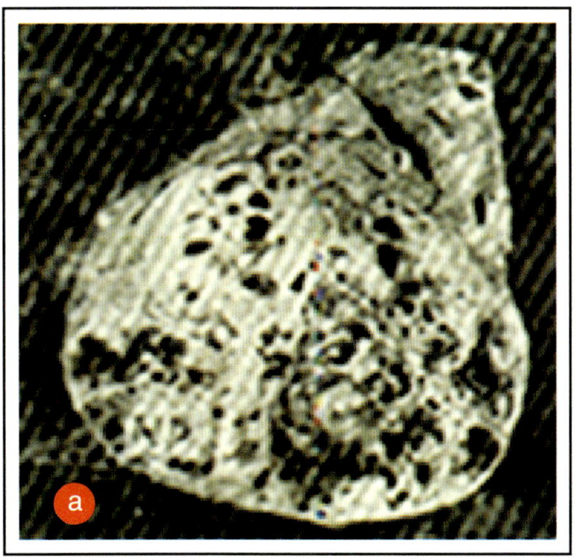

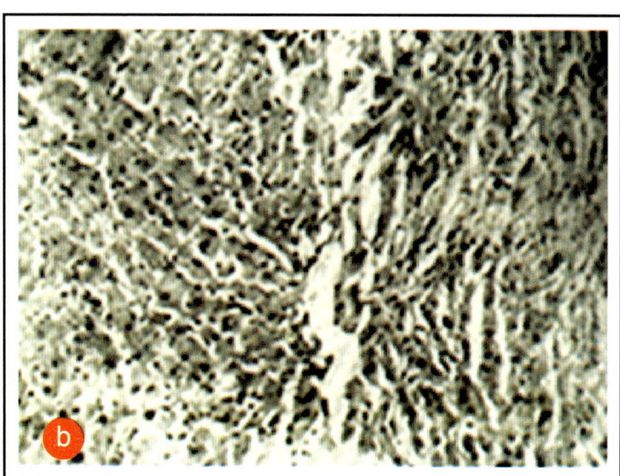

Figure 128: (a) Hepatocellular carcinoma with a small portion of normal liver from chital (*A. axis*). (b) Histopathological picture showing normal and neoplastic liver tissue. H& E, x 160 (Parihar & Tripathi, 1981).

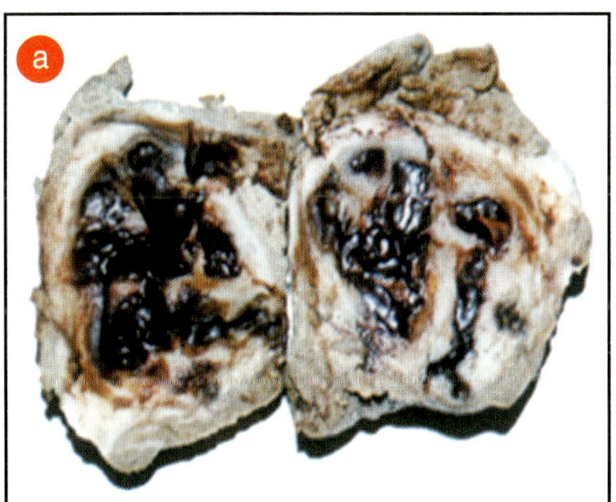

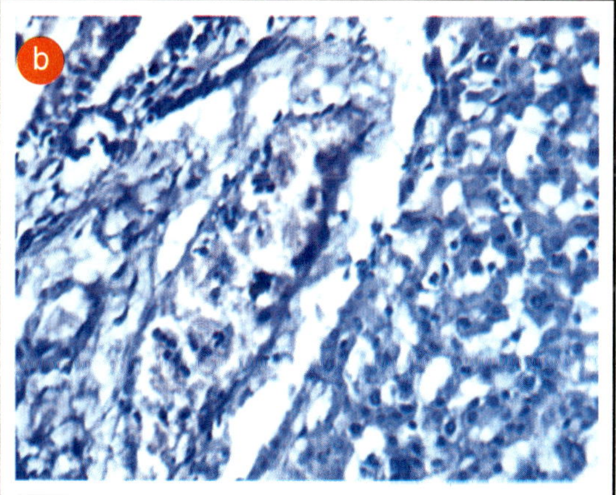

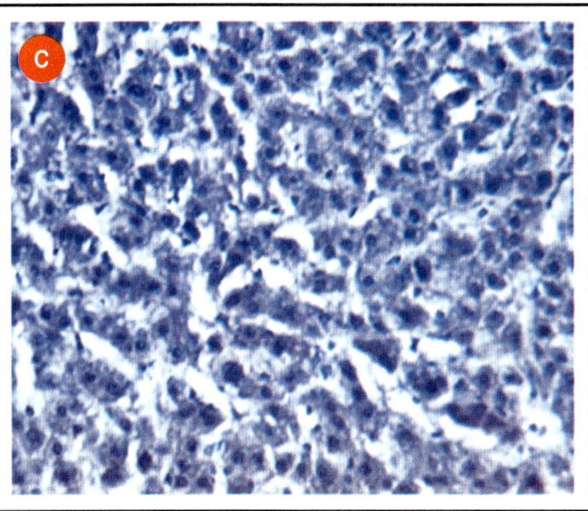

Figure 129 :Adenocarcinoma encountered in chital (*A. axis*) died in wild. (a) Cut opened nodular growth from liver. Photomicrographs of (a) showing: (b)Glandular cells with incomplete acini formation. H & E x 100 (c) Anaplastic and hyperchromic cells with numerous mitotic figures. H & E x 100 (Courtesy: Somesh Singh).

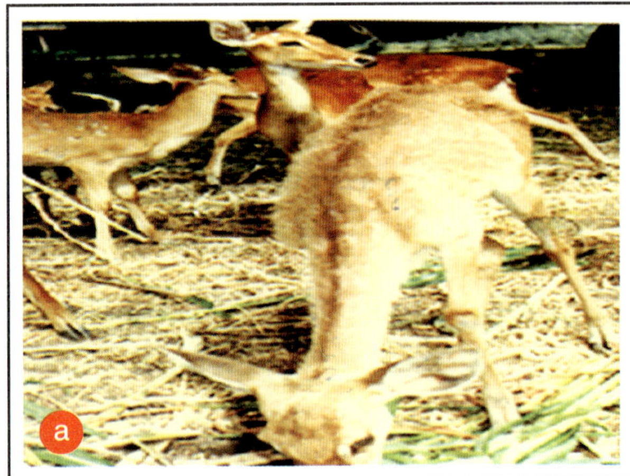

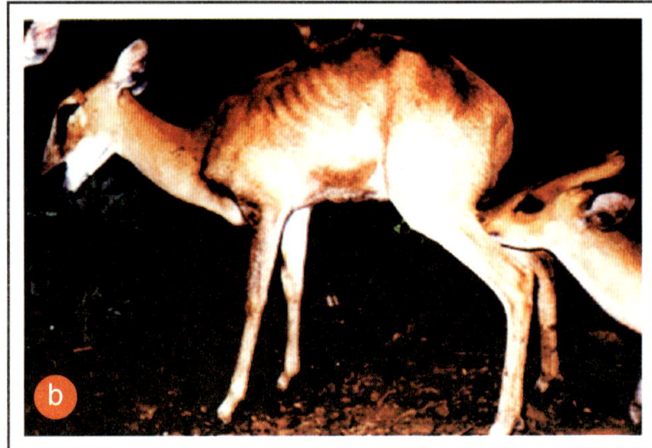

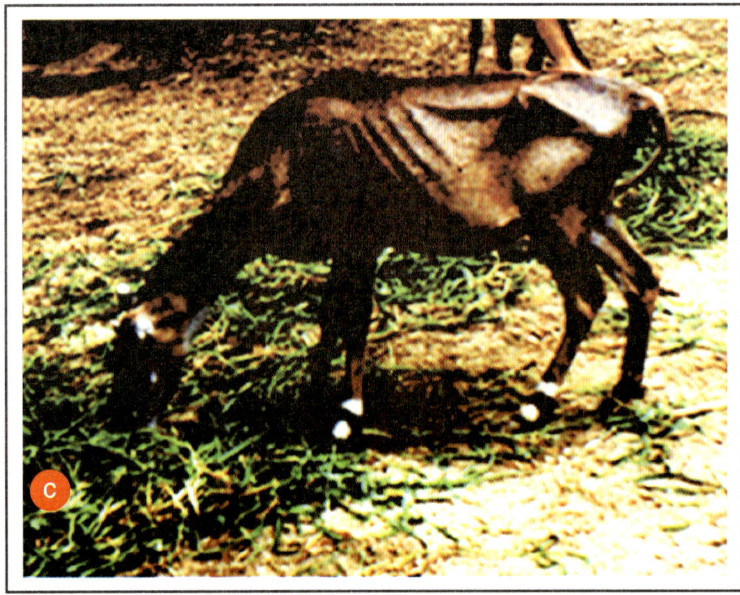

Figure 130 : Debilitated deer and antelopes: (a) Sangai deer (*C. eldi eldi*). (b) Chousingha (*T.quadricornis*). (c) Nilgai (*B. tragocamelus*). Note:Inadequate food availability due to agonistic behaviors of companions, besides tuberculosis and fasciolosis is attributed for such syndrome in captivity.

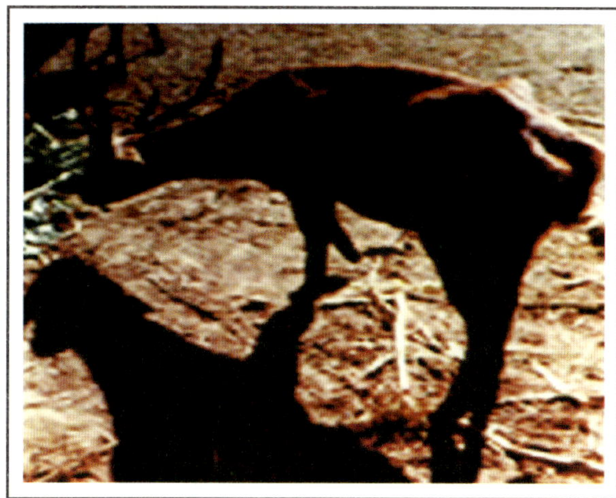

Figure 131 : Debilitated young adult male hog-deer (*A. porcinus*): Anorexia effect of immobilization with Xylazine HCl on different occasions.

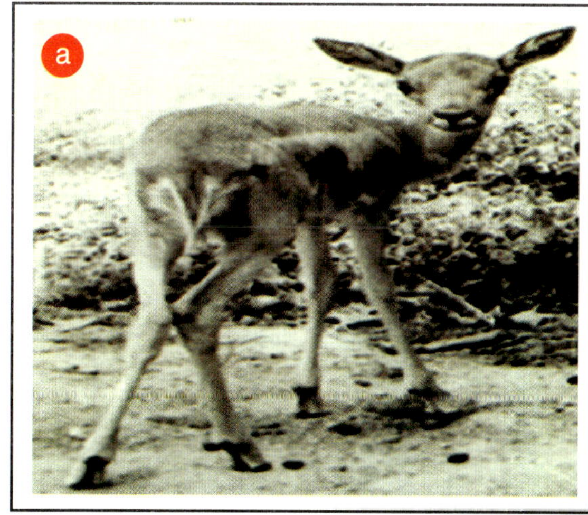

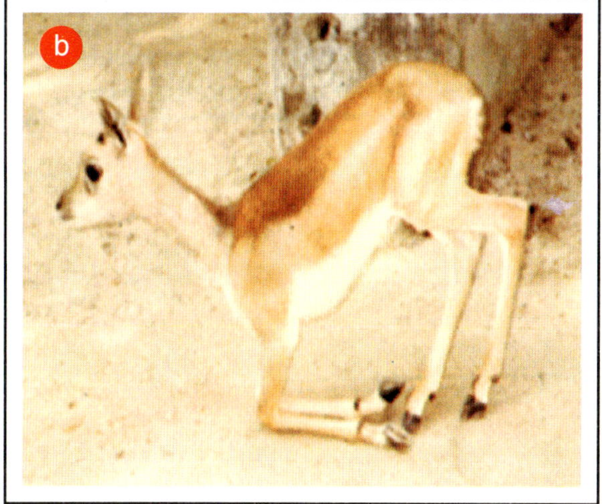

Fiurge 132 : (a) 79-day-old blackbuck (*A. cervicapra*) hand reared had developed knuckling of hock joints, (b) Sub-adult female blackbuck (*A. cervicapra*) unable to bear weight on fore limbs. Administration of calcium (Macalvit) cured the condition in two weeks.

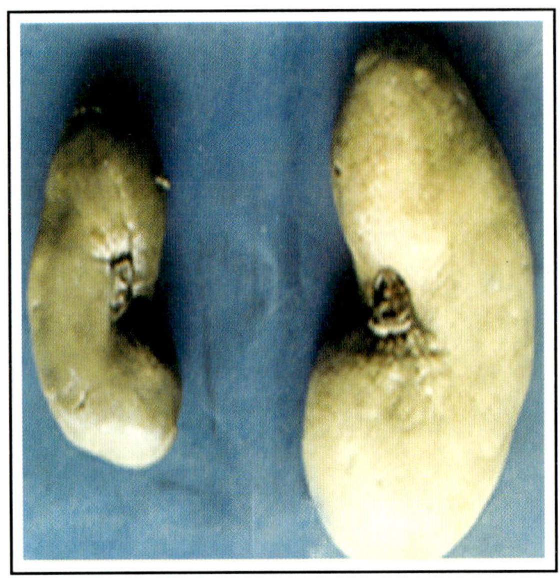

Figure 133: Photograph of hypertrophied right kidney of 6-month-old chital (*A.axis*) died at V.P.U., I.V.R.I., Izatnagar (UP.).

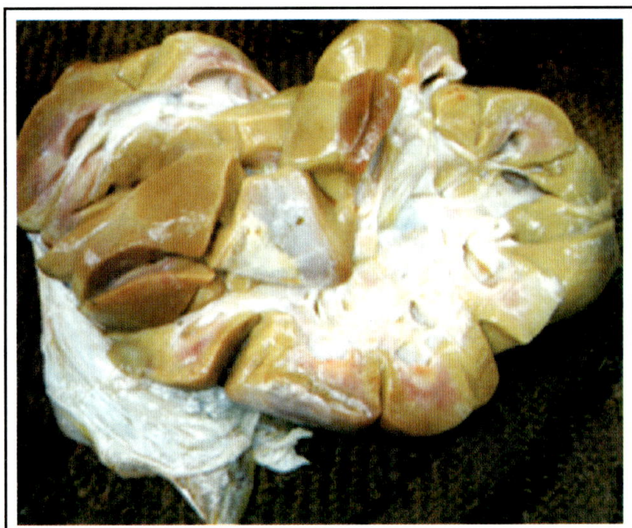

Figure 134: Photograph showing polycystic kidney in male gaur (*B. gaurus*). (Courtesy: Vishwanath, G.K. & Arun, A. Sha).

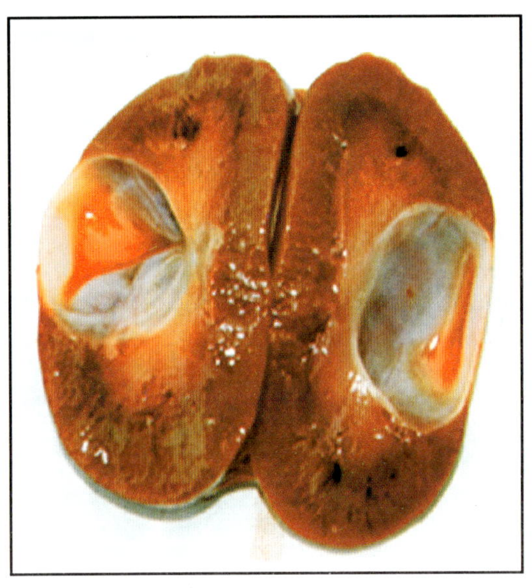

Figure 135: Photograph showing cystic left kidney of 6-yr.-old female hog-deer (*A.porcinus*) died at Z.G. Mysore (Courtesy: Nanjappa,K.A.).

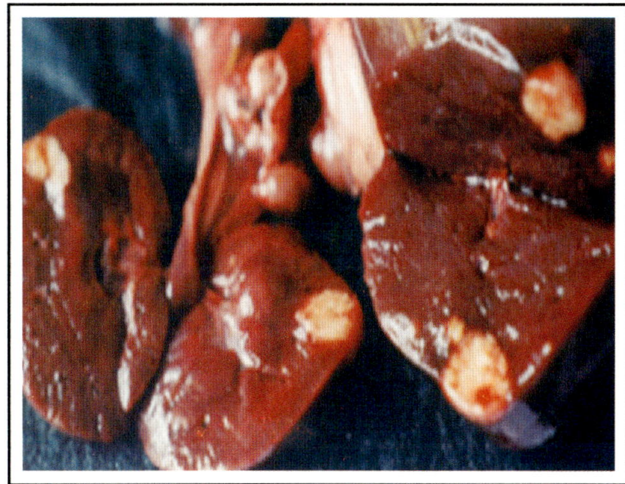

Figure 136:Photograph showing caseous tuberculous nodular lesions in the kidney of chousingha (*T. quadericornis*). (Courtesy: Suryawanshi,D.S.).

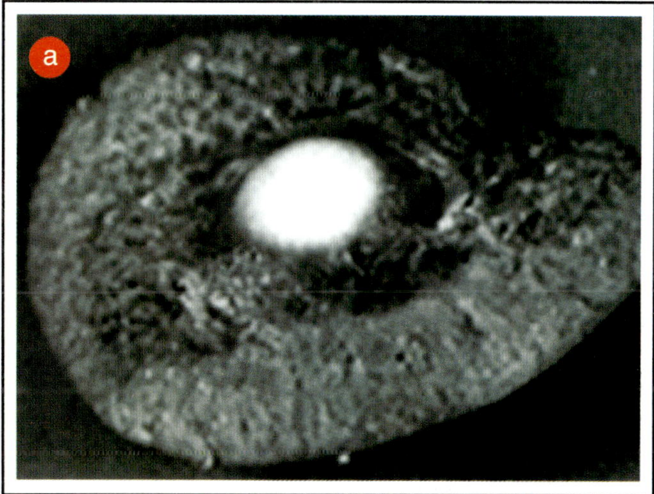

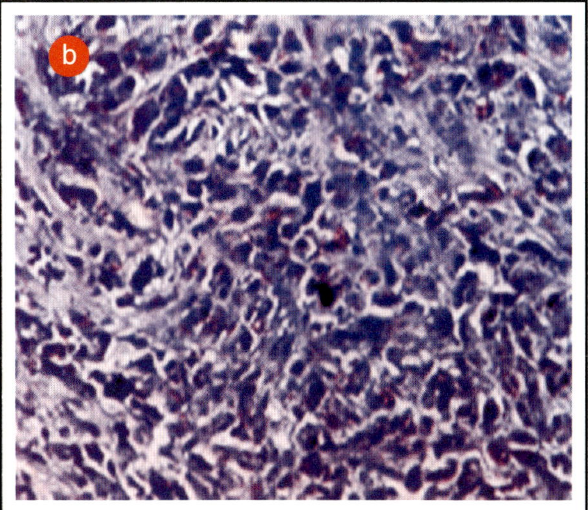

Figure 137: (a) Photograph of kidney of young adult chital (*A. axis*) showing tuberculous nodule in the medulla. (b) Photomicrograph of (a) showing lesions of tuberculous nephritis. H & E, x 400.

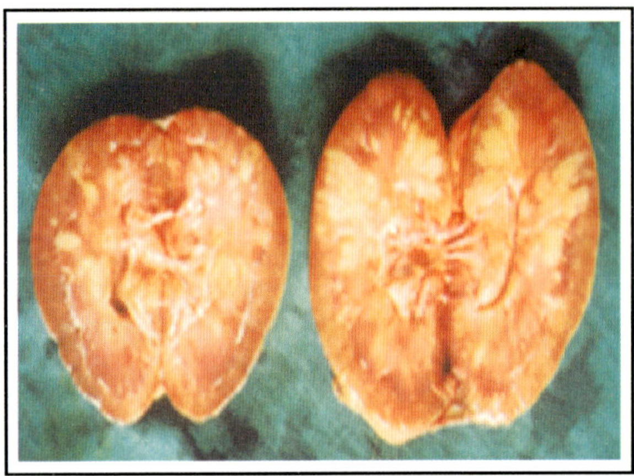

Figure 138: Photograph of kidney of blackbuck (*A. cervicapra*) showing suppurative nephritis. Note lesions in the cortex and medulla.

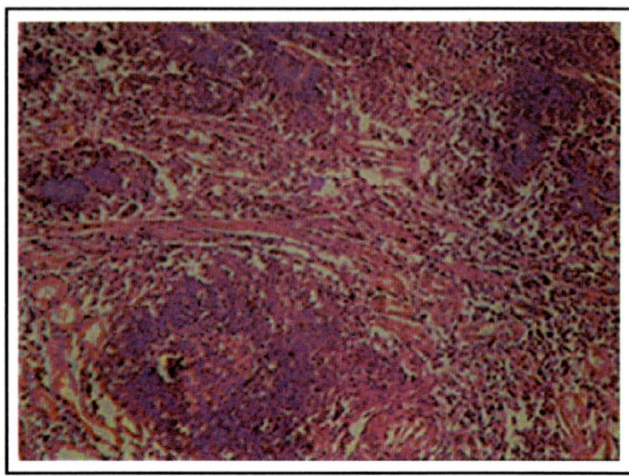

Figure 139 : Photomicrograph showing granulomatous lesions in the kidney of deer. H & E, x 100 (Courtesy: Dept.of Pathology, CVSc, Nagpur, M.S.).

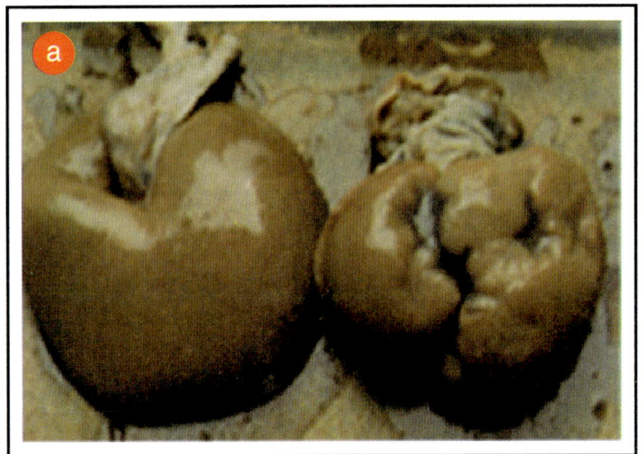

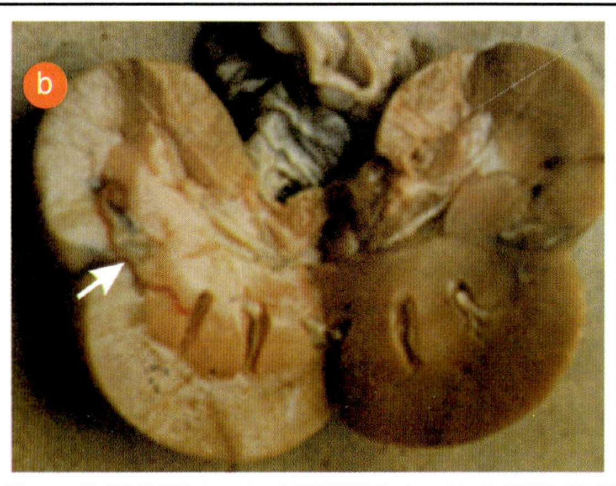

Figure 140 : Photograph of kidneys of blackbuck (*A. cervicapra*). (a) Left kidney normal but right kidney showed constricted and tortuous lesions on external surface. (b) On incision pelvis of right kidney showed presence of a *Dictophyma renale* (arrow).

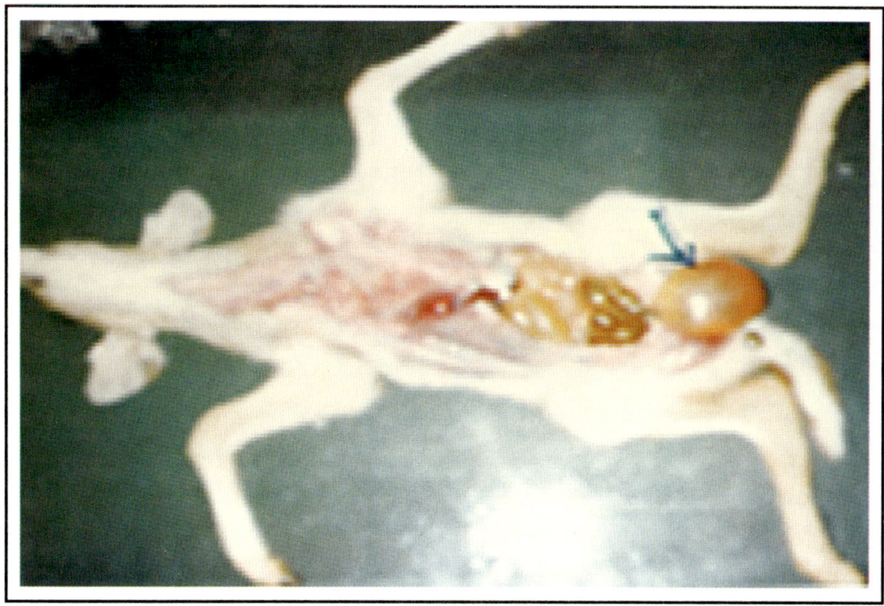

Figure 141: Photograph showing distended urinary bladder due to retention of urine in chital (*A. axis*) fawn died in Corbett National Park, Ramnagar, Uttarakhand.

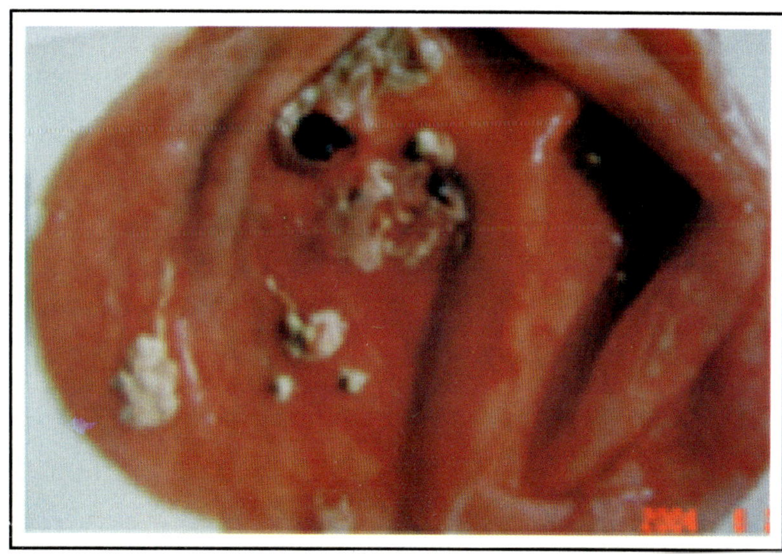

Figure 142: Photograph of urinary bladder of pigmy hog (*P.salvania*) died in captivity,showing oedematous and congested mucosa with ulcers and uroliths.

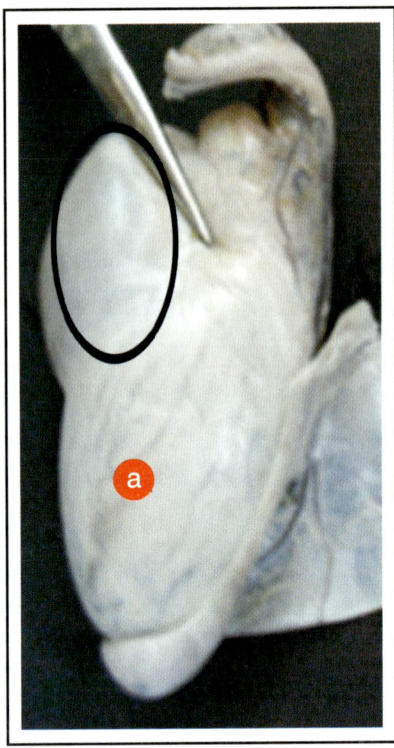

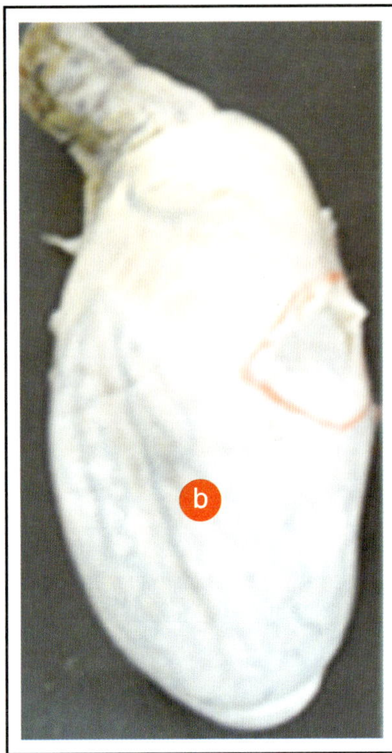

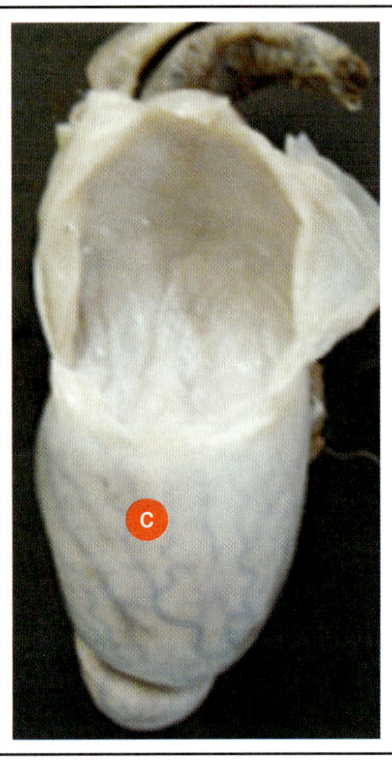

Figure 143: Restes anomaly encountered in adult sangai (*C. eldi eldi*) died at National Zoological Park, New Delhi. Photographs showing: (a) A large cyst in right testis. (b) A small cyst in left testis. The fluid of cysts was straw coloured, transparent and sterile. (c) Removal of sac showed a large depressed cavity due to absence of parenchymal substance in the fore half of right testis. There was also small depression in the left testis. Note: Animal had deformed antlers. [Also see integumentary system]

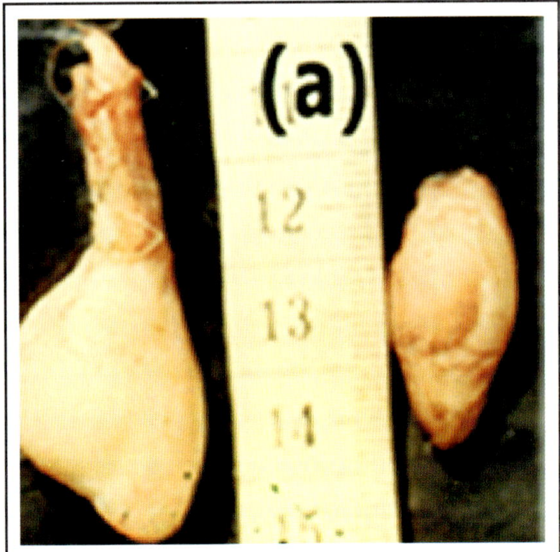

Figure 144: Photograph showing hypoplasia of right testis (600mg)and left testis was normal (3016 mg) in 4-month-old blackbuck (*A. cervicapra*) died in captivity.

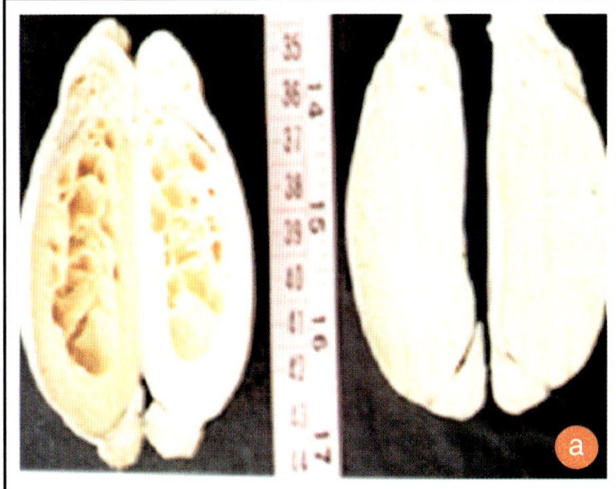

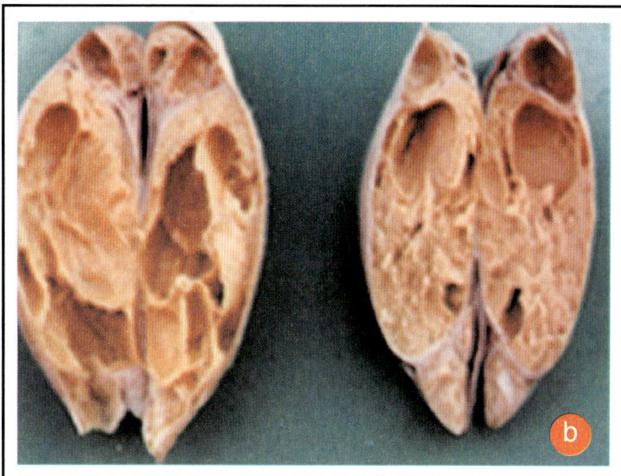

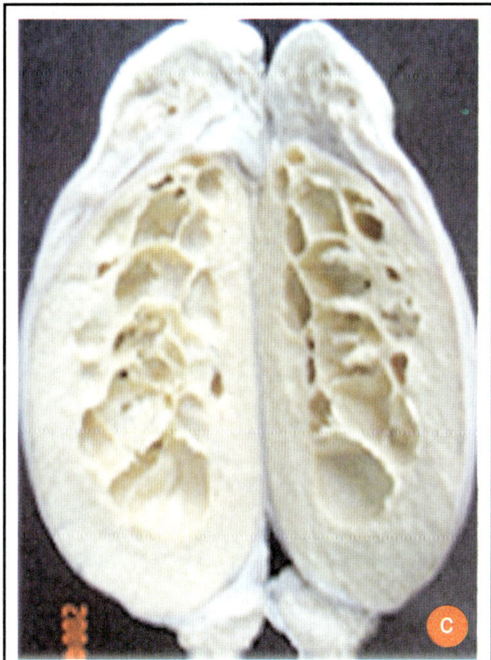

Figure145: Photographs showing cavitations in testes,due to absence of mass of convoluted seminiferous tubules and rete test is encountered one case each of: (a) blackbuck (*A.cervicapra*),(b) Goral (*N. goral*). (c) Nilgai (*B. tragocamelus*).

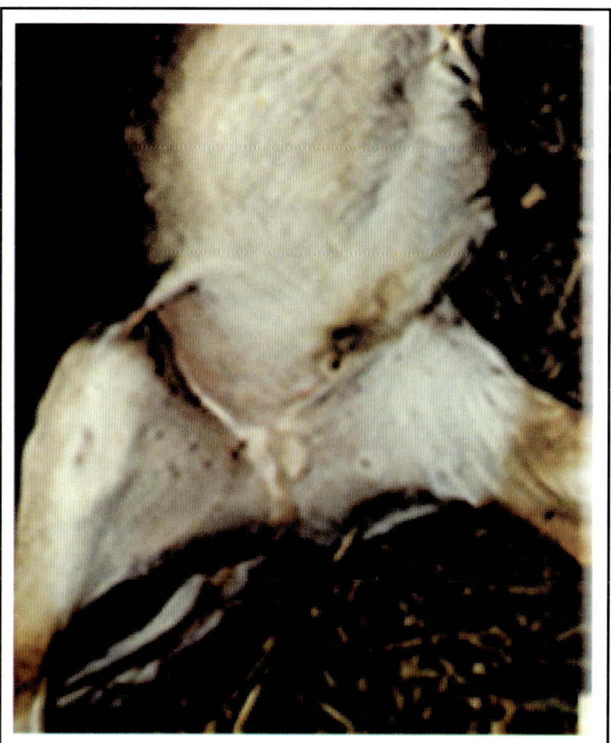

Figure 146: Photograph showing absence of right testis in a wild nilgai (*B. tragocamelus*).

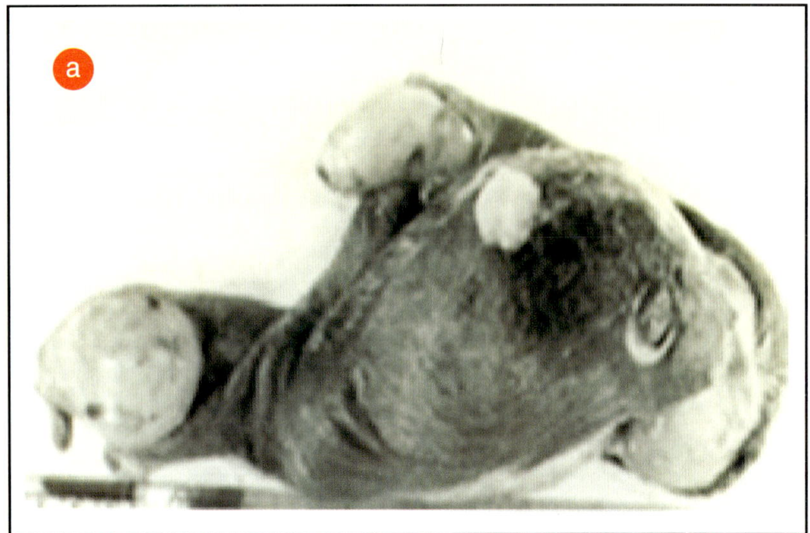

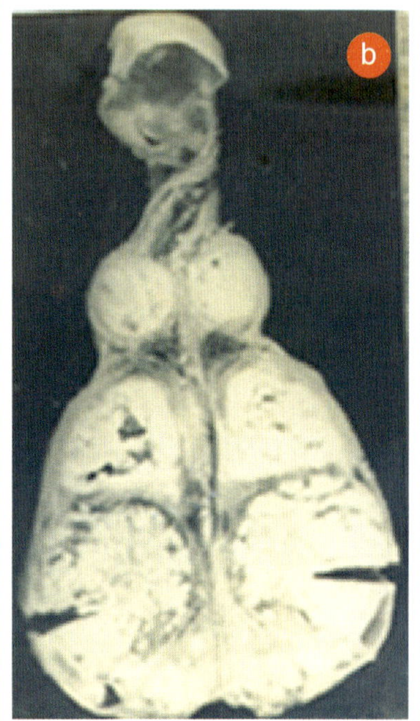

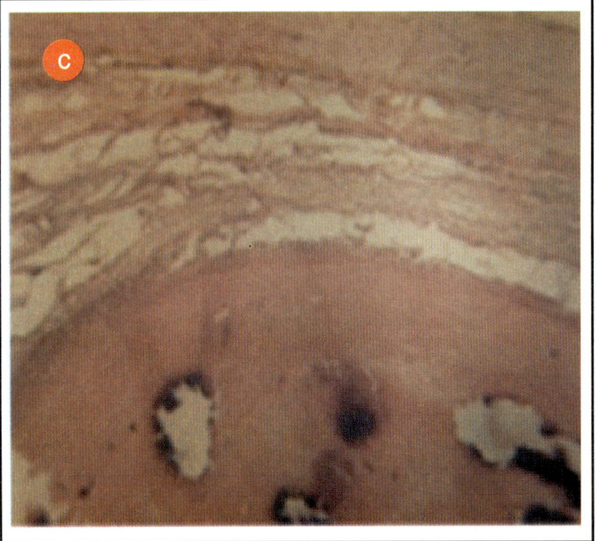

Figure 147: (a) Photograph showing a fistula in the enlarged testicle of blackbuck (*A. cervicapra*).Note discharge of pus through fistula. (b) Section of above testis showing concentrically laminated pus typical of onion scale like lesions caused by *Corynebactrium ovis*. (c) Photomicrograph of (b) showing focal areas of caseative necrosis and calcification surrounded by fibrous connective tissue.H & E,x28

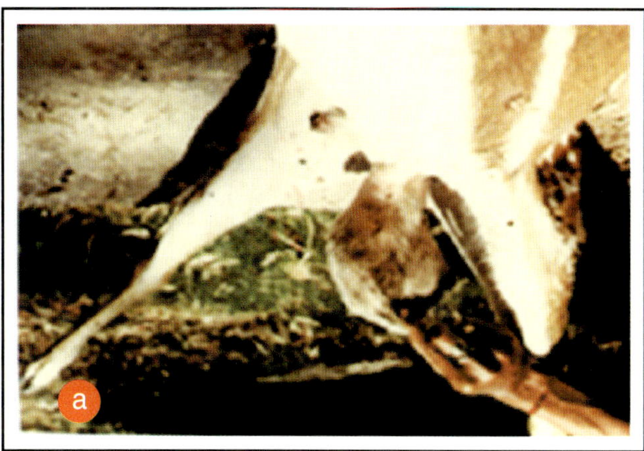

Figure 148: (a) Photograph of carcass of an adult chital (*A. axis*) showing enlarged testicles. (b) Cut open testes showing caseated tuberculous lesions.

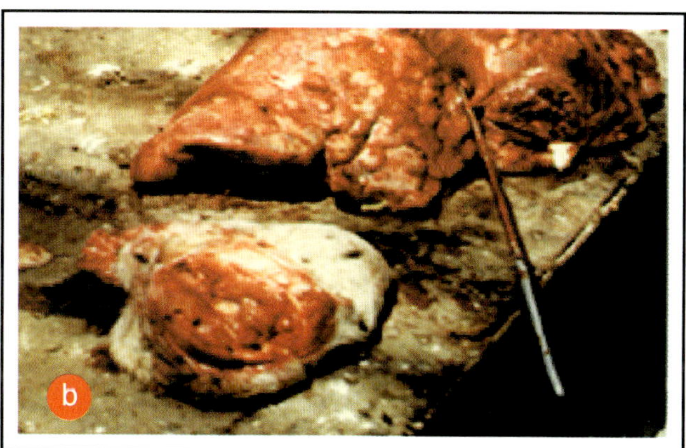

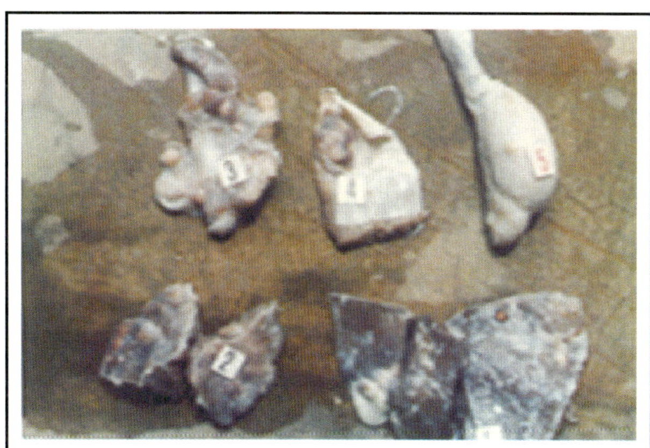

Figure 149: Photograph showing tuberculous lesions in testis and in other organs in chital (*A. axis*) died of generalized form of disease.

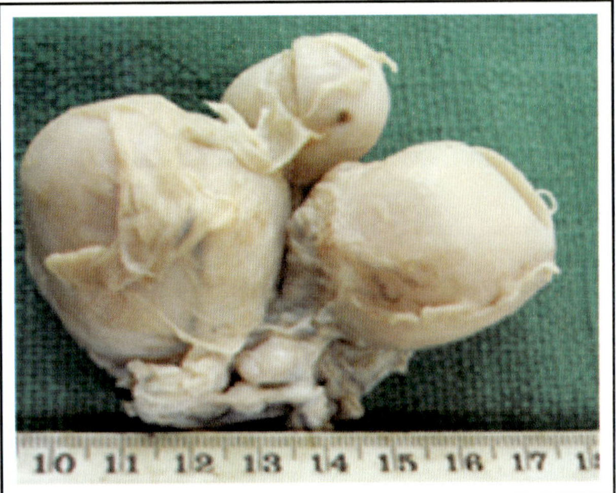

Figure 150 :Photograph of cystic ovaries and hydrosalphinx with adhesions encountered in serow (*C.sumatraensis*) died at Zoological Garden, Guwahati, Assam.

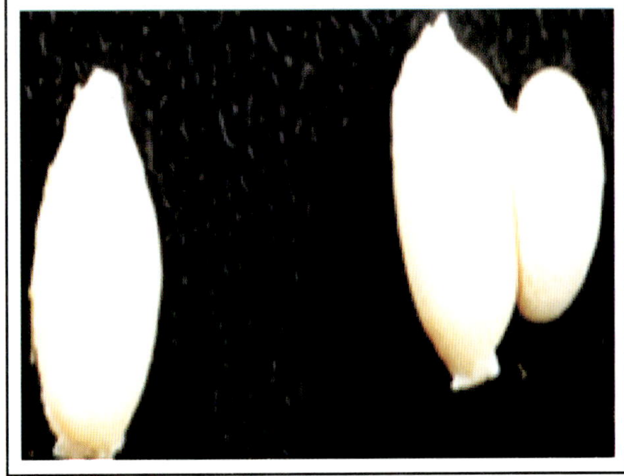

Figure 151: Photograph showing right normal ovary. The left ovary was having a growth in young adult female chital (*A. axis*).

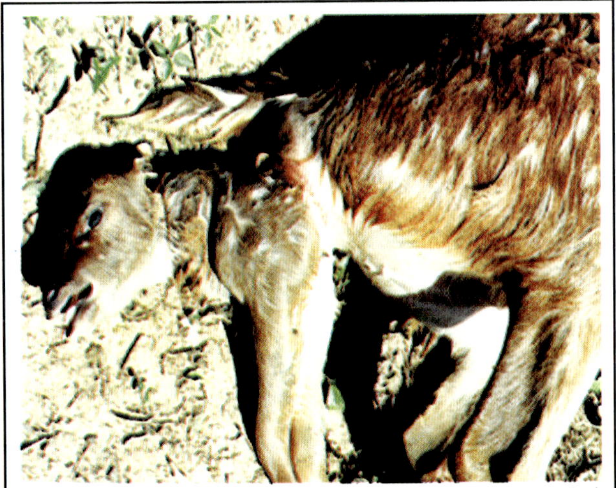

Figure 152: Photograph showing (a) foetus died due to dystocia in chital (*A. axis*). The foetus weighed nearly one ninth of the mother's body weight.

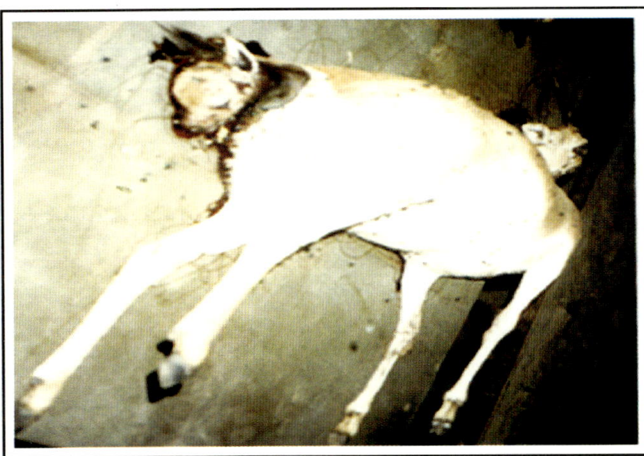

Figure 153: Carcass of blackbuck (*A. cervicapra*) doe (weighing 25 kg.)showing foetal dystocia due to large sized foetus(b.w 4.8 kg).

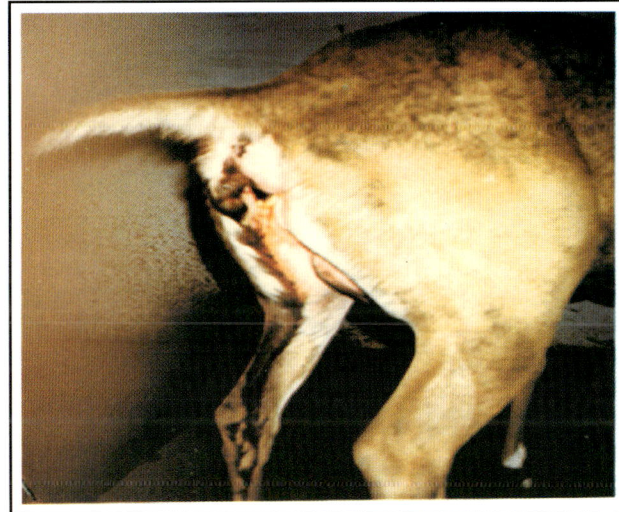

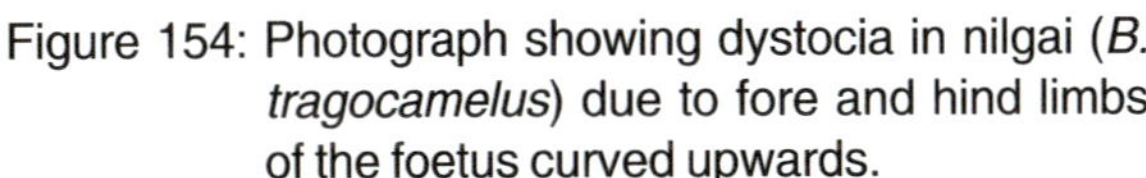

Figure 154: Photograph showing dystocia in nilgai (*B. tragocamelus*) due to fore and hind limbs of the foetus curved upwards.

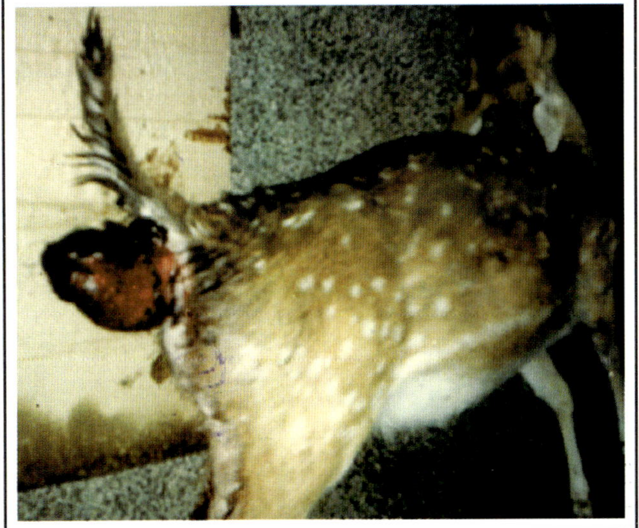

Figure 155: Photograph showing prolapse of uterus in a primiparus chital (*A.axis*).

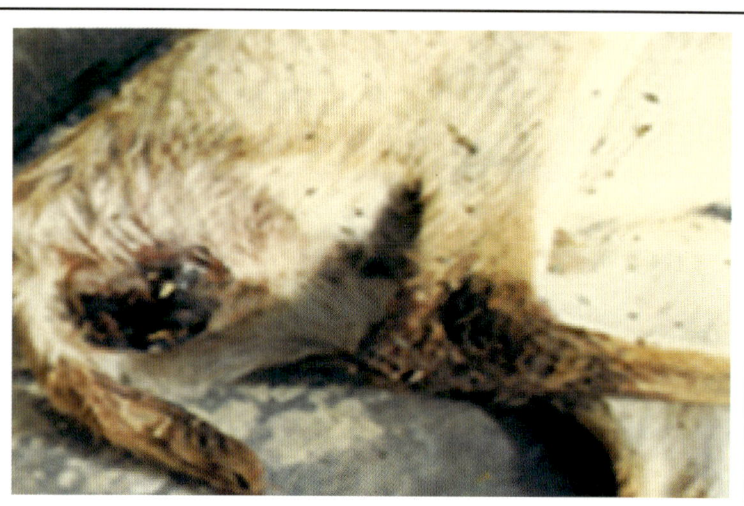

Figure 156: Photograph showing necrotic tuberculous lesion of vulva (vulvitis) of blackbuck (*A. cervicapra*).

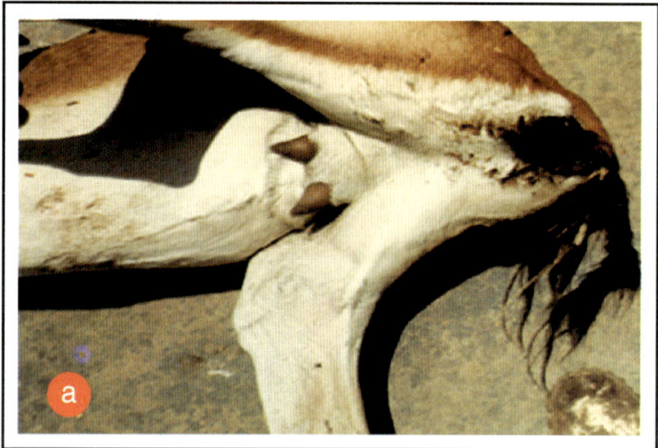

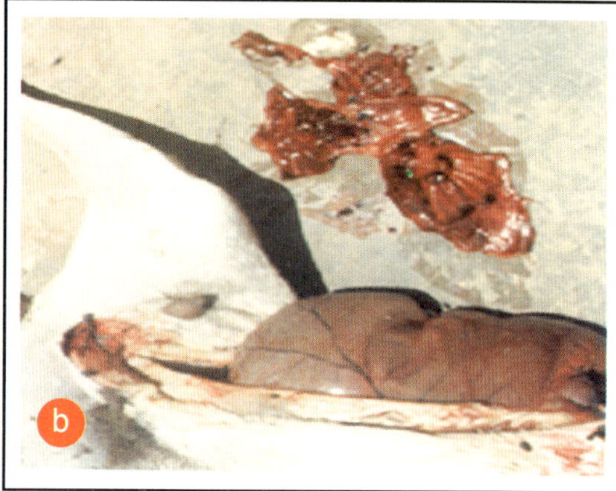

Figure 157: (a) Photograph showing vulvo-vaginitis with putrid discharge in chinkara (*G. gazella*) (b). Necropsy of (a) showed suppurative metritis and presence of lacerations.

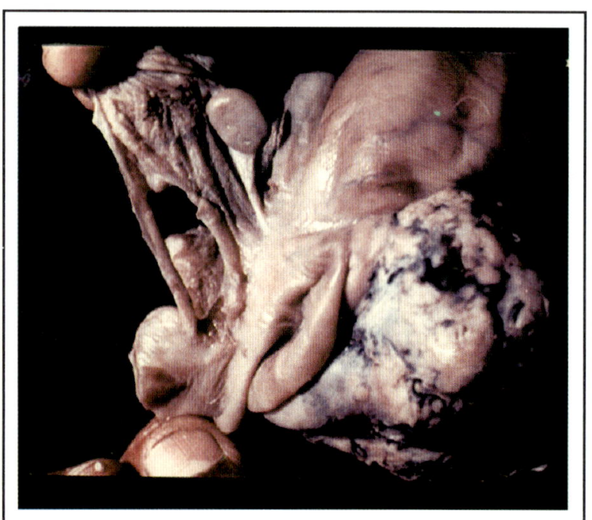

Figure 158: Photographs showing adenocarcinomatous growth in the uterus of an adult female hog-deer (*A. porcinus*).died in captivity.

Nervous System

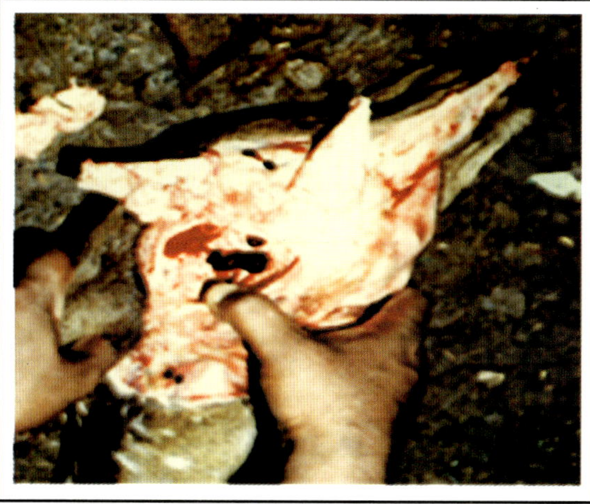

Figure 159: Photograph showing haemorrhagic clot in the brain of chital (*A. axis*) that collapsed in transportation crate after striking its head repeatedly against the crate walls.

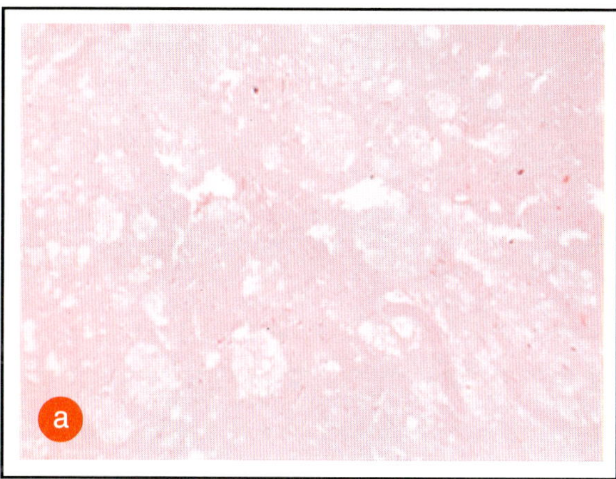

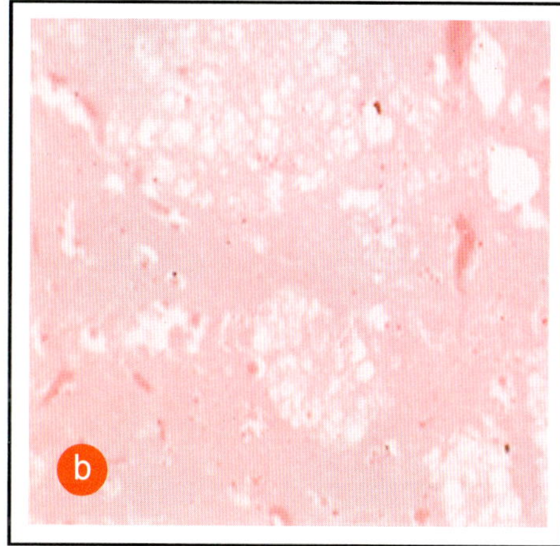

Figure 160 (a) Photomicrograph of brain of serow (*C. sumatraensis*) died in captivity showing lesion of encephalomalacia with congestion and demyelination. H&E, x 100 (b) Higher magnification of (a) H&E, x 400.

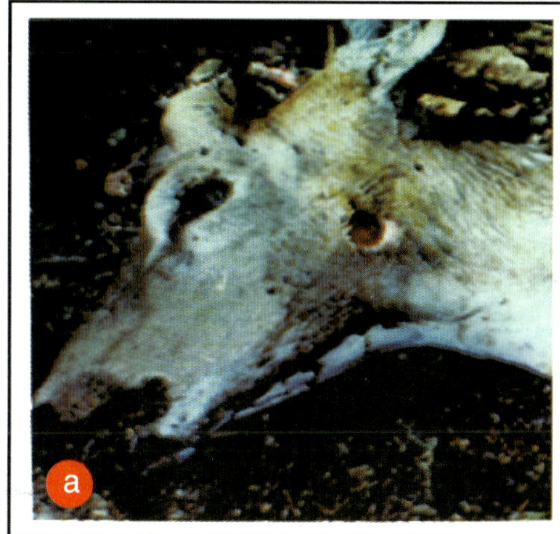

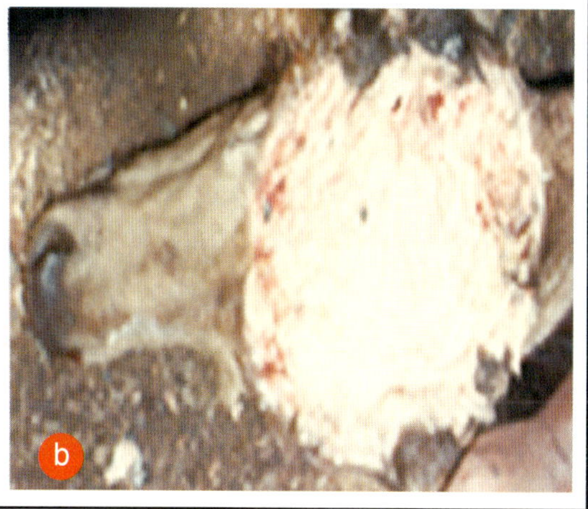

Figure 161: Photograph showing suppurative lesions in: (a) Parotid gland (pus cleaned) and (b) brain of chital (*A. axis*) died of generalized *Mycobacterium avium* infection.

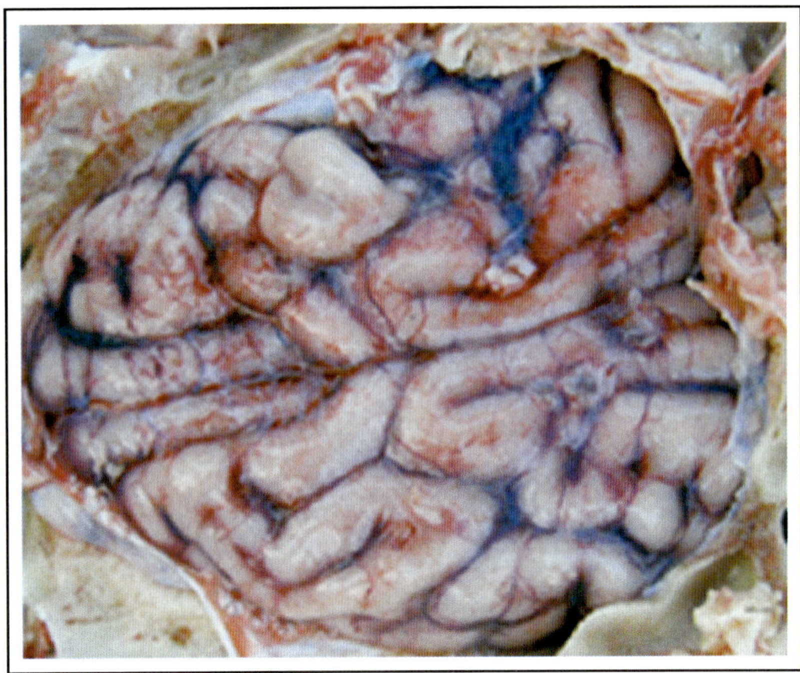

Figure 162: Photograph showing severe congestion of brain of wild boar (*S. scrofa*) died due to swine fever in Garumara NP. The case is cited under digestive system. (Courtsey: Anupam Rakshit)

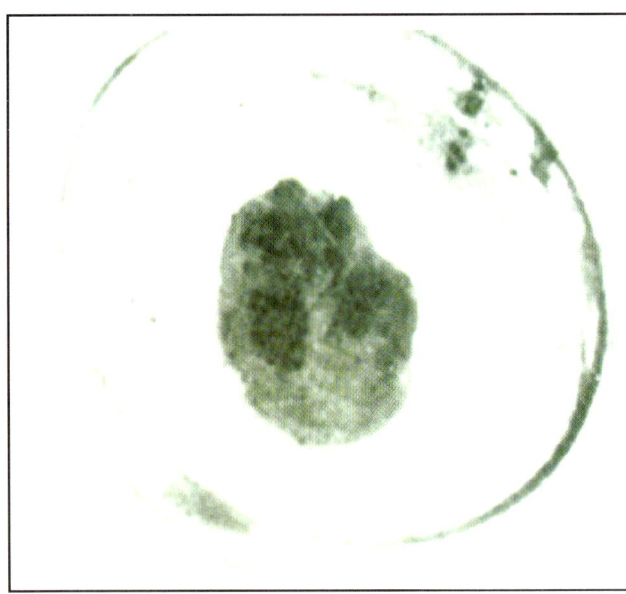

Figure 163: Photograph showing *Cysticercus tenuicollis* from the brain of oryx (*Beisa oryx*, an exotic sp.). It caused increase in intracranial pressure resulting in loss of vision and circling movement of the animal.

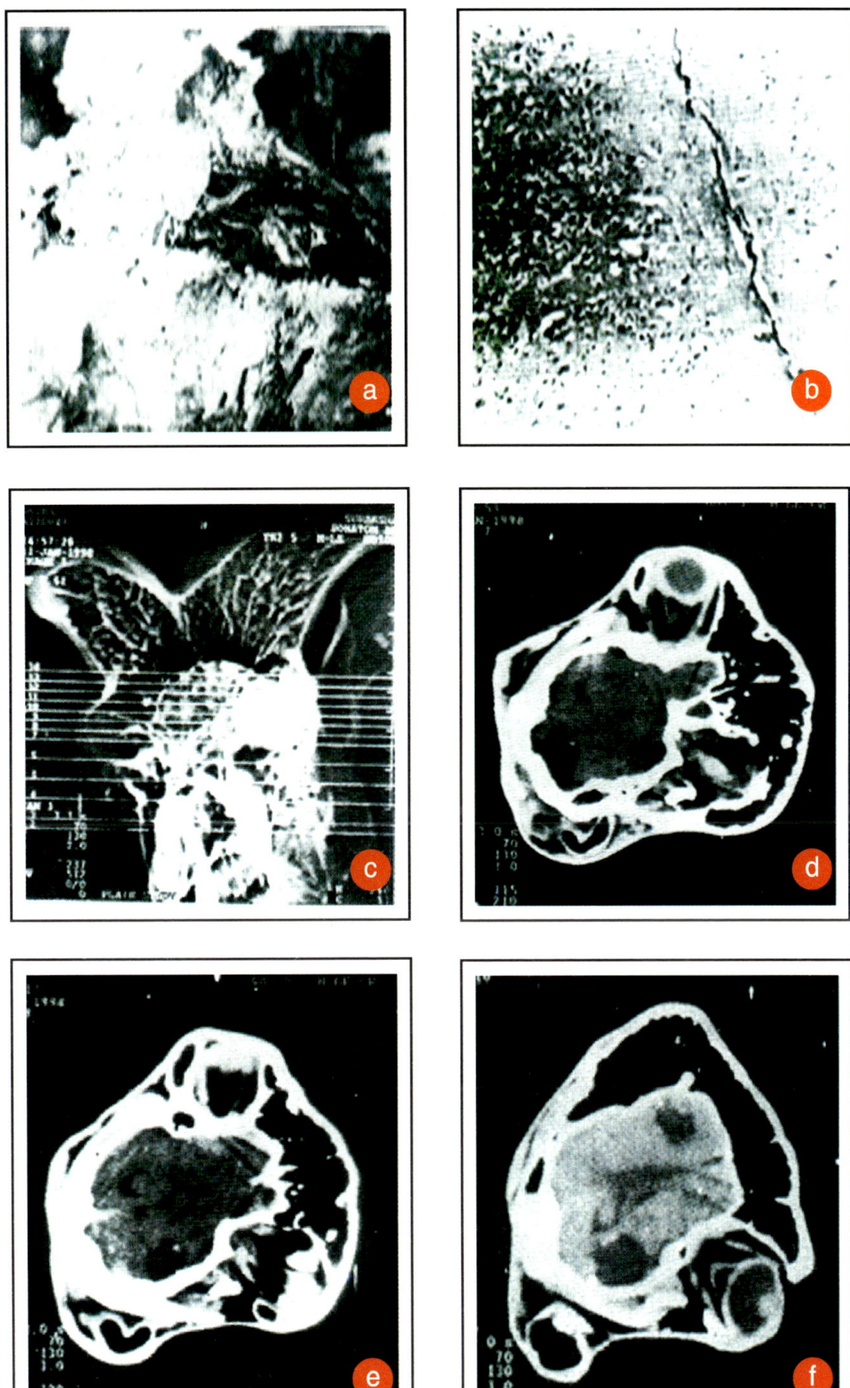

Figure164: Coenurosis in Himalayan tahr (*Hemitragus jemalahicus*). (a)Photograph showing *Coenurus cerebralis* (b)Photomicrograph showing vacuolation,demyelination and necrosis of nerve cells with evidence of heamorrhagic tract. H & E, x 400 (c) Topogram showing levels of CT sections of the animal.(d) Cystic lesion at the level of lower cerebellum on the left side.(e) Another cystic lesion in left temporal lobe(f) Cystic lesions in left parietal and right frontal region.(Chakraborty *et al.,* 1998). Photo with permission of the first author.

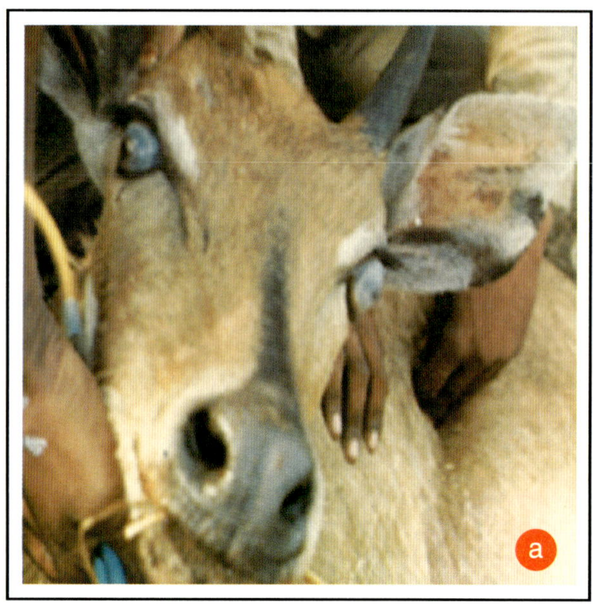

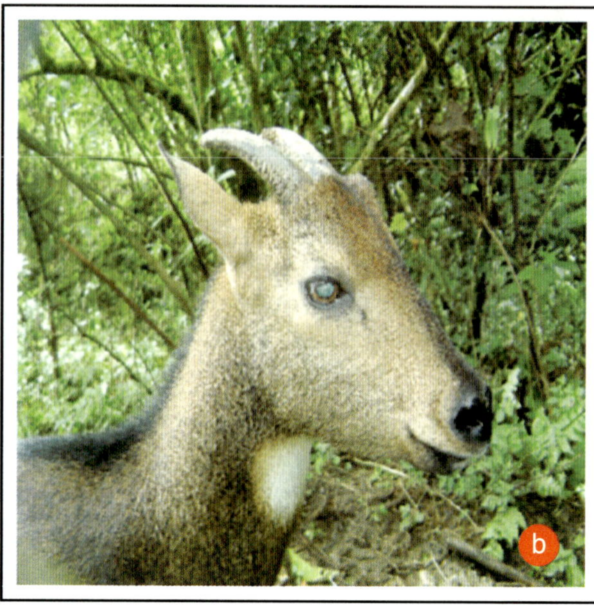

Figure 165: Corneal opacity in: (a) Male nilgai (*B. tragocamelus*) belonging to Sariska National Park, Rajasthan. Also animal had ear sore due to *Stephanofilaria* sp. infection. (b) Goral (*Nematofirus goral*) belonging to Zoological Garden, Sikkim. (Courtesy Shankar, K.S.M.)

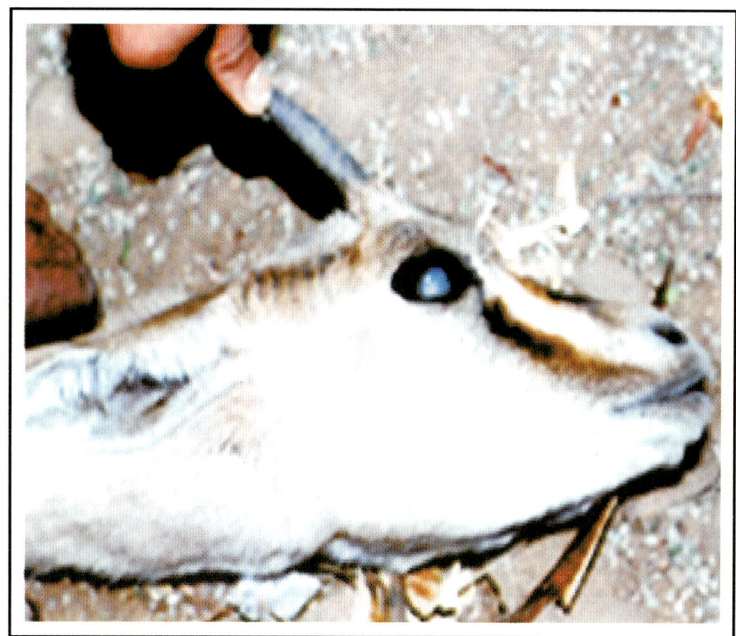

Figure 166: Corneal opacity in right eye of chinkara (*G. gazella*) belonging to Zoological Garden, Jammu. (Courtsey: Sudhan, N.A.).

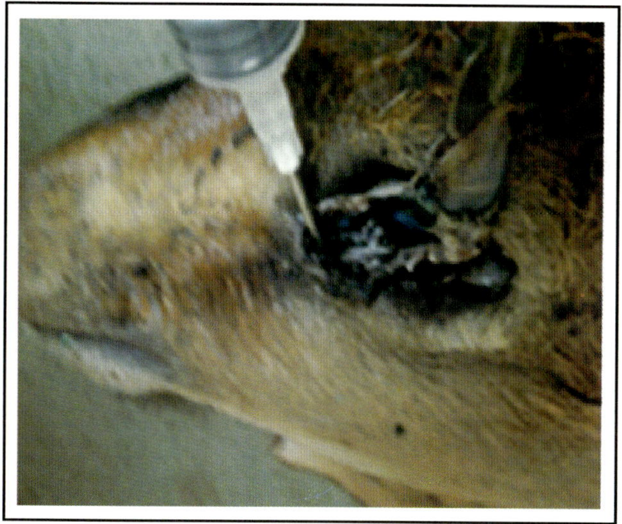

Figure 167: Photograph of head of chinkara (*G. gazella*) showing left eye damaged completely.

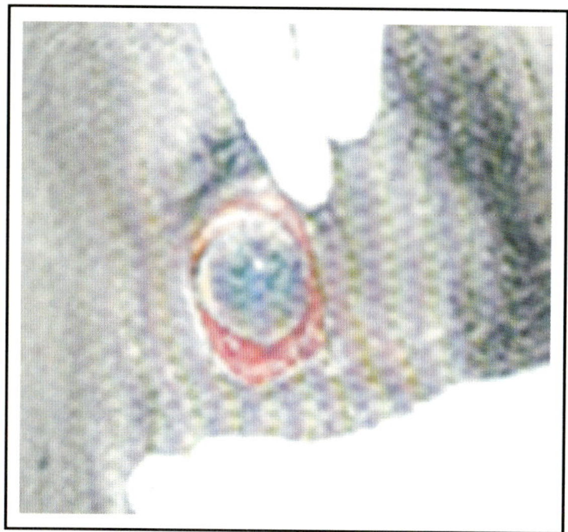

Figure 168: Photograph showing severe congestion of eye in pasturellosis in gaur (*B. gaurus*). The case is also referred under respiratory system.

Integumentary System

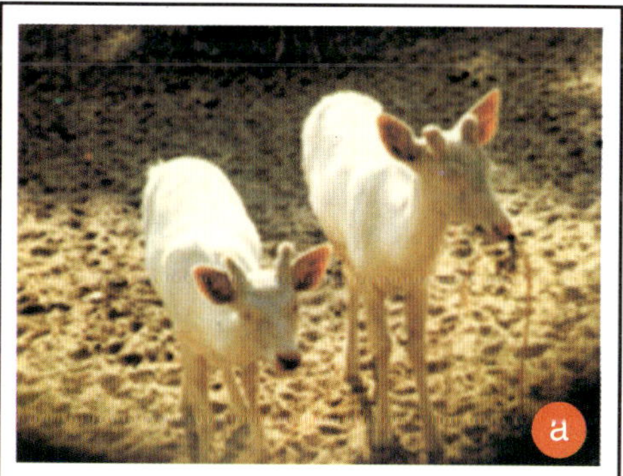

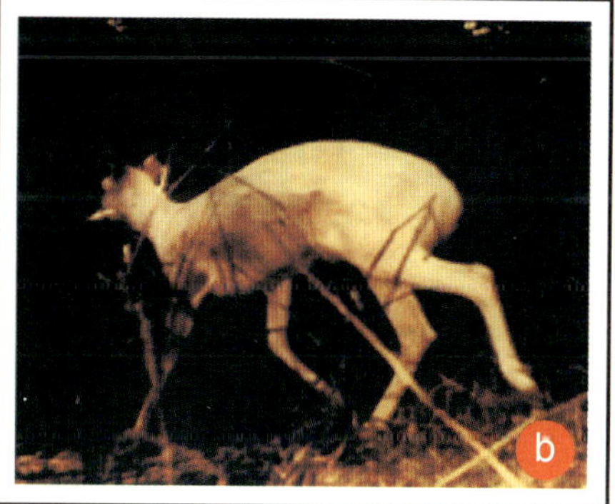

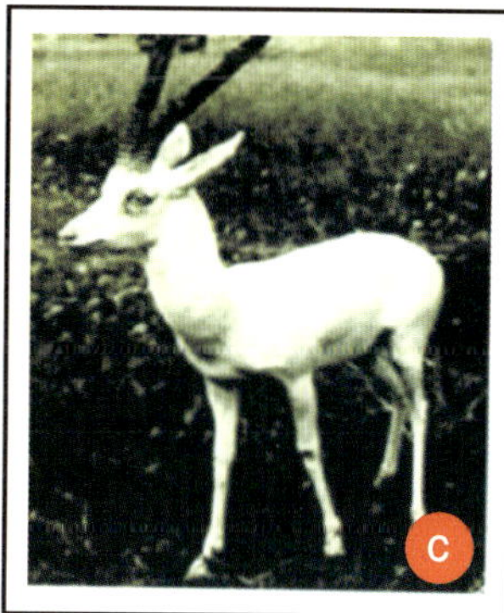

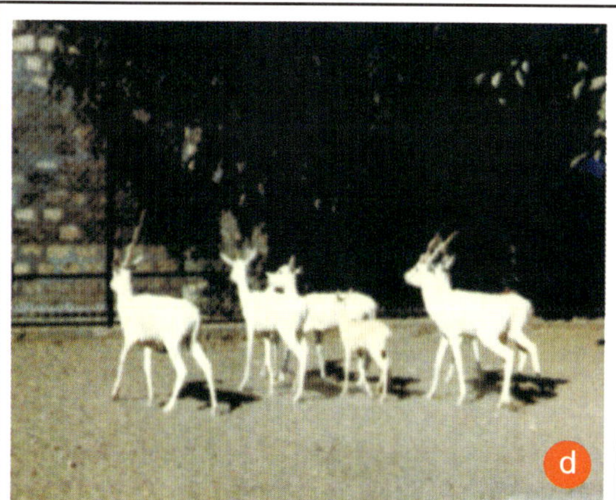

Figure169: Colour variants: (a) Albino chital (*A.axis*). Zoological Garden, Ahmadabad. (b) Predominant white colour barking deer (*M. muntjak*) at Zoological Park, Kanpur (U.P.). (c) Albino chinkara (*G. gazella*) at Zoological Garden, Ahmedabad.(d) A herd of White colour blackbucks (*A. cervicapra*). Zoological Garden, Bhilai (CG).

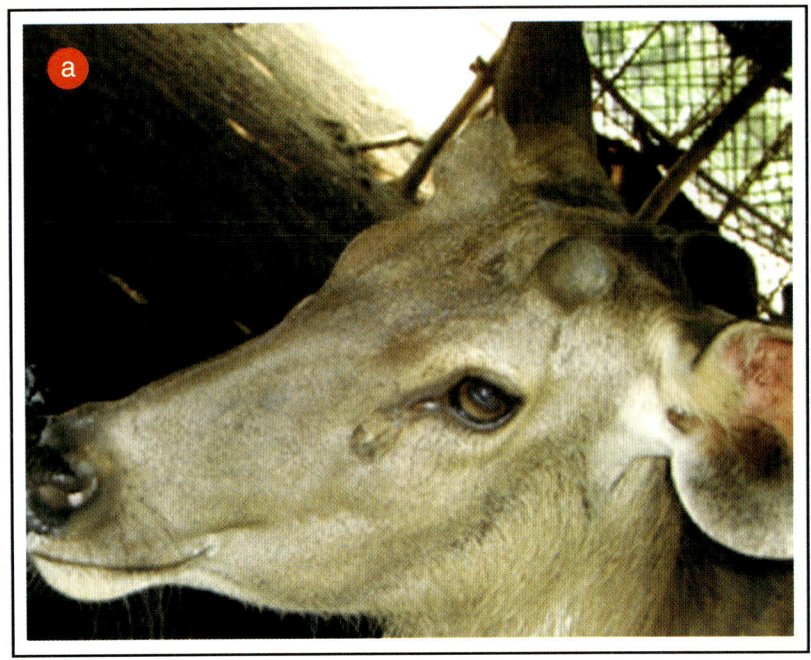

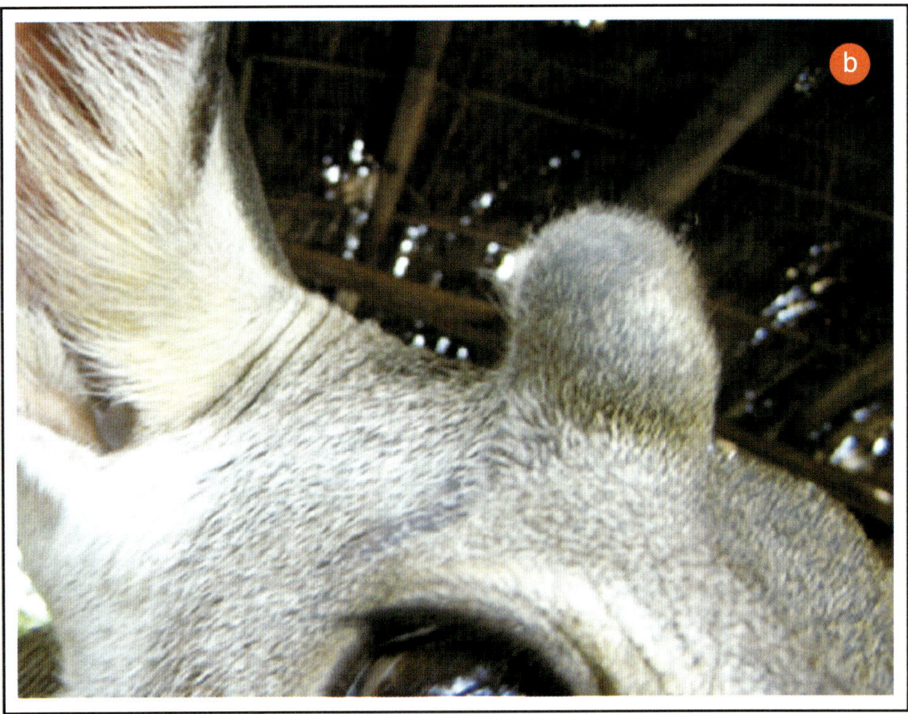

Figure 170: Photographs(a,b) showing small sized velvet covered antlers in female sambars (*C. unicolor*).

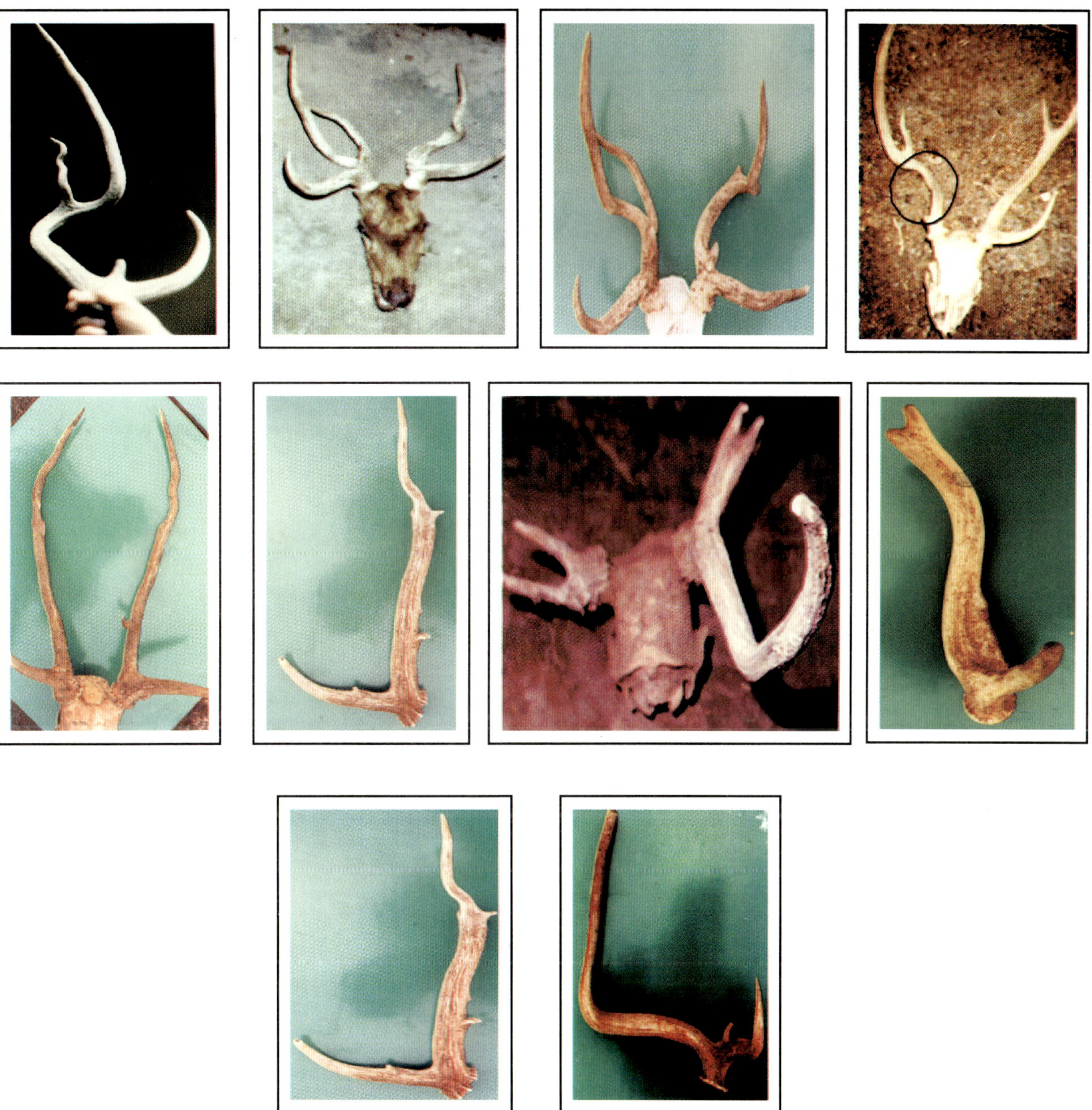

Figures 171 : Atypical shaped antlers of chitals (*A.axis*) from different zoological gardens.

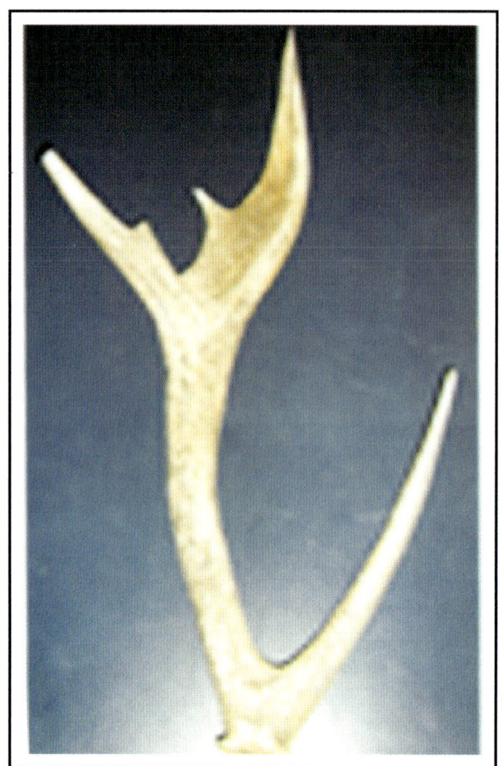

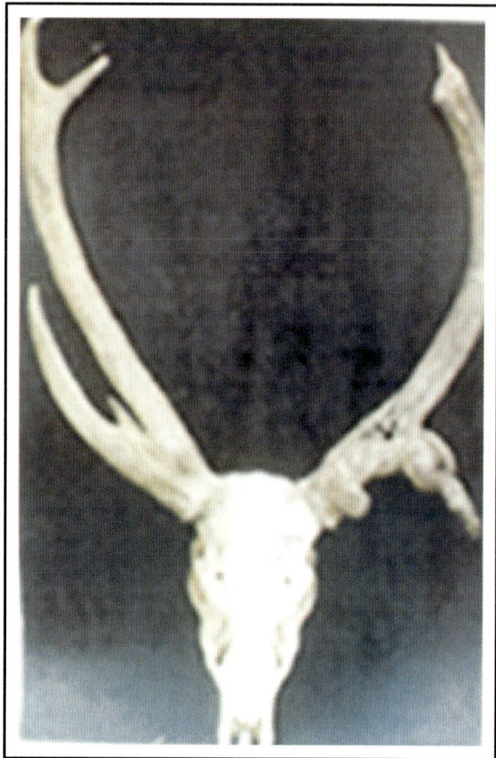

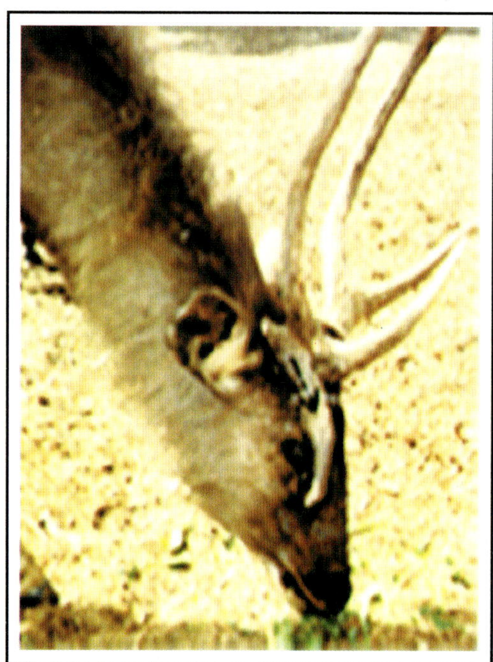

Figure 172: Photographs of atypical antlers of sambars (*C. unicolor*).

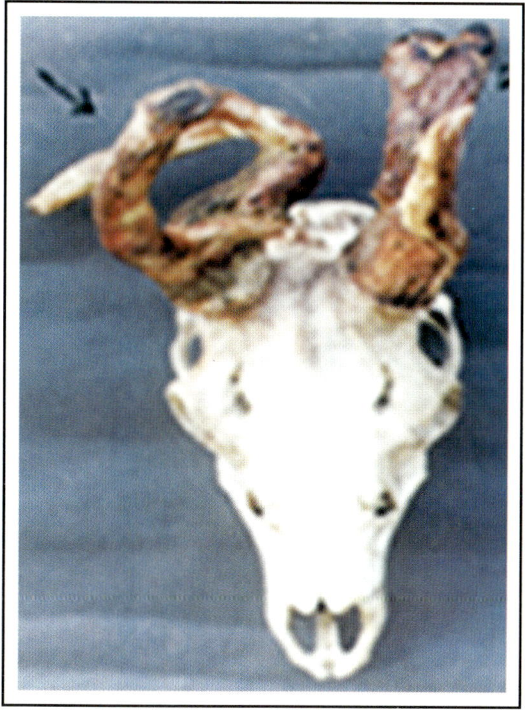

Figure 173: Atypical antlers in sangai deer (*C. eldi eldi*)

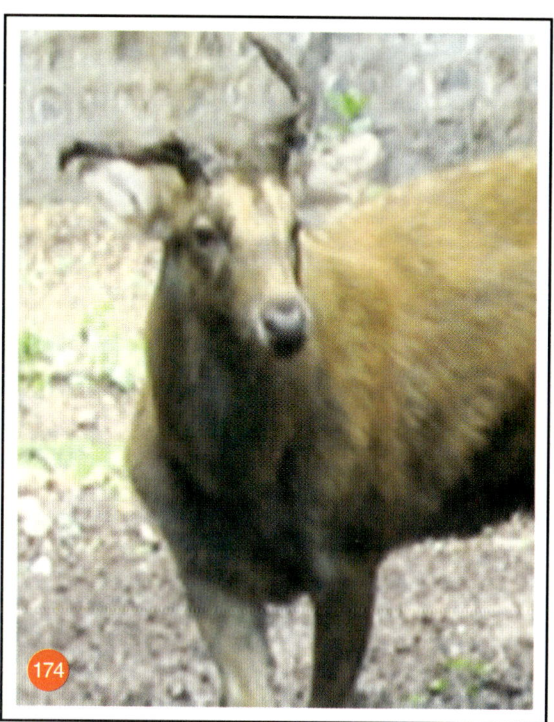

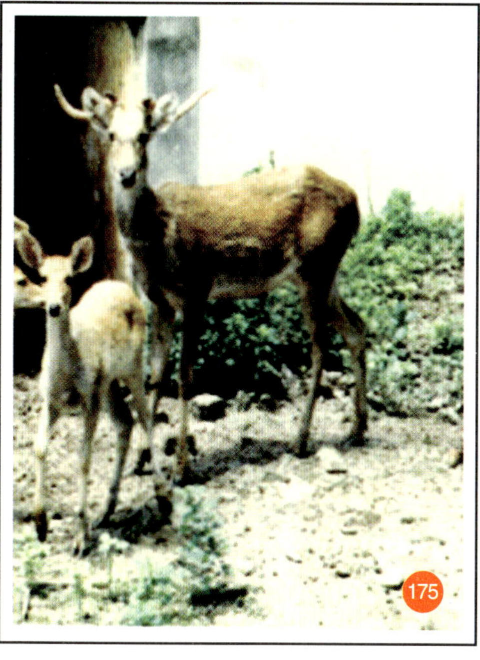

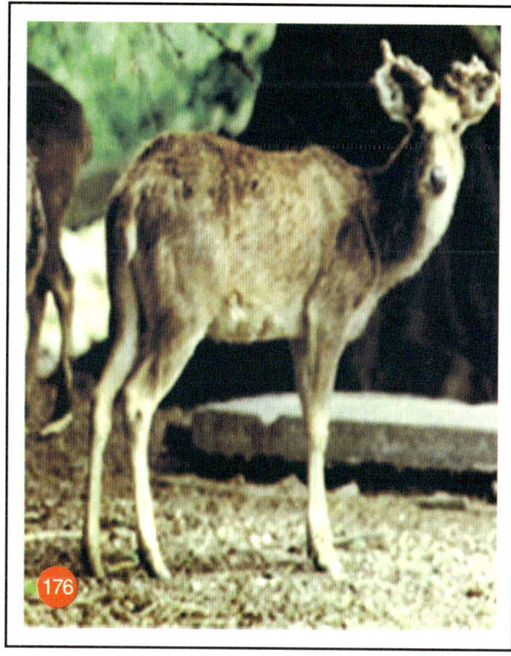

Figure 174-176: Irregularly grown antlers in barasingha (*C. d.duvauceli*). Each belonging to different captive facility.

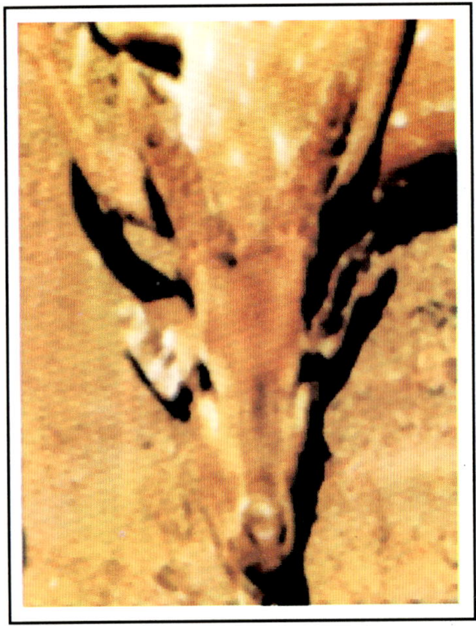

Figure 177: Atypical antlers in castrated chital (*A. axis*).

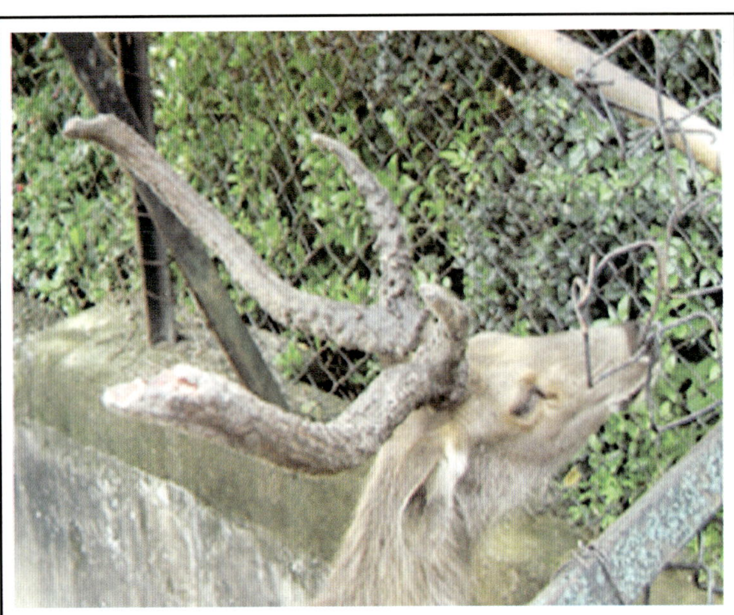

Figure 178 : Persistance of velvet in antlers of castrated sambar (*C. unicolor*)

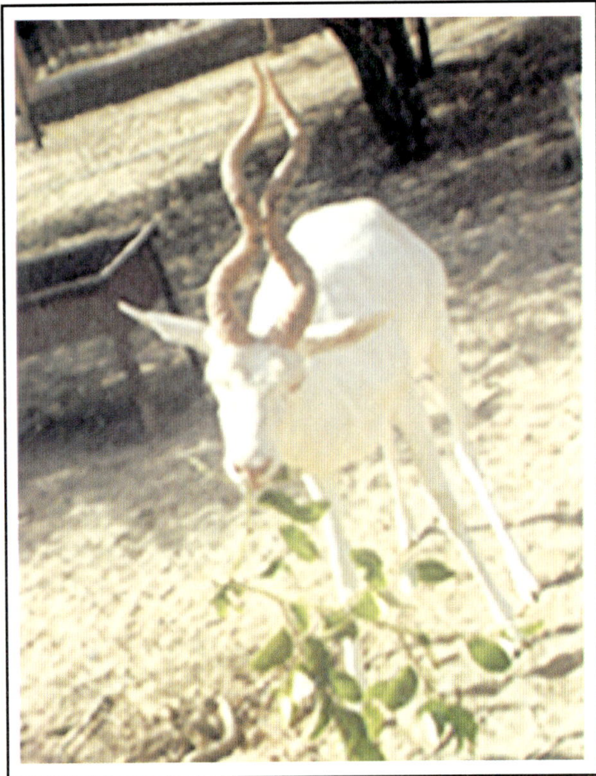

Figure 179: Photograph showing atypically curved horns in blackbuck (*A.cervicapra*).

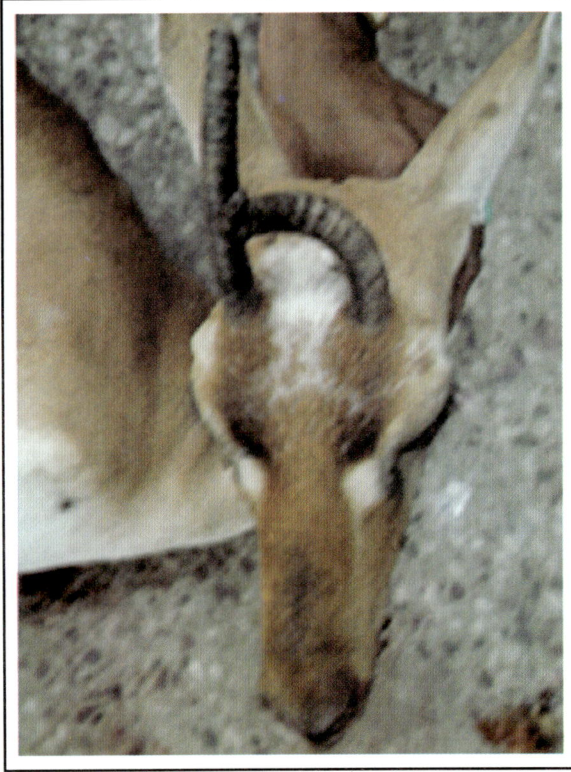

Figure 180: Photograph showing one atypically curved horn in female chinkara (*G. gazella*).

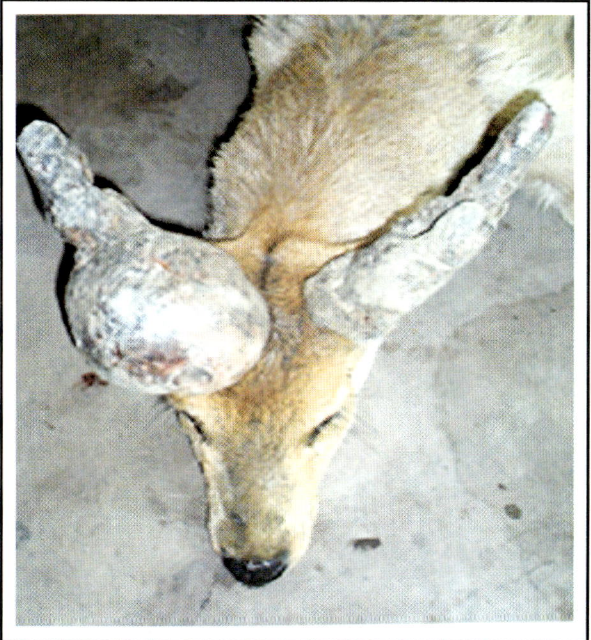

Figure 181: Right antler of hog-deer (*A. porcinus*) in velvet having developed a big abscess (Courtesy: Kishtwaria, R.S.).

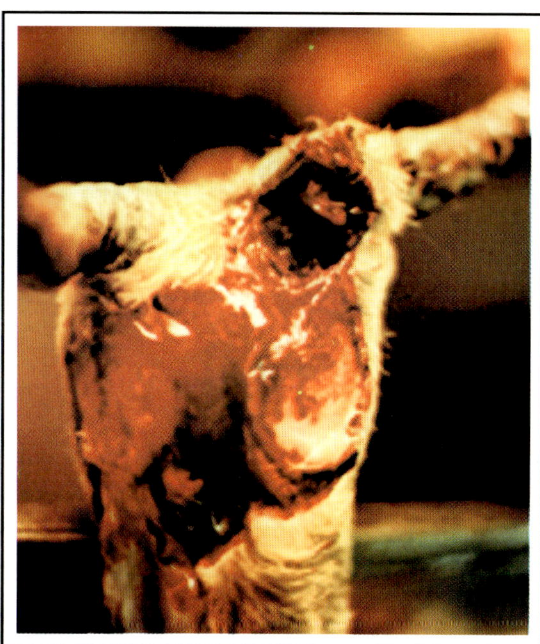

Figure 182: Photograph showing uprooted horn in blackbuck (*A.cervicapra*)caused during fighting with con-specific male.

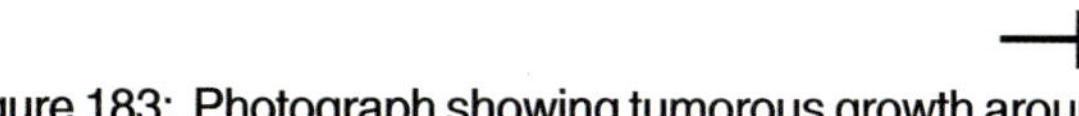

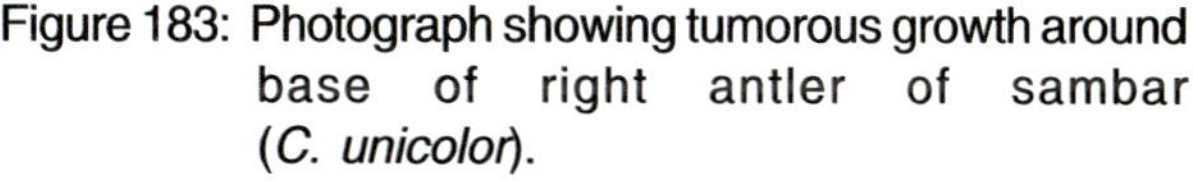

Figure 183: Photograph showing tumorous growth around base of right antler of sambar (*C. unicolor*).

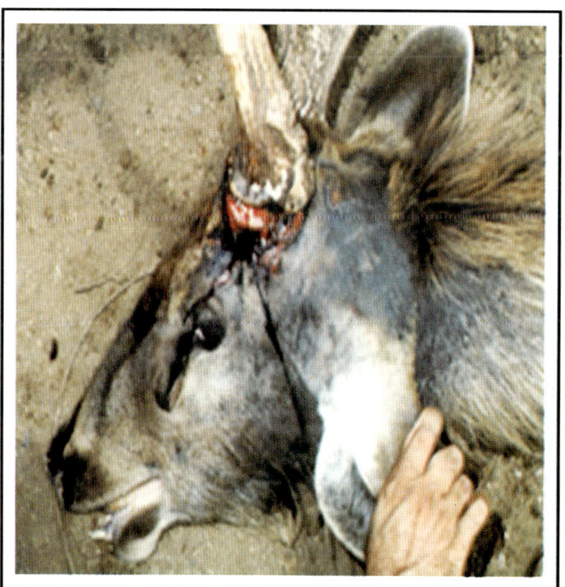

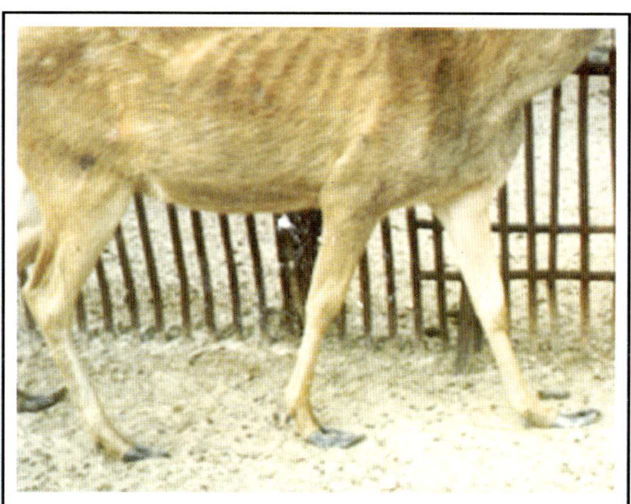

Figure184:Overgrown hooves in barasingha (*C.d.duvauceli*) belonging to Zoological Garden, Lucknow (U.P.).

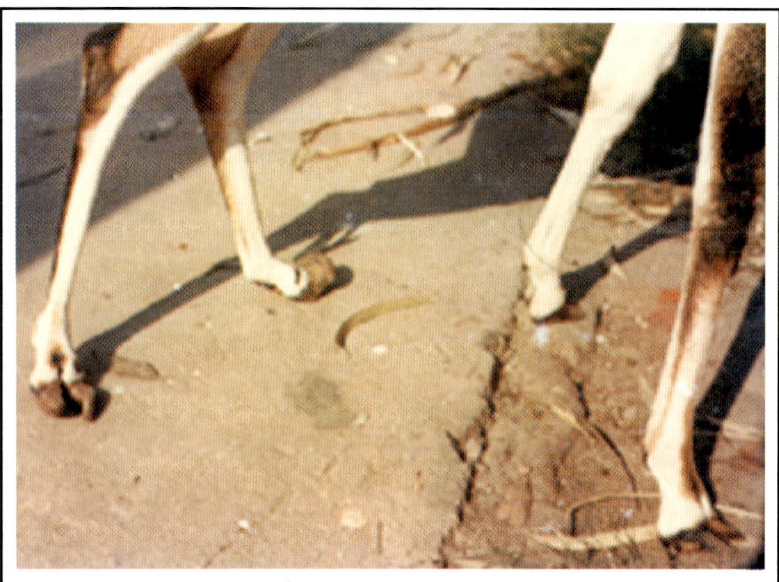

Figure 185: Deformed hooves in blackbuck (*A. cervicapra*).

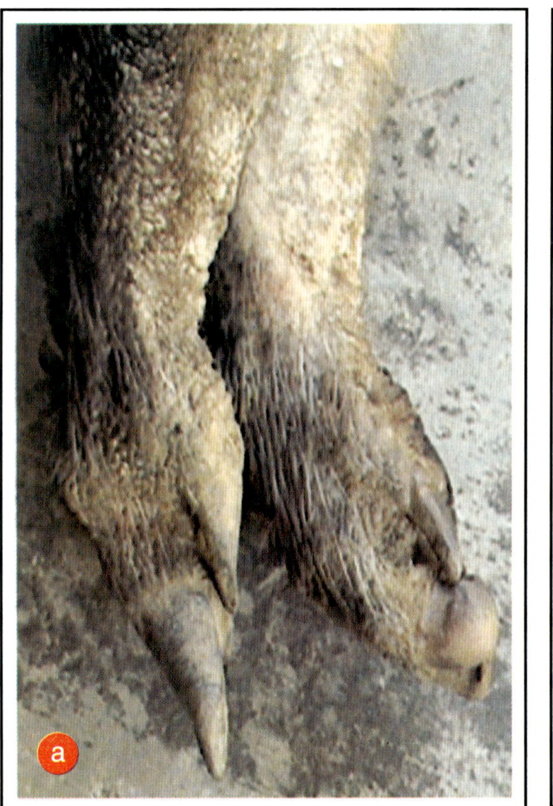

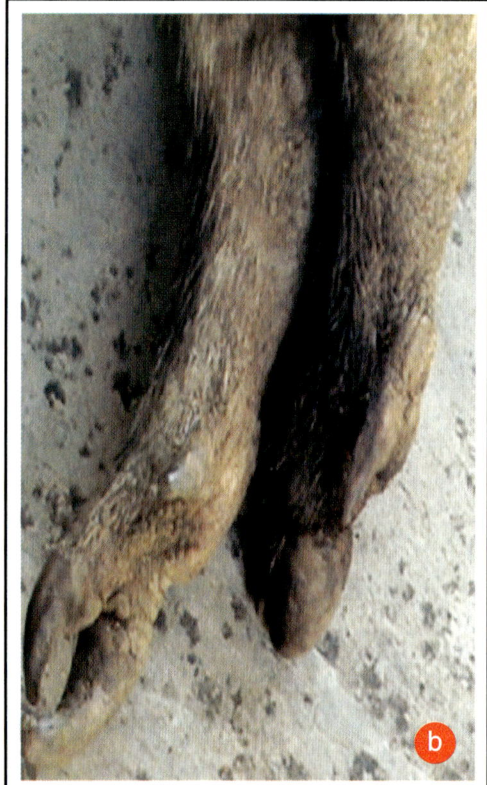

Figure 186: Photographs (a,b) showing deformed hooves in pigmy hog (*P. salvania*).

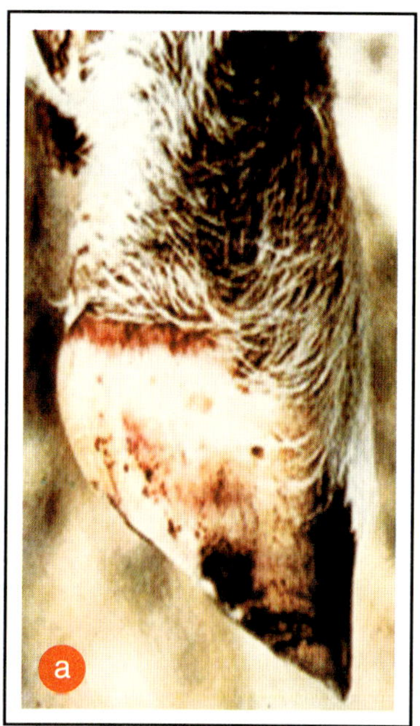

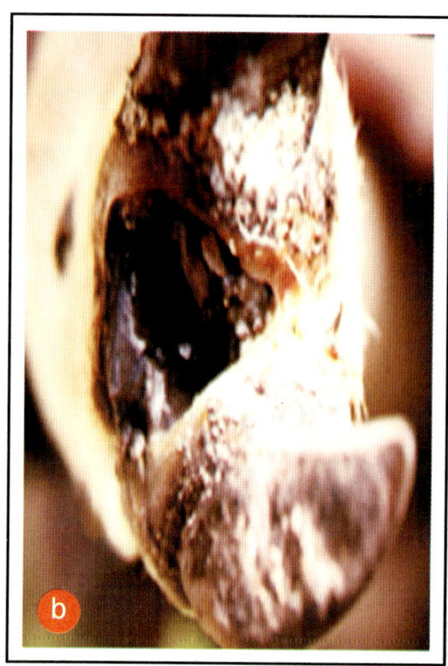

Figure 187: Photographs (a, b) showing foot rot lesions resulting into sloughing of hoof in deer in Bandipur National Park (Courtesy: Renukaprasad, C.)

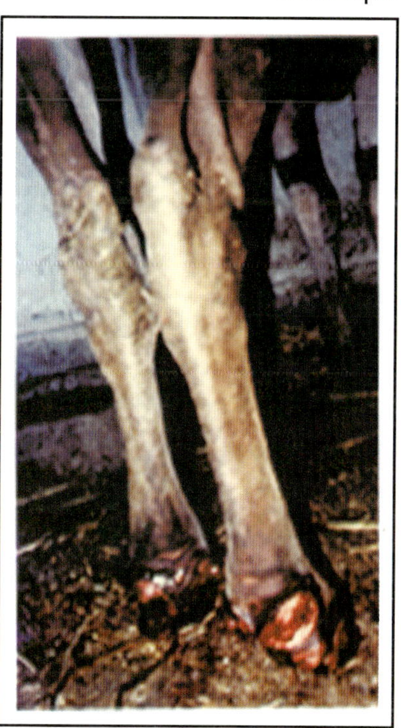

Figure 188: Photograph showing ulcerative lesions after burst of (FMD) vesicles in hind feet of captive eland (*Taurotragus oryx*, an exotic sp.).

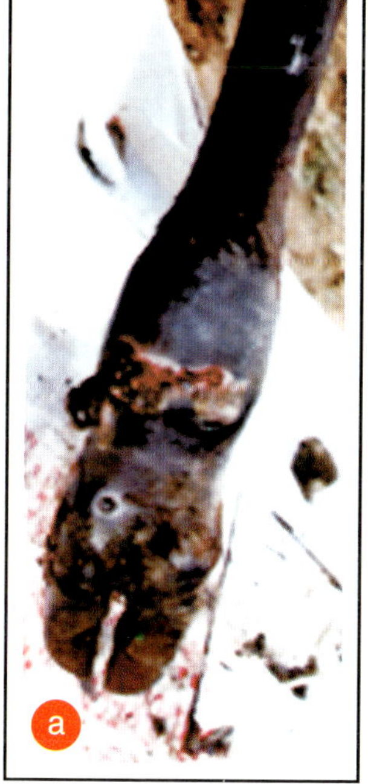

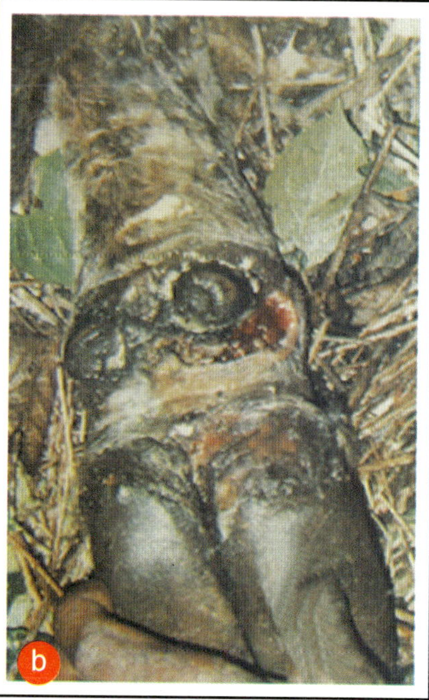

Figure 189: Photograph showing foot lesions in captive: (a) Nilgai (*B. tragocamelus*) affected with FMD-O serotype (Courtesy: Sudhan,N.A.).(b) gaur (*B. gaurus*) belonged to Zoological Park, Chennai (Courtesy: Dept. Wildlife Sci. Chennai, TN)

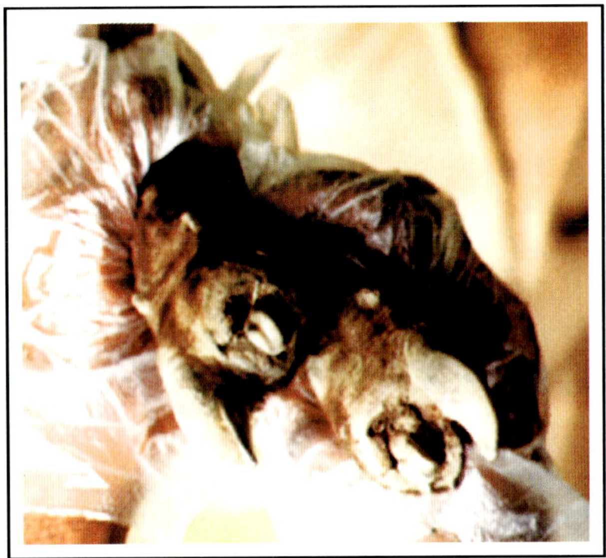

Figure 190: Photograph showing parakeratosis over the pastern joints and deformed hooves in wild hog-deer (*A. porcinus*) sequelae to FMD at Corbett Tiger Reserve, Ramnagar (Courtesy: Choudhury, B.).

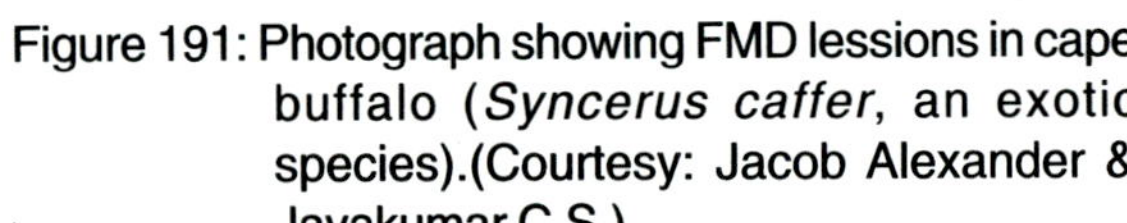

Figure 191: Photograph showing FMD lessions in cape buffalo (*Syncerus caffer*, an exotic species).(Courtesy: Jacob Alexander & Jayakumar,C.S.).

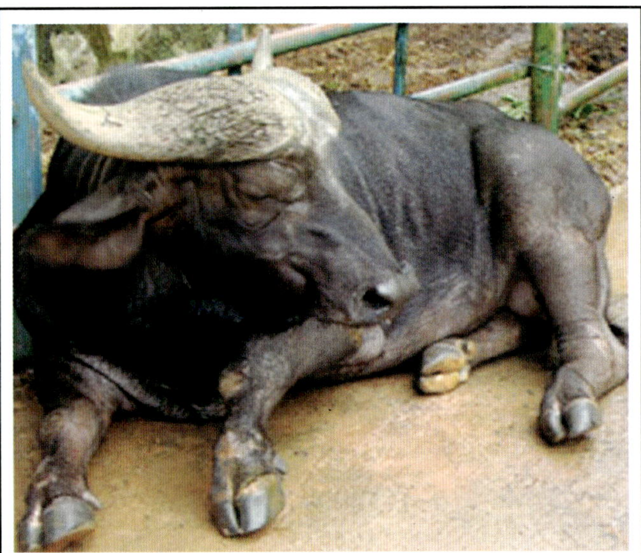

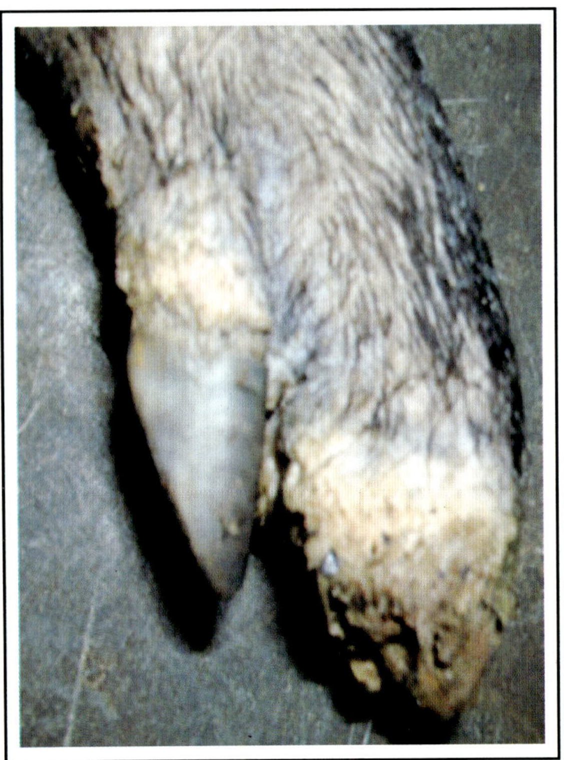

Figure 192: FMD foot lesion in wild boar (*S.scrofa*) caused due to FMD serotype 'O' (Courtesy: Jacob Alxenader, & Jayakumar,C.S.).

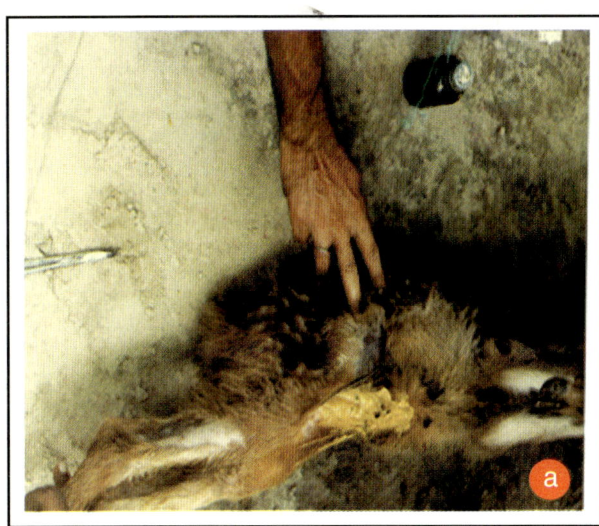

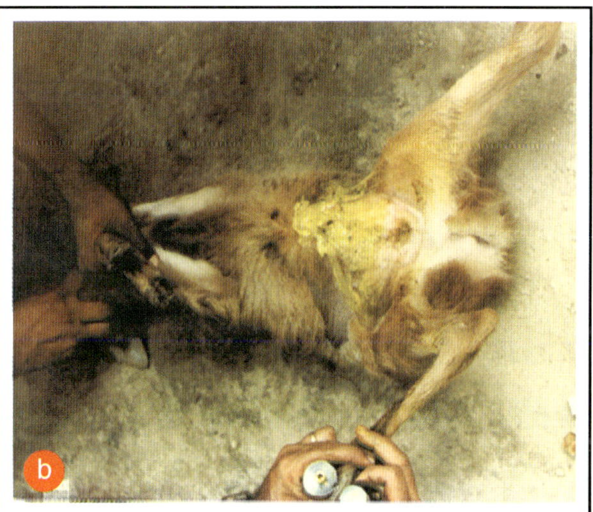

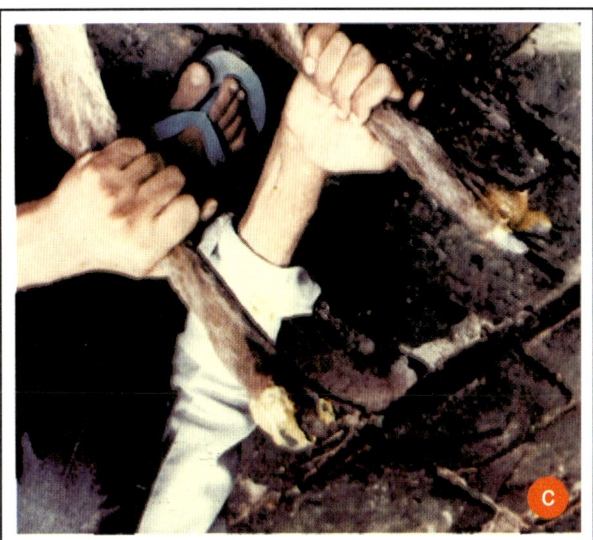

Figure 193: Photographs showing suppurative lesions at navel region(a,b) and coronary band of hindfeet (c) of sika deer (*Cervus nippon*,an exotic sp.) caused due to *Pseudomonas aeruginosa* infection.

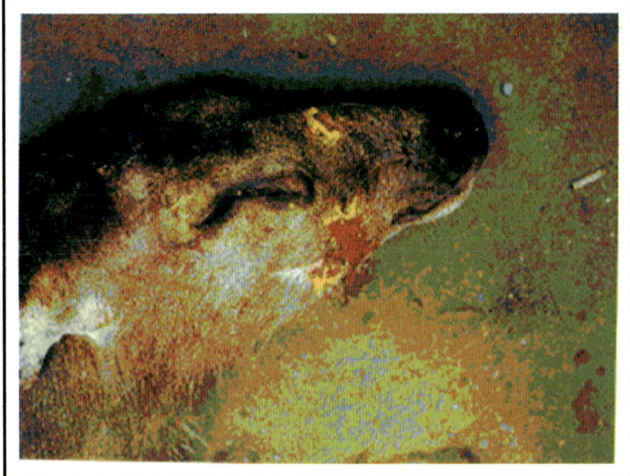

Figure 194: Sambar (*C. unicolor*) sustained abrasions and lacerations in head region during trapping (Courtesy:Nigam, P.).

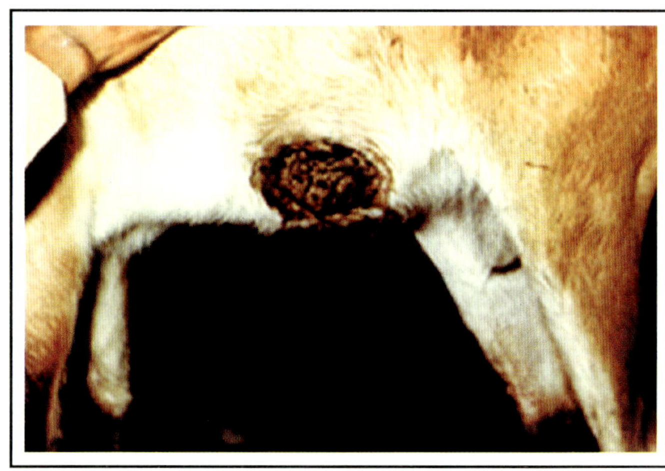

Figure195: Photograph showing chronic wound at left ventro-lateral aspect of abdomen of red lechwae (*Kobus leche leche*,an exotic antelope).

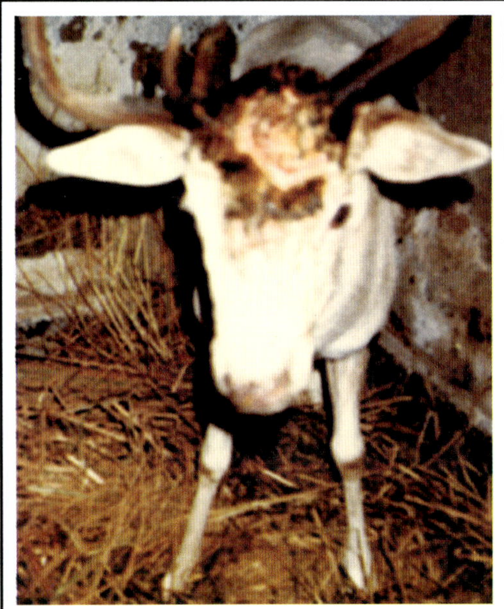

Figure 196: Photograph showing suppurative wound in the pole region of fallow deer (*Dama dama*,an exotic sp.) at National Zoological Park, New Delhi.

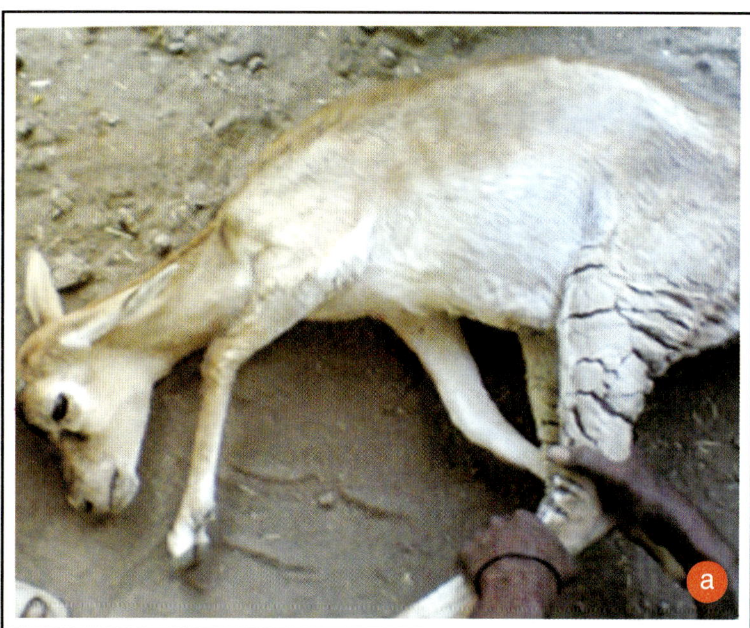

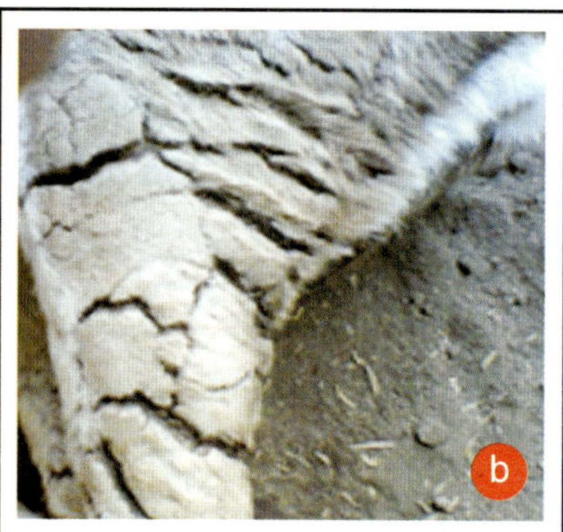

Figure 197: Blackbuck (*A. cervicapra*) carcasses (a, b) showing dry deep cracks in the skin mainly from thigh region to stifle joint.The condition was associated to zinc deficiency as a result of feeding mainly on lucerne. All 13 animals of the herd of 50 individuals had died in a period of three months in a captive facility located near Mumbai.(Courtesy : College of Vet. Sc., Mumbai).

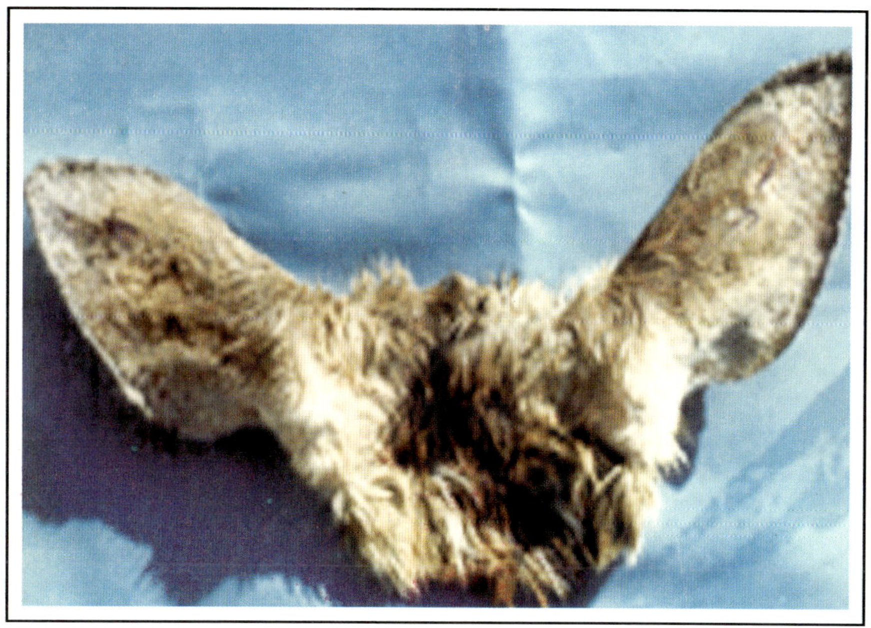

Figure 198: Photograph showing ear dermatitis (alopecia and small necrotic lesions) due to *Trichophyton mentagrophytes* infection in chital (*A. axis*) belonging to National Park, Dudwa of UttarPradesh.

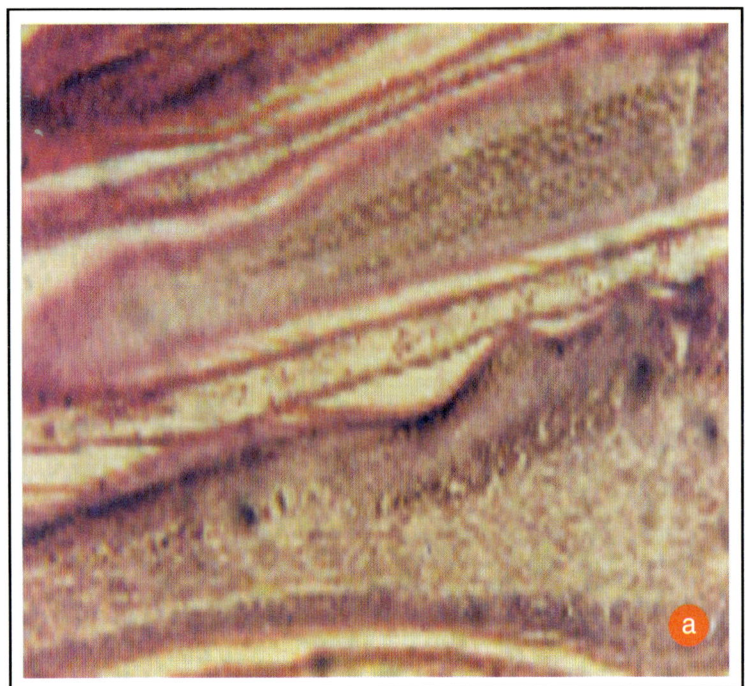

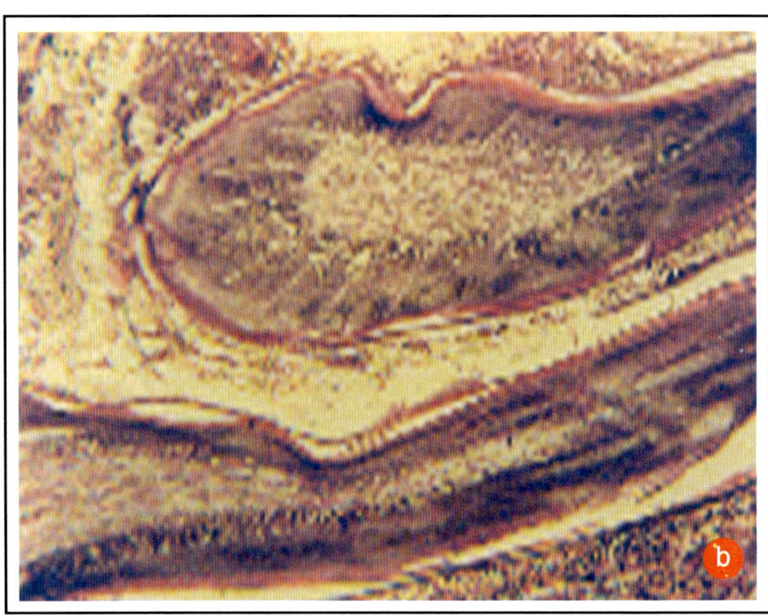

Figure 199: Dermatomycosis in hog-deer (*A.porcinus*).Photomicrographs showing: (a) Cavity formation and destruction of hair follicles with presence of fungal bodies. (b) Mosaic pattern of fungal spores in the hair follicle. H&E x150. (Courtesy: Bhowmik, M.K.)

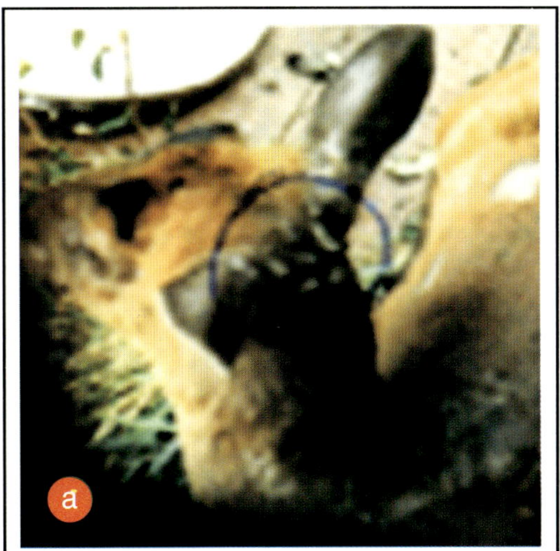

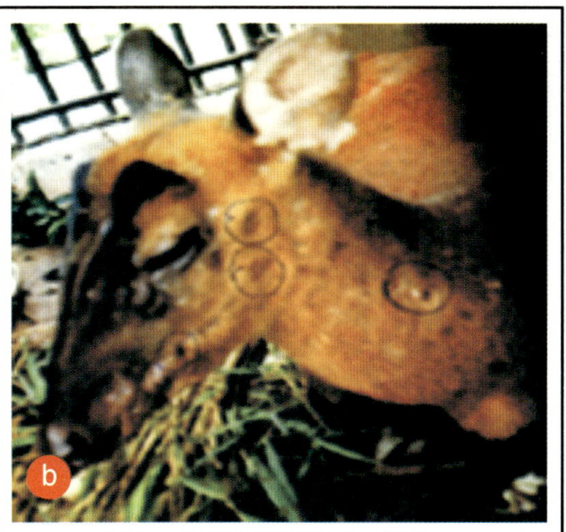

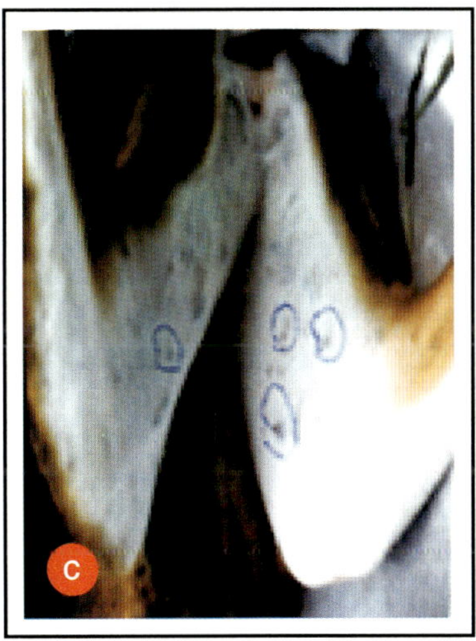

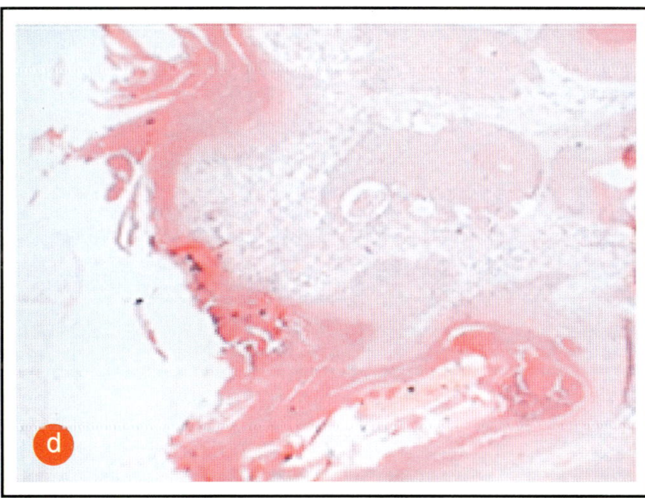

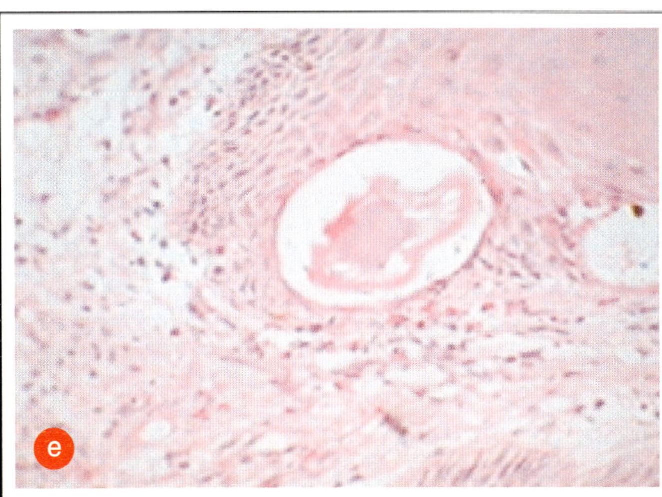

Figure 200: Photographs (a-c) showing dyskeratosis in barking deer (*M. muntjak*) at Zoological Garden Gangtok, Sikkim. Lesions included formation of small nodular growths on the back of the ear extended to pole (a), neck, face (b)and inner aspect of thighs(c). Photomicrographs(d, e) showing condition caused due to *Stephanofilaria assemensis* infection. (d) H &E,x100 (e) Higher magnification H &E, x400 (Shiva shanker & Chakraborty, 2005).

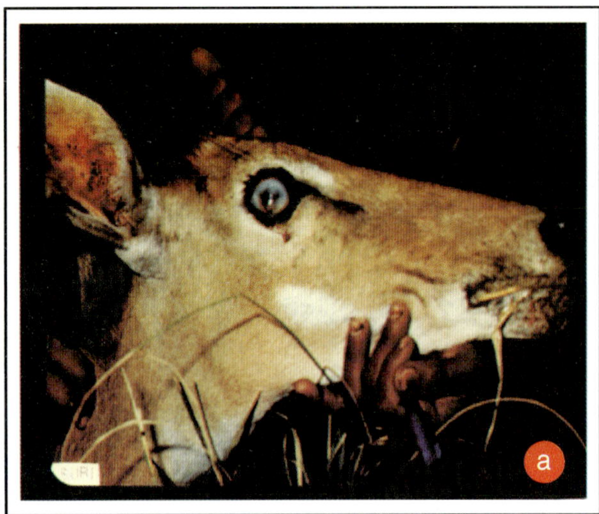

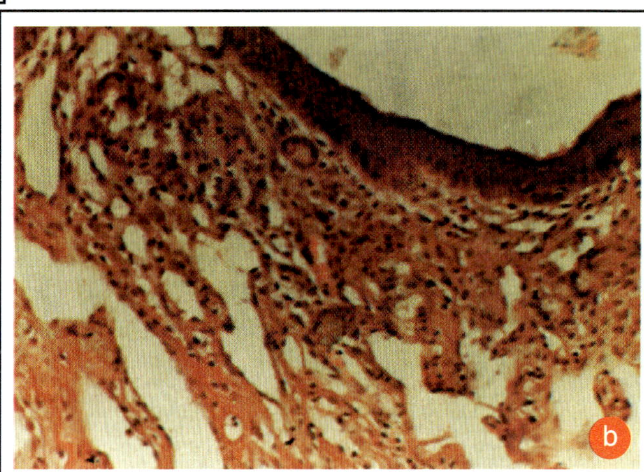

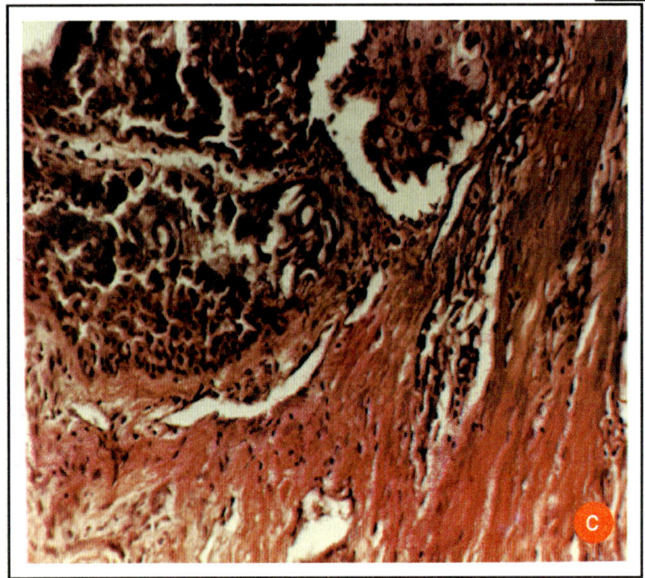

Figure 201: (a) Photograph showing ear sore lesion and corneal opacity in a male nilgai (*B. tragocamelus*) belonging to Sariska National Park, Rajasthan. Photomicrographs (b,c) showing ear lesions (a) related to *Stephanofilaria* sp. infection. H&E, x 400

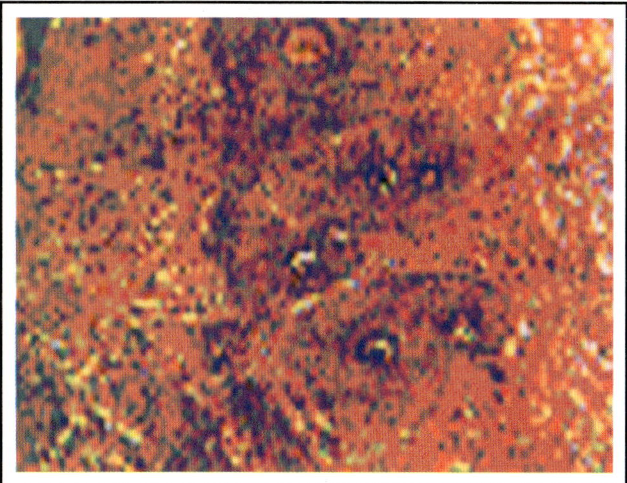

Figure 202: Photomicrograph showing chronic dermatitis and folliculitis with evidence of calcified mite (scabies)in hog-deer (*A. porcinus*).H&Ex100 (Courtesy: Bhowmik, M.K.).

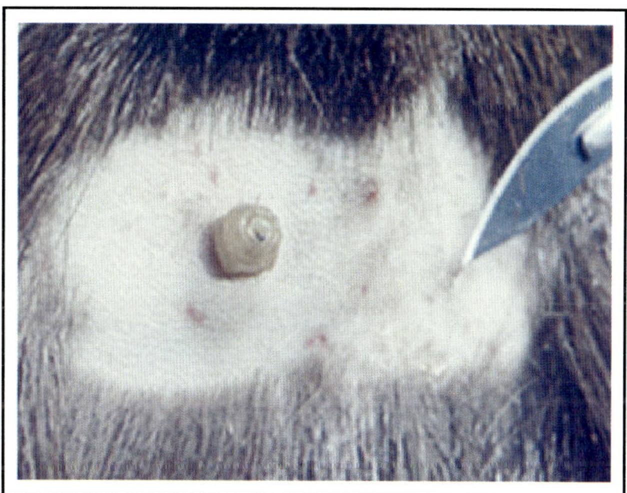

Figure 203: Photographs showing *Hypoderma dianna* protruding through skin of hog-deer (*A. porcinus*) belonging to Orang National Park, Assam

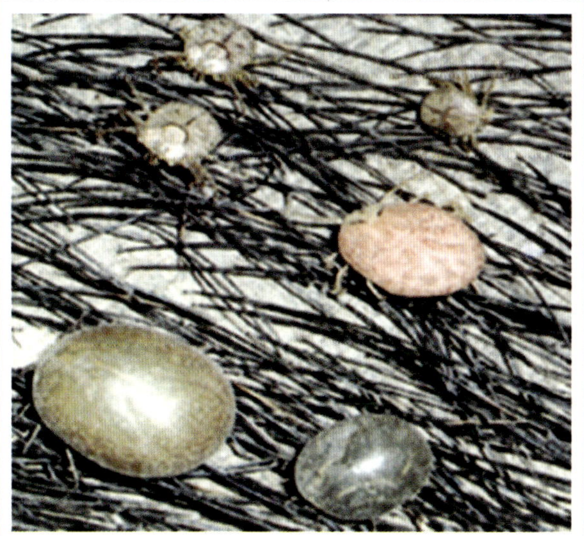

Figure 204: Ticks infestation in wild boar (*Sus scrofa cristatus*). Courtesy: Anupam Rakshit.

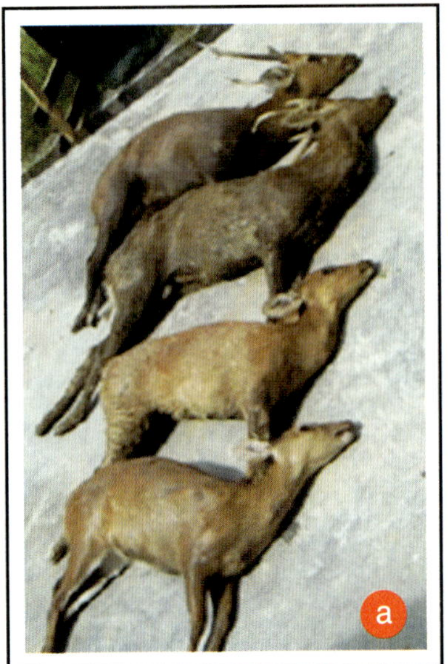

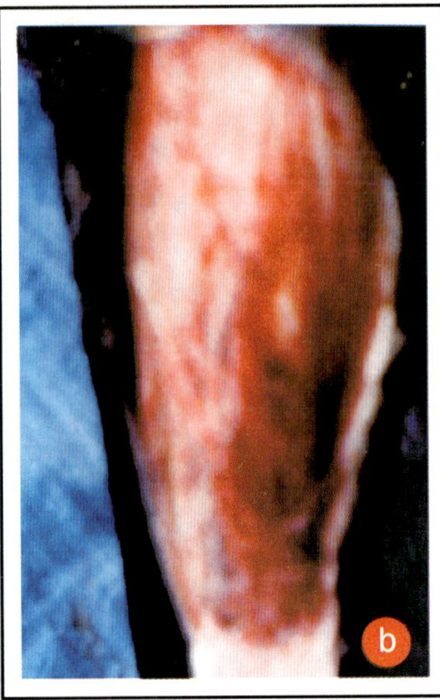

Figure 205: (a) Carcasses of hog-deer (*A. porcinus*). Animals had died of capture myopathy in effort to save them during flood in Kaziranga National Park, Assam (b) A specimen from (a) showing diffuse haemorrhages in subcutaneous tissue and muscles alleged to capture myopathy (Courtesy: Talukdar, A. & Choudhury, B).

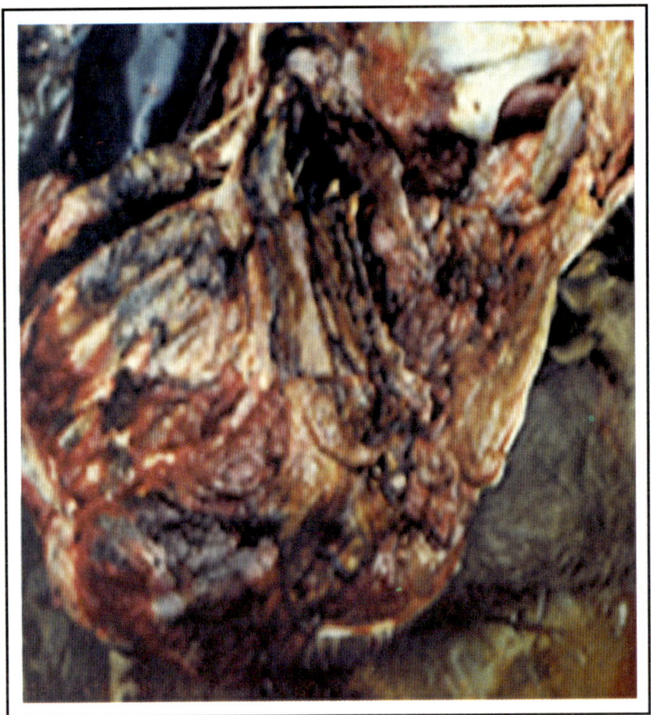

Figure 206: Photograph showing gangrenous myositis and cellulitis at shoulder joint in sambar (*C. unicolor*) at Zoological Garden, Assam.

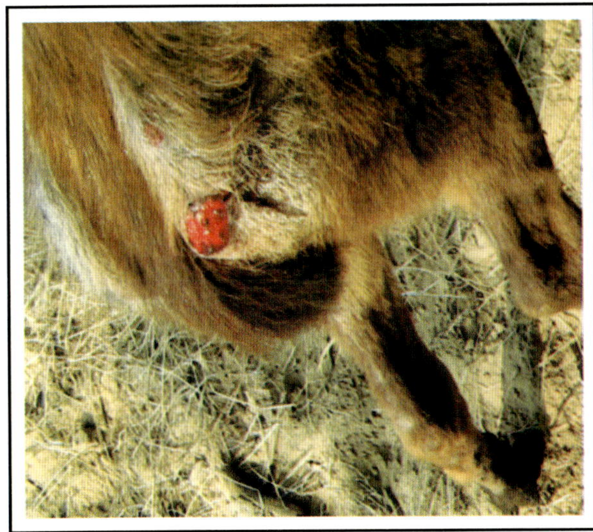

Figure 207: Deep lacerated wounds in sambar (*C. unicolor*) caused due to con-specific conflicts. (Courtesy: Kishtwaria, R.S.)

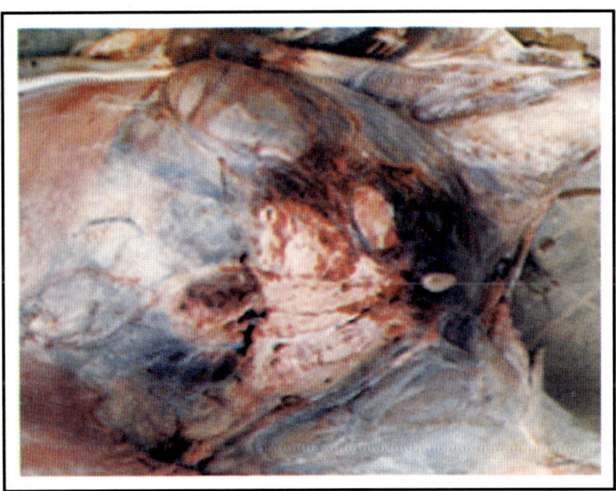

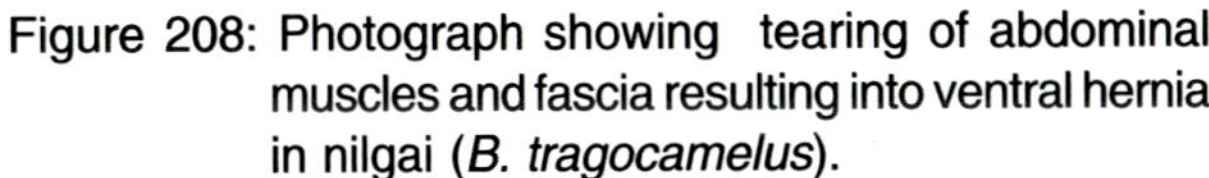

Figure 208: Photograph showing tearing of abdominal muscles and fascia resulting into ventral hernia in nilgai (*B. tragocamelus*).

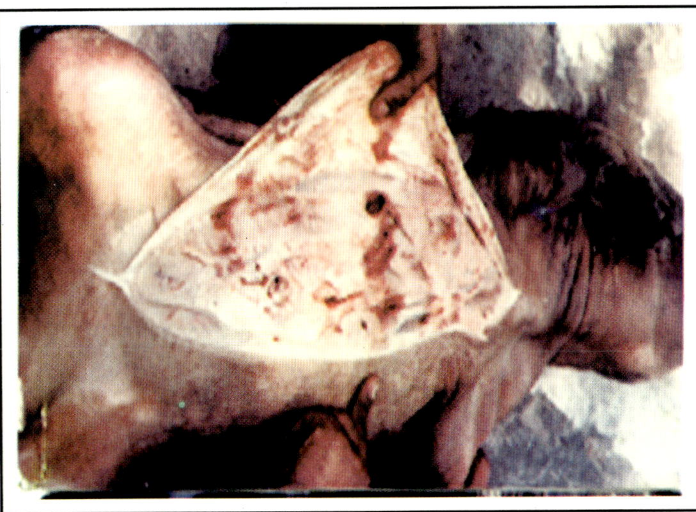

Figure 209: Photograph showing skin lacerations and muscle rupture in hippopotamus (*H. amphibius*, an exotic sp.) calf died due to treading by the male parent after birth in National Zoological Park, New Delhi.

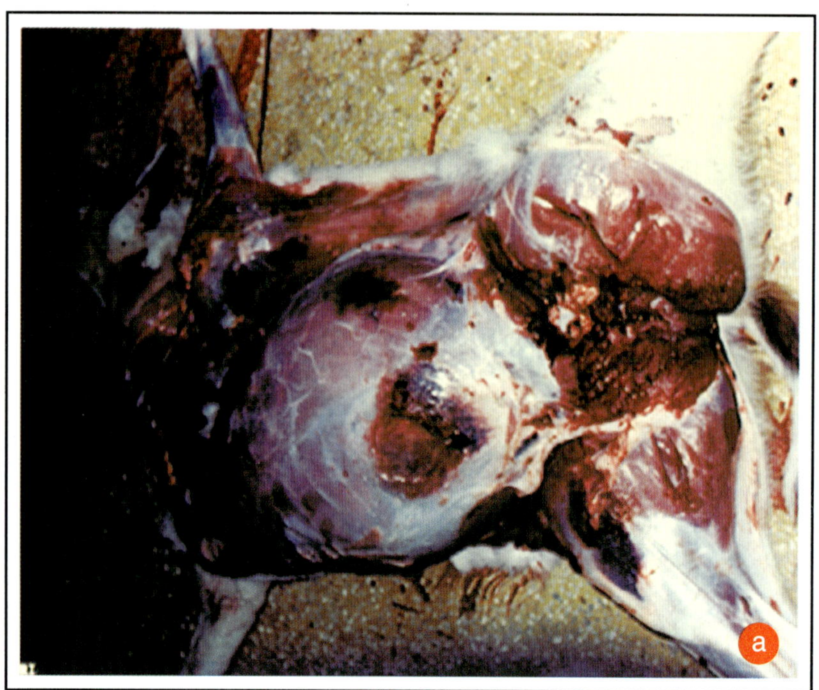

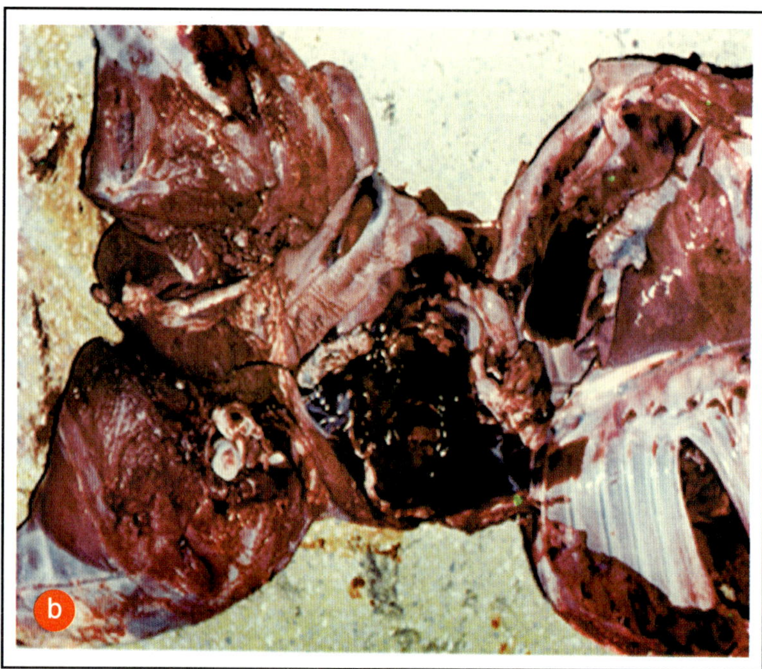

Figure 210: Photographs showing:(a) Rupture of abdominal musculature and (b) Note heavy bleeding from left kidney of a male chital (*A.axis*) caused due to goring by the stronger male companion.

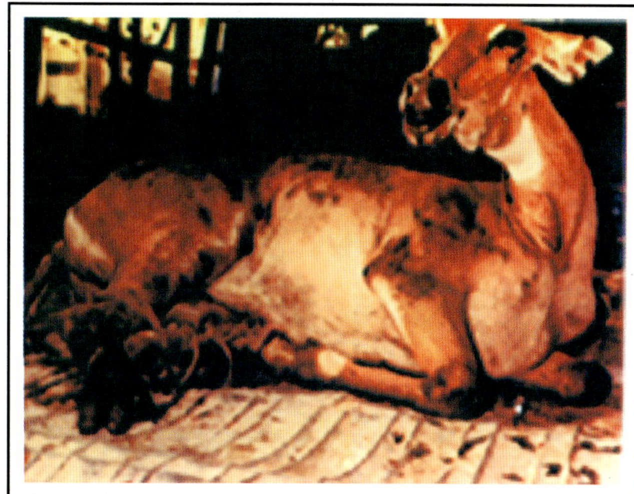

Figure 211: Severely injured adult female nilgai (*B. tragocamelus*),which collided with a truck on the forest road of Uttar Pradesh.

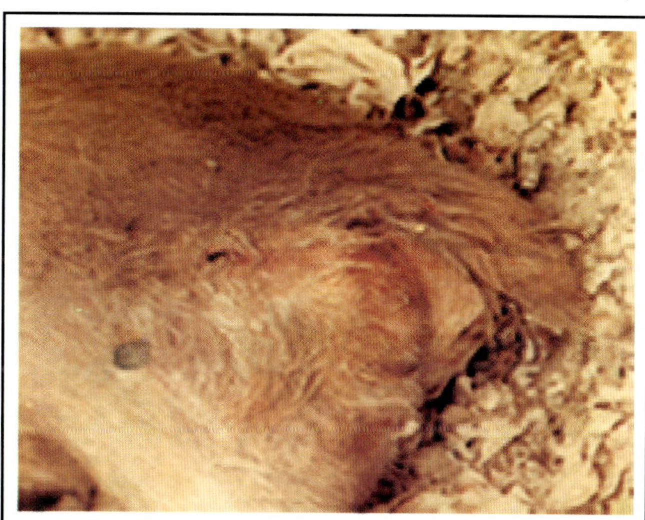

Figure 212: Swollen thigh muscle of hog-deer (*A. porcinus*) due to abscess formation, which occurred after a couple of days following tranquilization.It could be either due to contaminated dart needle or invasion of pathogen through the traumatized skin.

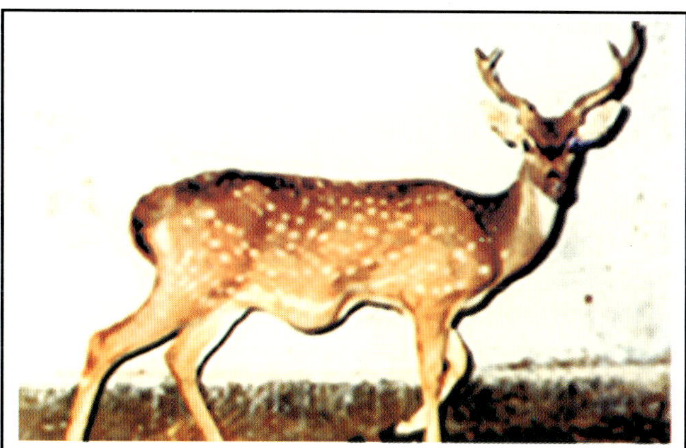

Figure 213: Photograph showing tuberculous abscess involving abdominal musculature on right ventro-lateral aspect in chital (*A. axis*).

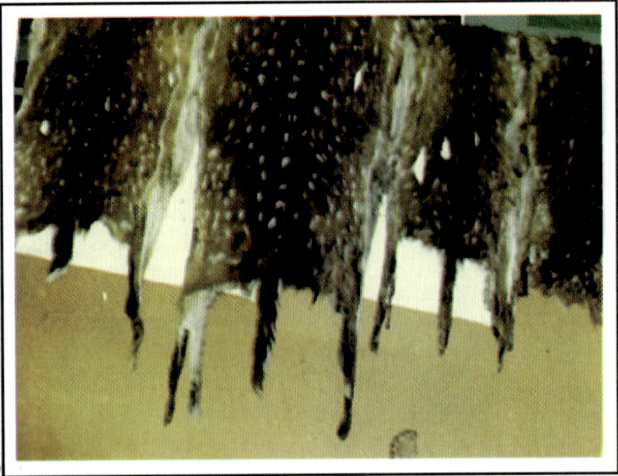

Figure 214: Photograph of skins of chitals (*A. axis*) showing bullet marks caused by poachers.

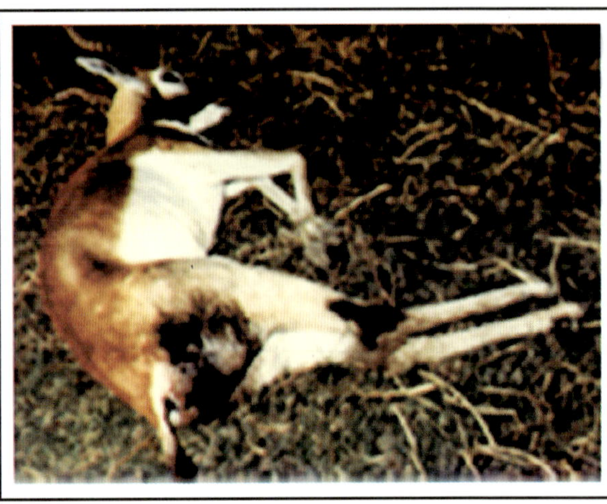

Figure 215: An adult male blackbuck (*A. cervicapra*) shot dead by poacher. Note bullet marks in the thigh muscles.

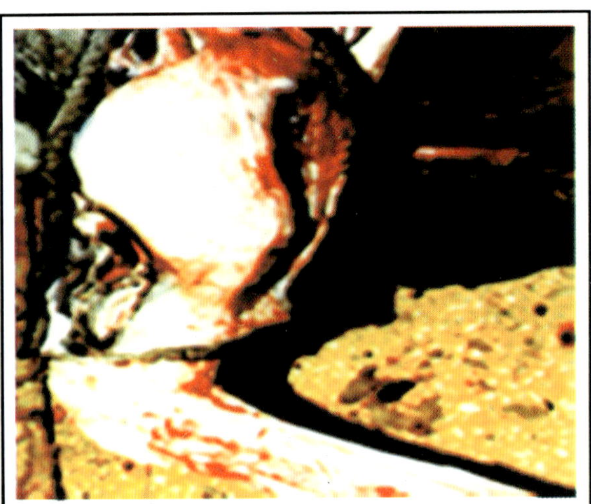

Figure 216: Photograph showing atrophy of hind leg muscles of an adult nilgai (*B. tragocamelus*) because hind limb being kept tied for prolonged period.

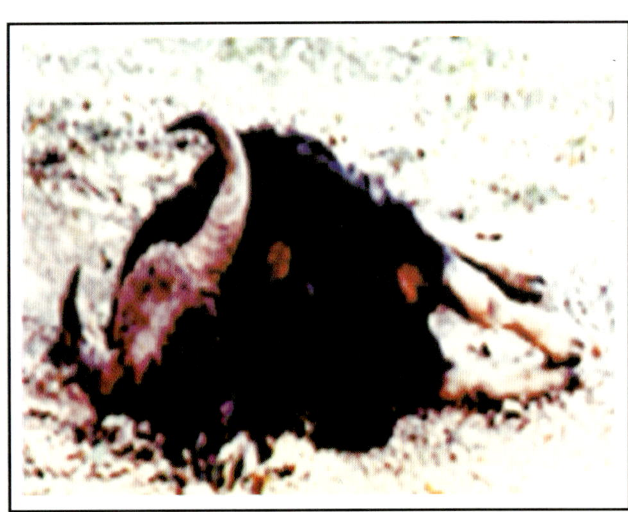

Figure 217: Carcass of gaur (*B.gaurus*) showing forest fire burn marks on left shoulder and dewlap.

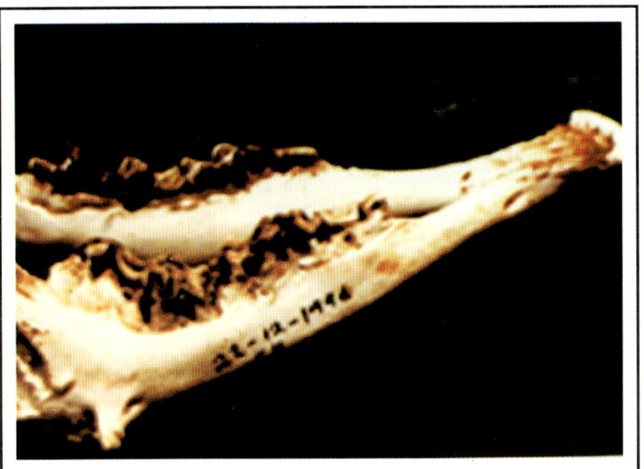

Figure 218: Photograph of chital (*A. axis*) mandible showing small growth on the latero-ventral aspect of right ramus. Note wear of cheek teeth.

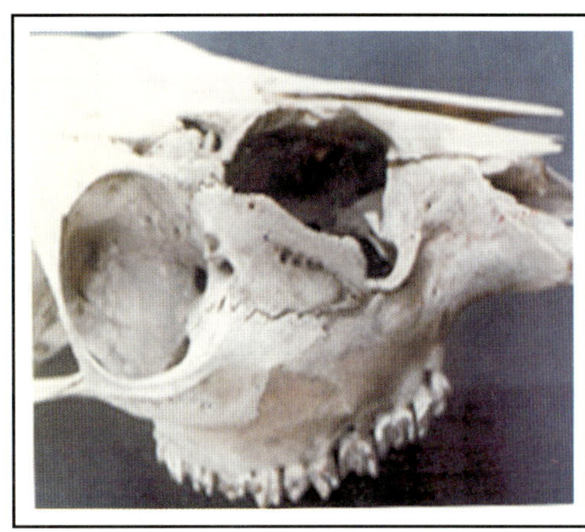

Figure 219: Photograph of skull of an adult male chital (*A. axis*) showing traumatically deformed maxillary bone, may be a result of same traumatic impact experienced in early life.

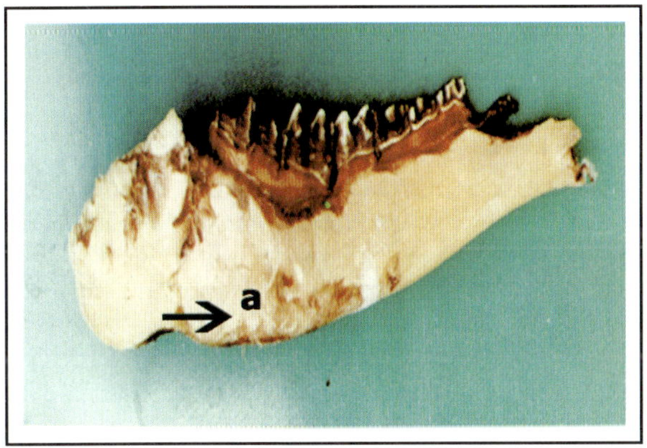

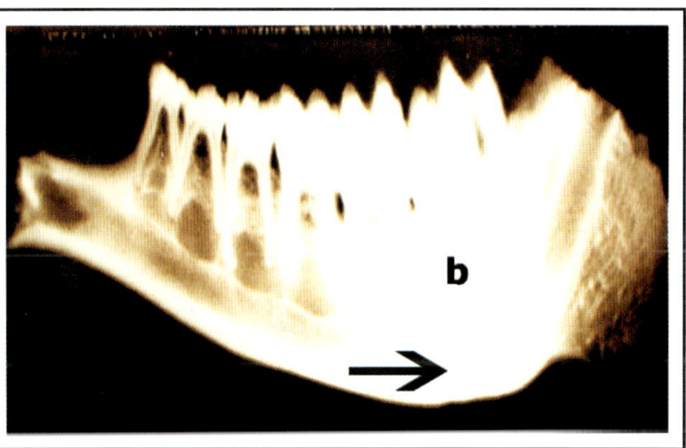

Figure 220: (a)Right ramus of chital (*A.axis*) marked for enlarged size. (b) Radiograph of (a) showing obliteration of mandible canal.

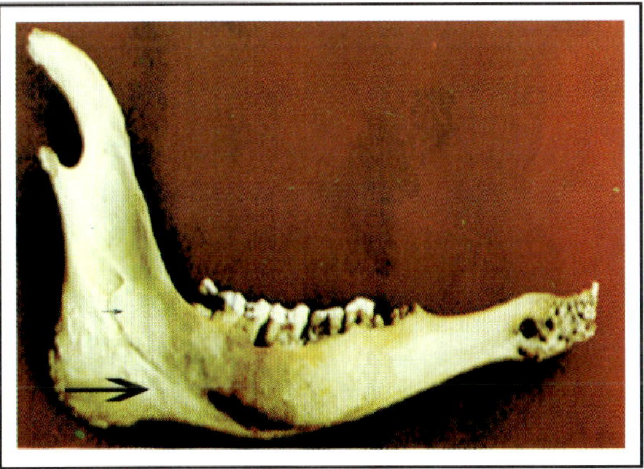

Figure 221: Lingual surface of left ramus of chital (*A.axis*) showing hyperostosis.

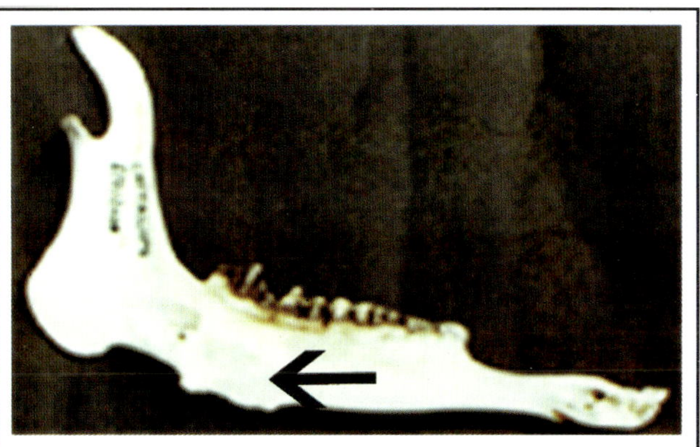

Figure 222: Lingual surface of left ramus of chital (*A.axis*) showing hyperostosis at the level of molar teeth extending from ventral border.

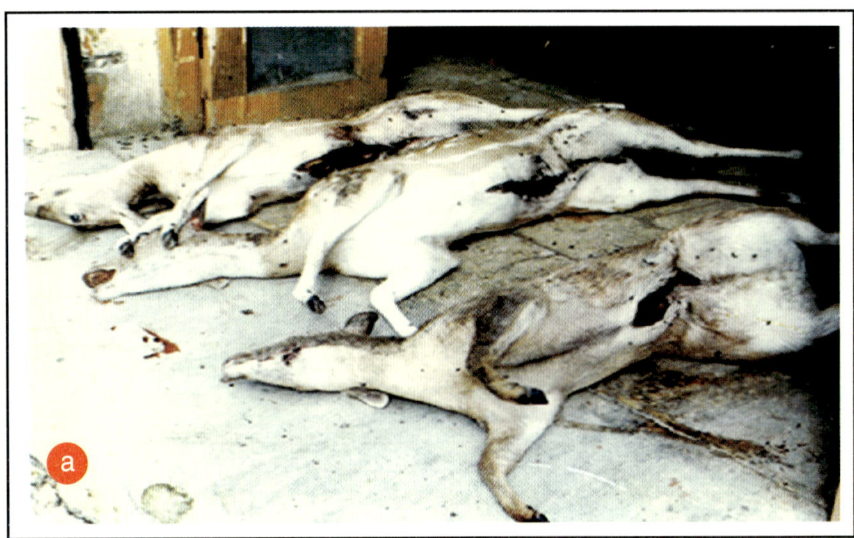

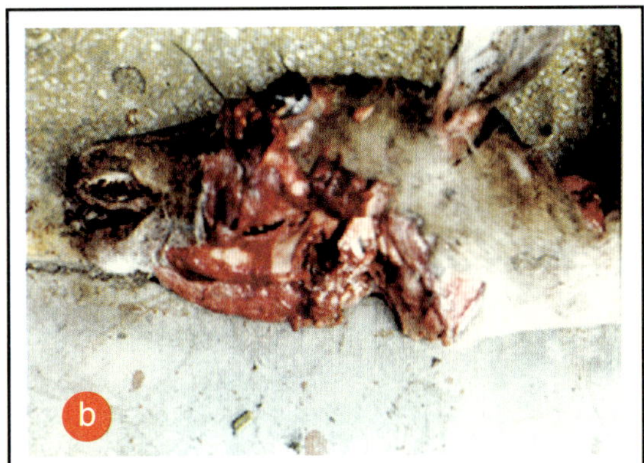

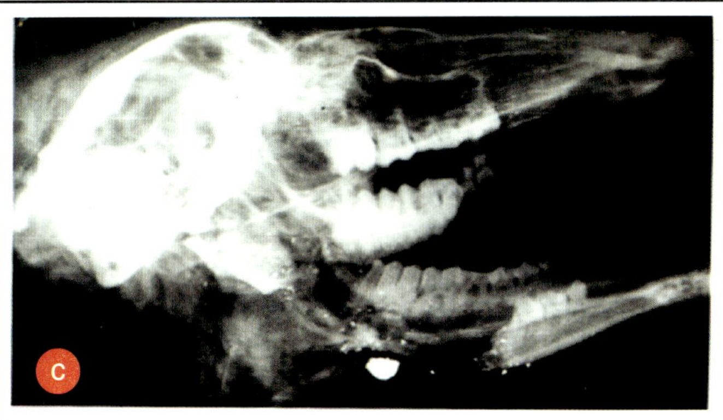

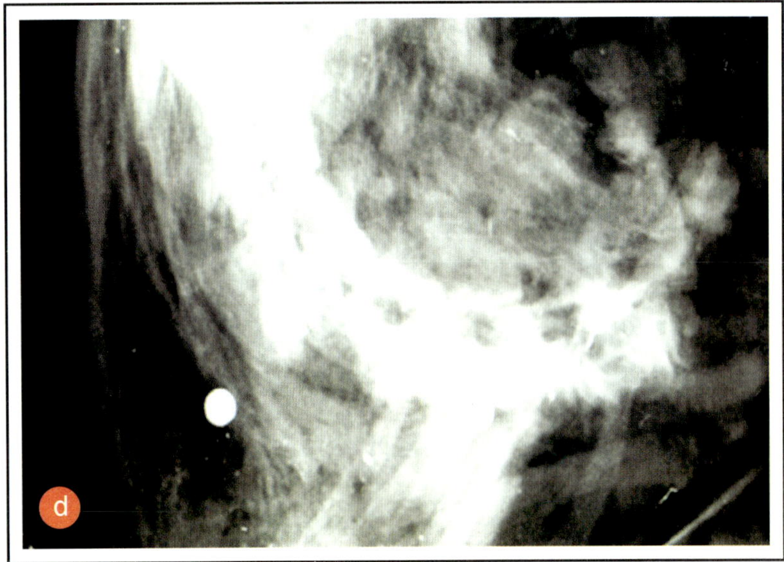

Figure 223: (a) Carcasses of chital (*A. axis*) and hog-deer (*A. porcinus*).(b) Head of hog-deer evidencing traumatized jaw. (c) Radiograph of (b) showing embedded pellets (white circular spot) in the lower jaw (causing fracture) and (d) in the cervical region.

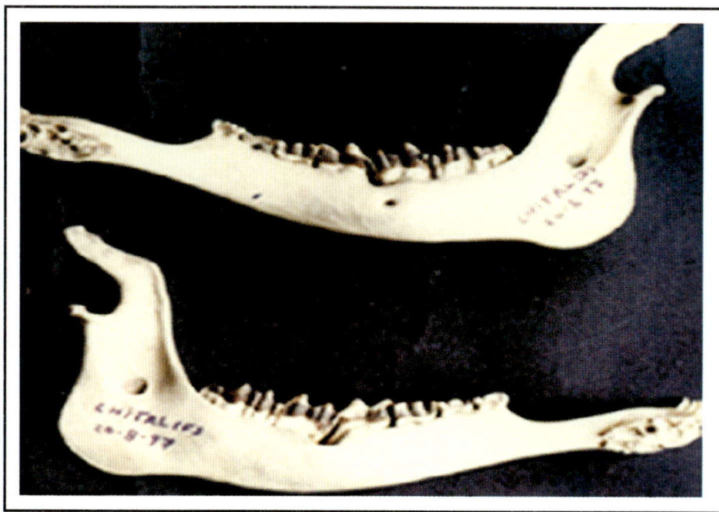

Figure 224: Lower jaw of chital (*A. axis*) showing recession of alveolar borders due to caries.

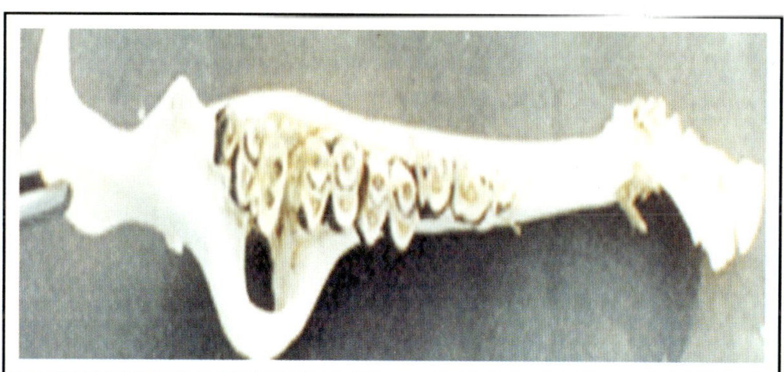

Figure 225: Photograph of lower jaw of chital (*A. axis*) showing necrotic lesion extending from teeth forming hole at the levels of 2nd premolar and 3rd premolar and third molar related to caries.

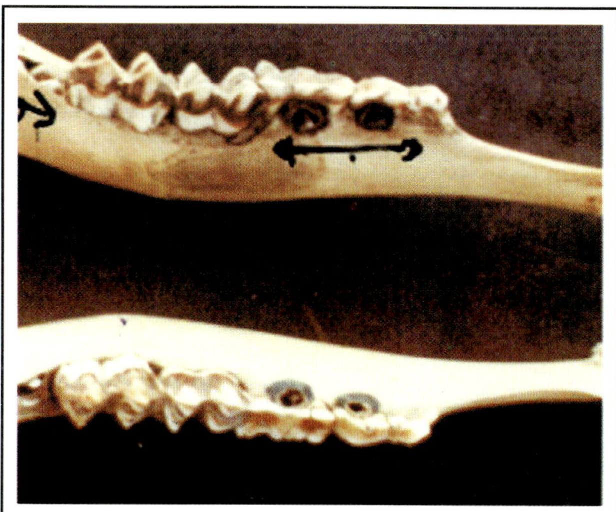

Figure 226: Photograph showing suppurative mandibular osteitis at the level of first and second molars in chital (*A. axis*).

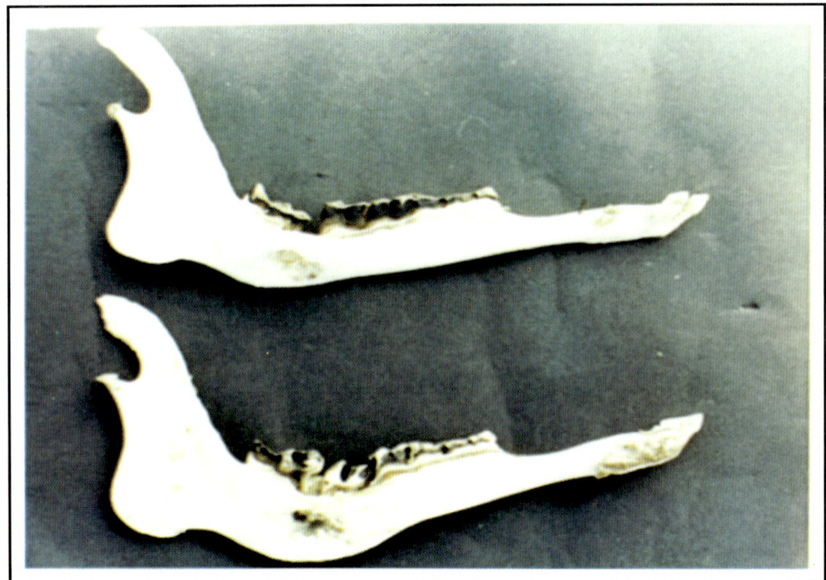

Figure 227: Photograph showing right mandible of chital (*A. axis*) affected with *Actinomyces* sp. infection. Note deformity of bone.

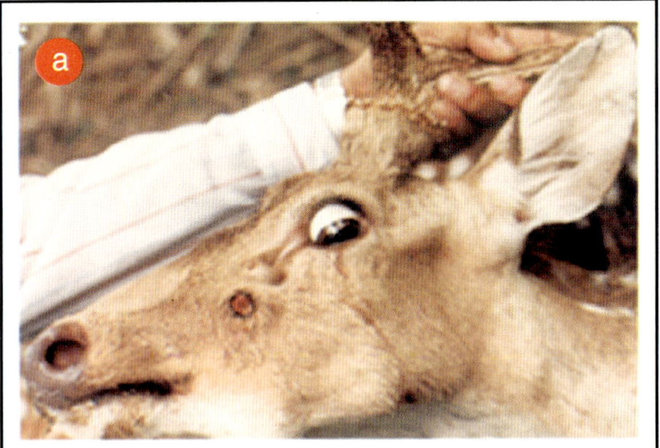

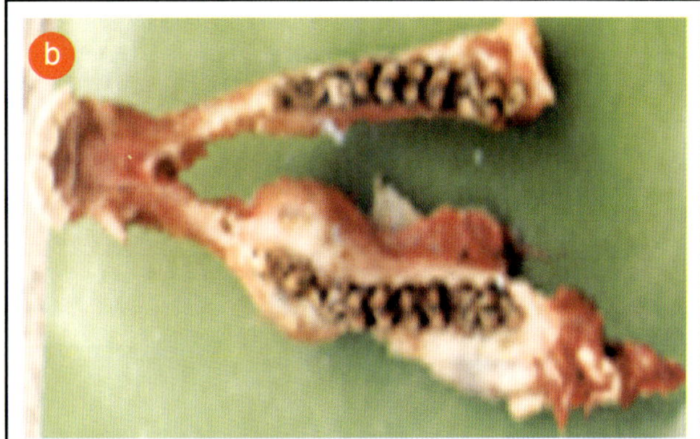

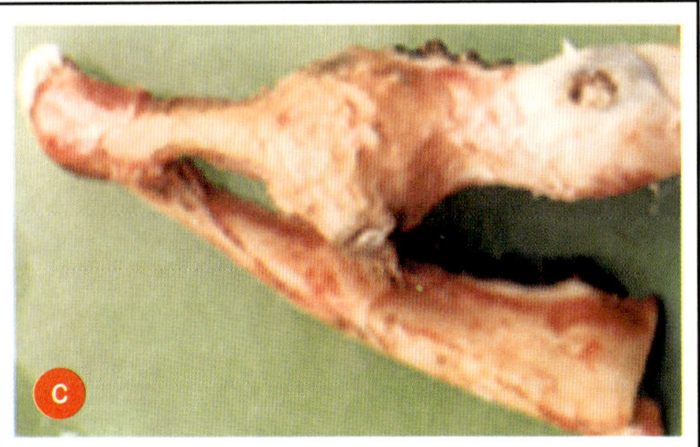

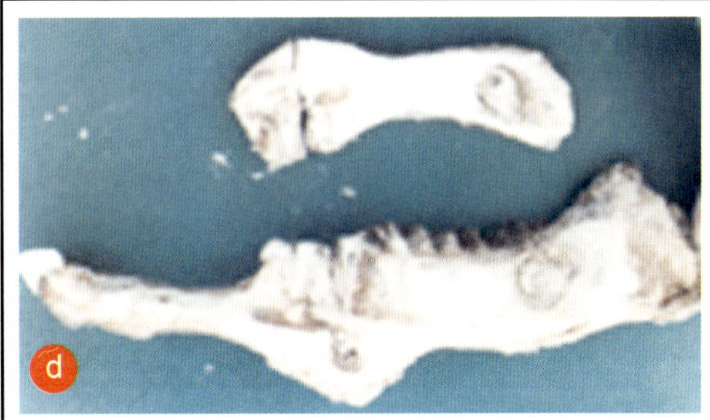

Figure 228: (a)Chital (*A.axis*) head showing mandibular osteitis due to *Staphylococcus aureus.* (b) Left ramus swollen of (a). (c) Latero-ventral aspects of (b) showing pus pockets. (d) The sliced affected ramus showing a large abscess below the level of premolars and another abscess below the last molar.

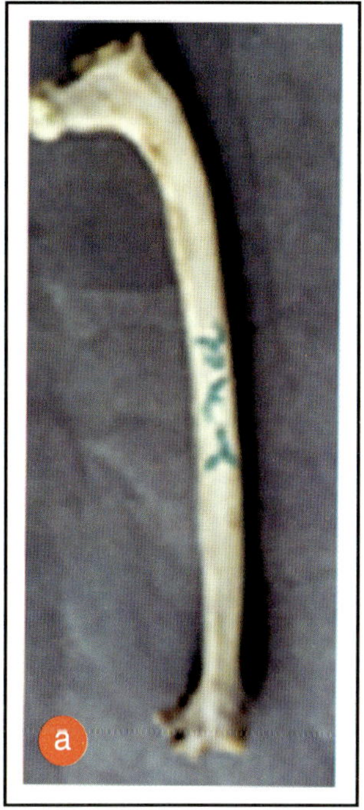

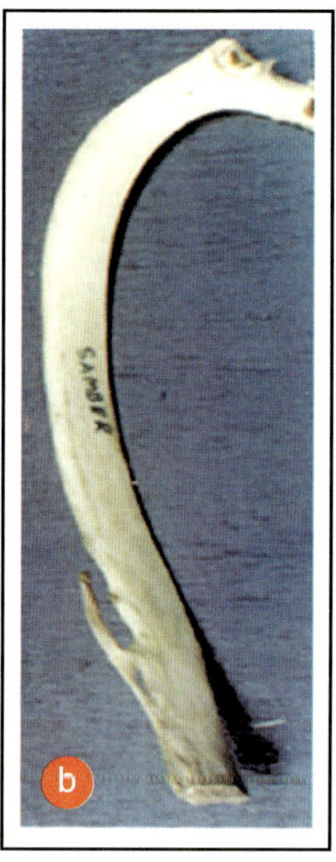

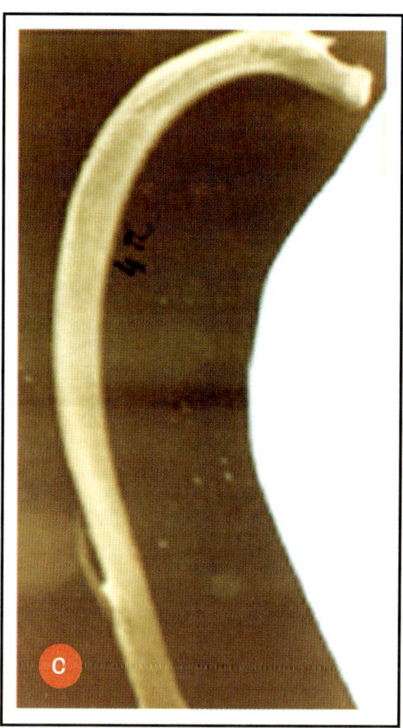

Figure 229: Ribs of sangai deer (*C. eldi eldi*). (a) Sternal end of 2nd left rib showing flaring. (b) Lower third of caudal border of 4th left rib revealed splinter and radiograph (c) showing its periostium origin.

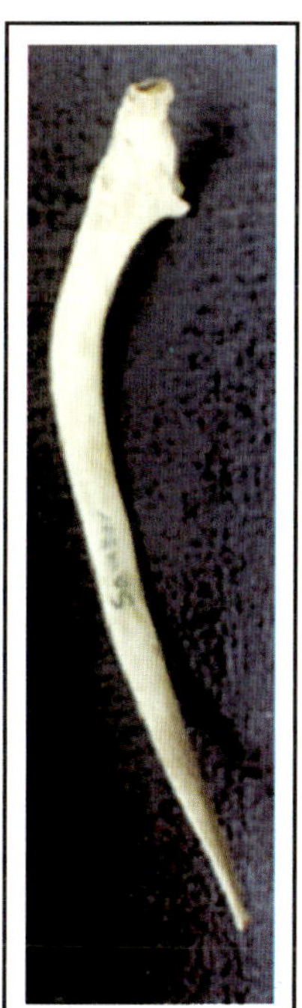

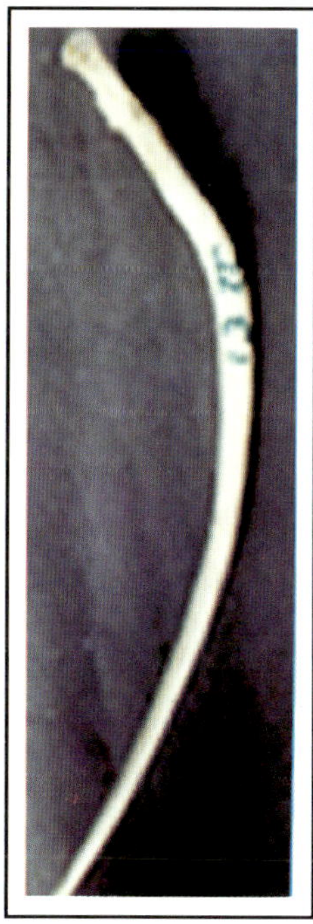

Figure 230: (a) Right 13 th rib of sambar (*C. unicolor*) smaller in size but proximally more flat than the left one(b).

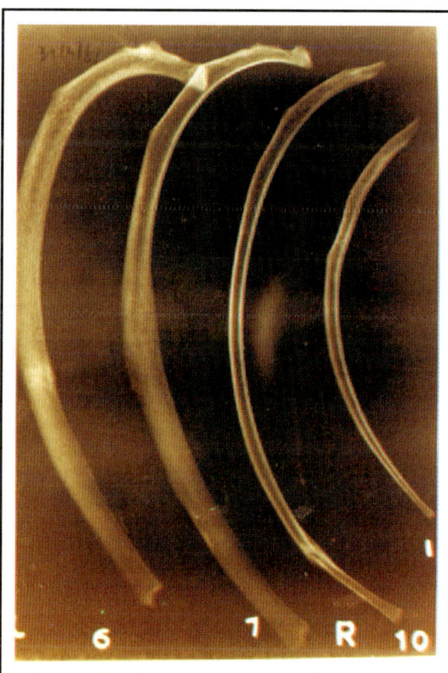

Figure 231: Radiograph of left 6th, and 7th and right 10 th ribs from sangai (*C. eldi eldi*) showed well organized healing of fracture.

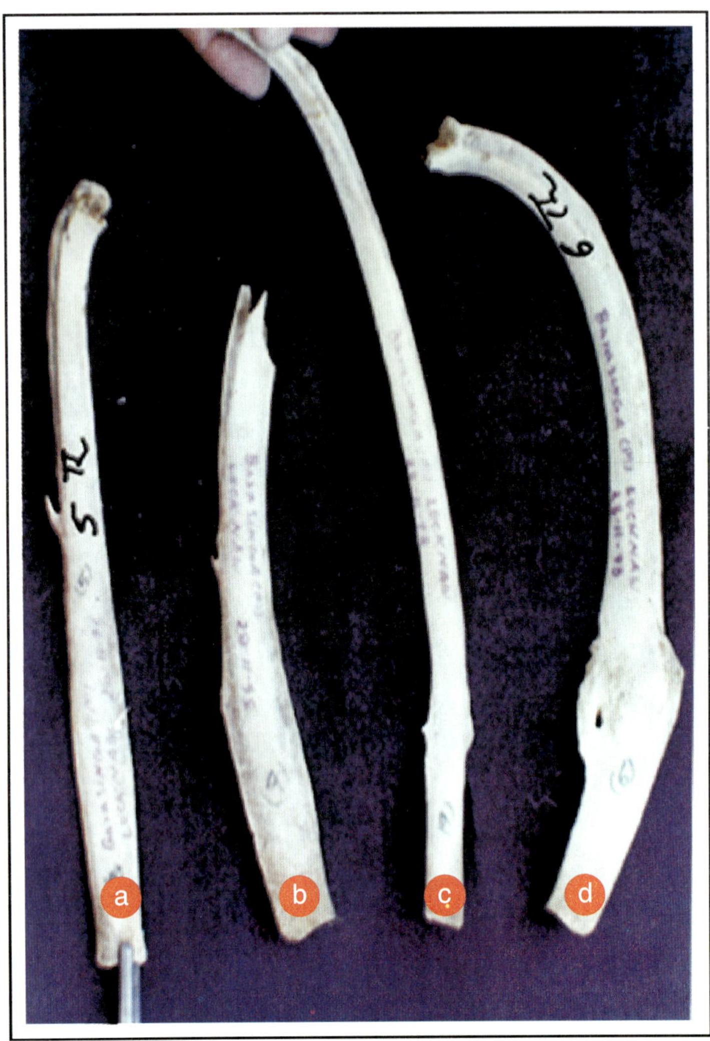

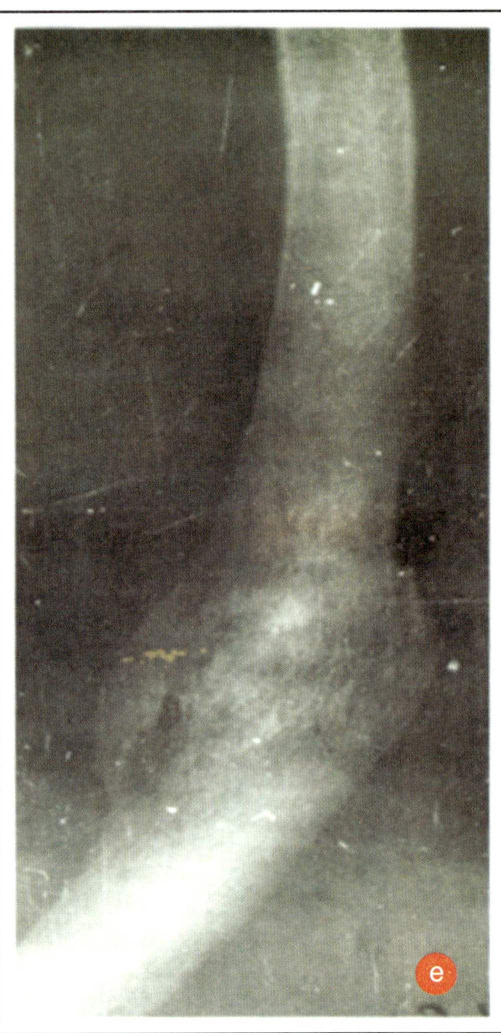

Figure 232 (a-c) Photograph showing a bony spur like structure at the middle of the caudal border of 1st, 5th and 7th ribs of male barasingha (*C. d. duvauceli*) died in the Zoological Garden, Lucknow(U.P.). (d) Sixth rib showing gross appearance of healed fracture and (e) radiograph of the same.

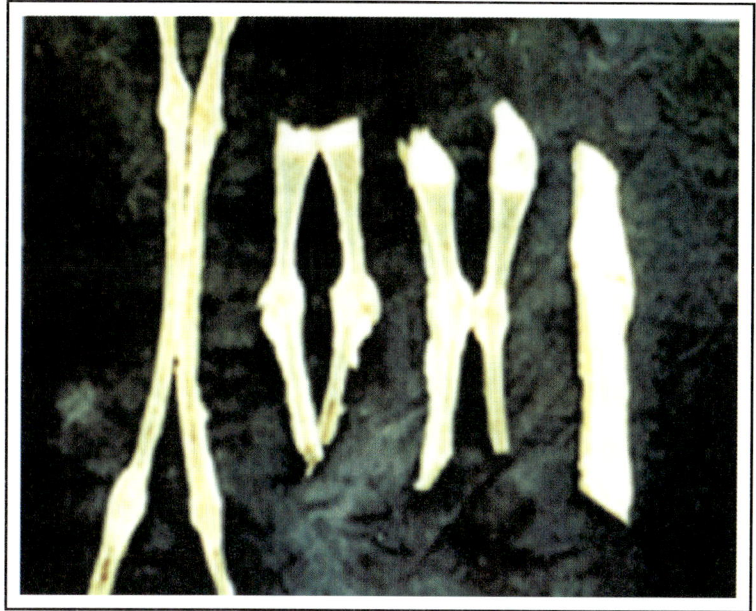

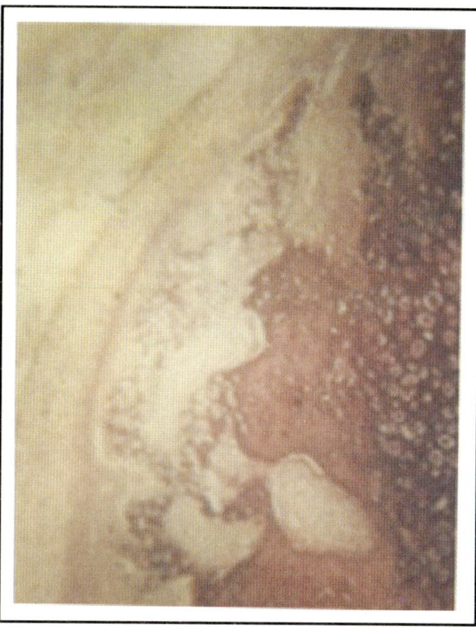

Figure 233: Photograph showing multiple cartilaginous exostoses (including osseous part) on the ribs from serow (*Capricornis sumatraensis*) died in Zoological Garden, Guwahati (Assam). (b) Histopathological changes were suggestive of osteochondroma. H&E, x 70

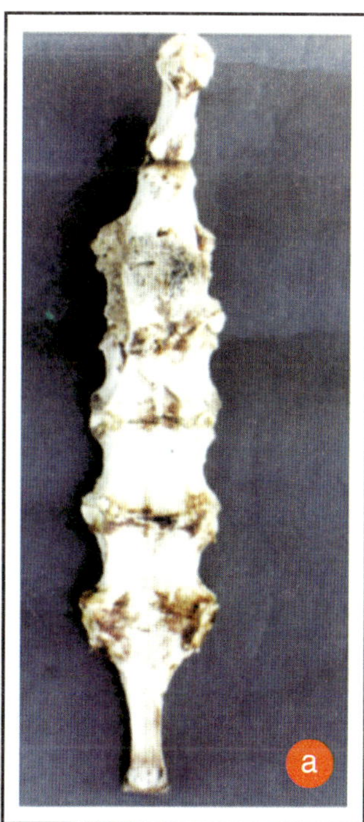

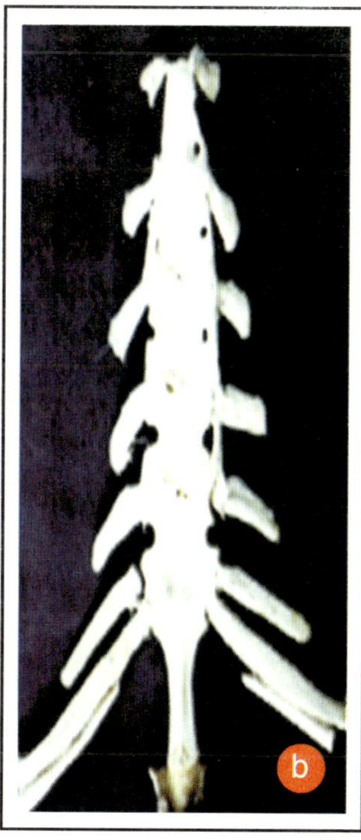

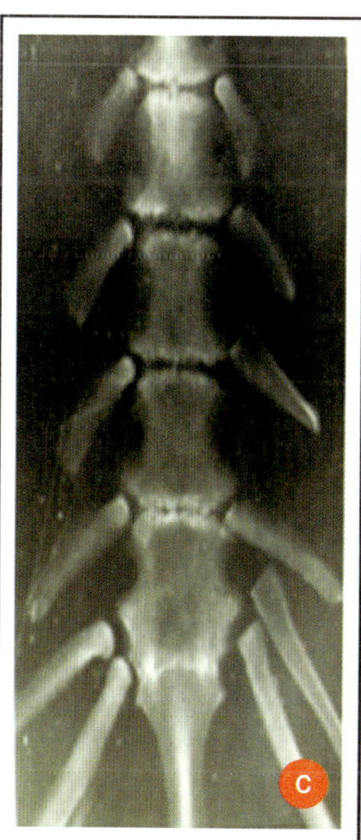

Figure 234: Photograph showing ossification of interstrenebrae cartilage discs in: (a) sangai (*C. eldi eldi*). (b) Barasingha (*C. d. duvauceli*). (c) Radiograph of sternum of (b) showing ossification of rib cartilages.

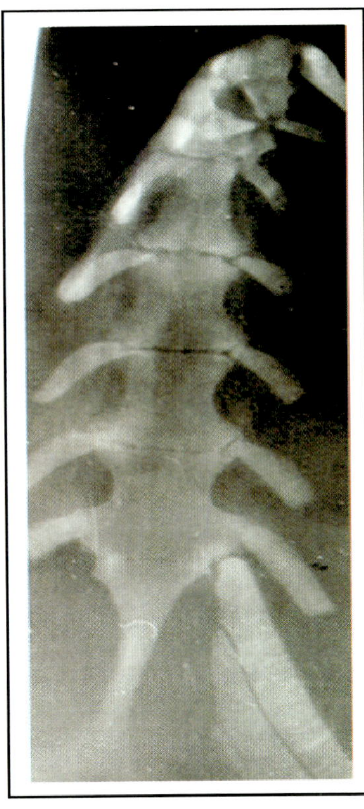

Figure 235: Radiograph showing deformed manubrium and ossification of interstrenebrae cartilage discs in blackbuck (*A.cervicapra*).

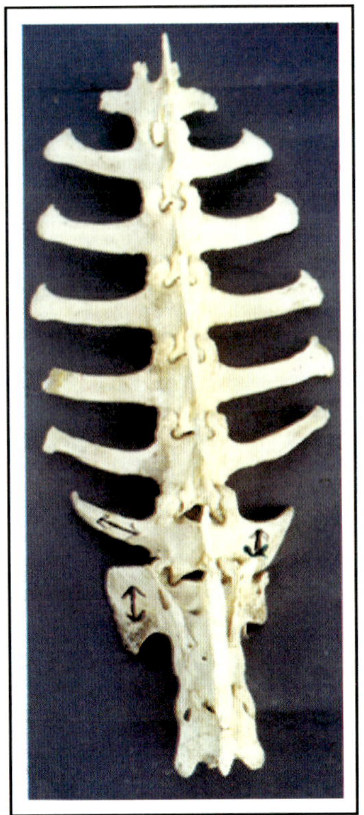

Figure 236: Photograph showing smaller but wider right transverse process of last lumbar vertebra than the left encountered in sambar (*C. unicolor*) died in captivity.

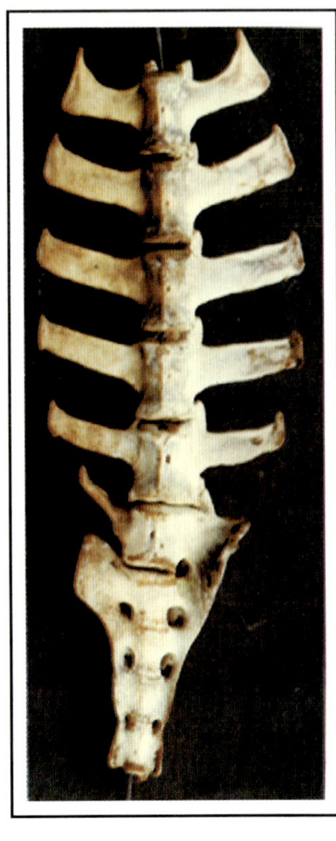

Figure 237: Photograph showing poorly developed right transverse process of the last lumbar vertebra of a wild blackbuck (*A. cervicapra*). Note left normal transverse process fused with the wing of sacrum.

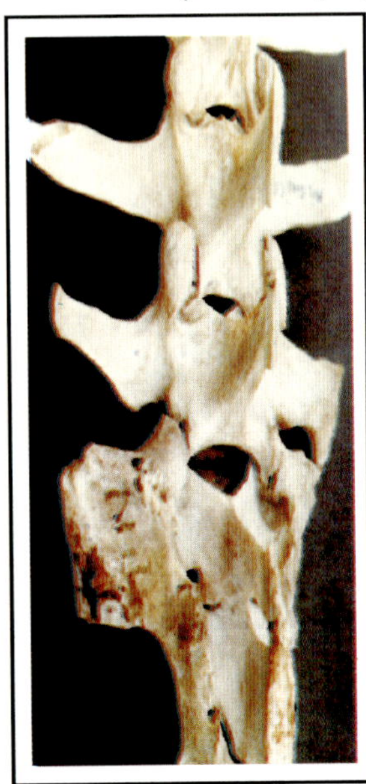

Figure 238: Photograph showing right transverse process of the last lumbar vertebra (*B.tagocamelus*) straight and double in width than its counter part encountered in wild nilgai.

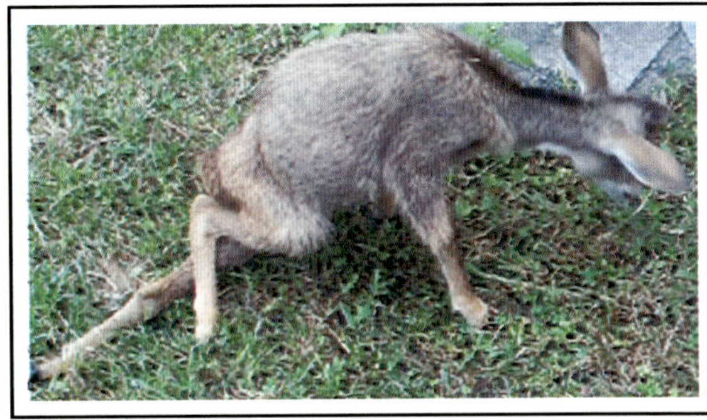

Figure 239: Photograph showing deformed hind limbs in a wild goral (*N. goral*) fawn.(Courtesy: Kishtwaria, R.S.).

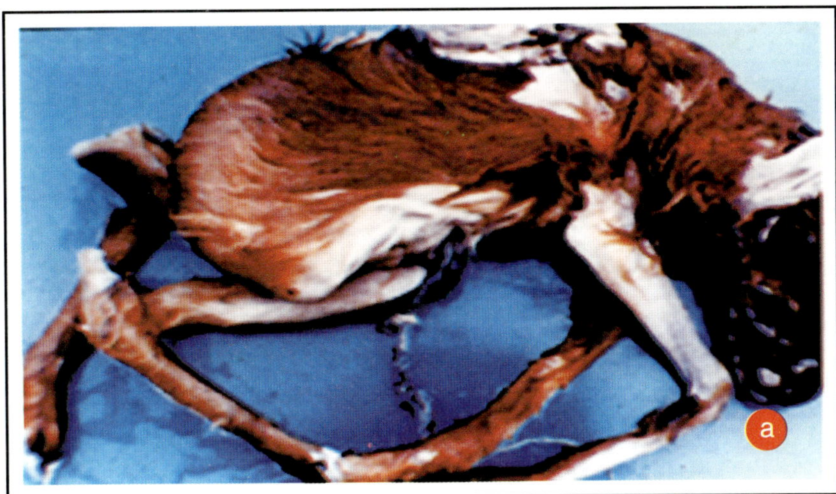

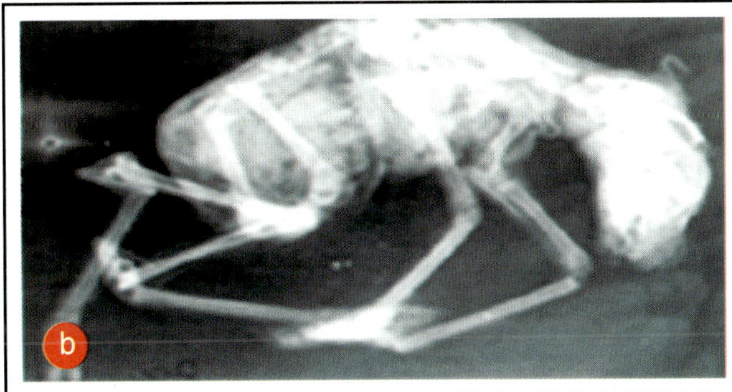

Figure 240: (a) Photograph of carcass of deformed stillborn sangai (*C. eldi eldi*) fawn. (b) Radiograph of (a) showing disproportionately longer legs and deformed vertebral column.

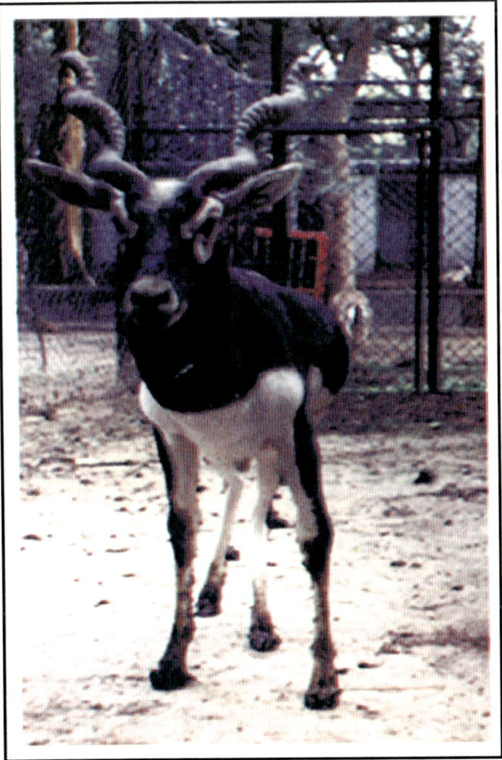

Figure 241: A rescued male blackbuck (*A. cervicapra*) in Zoological Park, Kanpur (U.P.) had both its fore legs set quite apart, straight and thicker with prominent sternum front and ribs cage. This anomaly could be akin to bilateral carpus varsus.

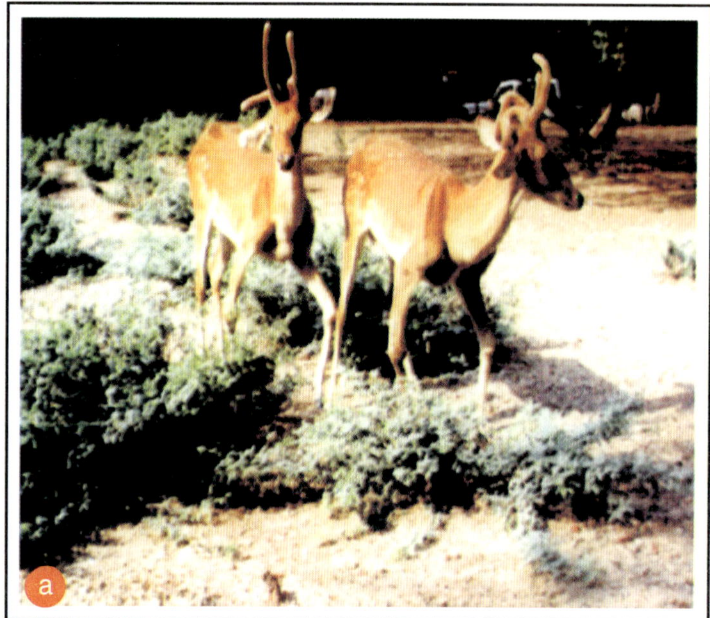

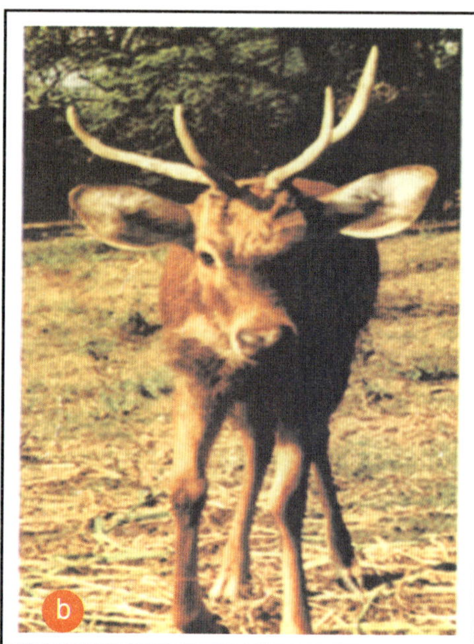

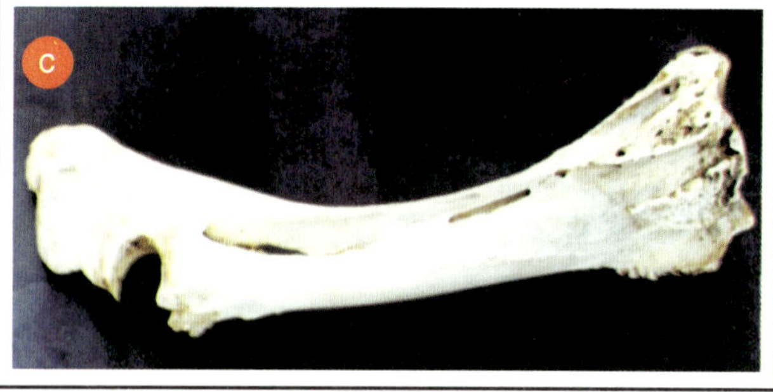

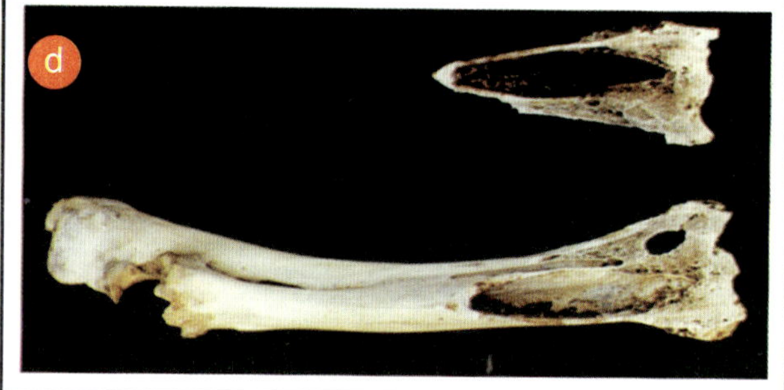

Figure 242: Photograph showing deformed forelegs in 3 adult male sangai deer (*C. eldi eldi*), which died later in National Zoological Park, New Delhi(a, b). Long bones from one of them showed exostoses of lower extremity of radius and ulna (c, d).

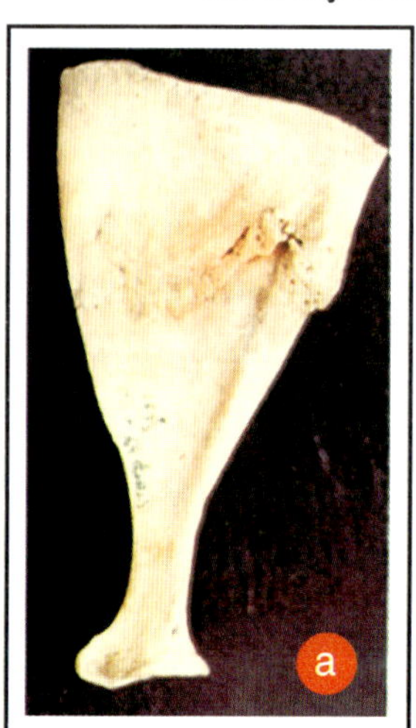

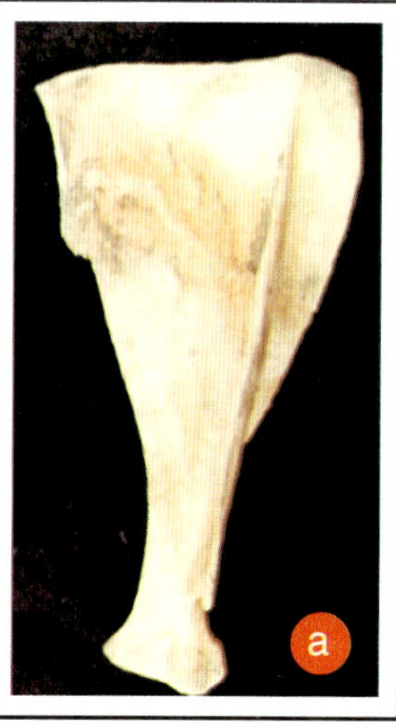

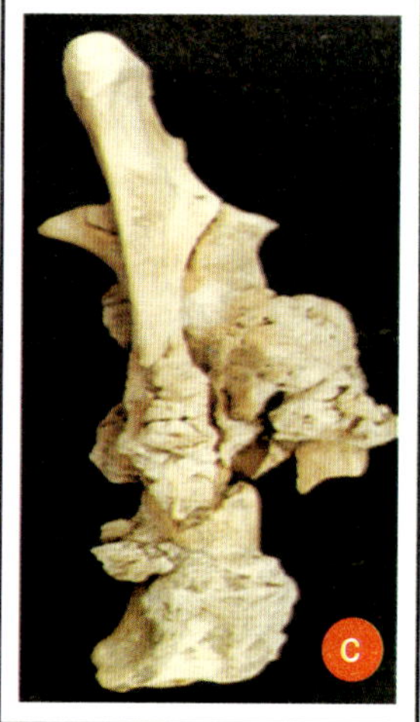

Figure 243: Photographs (a, b) scapula (lateral and medial surface views) and (c) radius and ulna of chital (*A. axis*) showing irregular and uneven healing process of their multiple fractures.

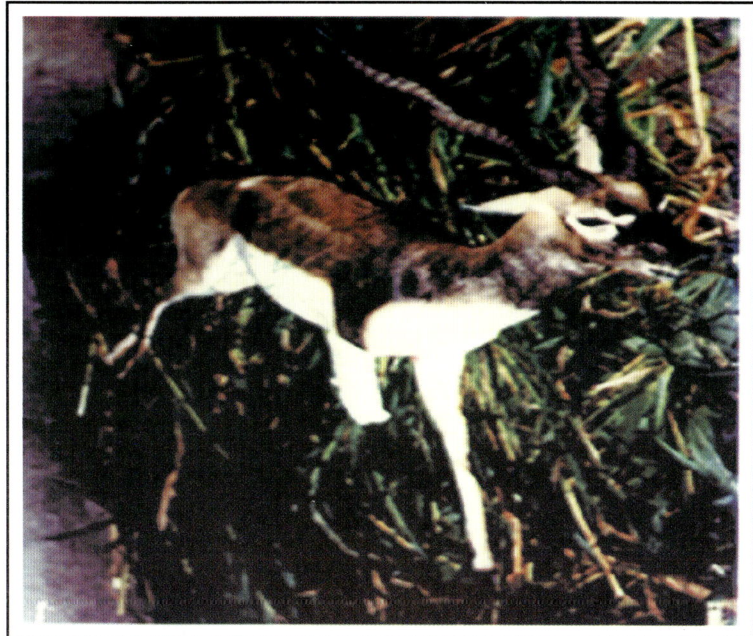

Figure 244: Infighting with companion male led to compound fracture of right fore limb in male blackbuck (*A. cervicapra*), which was amputated.

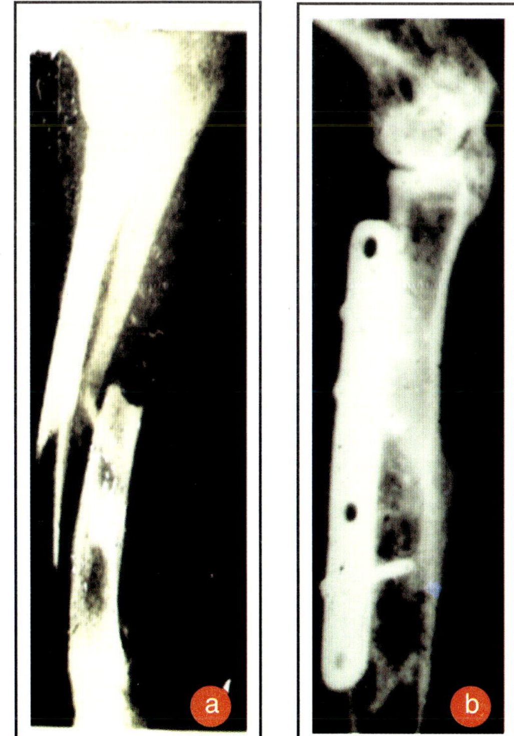

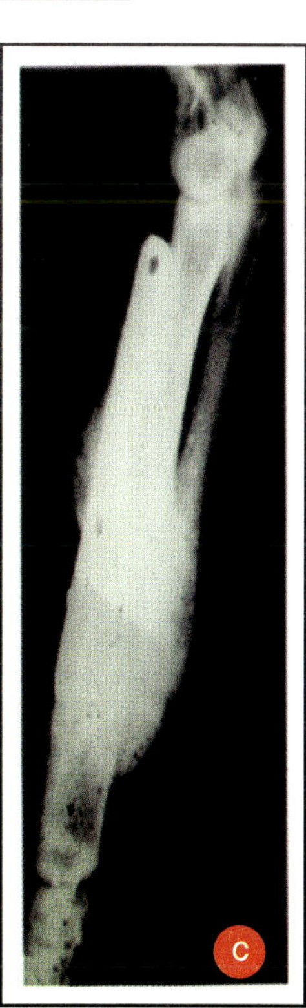

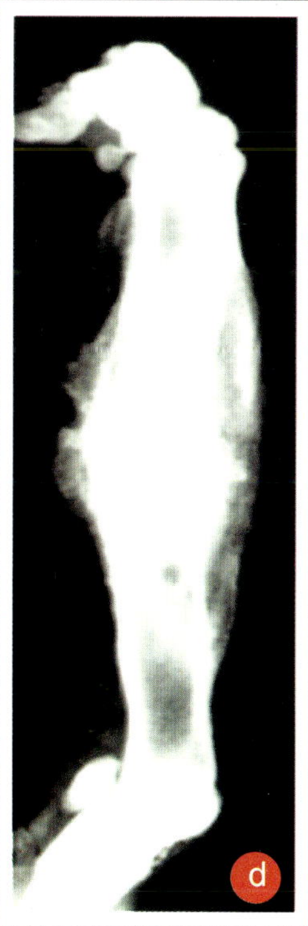

Figure 245: Radiographs showing:(a) Compound fracture in radius and ulna in semi-wild young female chital (*A. axis*). (b) Fixation of radius with bone plate and external immobilization with plaster cast. (c) Periosteal proliferation along the length of the plate and a well defined callus uniting fractured ends 90 days after surgical intervention. (d) After removal of the plate front view showing the remodeling of callus.

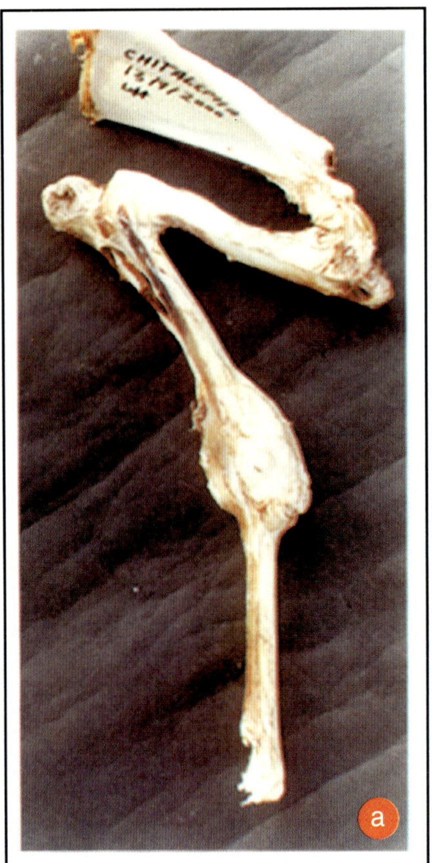

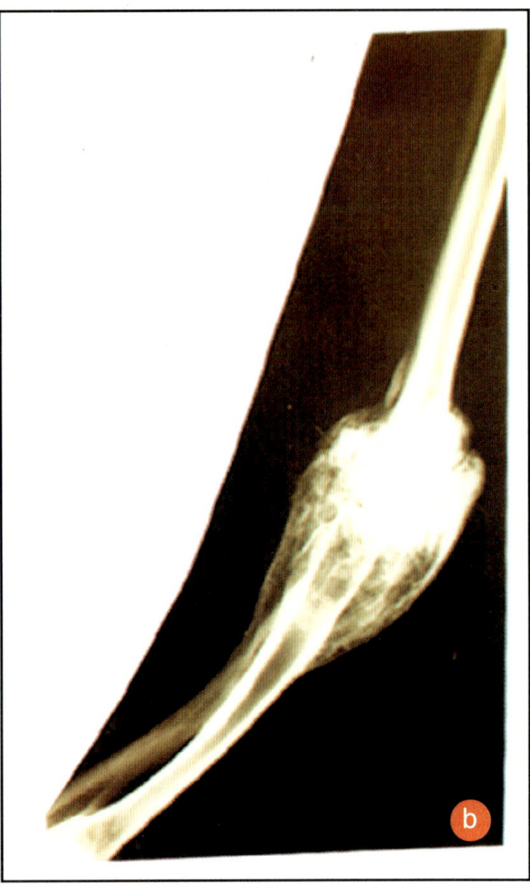

Figure 246: Photograph showing joints anomalies encountered in an adult male chital (*A. axis*) died in captivity: (a) Ankylosed carpal joint. (b) Fusion of carpal bones and suppurative process seen on slicing. Radiograph of (a) showing indistinct two rows of carpal bones and their union with the radius and ulna and head of metacarpal. The deformity led to fusion of all the three sets of articulations(radio-ulnarcarpal,intercarpal and carpo-metacarpal joints).

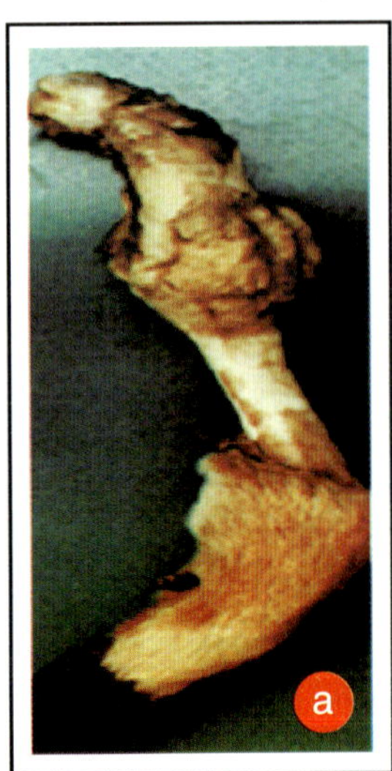

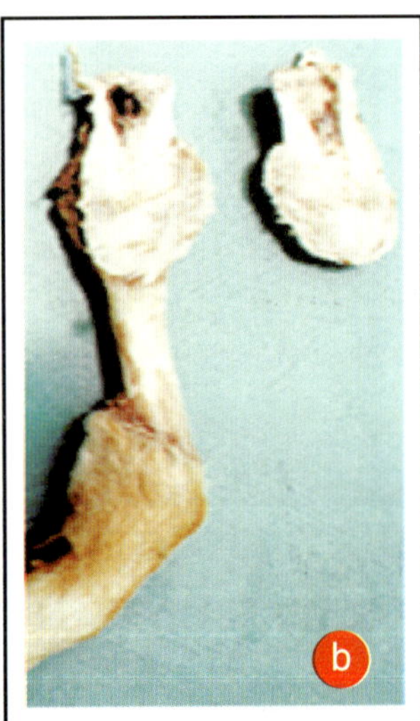

Figure 247: Photographs showing (a) swollen right radioulnar-metacarpal joint of chital (*A. axis*). (b) Longitudinal section of (a) showing complete fusion of their fracture ends and excessive bony deposition.

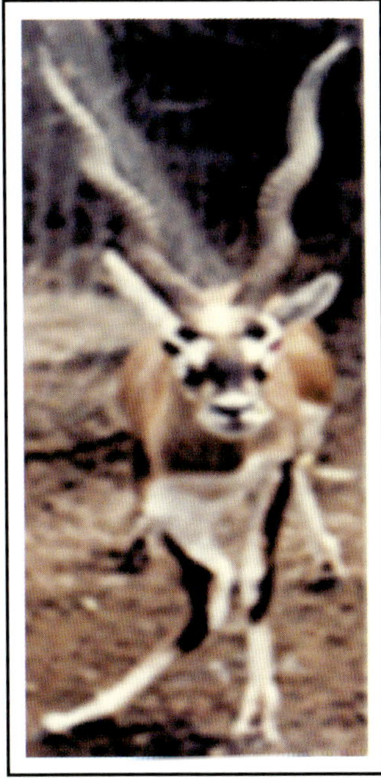

Figure 248: Photograph showing faulty healing of multiple fractures of fore right limb bones in a captive blackbuck (*A. cervicapra*),which led to disfiguration and ankylosis.

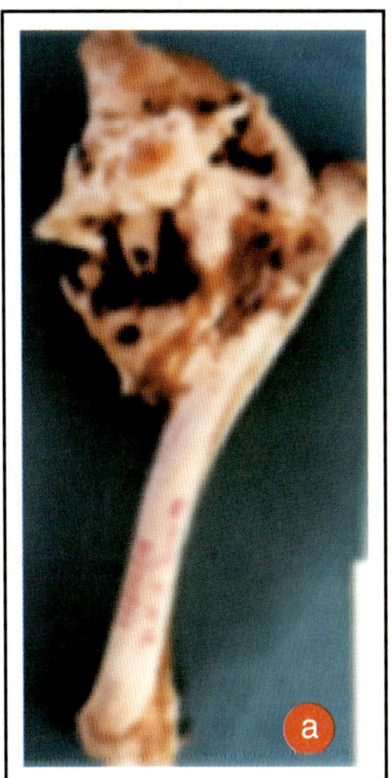

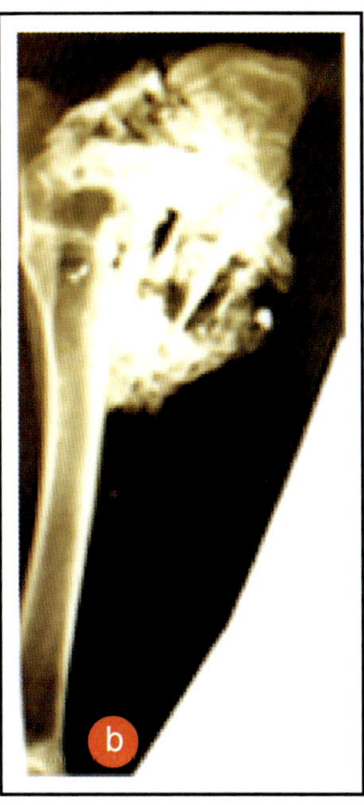

Figure 249: Faulty healed multiple fractures in radius and ulna, carpal joint and metacarpal bone encountered during necropsy of captive blackbuck (*A. cervicapra*).(b) Radiograph of (a).

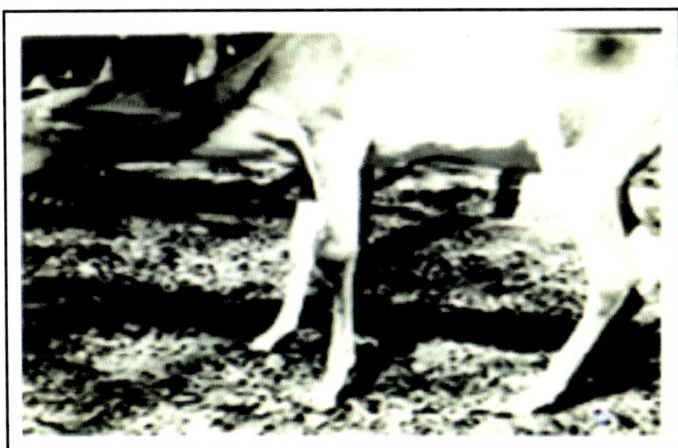

Figure 250: Photograph showing swollen left knee joint in captive blackbuck (*A. cervicapra*), which gets aggravated in every winter season.

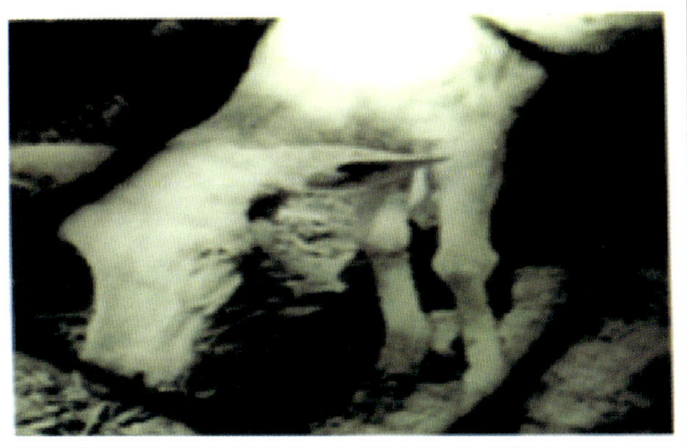

Figure 251: Both knee joints of fore limbs of a fallow deer (*Dama dama*, an exotic sp.) showing chronic arthritis.

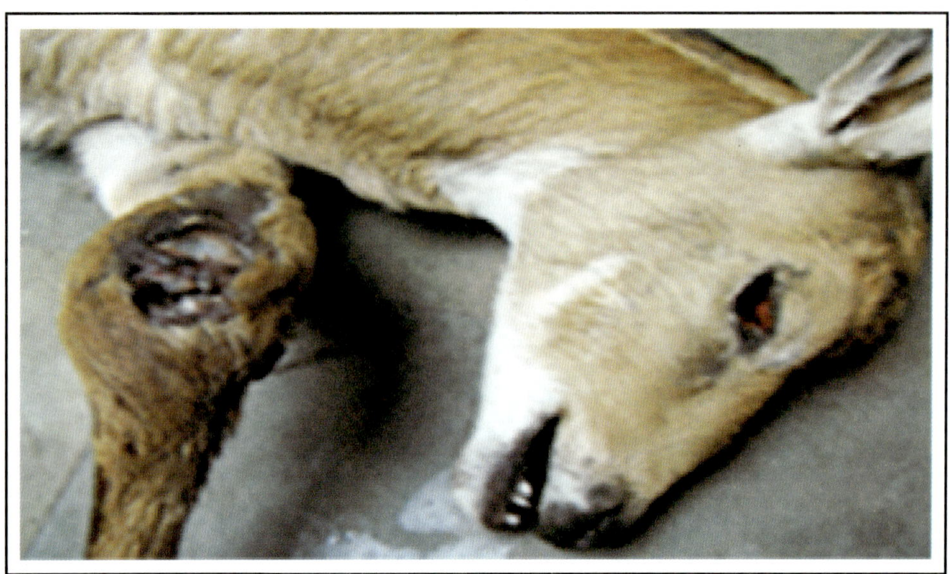

Figure 252: Affected left knee joint involving joint bones in a male nilgai (*B. tragocamelus*) calf.

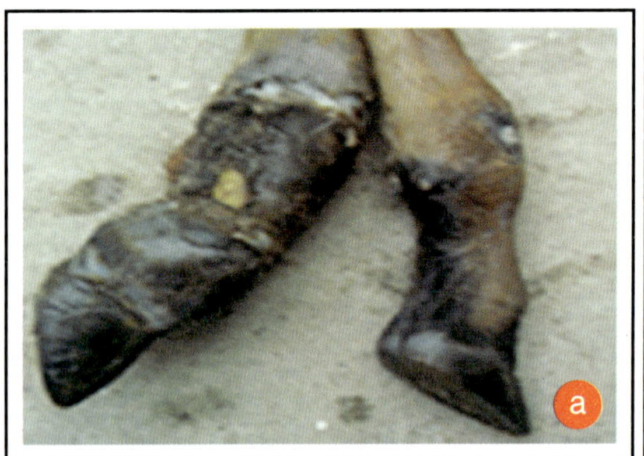

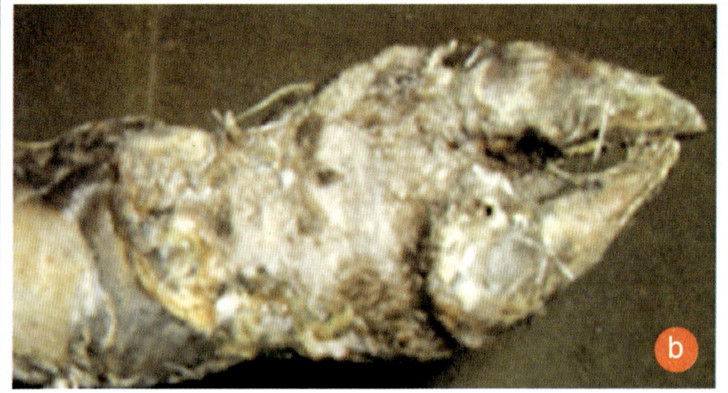

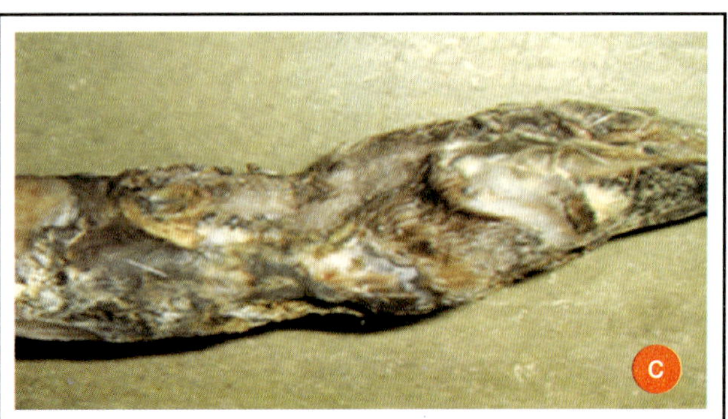

Figure 253: (a) Meto-carpo- phalangeal and interphalangeal joints showing suppurative lesions in a chinkara (*G. gazella*). (b) lesions of (a) showing from different surfaces of the joints involved.

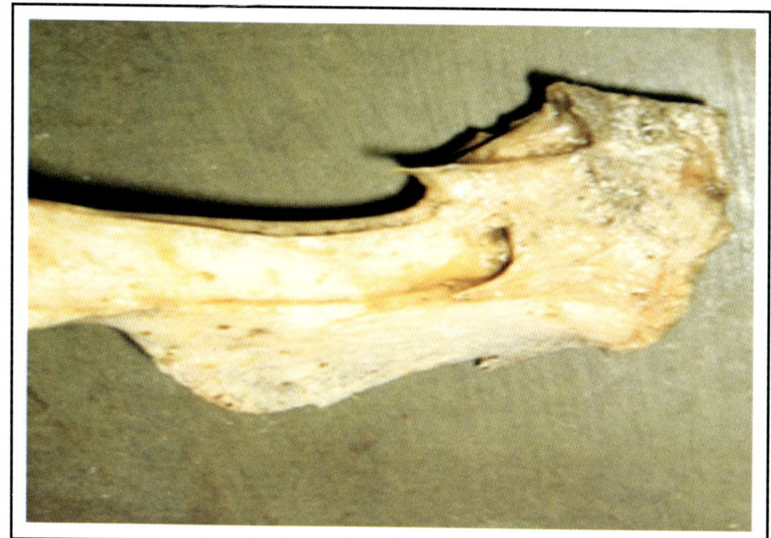

Figure 254: Photograph of plevis of blackbuck (*A. cervicapra*) died in captivity showing spiny exostosis at sacral end of left ilium.

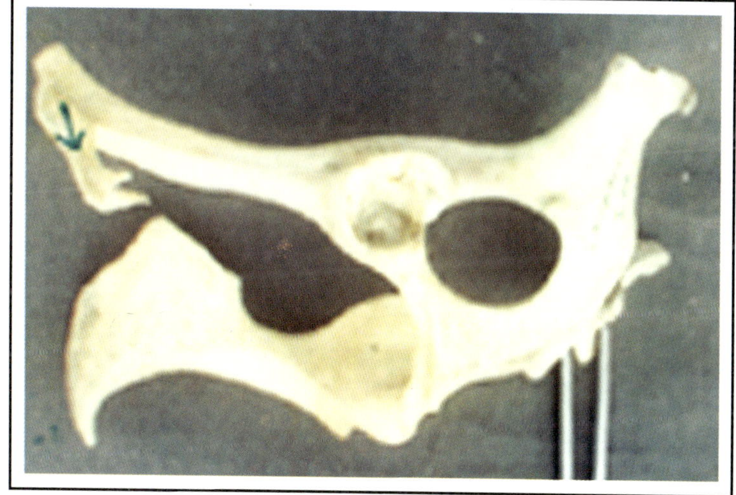

Figure 255: Pelvis of blackbuck (*A. cervicapra*) showing fork like spiny exostosis at the left tuber coxae.

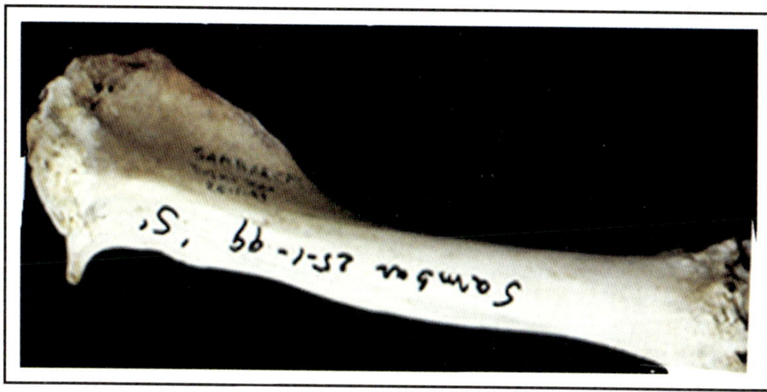

Figure 256: Photograph showing tibia of sambar (*C. unicolor*) having rod like growth of about 1 cm long developed from its head.

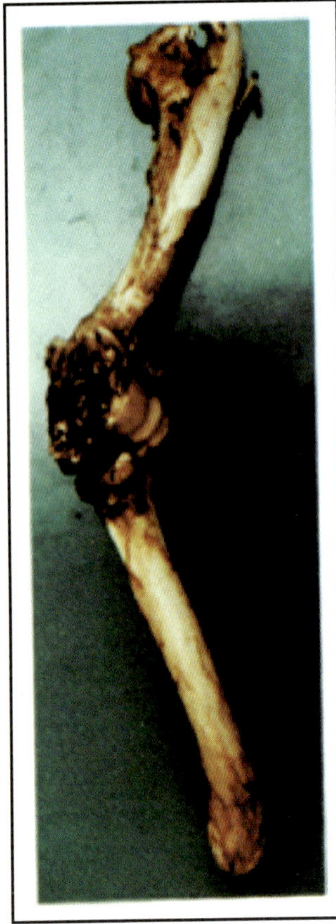

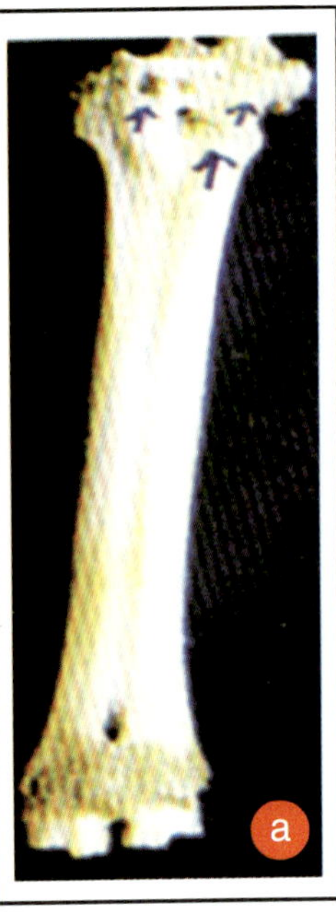

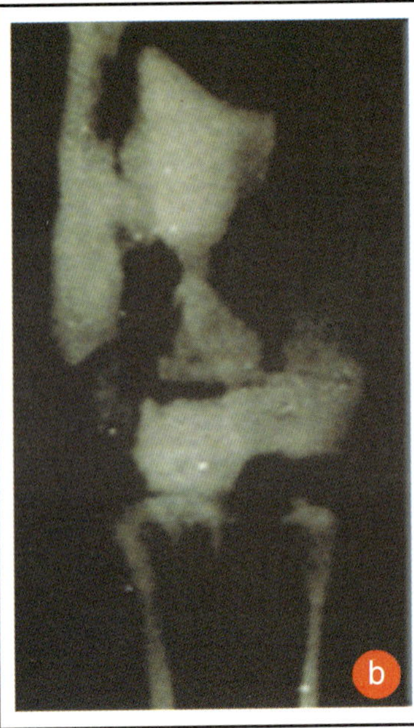

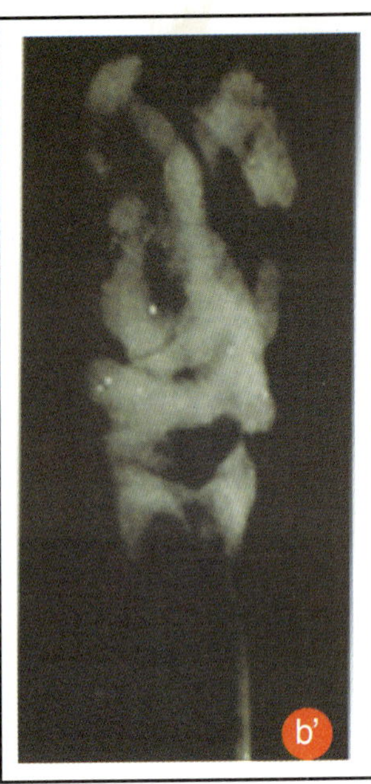

Figure 258: (a) Photograph showing tarsal bones (4+C/ 2+3) of sambar (*C. unicolor*) fused with each other and head at metatarsal bone.(b, b') Radiographs of (a)-front and dorso views.

Figure 257: Photographs showing proliferative growths around the tibio-metatarsal joint encountered in a chital (*A.axis*) died in captivity that had complaint of ankylosis.

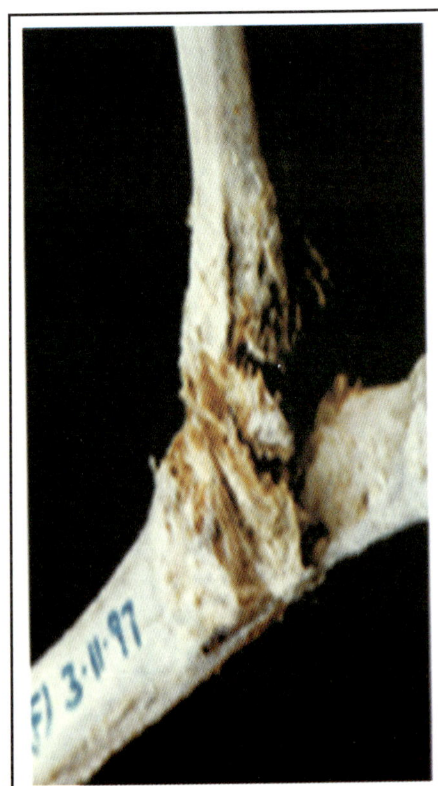

Figure 259: Cracks in the distal extremity of tibia, encountered during necropsy of 13-year old female hog-deer (*A. porcinus*). This could be due to unbearable stress of old age and body weight on her joint.

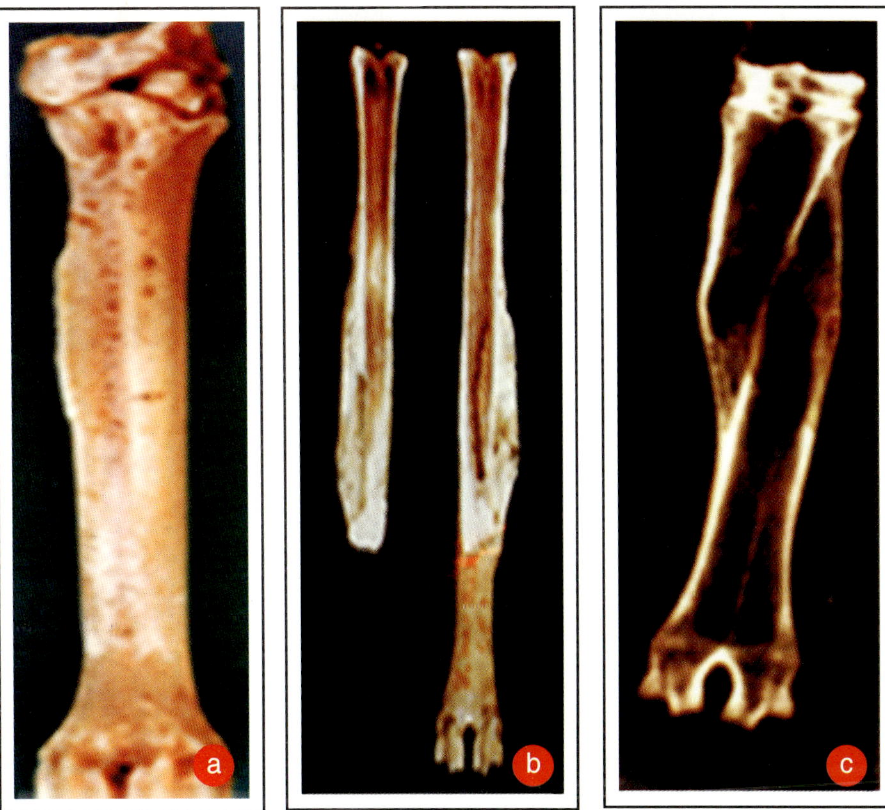

Figure 260: Photograph showing natural healing of fractures encountered during necropsy. (a) Metatarsal bone of chital (*A. axis*).(b) Metatarsal of goral (*N. goral*). (c) Radiograph of (b) showing proliferative new bone formation.

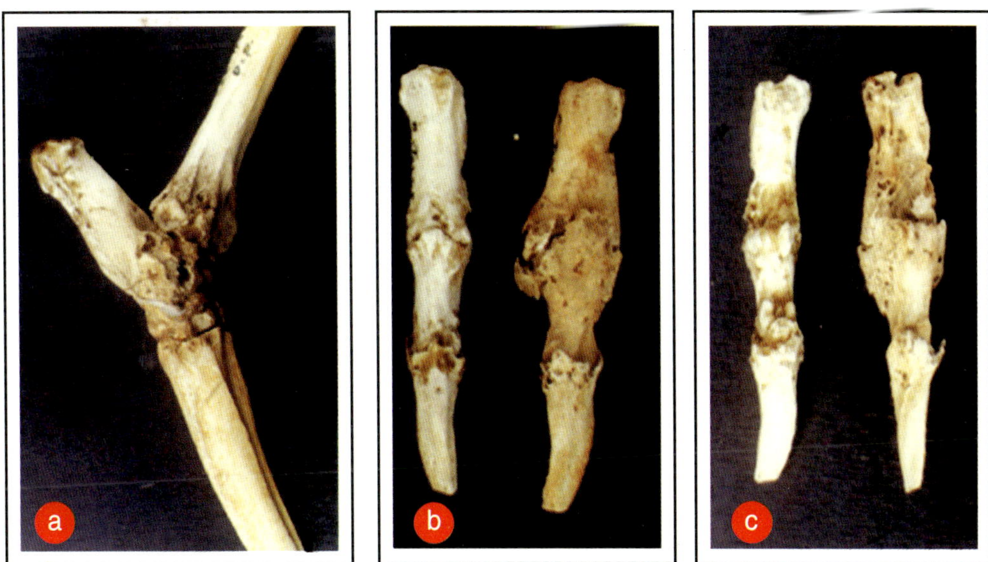

Figure 261: Photographs showing affection of stifle joint (a) and fusion of phalangeal joints (caused ankylosis) of both hindlimbs (b, b') encountered in 16 yr-old-male barasingha (*C.d. duvauceli*) that had complaint of arthritis.

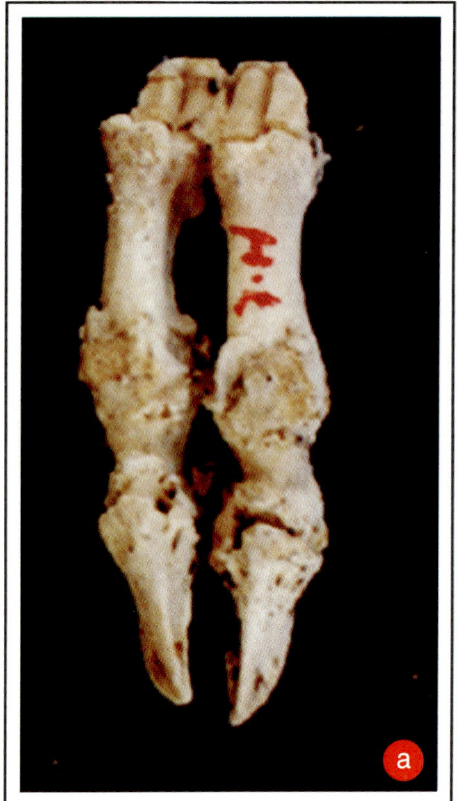

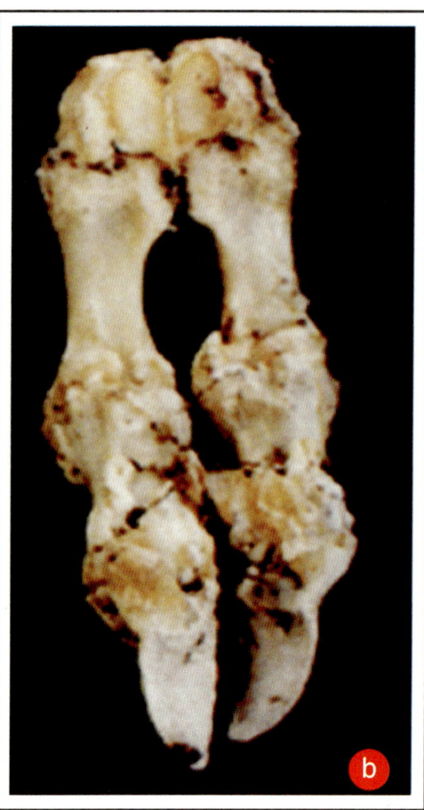

Figure 262: Photographs (a- Front view and b-Volar view) showing broken second phalanges of hind limbs of an adult blackbuck (*A. cervicapra*) in the process of natural healing resulted in uneven callus formation and ankylosis of interphalangeal joints.

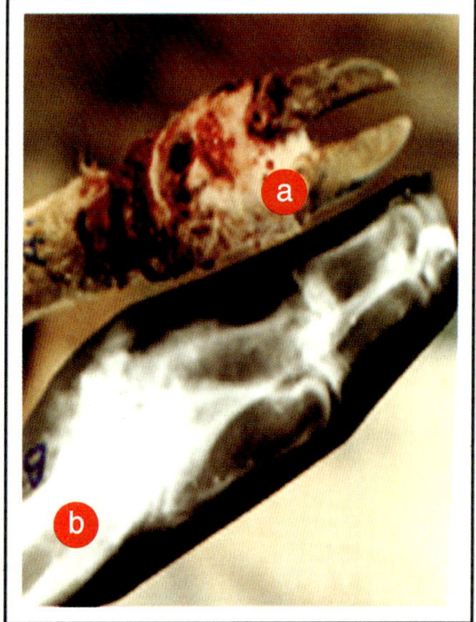

Figure 263:(a) Traumatized pastern joint of captive chital (*A. axis*) supervened by pathogen. (b) Radiograph showing ankylosed metatarsal-phalangeal joint due to new bone formation.

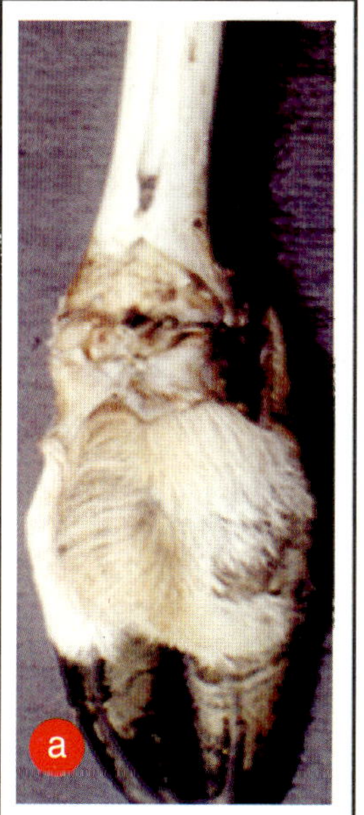

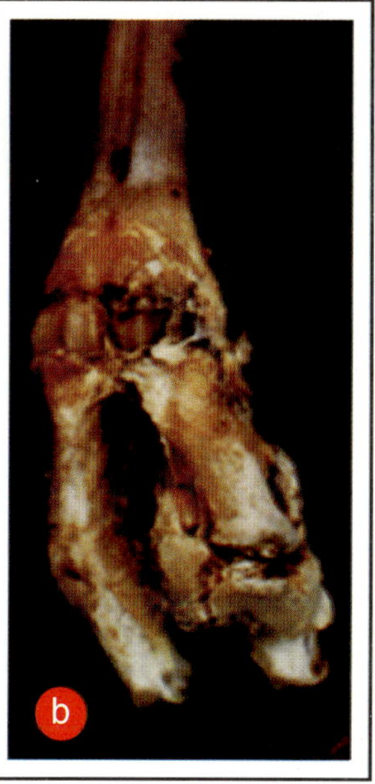

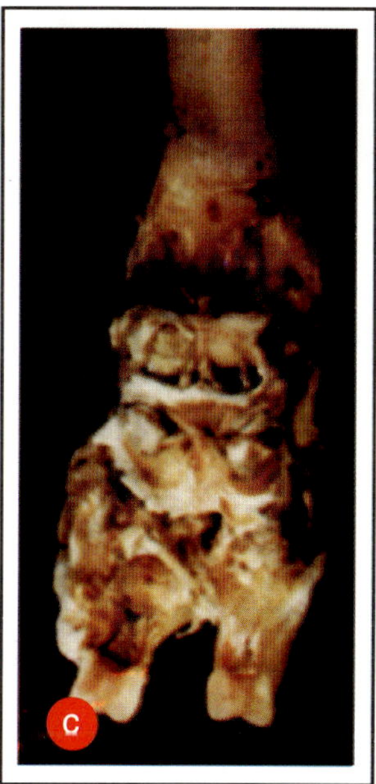

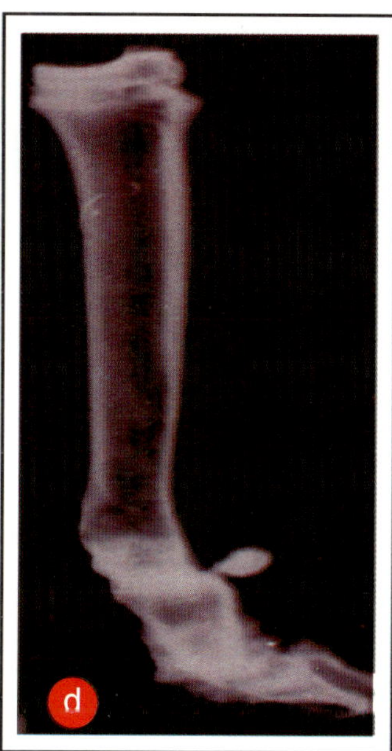

Figure 264: (a) Swollen left pastern in young adult chital (*A. axis*).(b) De-skinned (a) showing compound fracture. (c) Caudal aspect of (b) showing suppurative lesion. (d) Radiograph of (a) showing right interphalangeal joints fused.

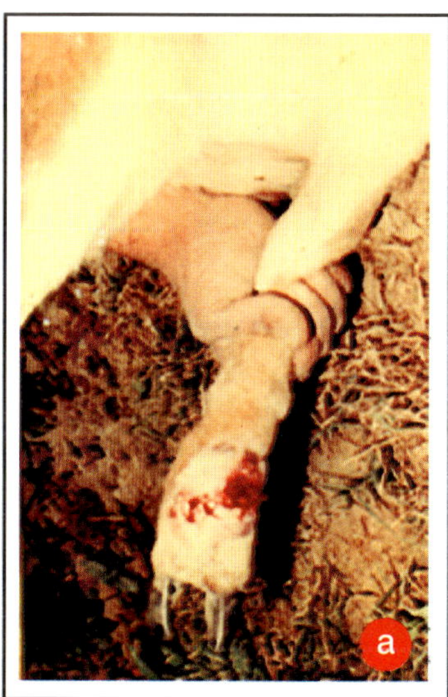

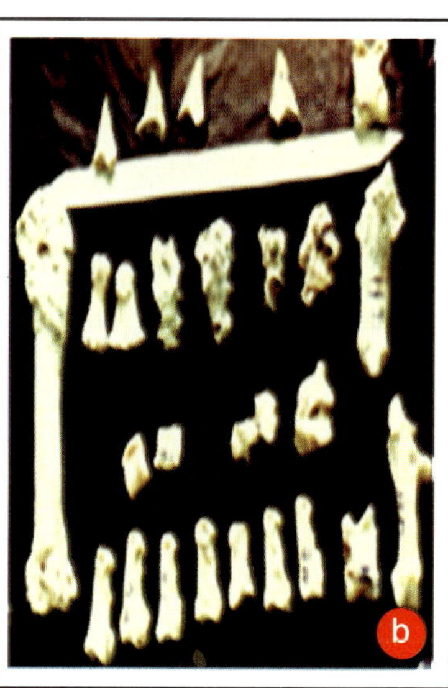

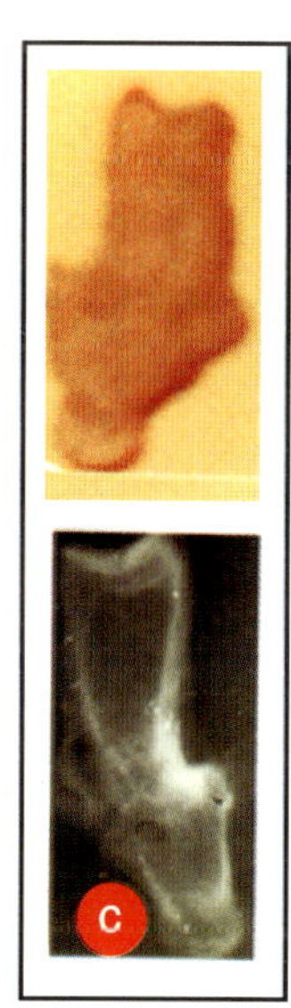

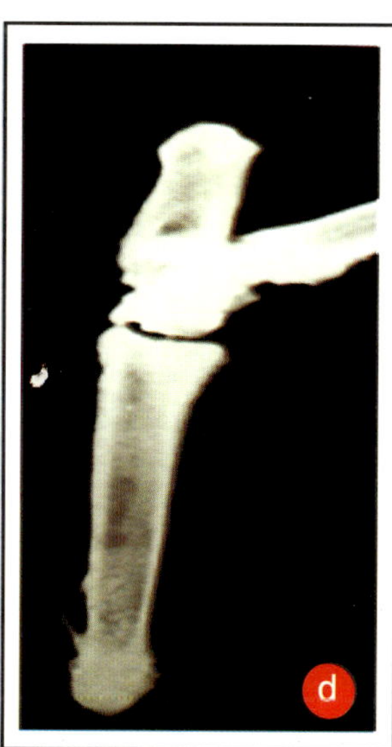

Figure265: (a) Pastern region of left leg of hog-deer (*A.porcinus*) lacerated due to tree stub and was further damaged by crows pecking.The crippled animal died after prolong illness.(b) Necropsy showed exostoses of phalanges, metatarsal and tarsals (not shown in sequence). (c) Distal end of one of the 1st phalanx fused with the proximal end of 2nd phalanx. (d)Radiograph also showing formation of a thin bow type growth extending from periosteum at distal fourth of metatarsal.

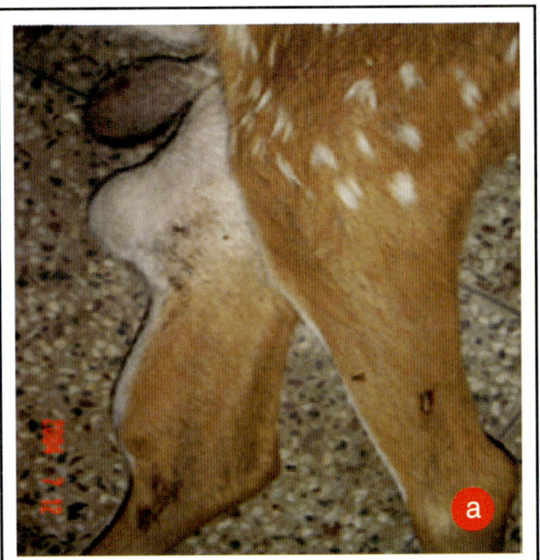

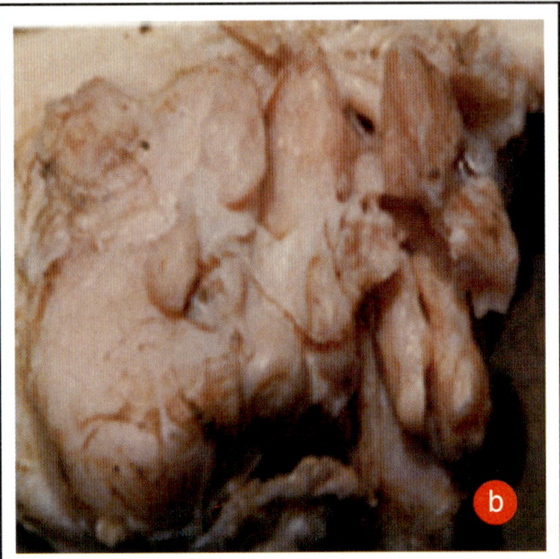

Figure 266: Cases of bone tuberculosis encountered in chitals (*A.axis*) died of generalized form of disease in captivity. Case (a) Right tibia showing tuberculous abscess. Case (b) Tuberculous lesion found involving stifle joint.

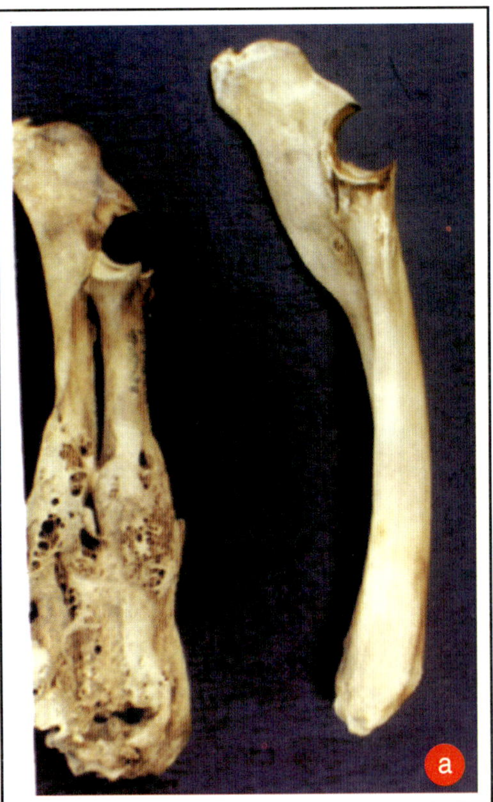

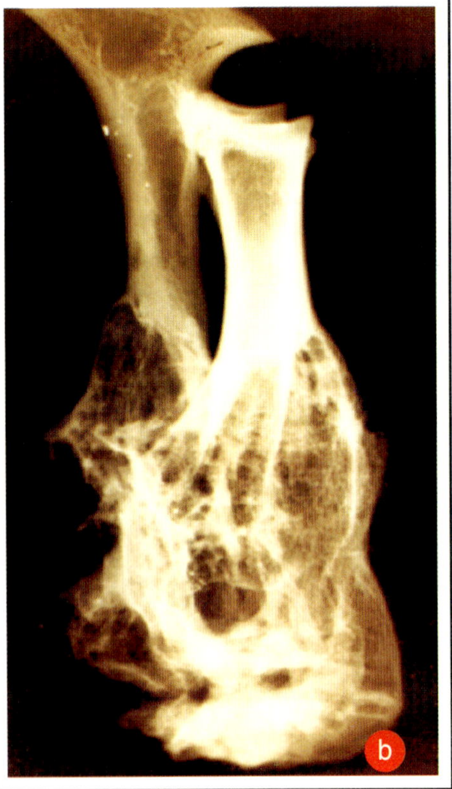

Figure 267: (a) Left radius and ulna of chital (*A. axis*) fused together in an irregular mass of tissue likely to be tumerous growth. The right ulna was enlarged in its proximal third. (b) Radiograph evidencing spongy mass suggestive of tumour.

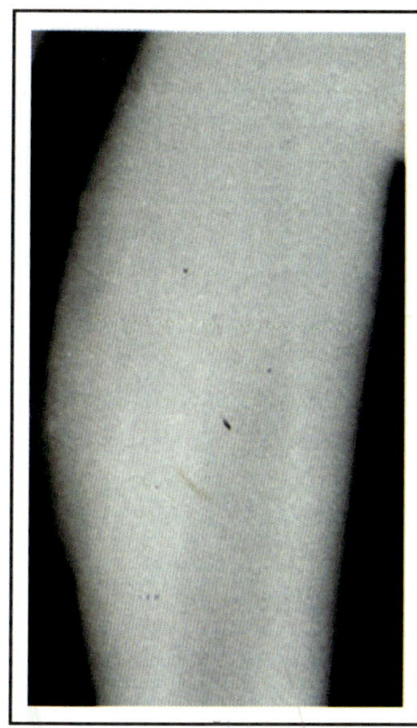

Figure 268: Radius bone of wild blackbuck (*A. corvicapra*) showing excessive thickening of periosteum. It appears to be a case of bone neoplasma.

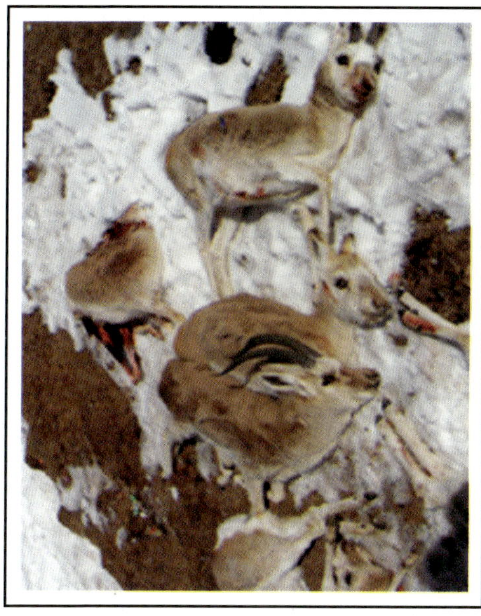

Figure 269: A picture shows the bodies of Tibetan gazelles that died during the snow disaster in Ganzi Tibetan Autonomous Prefecture in Southwestern China's Sichuan Province-norsang. [Photo: Tianfu Morning Post March 15, 2008]. Through: Wildlife Trust of India ERN Members dated April 4, 2008.

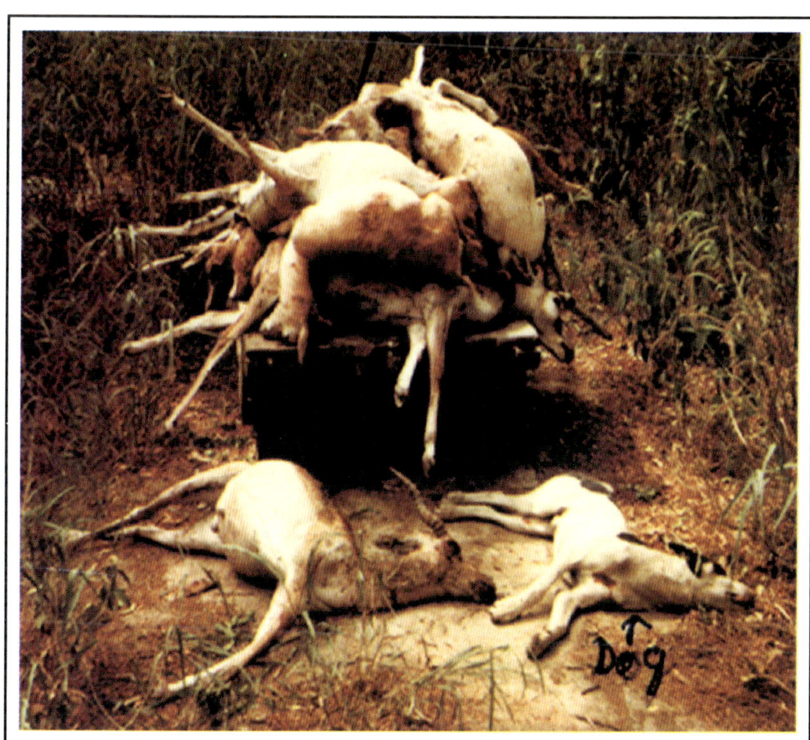

Figure 270: Blackbacks (*A. cervicapra*) victims of stray dogs in National Zoological Park, New Delhi.

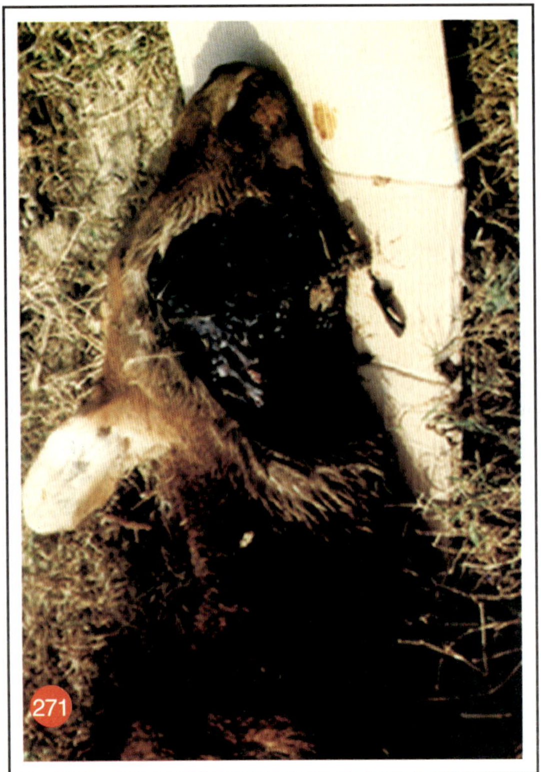

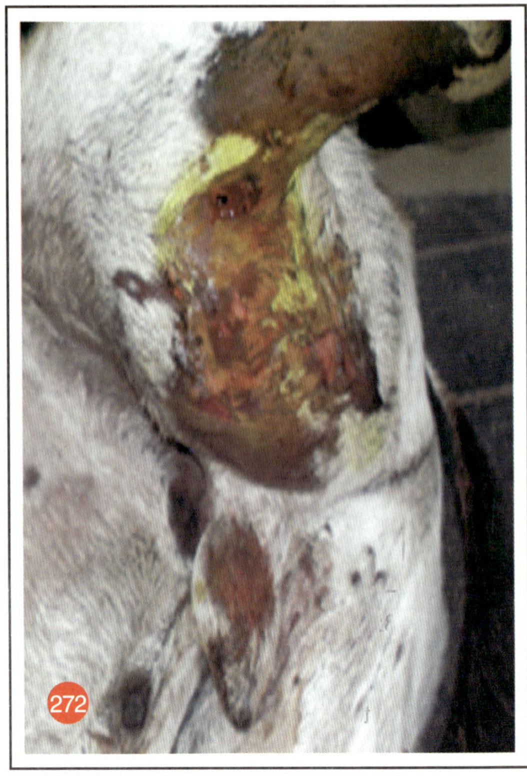

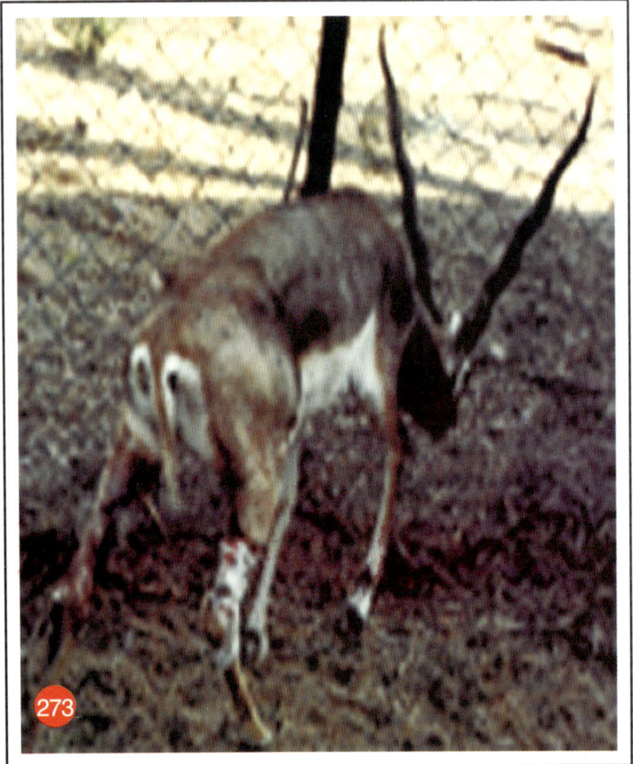

Figure 271-273: Biting wound caused by stray dog: (271) At the neck of an adult female hog-deer (*A. porcinus*) & (272) hind portion in chinkara (*G. gazella*). (273) The lone injured surviving blackbuck out of eight blackbucks (*A.cervicapra*) and chitals (*A.axis*) attacked by stray dogs during the night of 11 March,1995 in Z.G. Lucknow (U.P.).

References

Arora, B.M. (2003). Indian wildlife diseases and disorders. 1st Edition, Published by Association of Indian Zoo & Wildlife Veterinarians.

Chakraborty, T. *et al.* (1998). Spontaneous coenurosis in Himalayan tahr and markhor. *Indian J. Anim. Hlth.* 37:33-34.

Chauhan, P.P.S., Pande, B.P. and Singh, M. (1972). A new species of *Ashworthius* sp. from two wild ruminants with a note on associated lesions. *J. Helminth. 46*:140-155.

Nashiruddullah, N. *et al.* (2007). Recovery and pathology of *Dictyocaulus* species infection in lungs of a Kashmir red deer (*Cervus elephus hanglu*). Presentation in: *International Congress on Advances in Zoo & Wild Animals Health& Management, organized jointly by College of Vet Sc.&A.H.& AIZ&WV*, held from 26-27 April 2007 at SKUAS&T, Jammu (J&K).

Parihar, N.S. and Tripathi, J.C. (1981). Heptocarcinoma in a chital (*Axis axis*). *Indian J. Vet. Path.* 5:50-52.

Rao, A.T. and Acharjyo, L.N. (1992). Mortality in some Indian deer at Nandan Kanan *Indian J. Vet. Path.*16:120-21.

Rao, A.T and Acharjyo, L.N. (2003). Diseases of wild ruminants, published by A.T Rao 1021/44, Lingaraj Nager, Bhubaneswer - 751002

Singh, B. *et al.* (1981). Causes of mortality of some Zoo Animals. *Zbl. Vet. Med.* 28:596-602.

Sivashanker, M.K. and Chakraborty, A.(2005). Efficacy of ivermectin against stephanofilariasis in barking deer (*Muntiacus muntjak*). *Indian Wildlife Year Book.*4:65-68.

CARNIVORES

Introduction

The order-carnivore is represented by two suborders namely **Fissipedia**, which includes 8 families including 79 terrestrial species and Pinnipedia, which includes all the aquatic carnivore species. The table 2 presents common and endangered species and subspecies of suborder **Fissipedia** found in India. To present their clinico-pathological conditions, the chapter is divided in four sections as, large and medium cats, small cats (including civets), canids and hyena, and bears and panda due to their phylogenic relatedness.

Table 2: Common and endangered carnivore species and subspecies

SN	Family & Subfamily	Genus	Species/ subspecies
1	*Felidae*	*Panthera*	Tiger (*Panthera tigris tigris*); Lion (*Panthera leo persica*); Leopard (*Panthera pardus*)
		Uncia	Snow leopard (*Uncia uncia*)
		Acinonyx	Cheetah (*Acinonyx jubatus ventieus*)
		Neofelis	Clouded leopard (*Neofelis nebulosa*)
		(i) Felis (ii) *Profelis,* *(iii) Prionailurus* *(iv) Pardofelis* *(v) Otocolobus*	Jungle cat (*Felis chaus*); Desert cat *(Felis lybica ornata),* Flat headed cat (*F. planiceps* south- east asia *). (ii)* Golden cat (*Profelis temmincki*) (iii) Leopard cat *(Prionailurus bengalensis*) Fishing cat *(Prionailurus viverrina*) Rusty spotted cat *(Prionailurus rubinginosa*) (iv) Marbal cat *(Pardofelis marmarata*). (v) Pallas cat (*Otocolobus manul*)
		(i)*Caracal* (ii) *Lynx*	(i)Caracal (*Caracal caracal*) (ii) Lynx (*Lynx lynx*)
2	*Viverridae* *(a) Viverrinae*	(i) *Viverra* (ii) *Viverricula*	(i) Large Indian civet (*Viverra zibetha*),Malabar civet (*Viverra megashila*)(ii) Small Indian civet (*Viverricula indica*).Spotted linsang (*Prionodon pardicolor*)
	(b) Paradoxurinae	*(i)Paradoxurus* (ii) *Paguma*	Toddy cat / Small Indian civet(*Paradoxurus hermaphroditus*),Brown palm civet (*Paradoxurus jerdoni*) (ii) Himalayan palm civet/Masked palm civet(*Paguma larvata*)
		Arctictis	Binturong/Bear cat (*Arctictis binturong*)
3	*Canidae*	(i) *Canis;*(ii) *Vulpes* (iii) *Cuon*	(i) Wolf (*Canis lupus papillipus* and *Canis lupus chenco*), Jackal (*Canis aureus*), (ii) Red fox (*Vulpes vulpes montana*); Common fox (*Vulpes vulpes bengalensis*) (iii) Wild dog (*Cuon alpinus*)
4	*Hyaenidae*	*Hyaena*	Striped hyena (*Hyaena hyaena*)
5	*Ursidae*	*Melursus, Ursus, Selenarctos, Helarctos*	Sloth bear (*Melursus ursinus*); Brown bear (*Ursus arctos*); Himalayan bear (*Selenarctos thibetanus*); Malayan sun bear (*Helarctos malayanus*)
6	*Procyonidae*	*Ailurus*	Red panda (*Ailurus fulgens fulgens, A. fulgens satyani*)
7	*Mustelidae* *(a) Lutrinae*	*Lutra*	Common Otter (*Lutra lutra*) Smooth Indian Otter (*Lutra perspicillata*) *Clawless/Small claw otter (*L. capensis/cinerea*)
	b) *Mustelinae*	*Marten*	Stone marten (*Martes sibirica/M. foina*) Yellow throated martens (*M. flavigula*)
		Mustela	Himalayan weasel (*Mustela (weasels) sibirica*), Pale weasel (*Mustela altaica*), Yellow bellied weasal (*Mustela kathiah*) Ermine (*Mustela erminea*) Striped back weasel (*M. strigidorsa*)
8	Herpestidae	*Herpestes*	Common mongoose (*Herpestes edwardsi*)

(a) Large & medium cats: Of the 36 species of cats known in the world, 15 are found in India. Of these, tiger (*Panthera tigris tigris*), Asiatic lion (*P. leo persica*), snow leopard (*Uncia uncia*) and leopard (*P. pardus*) are the large ones and the clouded leopard (*Neofelis nebulosa*) medium (most taxonomists include it under small cats).The unique Indian species dwell in Indian natural habitats and maintained in captivity. Except the common leopard (*P. pardus*) all are critical endangered species. The presentation of their clinico-pathological conditions follows the same order as that of artiodactylid species.

Developmental anomalies : Cleft palate **(Figure 305)**, hernia **(Figure 306)**, bifid teeth (**Figure 307)**, absence of kidney **(Figure 366)**, improper sized fetuses in a litter **(Figure 394)**, exencephaly/ meningoencephalocele **(Figure 399)**, stump tail **(Figure 435)**, rickets **(Figure 436)** are some of the congenital anomalies encountered in large cats illustrated. The amber body hair colour with black strips is the normal colour tiger. Birth of white tigers **(Figure 408)** and lions **(Figure 410)** and black leopards **(Figure 409)** is well known genetic aberrant of normal colour. However, finding of wild tigers with different shapes and sizes of strips **(Figure 408)** and in leopard (*P. pardus*) with abnormal colour rosette spots **(Figure 409b)** is genetic curiosity. The body colour of hybrid specimen differs in stripes colour as well as size too **(Figure 410 b).**

Eco-husbandry associated health hazards : Many tiger reserves registered mortality in tigers on account of infighting. Diagnosis of such cases is based on presence of numerous lacerated wounds in the region of neck, face, head and even complete damage of eye inflicted by the claws and canine teeth. Presence of clotted blood trailing from the wounds and pugmarks of two different animals substantiate the provisional diagnosis perceived. It gets confirmed when necropsy encounters tearing of underneath musculature caused due to claws penetration. In such conflicts at times fracture of skull bones and vertebrae **(Figures 443,447 to 448)** may be caused. Poachers always try to collect unblemished skins of the large cats to fetch more. The use of special trap of wire nettings or snares designed to trap a large cat at times severe its leg and warrants surgical intervention **(Figures 451- 453)**. Usually villagers do not lay trap, shoot or adopt course of electrocution **(Figure 418)** or poisoning to wipe out the dangerous beast that spills over from their territory until they harm them and their livestock persistently and forest management decision is delayed. At times news papers carry story of wild tigers and leopards death are alleged to colliding with motor vehicles **(Figure 450)**. Such accidents are only possible when tiger move from its core area and reaches to busy traffic roads during dusk or dawn hours of foggy winter. There are about 9000 open-wells within 6 km periphery surrounding the Gir Forest. They are said to be "Watery Graves", as these wells are without boundary walls, therefore lions and other wild animals accidentally fall into and die due to drowning asphyxiation **(Figure 286)**.

In captivity traumatic injuries include lacerations, contusions, and wound that result often in mating, restraint stress in squeeze cage and translocation. Keeping of large cat in unhygienic conditions often deteriorates concealed injuries such as in the toes and foot sole **(Figures 423,425).** Cases of pneumonoconosis in lions are comparatively more **(Figures 288a-c)** than other large cats. Ingestion of long bone pieces with beef at time may cause severe damage to oesophagus, stomach and intestine **(Figures 321-322)**, which is mainly due to penetration of sharp ends of bones into the mucosa. Obstruction of intestine due to hairballs formation owing to body licking habit of the cats is not uncommon. Ulcerative lesions in the stomach **(Figure 327)** of a siberian tiger (*P. t. altacia*) died in captivity were studied and were related to NTN. During necropsy Stomach ulcers in Indian tigers (*P. t. tigris*) and lions (*P. leo*) died in captivity were also noticed **(Figure 328**) but without relating to any specific factor(s).

Laxation of eye lens and corneal opacity are clinically diagnosed ophthalmic problems in large cats **(Figures 402 to 406).** In one young adult tiger development of corneal opacity was observed and treatment (administration of Vit. A, and instillation of medicine) yielded no result.

Nutritional and metabolic disorders: Nutritional problem in snow leopards (*Uncia uncia*) in captivity are reported. About congenital rickets is referred under musculoskeletal disorders. Chemical analysis, and radiological examination related to morphological changes in the different long bones and vertebrae observed in a debilitated jaguar (*Panthera onca*, an exotic sp.) died in captivity due to osteomalacia **(Figure 441)**. Cases of hyperostoitic growths in skeletal elements due to unknown etiology are often encountered in large cats **(Figures 437-440).**

However, their relatedness to nutritional or metabolic factors or any other cause remained undetermined. Workers have made little attempt to study the pathology of longevity/ senility on the hematopoietic system, endocrine glands **(Figure 466)** and metaplastic changes in cartilages of inter sternebrae, ribs, scapula, which may get ossified in old age.

Diseases. (A) Infectious & Parasitic: Unfortunately disease investigation works are sketchy despite rapid declining of populations of large cat species from the nature reserves. Morbidity and mortality data garnered show parasitic diseases were encountered more frequently than other diseases, particularly in tiger.

(a) Cardio-vascular system: Collibacillosis (*E. coli*) septicemic lesions have been recorded in two leopard (*P. pardus*) cubs died in captivity **(Figure 274)**. *Pasteurella multocida* was isolated from a sick wild tiger (*P. tigris*) and in captive snow leopards (Arora, 2003). However, pictorial documentation of disease lesions could not be presented. In captive tigers (*P. tigris*) heavy losses have been experienced due to trypansomiasis **(Figure 276)**. *Babesia sp* infection has also been diagnosed in captive tigers **(Figure 275)**. *Ehrlichia* infection **(Figure 277)** has been demonstrated in Asiatic lion (*P. leo persica*). But its clinical importance is yet to be established. Histopathological examinations accidentally may find cardiac muscle infested with sarcocyst **(Figure 278)**. Necropsy of a debilitated wild tiger (*P. tigris*) showed large numbers of heartworms *Dirofilaria immitis* clogging the right ventricle of heart **(Figure 280).** Such cases have also been registered in large cats in captivity **(Figure 279a,b).** Animals died of *D. immitis* infection had also severe parasitic gastrointestinal lesions caused by other nematode species.

(b) Respiratory system: Carnivores in general are refractory to tuberculosis (Tb). Granulomatous and pearl shaped pulmonary lesions have been encountered in large cats **(Figure 296a,b)** died in captivity. Necropsy of an adult debilitated wild tigress (*P. tigris*) turned man-eater when shot dead showed complete damage of her lungs due to *Paragonimus westermanii* **(Figure 298).** Several cases of pulmonary paragonimosis have been recorded in large cats. Histopathologic examination of lung specimen from leopard (*P. pardus*) encountered *Filariodes osleri* **(Figure 301)**.

(c) Digestive system: Of the viral diseases affecting large cats, high incidence of feline panleucopenia (FPL) has been recorded in neonates died in captivity. **Figures 330 and 331** present microscopical intestinal lesions of FPL in tiger cubs died in two different captive facilities. Calcivirus infection was related to stomatitis **(Figure 318)** in a hybrid lion (*P. leo*). Inclusion body hepatitis (IBH) has been diagnosed in leopards (*P. pardus*) died in captive facilities **(Figures 350)**. Although several cases of rabies in large cats are registered but neither clinical nor pathological illustration could be arranged. Clinical cases of parasitic gastroenteritis are frequently registered in young large cats from the zoological collections. The important case presented were lesions of nodular growths in oesophagus **(Figure 342)** of leopard (*P. pardus*) due to *Spirocercus lupi* and in the intestine of tiger (*P. tigris*) due to *Galonocus pernisiosus* **(Figure 340).** Large cats in captivity and wild do suffer from severe gastritis and or gastroenteritis due to *Gnathostomum spinigerum* infection. The nodular lesions were the important findings encountered in the stomach and intestine of tigers (*P. tigris*) died in wild and in captivity **(Figures 344-347).**

Miscellaneous: A variety of hepatic problems such as jaundice, cirrhosis, cystic liver, in large cats were presented but mostly with unspecified etiology **(Figures 348,351-35, 336)**.

(d) Urinary system: In large cats most of the pathological conditions of urinary system diagnosed are based on gross and or histological findings. Nephritis and cystitis are not uncommon in large cats. Lesions such as pyelonephritis and glomerulo-nephritis (**Figure 372 a,b**) in tiger (*P. tigris*), suppurative nephritis **(Figure 373)** in lion (*P. leo*), and interstitial nephritis **(Figure 375)** in panther (*P. pardus*) encountered are presented. Chronic interstitial nephritis due to leptospiral infection **(Figure 377)** claimed death of tiger (*P. tigris*) in captivity**.** Lesion of hard, thickened uneven gritty growth diagnosed as granulomatous cystitis **(Figure 379)** in leopard (*P. pardus*) could not be related to any specific etiology. Cystitis in leopard (*P. pardus*) marked with necrosis and calcification in the mucosal layer of urinary bladder **(Figure 380).** Pyaemic cystitis **(Figures 381,382)** related to bacterial infection is presented one case each in leopard (*P. pardus*) and puma (*Panthera concolor*, an exotic sp.) died in our zoos.In latter case *Streptococcus* sp.was isolated from the chronic lesions in the urinary bladder of the animal.

(d) Nervous system: Rabies in tigers and lions has been encountered. Mild to severe congestion of brain is usually observed in rabies. For differential diagnosis, clinical history and traumatic injury are considered. No disease case has been included.

(e) Sense organs: Though infectious conjunctivitis and keratitis are clinically encountered but no specific case report is illustrated in this publication. A single case neoplasm-epidermoid carcinoma is documented **(Figure 407)**.

(f) Integumentary system: Histological demonstration of filamentous and yeast form of organisms of *Candida tropicalis* **(Figure 426)** was considered as causative agent for dermatitis in a hybrid lion (*P. leo*) cub. Ecto parasitic infestation in large cats includes both hard and soft ticks **(Figure 427)**. Severe ectoparastic dermatitis in a captive leopard (*P. pardus*) was treated with ivermectin **(Figure 428).**

(g) Musculo-skeletal system: Multiple hyperostetic growths involving long bones, vertebrae and ribs and sternum were diagnosed in three adult tigers in zoos **(Figures 461, 462)**.

(B) Neoplasms : Comparatively in captivity incidence of neoplasm in large cats is more than their free living counterparts, which may be due to fact that they have more longevity. A chapter on occurrence of neoplasms in Indian wildlife is included in the publication Indian Wildlife diseases and Disorders by Arora (2003). The gross and histopathological diagnoses of certain neoplasms included in table 3

Table 3: Recorded cases of neoplasm in large cats

Species	Source of specimen	Diagnosis (and criteria)
Hybrid lion (*P. leo*), Asiatic lion (*P.leo persica*)	Zoological Parks/Gardens	Figure 281: Histiocytic cell sarcoma of heart Figure 303: Adenomatosis of lung Figure 360: Adenocarcinoma of intestine Figure 363: Metastasis of carcinoma in mesenteric lymph nodes (and lungs) Figure 365: Haemangiosarcoma. The growths were attached to mesentery Figure 384: Adrenocortical carcinoma
Tiger (*P. tigris*)	All from captivity except case Figure 366 which was from wild	Figure 283: Mesothelioma on spleen Figure 304 :Adenocarcinoma of lung Figure 320: Squamous cell carcinoma of oral cavity Figure 364: Mesothelioma of mesentery Figure 395: Mammary gland adenocarcinoma Figure 396: Leiomyoma of uterus Figure 407: Epidermoid carcinoma of eye lid
Leopard (*P. pardus*)	Zoological Parks/Gardens	Figure 319: Fibropilloma oral cavity. Figure 357 to 358: Papilloma of stomach Figure 359: Leiomyoma at the base of duodenum Figure 361: Cholengiocellular carcinoma Figure 362: Adenocarcinoma of liver

Lipomatosis was encountered in imported cheetah (*Acinonyx jubatus*) died in captivity **(Figure 285)**. Radiograph of ulna from a wild sub-adult tigress (*P. tigris*) showed increased dimension mainly in its distal third with increased density due to thickening of the cortex extending focally in the middle due to oeteolytic changes possibly of osteoma **(Figure 463)**. Left ulna and radius of an adult wild tiger showed periostial growth, suggestive of a tumour **(Figure 464)** however, due to non availability of specimens the growth remained undermined for specific entity.

(b) Small cats & Civets: Table 1,lists native species of small cats under subfamily *Felinae* of the Family *Felidae.* Indian Zoological Gardens/ Parks mostly have leopard cat, jungle cat and fishing cat rescued from jungle. Civets belonge to family *Viverridae* and are strikingly different from cat species but possess certain resembles to them hence for convenience their pathological conditions are dealt together. Among the civet species, common civet (*Paradoxurus hermaphroditus*), small Indian civet (*Viverric ula indica*) and large Indian civet (*Viverra zibetha*) are represented more frequently in captive facilities, than binturong (*Arctictis binturong*), since they are rescued routinely from in and around the human habitations.

Developmental anomalies : Rarely albino or semi-albino **(Figure 500)** of common palm civet (*Paradoxurus hermaphroditus)* are seen in captivity. The important congenital anomalies illustrated include, cleft palate **(Figure 476)** and meningeoencephalocele in leopard cat (*P. bengalensis*) kitten **(Figure 498)** born in captivity, presence of gall bladder on the parietal surface of liver **(Figure 477a)** instead of visceral surface of right median lobe in a young fishing cat (*P. viverrinus*) and absence of gall bladder in common civet **(Figure 477b)**.

Eco-husbandry associated health hazards. The leopard and jungle cats and civets are usually active in the very early and late evening in search of food. In pursuance they move fast, straight through and often either get trapped in some abandoned human and animal dwelling structures, or while crossing roads get crushed under the speedy vehicles. Certain such cases were photographed **(Figure 507)**. However, losses on account of wild fire and flood in wild cats and civets remained unrecorded.

In captivity, the major physical health problems are related to injuries in leopard cats. Often the keepers are unable to explain about these whether they occurred due to infighting or piercing of any sharp projection/ fence wire ends of the enclosure **(Figures 501 to 502)**.

Nutritional & Metabolic disorderes: These are hardly been studied seriously in small cat and civet species. There are two such reports, one is based on clinical observations of limbs paralysis related to vitamin B_1 deficiency **(Figure499)** and other on histopathological diagnosis related to amyloidosis and diabetes **(Figure 486)** in large civet species (*Z. zebatha*). Presence of large amount of foreign matter in the stomach **(Figure 481)** of leopard cats allude to either non availability of optimum food or animal had some teeth anomalies such as heavy wearing or loss of teeth **(Figures 478, 479)** cutting up meat in cats and teeth in civets for cutting up meat and grinding of vegetable substances.

Diseases. (A) Infectious & Parasitic: In captivity course of illness in small cats is difficult to record because of shy nature of the animals. Investigation of death cases mostly remains to gross postmortem examinations. For example, documentation of fibrinous pericarditis in small Indian civet cat **(Figure 469)**, fibrinous bronchopneumonia **(Figures 473)** in leopard cat (*P. bengalensis*), haemorragic lesions in stomach **(Figure 480)** of fishing cat (*P. viverrinus*), leopard cat (*P. bengalensis*) and Jungle cat (*Felis shaus*) remained unexplained**,** Haemorrhagic gastro-intestinal lesons in a fishing cat(*P. viverrinus*), enteritis in small Indian civet **(Figures 483),** suppurative hepatits in common civet **(Figure 488)** and pyelonepharitis(**Figure 495**) in jungle cat (*F. chaus*) were attributed for infectious etiology.. Pyogenic foci in the liver, spleen (leading to peritonitis) attributed to *E. coli* infection **(Figure 487)** in small Indian civet (*V. indica*).Rabies in wild civet has been recorded (Arora, 2003). Toxoplasma schizont **(Figure 474)**in the lung of common civet (*Paradoxurus* sp.) was found**.**

Pulmonary infection of *Filariod osleri* **(Figure 475)** has been documented in a leopard cat (*P. bengalensis*) died in captivity, which appears to be the first report. A case of severe parasitic gastritis in Golden cats has illustrated **(Figure 484)**. Necropsy examination of a wild cat (*Fels chaus*) showed severe gastritis marked for nodular lesions caused by nematode sp. and formation of aneurysm in the duodenum due to tapeworm **(Figure 485).**

Fungal dermatitis was clinically diagnosed in a common in civet, lesions were mainly on its tail and legs **(Figure 503).**

(B) Neoplasms : Detailed gross and histo-pathological lesion of hepatic lipidiosis in a leopard cat (*P. bengalensis*) died in captivity is presented **(Figure 490).** Growths from liver of binturongs (*A. binturong*) died in captivity were diagnosed as cholangiocellular carcinoma and hepatocellular carcinoma one case each **(Figures 491, 492)**. Typical reactions in case of former include papillary projection on the biliary epithelium and metastatic lesions in the spleen **(Figure 493)** too. Animal had also lesions over the body, involving neck, shoulder and hind limb **(Figures 504)**. A case of Granulosa cell tumour **(Figure 497)** of the ovary was recorded in the small Indian civet (*V. indica*)died in captivity

(c) Canids & Hyena: Table 1 furnishes wild species and subspecies of Family *Canidae*. Family *Hyenidae* includes only one species, striped hyena (*H. hyaena*) existing in the country, which in built (legs and feet anatomy) and general appearance suggest its relationship with dog- member of family *Canidae*. It is scavenger by profession and food by scent. Therefore information on their health problems encountered in canid species and hyena are presented together.

Development anomalies: A pair of albino jackals (*C. aureus*) was collected from wild and lodged in Zoological Garden, Kolkota **(Figure 533).** During our studies we have not come across any form of congenital anomaly in canid species as well as in hyena.

Eco-husbandry associated health hazards: In captivity traumatic injuries in hyenas (*H. hyaena*) and jackals (*Canis aureus*) are mostly owing to infighting, when detected very late may prove fatal **(Figures 534- 536**). Leg fracture in hyena (*H. hyaena*) takes long time to cure **(Figure 538)**. Jackal (*C. aureus*) and hyena (*H. hyena*) are nomad, move in the din and dusk period in pursuits of their foods requirements at times while crossing the traffic roads, get collided with speedy vehicles and are crushed **(Figure 550)** as their sense of hearing compared to sense of smelling is poor. Wolf (*Canis lupus*) has been alleged to child lift hence often-fell victim of man. Wild dog (*Cuon alpinus*) is most endangered species. Its die offs in the wild are inadequately studied. In early January 2008, malicious DDT poisoning has claimed death of 16 wild jackals (*C. aureus*) in Uttar Pradesh **(Figure 549)**.

Nutritional and metabolic disorders: Mineralization (calcification and ossification) of in the aorta **(Figure 508)** of wild jackal (*C. aureus*) and in lung **(Figure 509)** of a wolf (*C. lupus*) died in captivity was diagnosed. In the above mentioned wolf and in a red fox (*Vulpes vulpes*) Jaundice was diagnosed **(Figures 521, 522)**.

Teeth wearing is more common in hyena as compared to canid species. Cases of loss of teeth marked by absence of alveolus in all the three canid species **(Figure 516 - 518),** which allude to that due to some traumatic impact teeth were lost earlier. Osteoporotic lesions extending from the level of symphysis to horizontal portion of both left and right mandible rami **(Figure 542)** were found in a hyena (*H. hyaena*) died in captivity.

Diseases. (A) Infectious & Parasitic: Mortalities in respect of infectious and parasitic etiologies in canid species and hyena are poorly studied. Infectious canine hepatitis, rabies, trypanosomiasis are known to cause heavy losses in them. But due to some technical difficulties we could not make out pictures of the findings. Occurrence of heart worm- *Dirofilaria immitis* causing dilation of right ventricle in captive fox (*V. bengalensis*) been reported**.** Lesions of lymphoid depletion **(Figure 523)** in spleen in wild dogs (*C. alpinus*) remained unspecified

A case croupous pneumonia (grey hepatization) in jackal (*C. aureus*) died in captivity was found where all the lobes were enlarged and solid and sink in water **(Figure 512)**.

Certain disease conditions such as enteritis **(Figures 513, 520)**, hepatitis **(Figures 524-525)**, and nephritis **(Figures 526-527)** diagnosed based on pathological findings are documented. Some of them are further detailed as follows. Suppurative hepatitis **(Figure 524)** was found in common fox (*V. bengalensis*) and hepatitis marked with infiltration of mononuclear cells in perivascular area, sinusoidal distension and congestion **(Figure 525)** in wild dog (*C. alpinus*) died in captivity. Tubular degeneration and necrosis (**Figure 527)** due to infectious etiology can not be ruled out.

In hyena (*H. hyaena*) that died in captivity, necrotic lesion in maxilla (**Figure 543**) and spondyloarthopathies **(Figure 544)** were important findings. Their details are included in the publication "Indian Wildlife Diseases & Disorders" by Arora (2003). In case of latter in addition to vertebrae, proximal portions of radius and ulna were affected, and their radiographic examination showed degenerative changes suggestive of osteoarthritis **(Figure 547).** Formations of excrescences **(Figure 546)** round the extremities of long bones are not uncommon

(B) Neoplasms: Cases of neoplasm presented hailed from the zoo specimens. Gross and histopathological features of melanosarcoma of lung **(Figure 514)** encountered in hyena (*H. hyena*) are detailed. The lung specimen from wolf *(Canis lupus*) showing small pin head to lancet sized hard raised foci which were the lesions diagnosed for alveolar cell carcinoma **(Figure 515)** with metastatic lesions on the ventral aspect of abdomen. The animal's liver was anaemic. Lymphosarcoma in kidneys was diagnosed in hyena (*H. hyaena*) died in captivity. The gross lesions were nodular elevations on their surfaces. Lymphoid tumour cells replacing the cortical tubules of the kidney were histological changes (**Figure 528**).

(d) Bears & Red panda: Table 1 includes common and endangered Asian species of bears belonged to *Family Ursidae* known in Indian limits. Our zoos have mainly two bear species namely; sloth bear (*Melursus ursinus*) and Himalayan black bear (*Salenarctus thibetanus*). Malayan bear *(Helarctos malayanus)* and brown bear *(Ursus arctoss*) number in wild is also dwindling and only few are present in certain zoos. The rescue centers mainly house sloth bears. In nature the onset of hibernation in bear species correlates with the commencement of winter season in temperate region, when food resource availability is constraint and also depends upon endogenous hypophyseal and hormonal influences. Based on molecular studies of the red panda (*Ailurus fulgens*) some workers have placed this in the family *Ursidae.* But others still hold that red panda is primitive procyonid. Chinese Giant panda *(Aailuropoda melanoleuca)* is not found within Indian limits.

Developmental anomalies: A Himalayan bear (*Selenarctos thibetanus)* in a zoo marked for white hair skin patch on the nose and other parts of the body **(Figure 588).** A female albino white sloth bear (*M. ursinus*) has been caught from Madhya Pradesh Jungles and lodged in a State zoo **(Figure 589).** The bone developmental anomalies such as hypertrophy and atrophy of transverse processes of vertebrae encountered in bears **(Figures 599,600)** could be acquired anomalies in postnatal life.

Eco-husbandry associated health hazards: Rarely inter species conflicts in wild are reported. Fatal intra species conflicts in adults are often registered based on the zoo keepers report but rarely such event are photographed **(Figures 591, 593)**. Infighting occurs only when either two unacquainted individuals are mixed accidentally or deliberately during breeding or when there is more number of males and females housed together in an enclosure. To manage injury/ wound **(Figures 562, 578a, 591-592)** because of animal non-cooperative behaviour is the major constraint and needs prolonged care. Restraint of bear by nose ring also causes severe damage to nose and snout skin **(Figure 553)**. Himalayan black bear *(S. thibetanus thibetanus*) has adopted and breed well in certain zoos located in tropical environment like Udaipur, Delhi, Guwahati, Kanpur, Chandigarh, Chennai, but if housed in bare exhibits heat stroke cases are likely to occur. A case of heat stroke in Malayan bear (*H. malayanus*) in National Zoological Park Delhi was registered. Necropsy showed blood clots in the brain of red panda (*A. fulgens*) died in a captive facility located in tropical environment alludes that the animal might had fallen from height due to heat stroke **(Figure 583).** Pollution hazard is evident by findings of pulmonary pneumonoconosis **(Figure 554a,b)** in red panda (*A. fulgens*) and sloth bear (*M. ursinus*) died in captivity. Aspiration pneumonia **(Figure 555)** claimed death of a sloth bear (*M. ursinus*)

The cases of teeth anomalies presented in bears include heavy wear **(Figure 560)** and loss of central pair of incisors **(Figures 561).** The miscellaneous directly or indirectly management associated health problems in bear are stomach ulcers (**Figure 566),** intestinal intussusception **(Figure 567)**, scrotal hernia **(Figure 579)**.

Nutritional and metabolic disorders: Intimal thickening of the aorta related to atherosclerosis in sloth bear (*M. ursinus*) died in captivity **(Figure 551)**. A case of limb paralysis is put on record but without expounding its raisen d'etre. Nutritional factor cannot be ruled out. Cases of corneal opacity in bears portrayed **(Figure 585-586)** are not uncommon in zoos. Such cases too need to be studied from nutritional, senility and infectious etiologies involvement point of view. Alopecia in a sloth bear (*M. ursinus*) was related to food toxicity **(Figure 596**).

Diseases. (A) Infectious & Parasitic: Pulmonary tuberculosis **(Figures 557 to 558)** was encountered in sloth bears (*M.ursinus*) dying in captivity. Hepatic tuberculous lesions exclusively are rare finding. Both bovine and human types of *Mycobacterium tuberculosis* are reported. Among the viral diseases, Canine infectious hepatitis (ICH) in a black bear *(Ursus americanus)* died at Agra Bear Rescue **(Figure 572)** and Panleucopenia **(Figure 573)** in red panda (*A. fulgens*) died at Darjeeling Zoological Garden appear to be the first reports. Agra Bear Rescue Facility had experienced death of 14 sloth bears (*M. ursinus*) due to rabies **(Figure 584)** between June–August 2003. *Clostridium perferingens* type 'D' is recorded in bears (Arora, 2003). Parasitic pneumonia **(Figure556)** in red panda (*A.fulgens*) and severe parasitic gastro-enteritis in sloth bear often proves fatal **(Figure 569)** if not treated timely. Occurrence of taeniosis in sloth bears (*M. ursinus*) is reported to be high in Bear Rescue Centre,

Bannerghatta. Cases of hepatic degeneration **(Figure 570),** suppurative hepatitis **(Figure 571),** chronic interstitial nephritis **(Figure 577),** orchitis **(Figure 578b),** keratitis **(Figure 586)** were the important infectious conditions encountered in bear species maintained in captivity. Severe ecto-parasitic dermatitis has been marked for alopecia in bear (**Figure 594**) and in red panda **(Figure 595).**

(B) Neoplasms: We have not come across any finding of neoplasm from the wild bears. **Table 4** includes certain documented cases of neoplasm encountered in bears died in captivity.

Table 4: Recorded neoplasms in bears died in captivity

Species	Organ involved	Neoplasm	Remark
Himalyan black bears (*Selenarctos thibetanus*)	Case (i) Lung Case (ii) Liver Case (iii) Testis	(i&ii) Adenoncarcinoma **(Figures 559,574)** (iii) Haemangioma **(Figure 580)**	In case (iii) keratinized squamous cell carcinoma was also diagnosed
Malayan bear (*Helarctos malayanus*)	Mammary gland	Mammary tumour **(Figure 581)**	Histopathological changes not presented
Himalayan brown bear (*Ursus arctos isabellinus*)	Liver	Mixed hepatocellular and intrahepatic bile duct carcinoma **(Figure 575)**	Growth was yellowish-white to gray nodular measuring 24x25x23 cm and weighing about 14 kg.
Sloth bear (*M. ursinus*)	(i). Gall bladder (ii). Canine, maxilla and upper lip	(i) Cholangiocellular carcinoma **(Figure 576)**. (ii) Benign osteoblastoma **(Figure 598)**	

(a) Large Cats

Cardio-vascular System

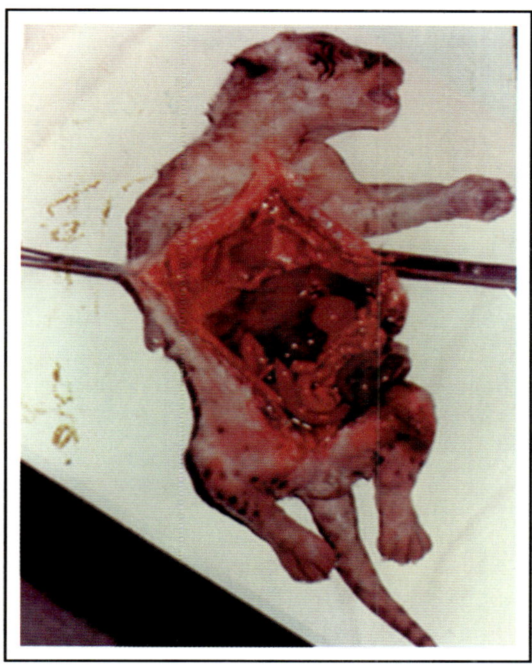

Figure 274: Photograph of one leopard cub (*P. pardus*) out of the two died of septicaemia attributed for *E. coli* infection showing congestion of viscera.

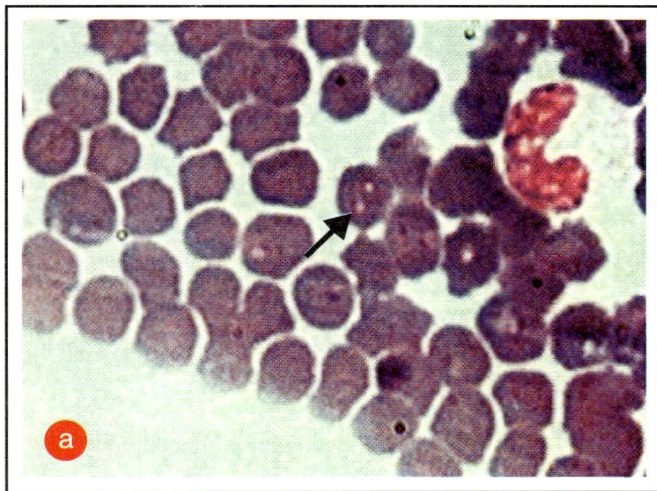

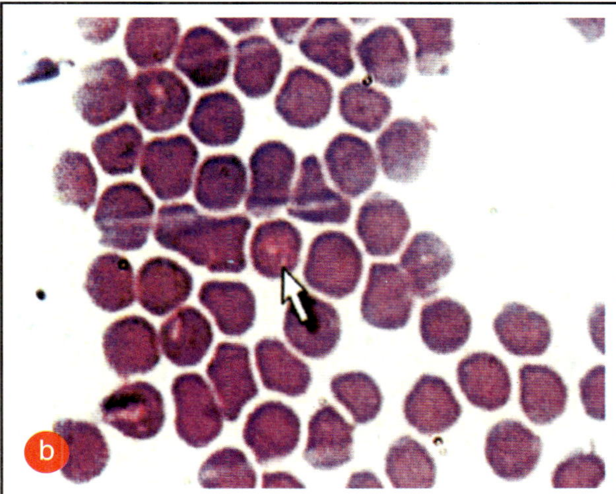

Figure 275(a,b): Blood smear from a sick tiger (*P. tigris*) belonged to Chhatbir Zoological Park,Chandigarh showing *Babesia* sp. (Arrow) Giemsa x 1000.

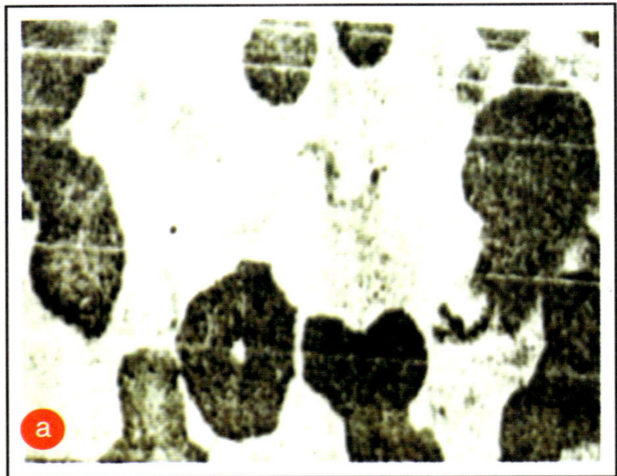

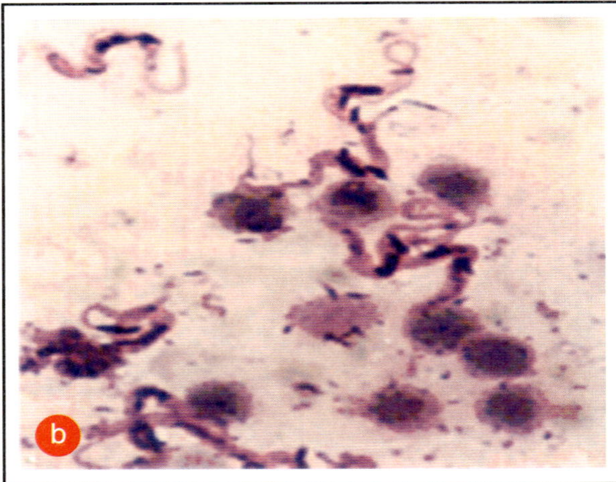

Figure 276: Blood smears showing *Trypanosoma evansi* . (a) Jaguar (*Panthera onca*, an exotic sp.) x 3200 (Sen and Chowdhuri ,1968). (b) Tiger, *(P. tigris)*. Giemsa x 1000. (Courtesy: Harish, B.R.).

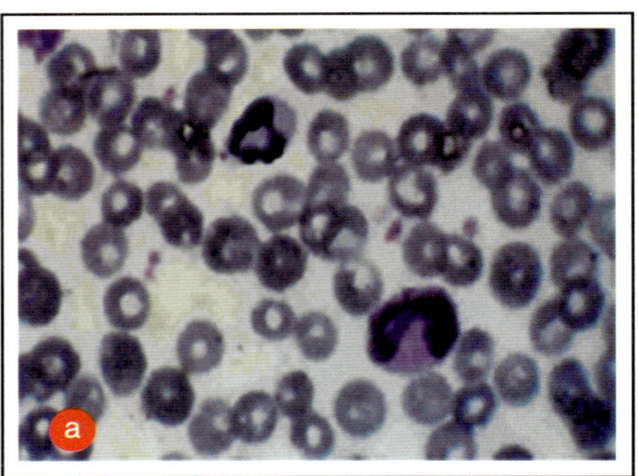

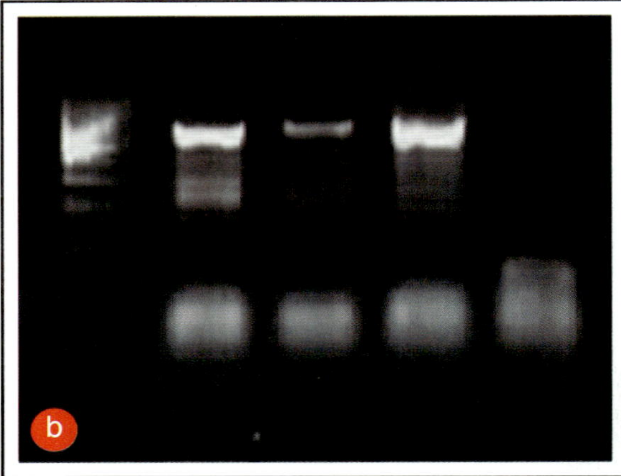

Figure 277: (a) Blood smear from captive Asiatic lioness (*P. leo persica*) suffering from endometritis, showing *Ehrlichia* infection. (b) The PCR based diagnosis revealed the presence of *Ehrlichia* sp. by OPM method. (Courtesy: Jani, R.G.).

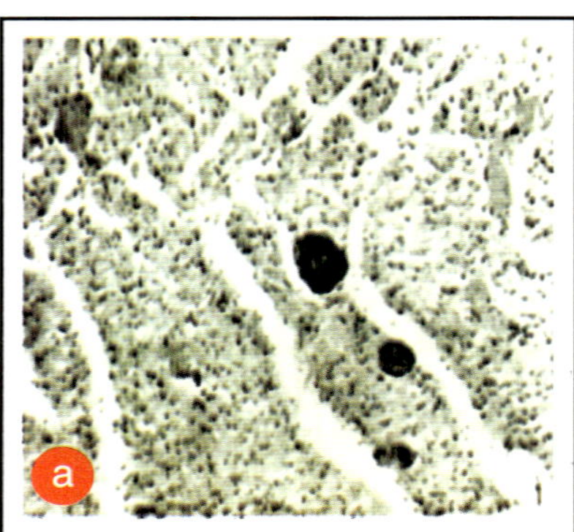

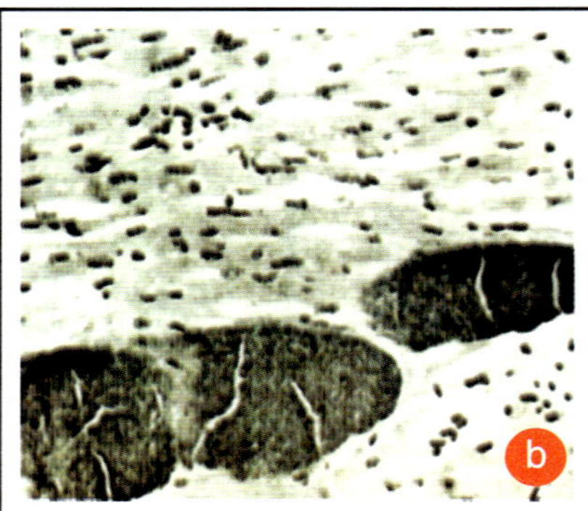

Figure 278: Photomicrograph showing:(a) Cross section of sarcocystis in cardiac muscle of wild leopard shot died in Ramnagar, Uttarakhand.H&E, x100 (b) Longitudinal section of sarcocystis showing sarcolema and tropozoites. H&E,x250 (Somvanshi *et al.,* 1987).

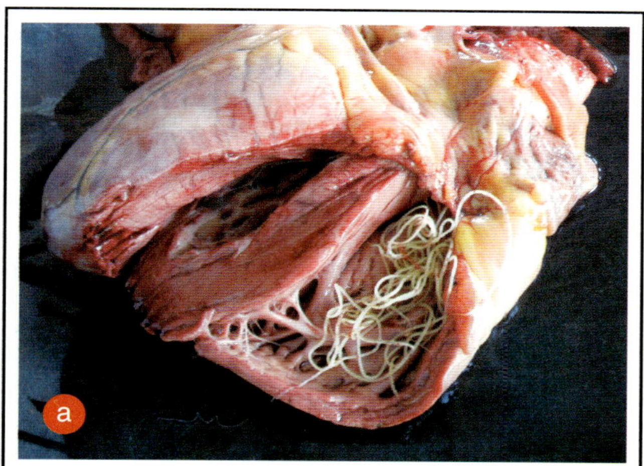

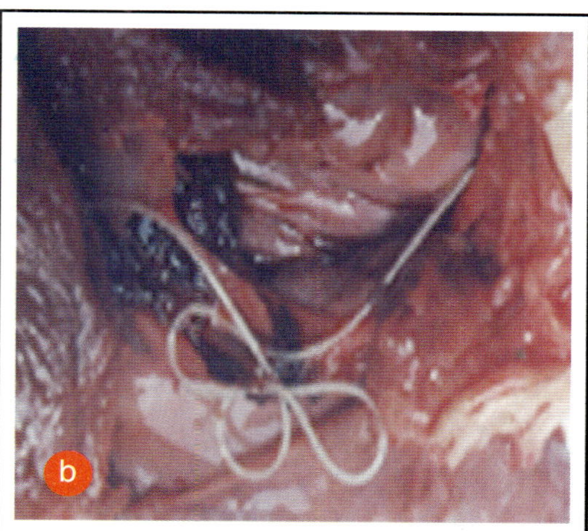

Figure 279: Photographs showing *Dirofilaria immitis* in the right ventricle of: (a) Tiger (*P. tigris*) Courtesy: Panda S.K. and Nath, I. (b) Lion (*P. leo*) died in captivity.

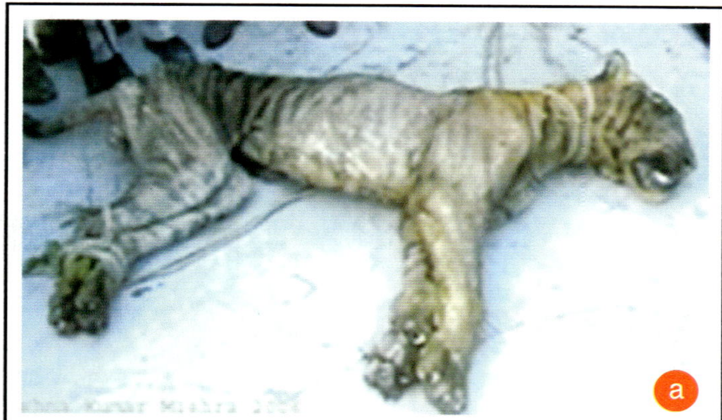

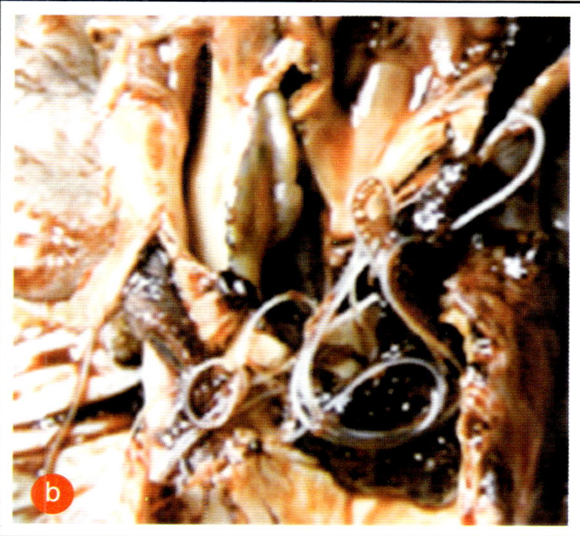

Figure 280: (a) Tigress (*P. tigris*) was shot dead officially. (b) Its necropsy (at IVRI) showed presence of large number of heartworms - *Dirofilaria immitis*. The case is also referred under digestive system.

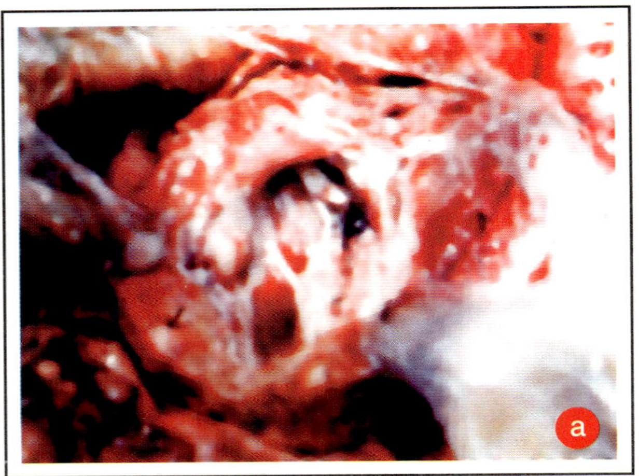

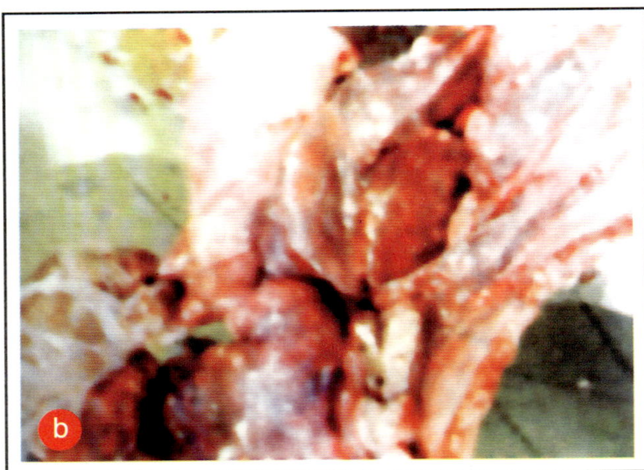

Figure 281: Photographs showing : (a) Nodular growths in heart of lion (*P. leo*) diagnosed as histiocytic cell sarcoma. (b) Enlarged mediastinal lymph nodes and nodular growths in lungs (Sharma *et al.*, 2004).

Haematopoietic Organs - Spleen

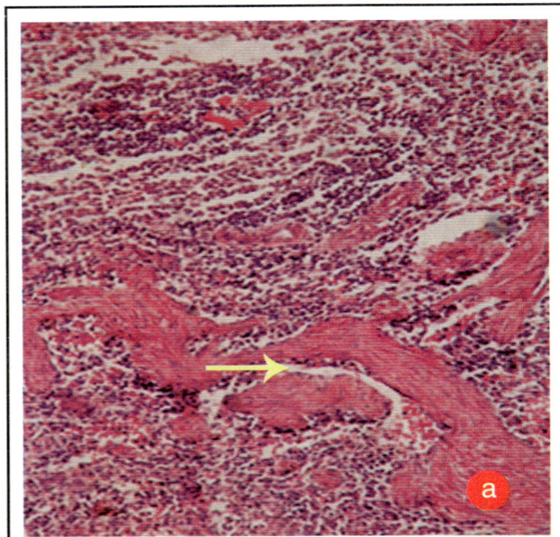

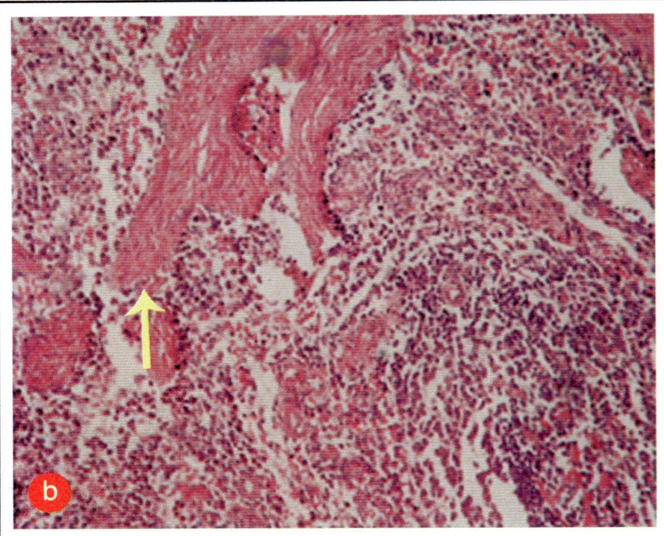

Figure 282: Photomicrographs (a,b) of spleen of panther (*P. paruds*) showing haemorrhages and congestion (Courtesy: Dept.of Vet. Pathology, CVSc. Nagpur, M.S).

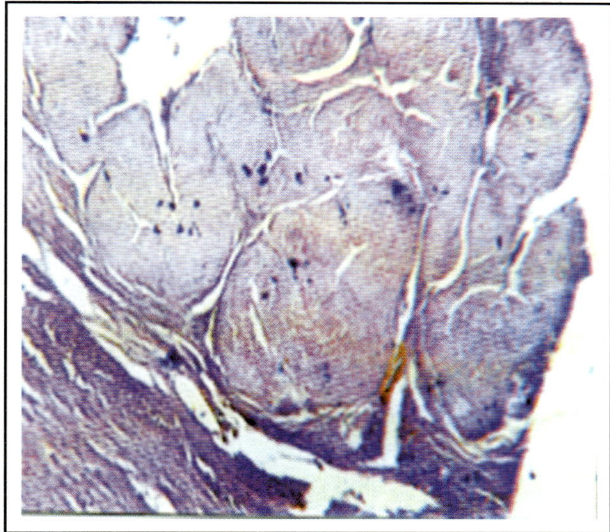

Figure283 : Photomicrograph showing mesothelioma on spleen of tiger (*P. tigris*) died in captivity . H&E, x 40 (Nashiruddullah *et al.,* 2007).

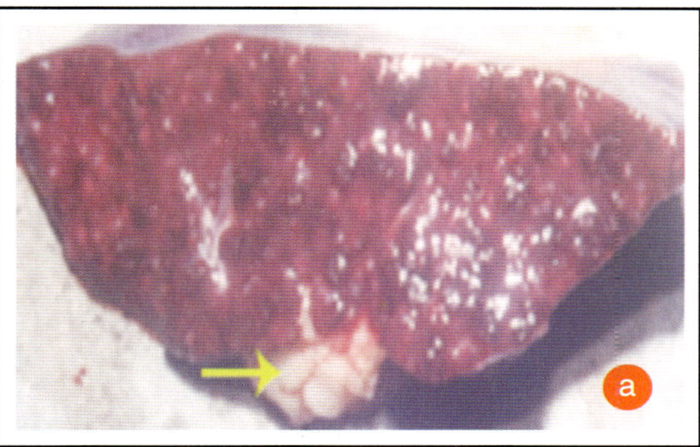

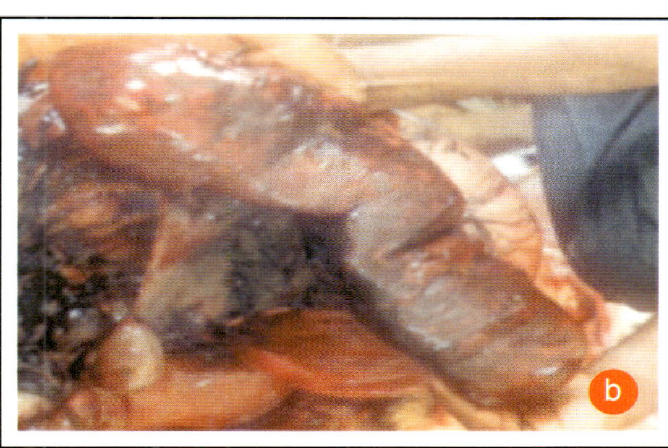

Figure 284: (a) Photographs of lymphosarcoma of spleen of: (a) Tiger (*P. tigris*) died in captivity. (Courtesy: Suryawanshi, D.S.). (b) Leopard (*P. pardus*) died in captivity. (Courtesy: Dept, of Pathology, C,V.Sc, Tirupati, A.P).

Figure 285: Lipomatosis of spleen encountered in cheetah (*Acinonyx jubatus*), which suffered from haematuria and prolonged illness at National Zoological Park.(a) Photograph showing multiple focal lipomatus growths in spleen.(b) Photomicrograph showing peripheral area of the lipomatous growth containing many vacuolated fat cells of variable sizes. H&E, x 100 (Parihar *et al.*, 1976).

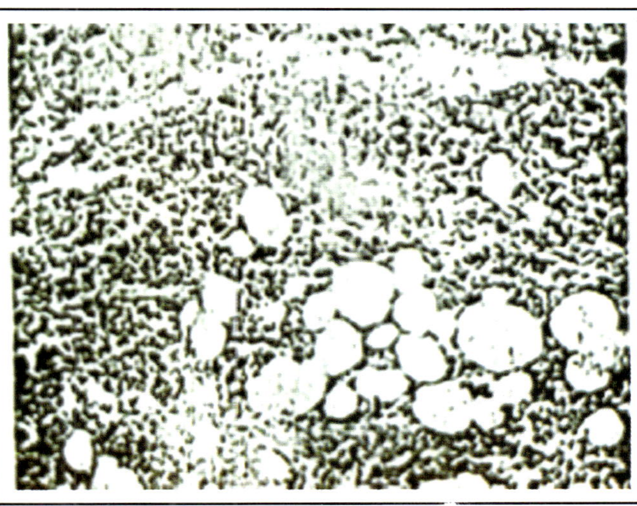

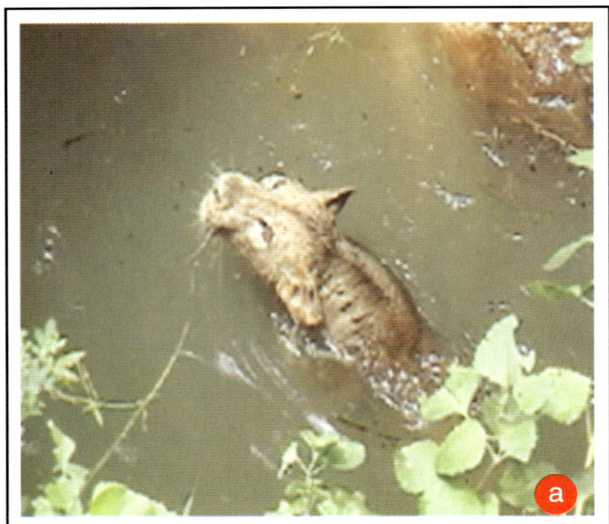

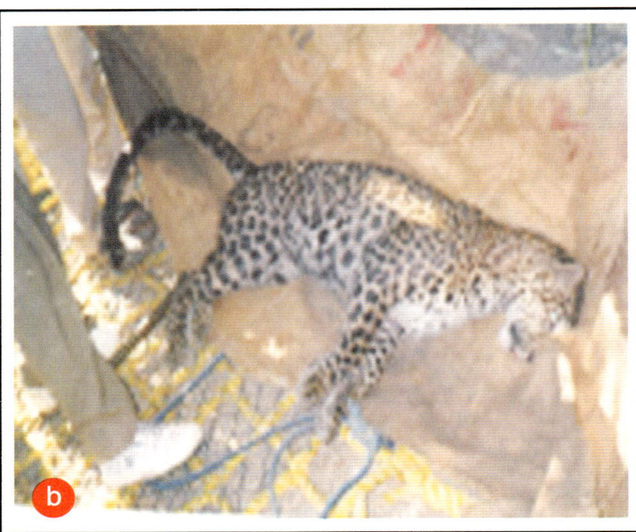

Figure 286: Photographs showing (a) Asiatic lion (*P. leo*) fell in the well in Gir forest (Courtesy: Kishore Kotecha). (b) Leopard (*P. pardus*) fell in the well in Gir forests (Courtesy: R.G. Jani).

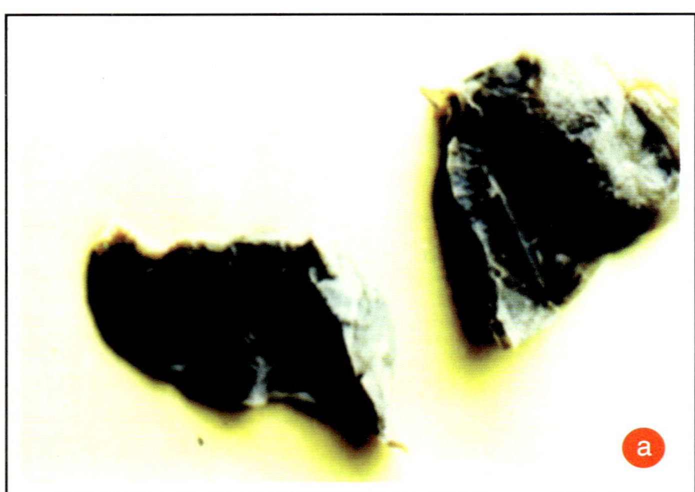

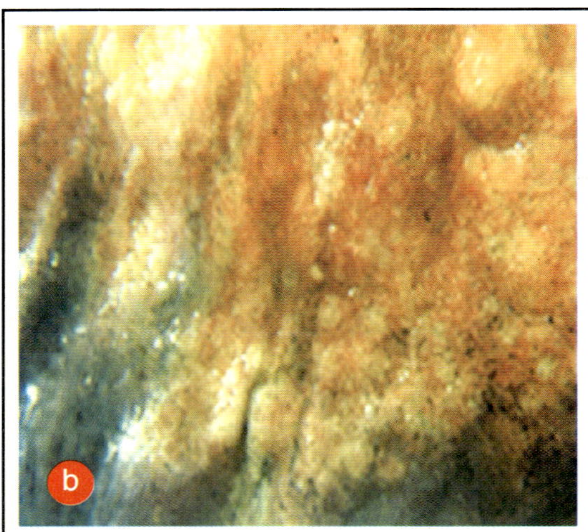

Figure 287: Photograph showing pneumoconiosis in: (a) Leopard (*P. pardus*) died in wild. (b) Tiger (*P. tigris*) died in Zoological Garden,Guwahati, Assam.

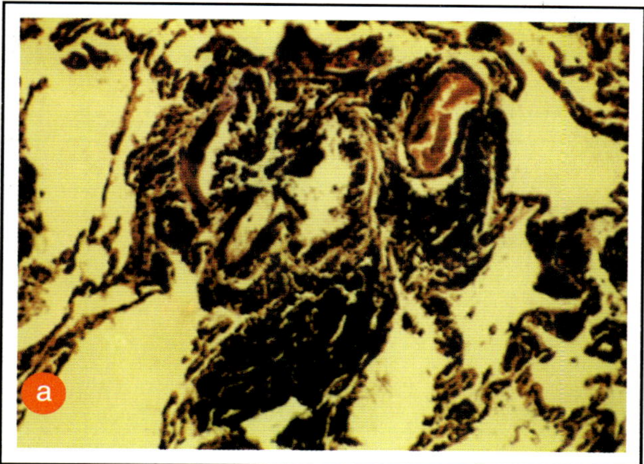

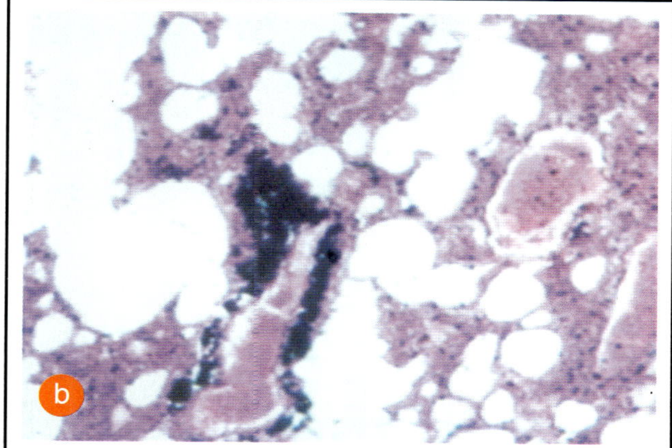

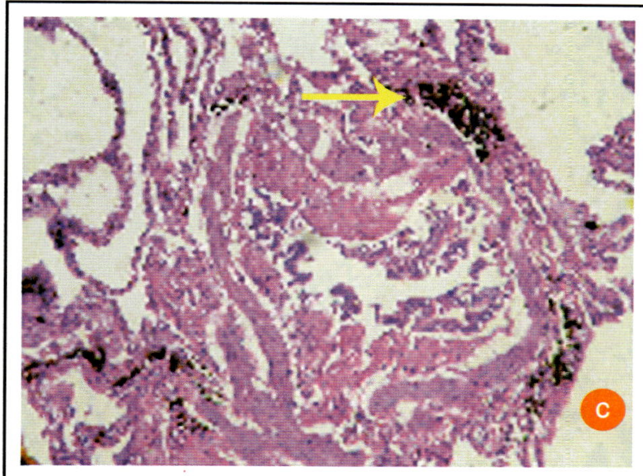

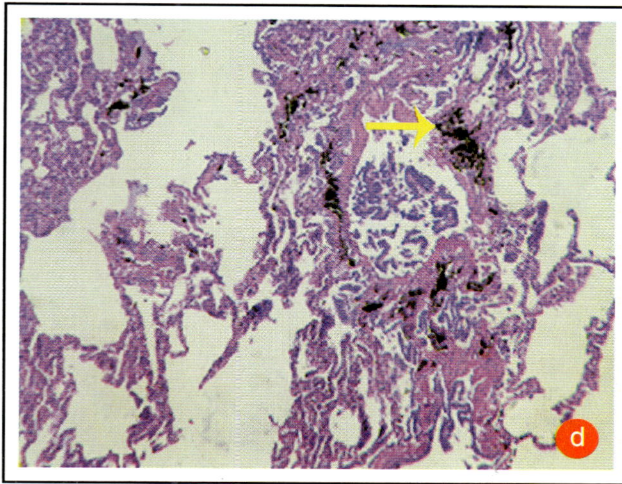

Figure 288: (a) Photomicrographs showing large granular deposits of carbon particles adjacent to bronchioles in lions (*P. leo*). (a) H&EX160 (Patil, 2002). (b) H & E, x 200. (Courtesy: Suryawanshi, D.S.),(c) H& E, x100 and (d) H& E, x 160. (Courtesy: Dept.of Vet. Pathology, C.V.Sc. Nagpur, M.S).

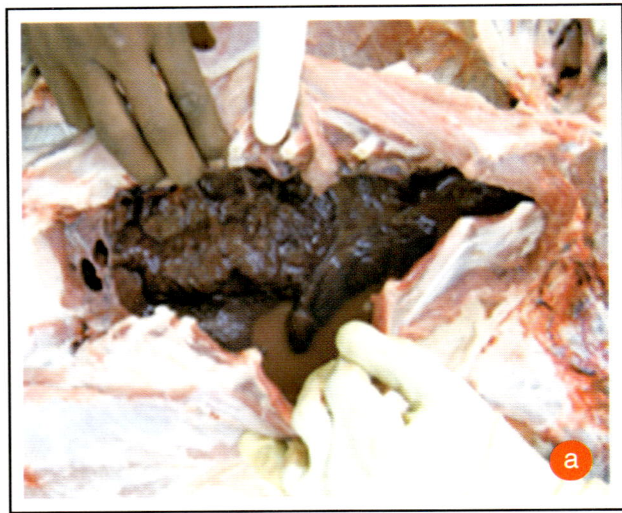

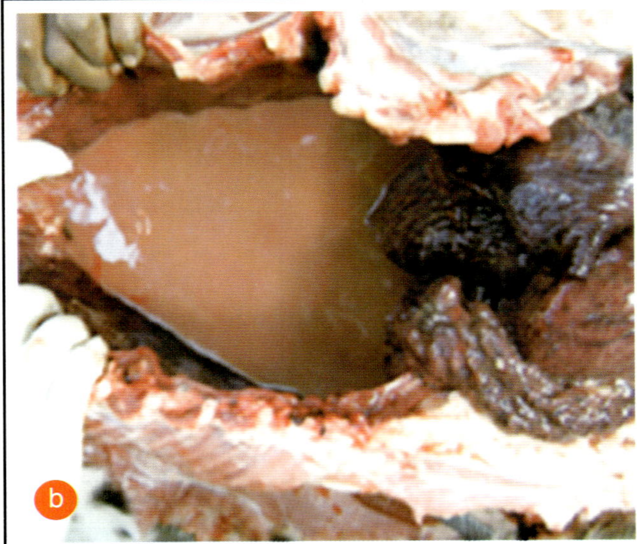

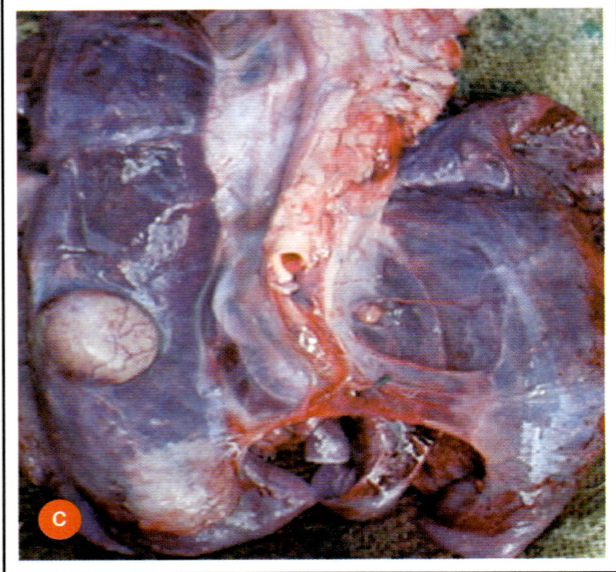

Figure 289: Photographs (a, b) showing hydrothorax in panther (*P. pardus*) died in Zoological Park, Kanpur (U.P.) Note sero-sanguineous fluid in thoracic cavity.(c) Abscess in the lung of lion (*P. leo* hybrid) died at Rescue Centre, of Zoological Park, Chennai, TN. (Courtesy: Thirumurugan, R.).

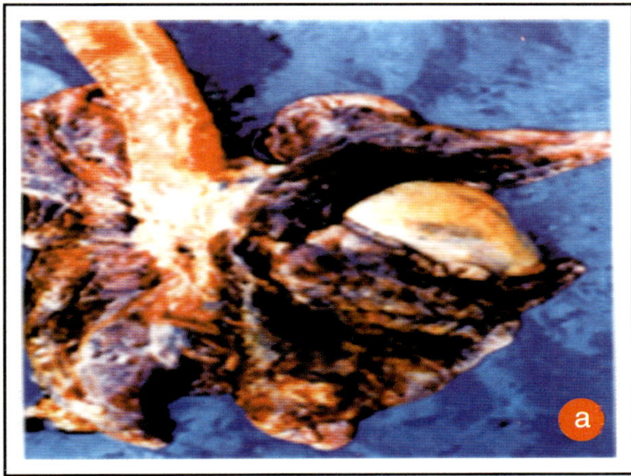

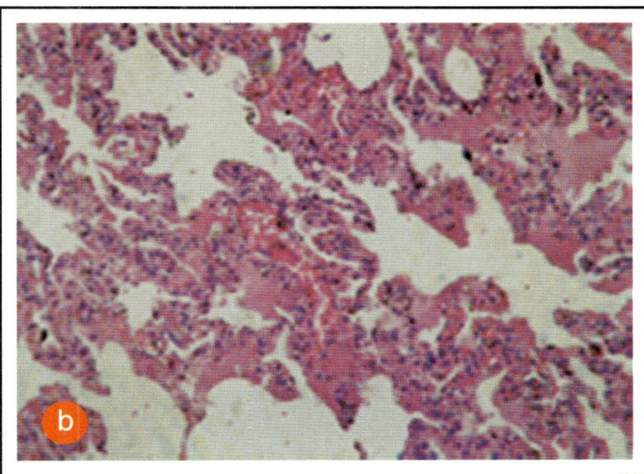

Figure 290: (a) Photograph of lung of panther (*P. pardus*) showing hemorrhages and oedema (Courtesy: Dept.Wildlife Sci., C.V.Sc, Chennai, T.N). H & E, x 100 (b) Photomicrograph of lung of panther (*P. pardus*) showing haemorrhages and oedema(Courtesy: Dept. of Pathology, C.V.Sc., Nagpur,M.S).

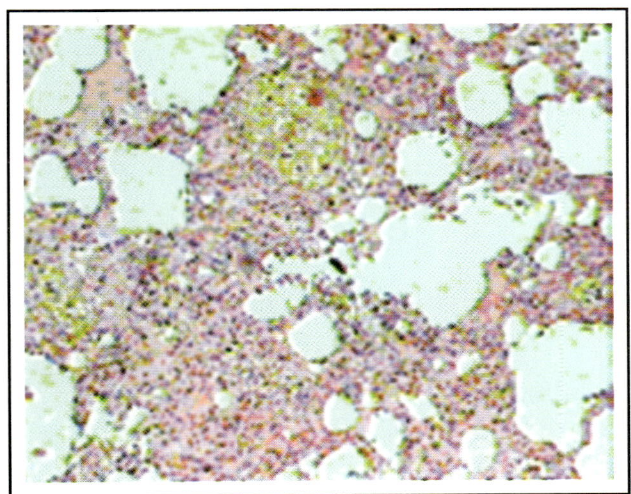

Figure 291: Photomicrograph of lung from tiger (*P. tigris*) showing interstitial pneumonia. H & E, x 100 (Courtesy: Dept.Wildlife Science, CVSc, Chennai, T.N).

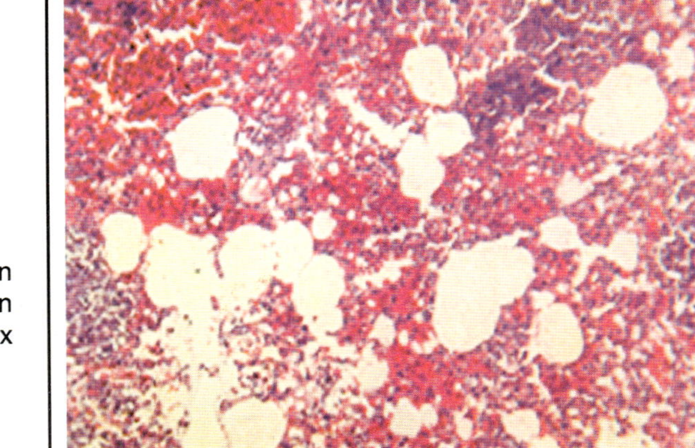

Figure 292: Photomicrograph showing pneumonic lesion in clouded leopard (*N. nebulosa*) died in Zoological Garden,Guwahati, Assam. H & E x 100.

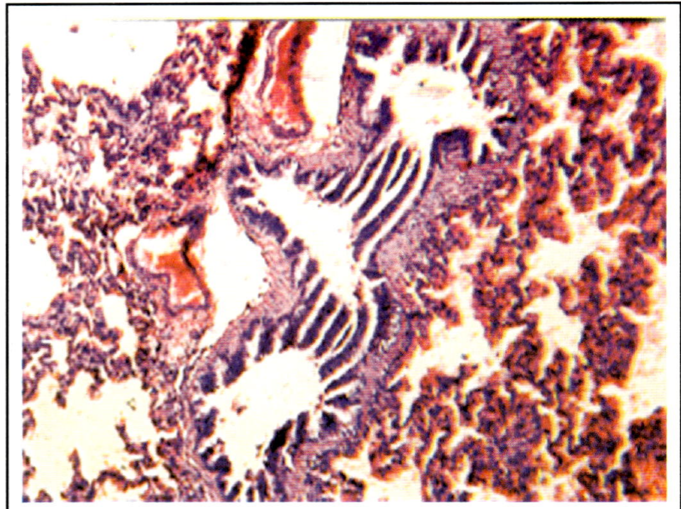

Figure 293: Photomicrograph showing pneumonic lesion in leopard (*P. pardus*) H & E x 100. Note the hyperplastic bronchiolar epithelium (Nashiruddullah *et al.,* 2007)

Figure 294: Photomicrograph showing fibrinous pneumonia in tiger (*P. tigris*) died in Zoological garden, Guwahati, Assam. Note fibronous casts mixed with mononuclear cells in the alveolar lumen. H & E x 100. (Nashiruddullah *et al.*, 2007)

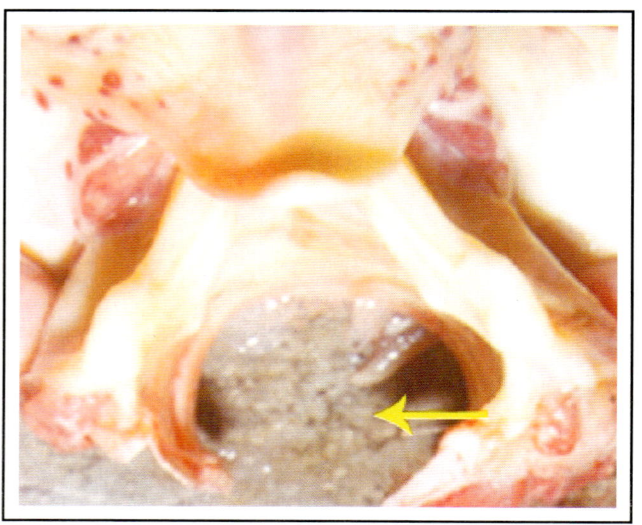

Figure 295: Photograph showing necrotic laryngitis in tiger (*P. tigris*). The animal had died of leptospiral infection. (Courtesy: Suryawanshi, D.S.).

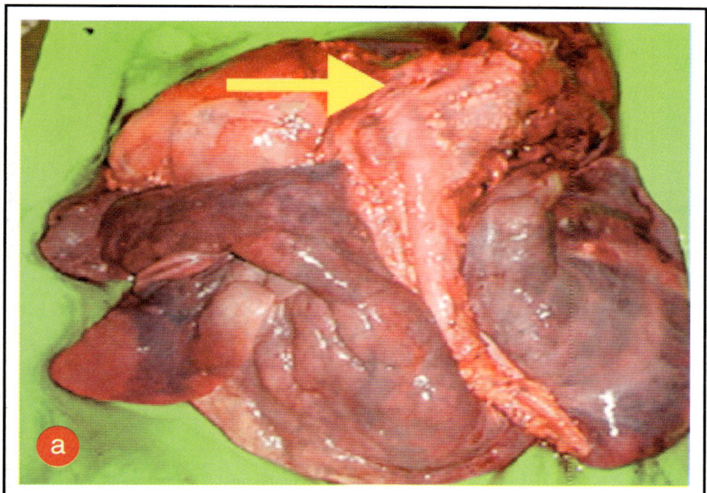

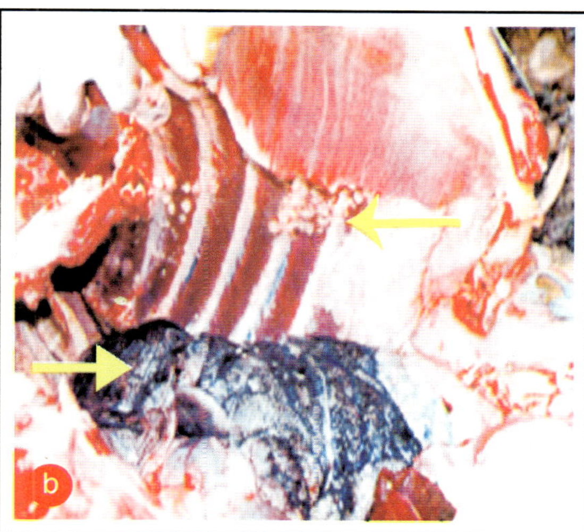

Figure 296: Photographs showing clusters of small pearl like tuberculous nodules (a) on the lung surface of tiger (*P. tigris*) and (b)adhered on the chest wall and also a few in the lung of lioness (*P. leo*) died in Zoological Park, Chennai (TN). Note severe anthracosis observed concurrently. (Courtesy: Dept of Wildlife Sc.,C.V.Sc & Thirumurugan, R.).

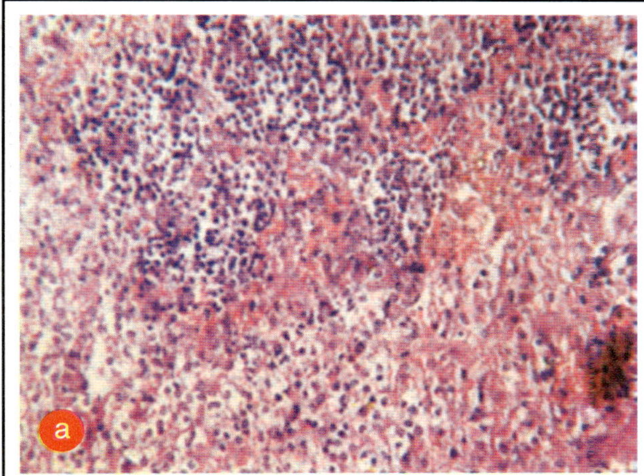

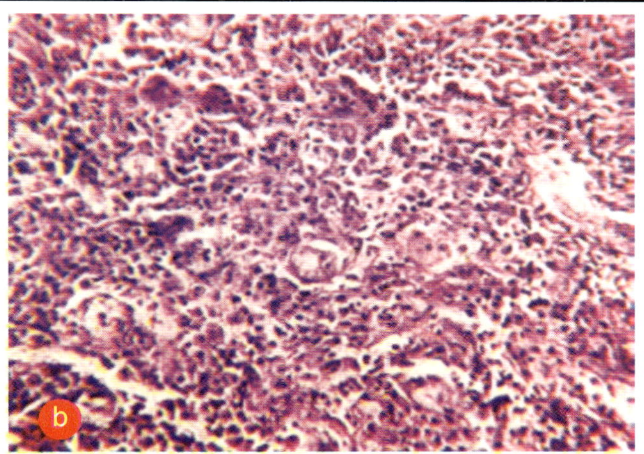

Figure 297: (a, b) Photomicrograph of lung of lion (*P. leo*) died in captivity showing granulomatous pneumonia associated to tuberculosis. (a) H&E, x100 (b) H&E, x 400 (Nashiruddullah *et al.*, 2007).

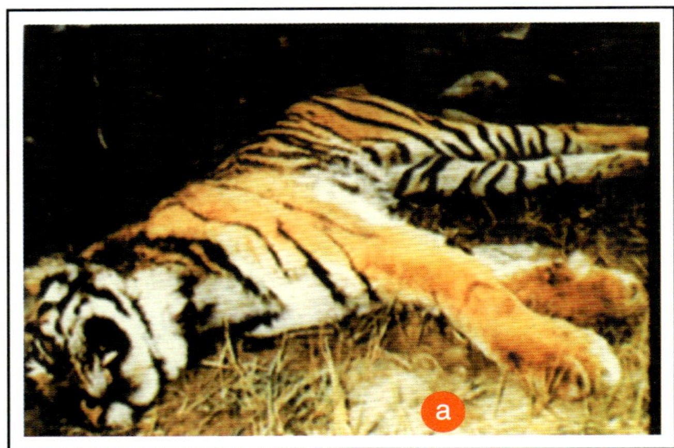

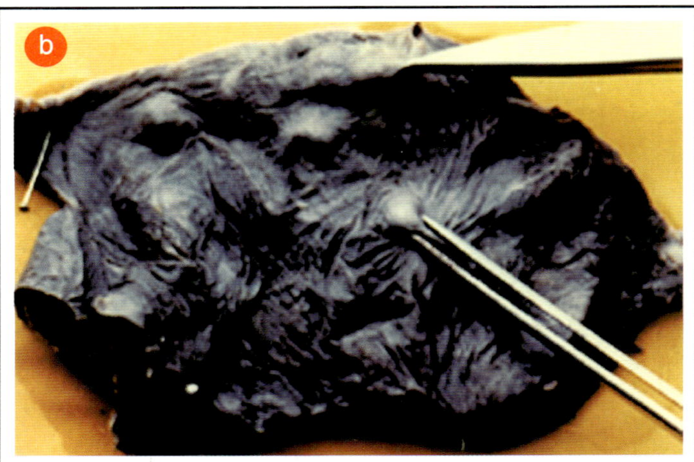

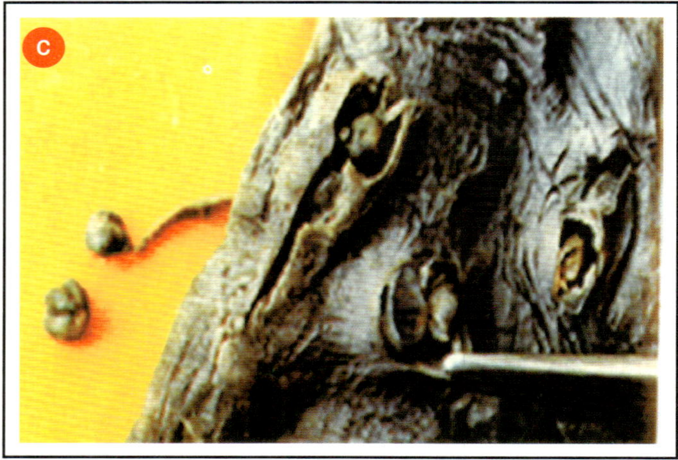

Figure 298: (a) Debilitated tigress (*P. tigris*) of Corbett National Park,Ramnagar (Uttarakhand) was shot dead when stealthily attacking the sleeping workers at the campus. (b) Necropsy showed parasitic cystic nodules in lungs. (c) Cut opened cysts showing *Paragonimus westermanii* in pairs. The case is also referred under digestive system.

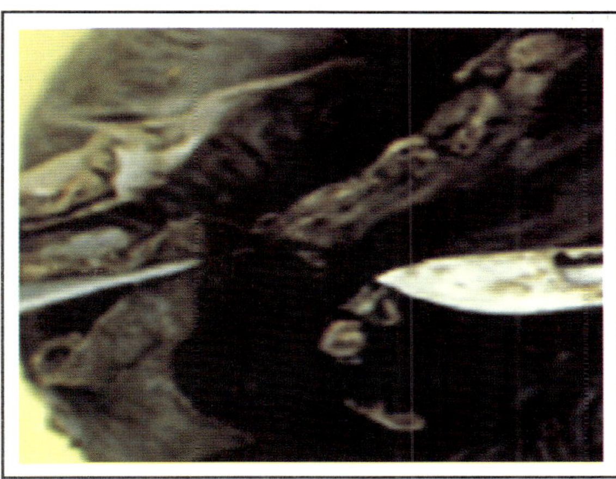

Figure 299: *Paragonimus westermanii* cysts in the lungs of leopard (*P. pardus*) died in the Corbett National Park, Ramnagar, Uttarakhand.

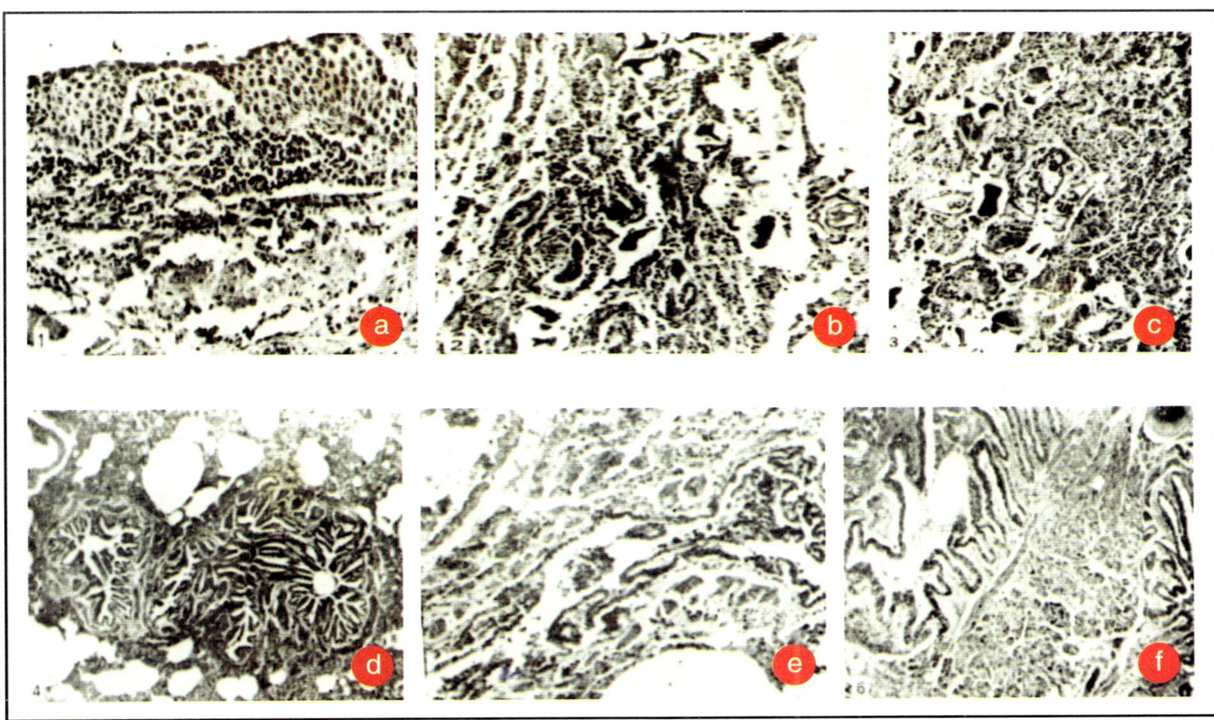

Figure 300: Bronchial hyperplasia in wild tiger (*P. tigris*) attributed to *P. westermanii* infection. Photomicrographs showing: (a) Metaplastic changes of bronchial lining. H&E, x 139. (b) Termination of parasitized bronchus into alveolar duct and parasitic eggs in the alveoli.H&E, x 80. (c) Parasitic structures in pulmonary tissue in other focus. H&E, x 80 (d) Heavy papillary infolding of epithelial lining of bronchioles H&E,x71. (e) Hyperplastic epithelium forming folds and projections in the bronchiole and alveolar duct. H&E, x71. (f) Large glandular areas containing acini in bronchial walls beyond muscle bundles. H&E,x81 (Parihar and Shrivastava, 1988).

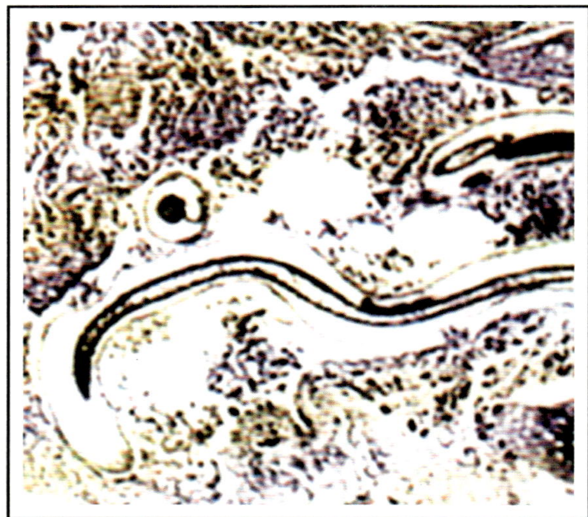

Figure 301: Photomicrograph showing *Filariodes osleri* in pulmonary tissue of wild leopard (*P. pardus*).

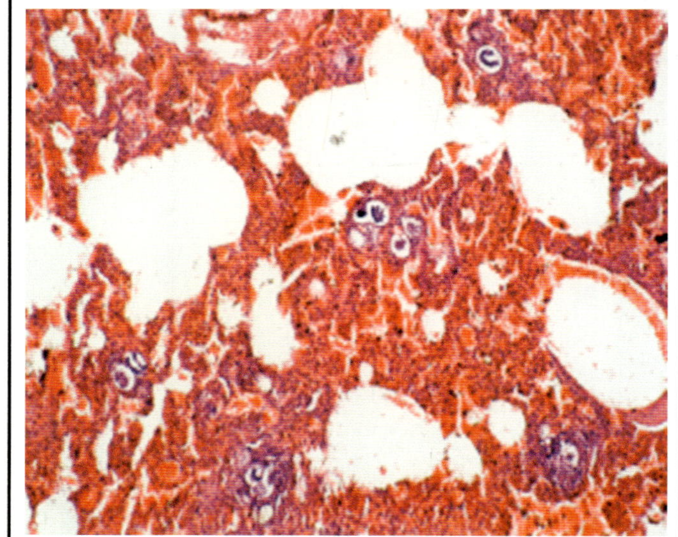

Figure 302: Photomicrograph of lung of panther (*P. pardus*)showing cross section of nematode parasite. H&E, x 10. (Courtesy: Singh, R.).

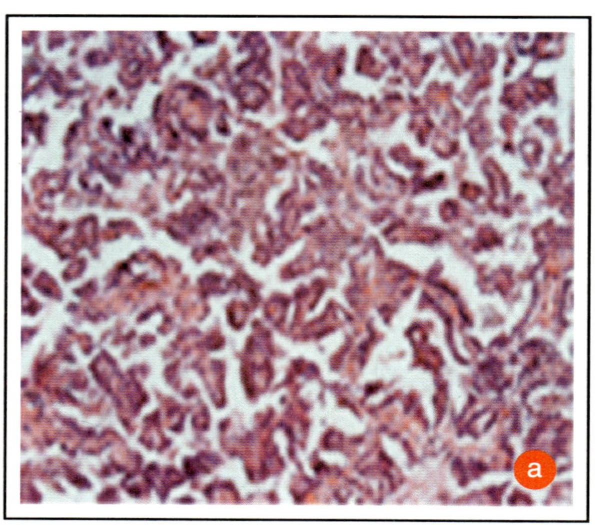

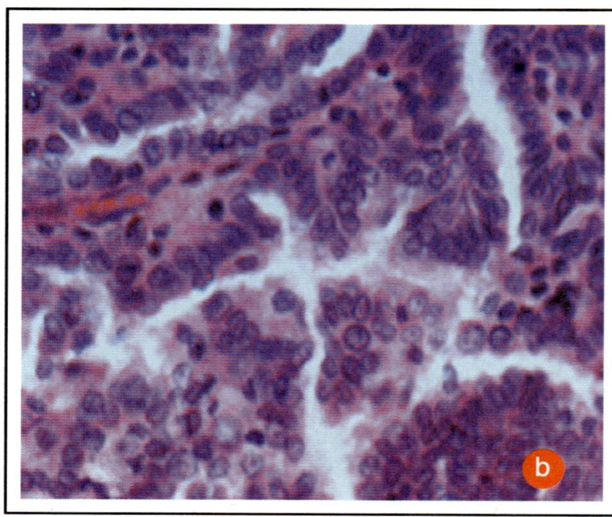

Figure 303: Photomicrograph of lung of lion (*P. leo*) died in captivity showing pulmonary adenomatosis. (a) H&E,x100 (b)H&E,x400 (Courtesy: Gupta, V.K.).

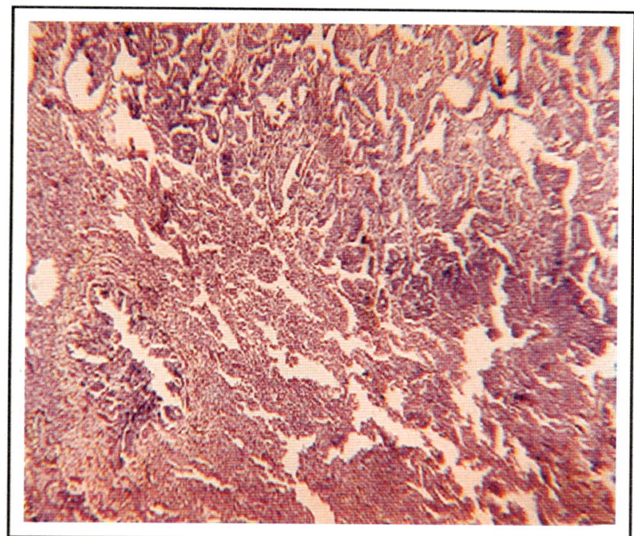

Figure 304: Photomicrograph of lung of tiger (*P. tigris*) showing adenocarcinoma (metastasis from mammary gland).H & E x 100 The case is also referred under reproductive system.

Digestive System

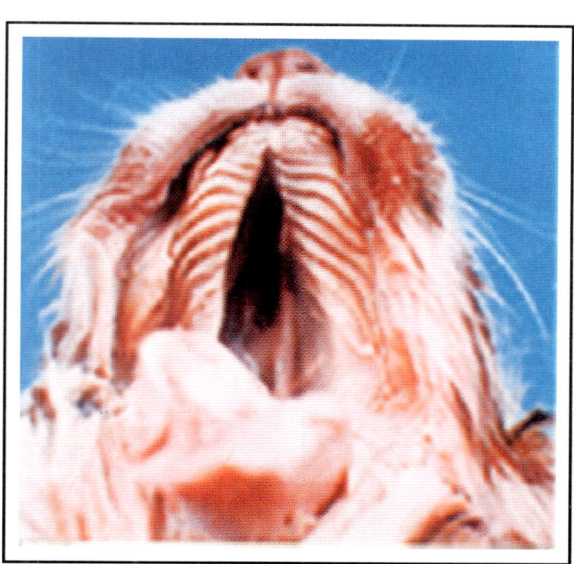

Figure 305: Photograph showing cleft palate in white tiger (*P. tigris*) cub died at National Zoological Park, New Delhi.

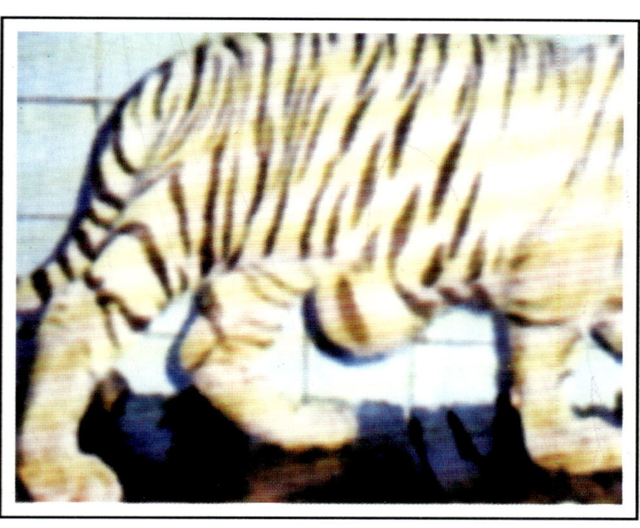

Figure 306: Photograph showing congenital umbilical hernia in white tiger (*P. tigris*) cub at National Zoological Park, New Delhi.

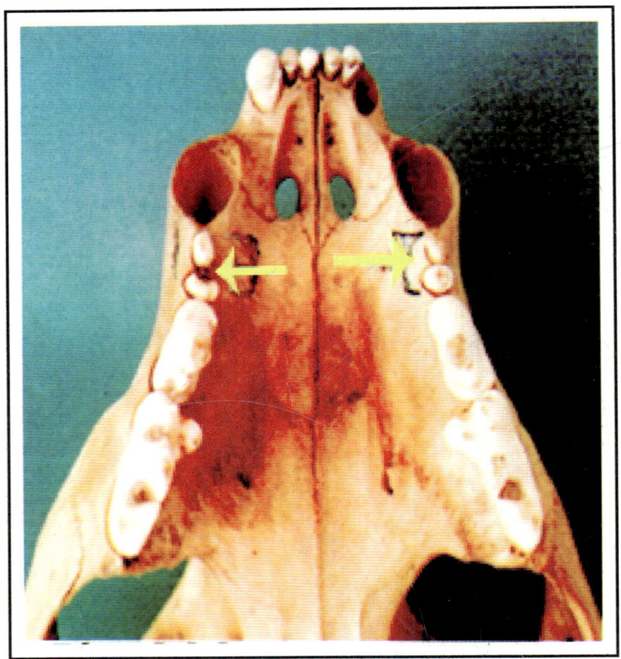

Figure 307: Skull of leopard (*P. pardus*) showing presence of bifid first premolar in both sides.

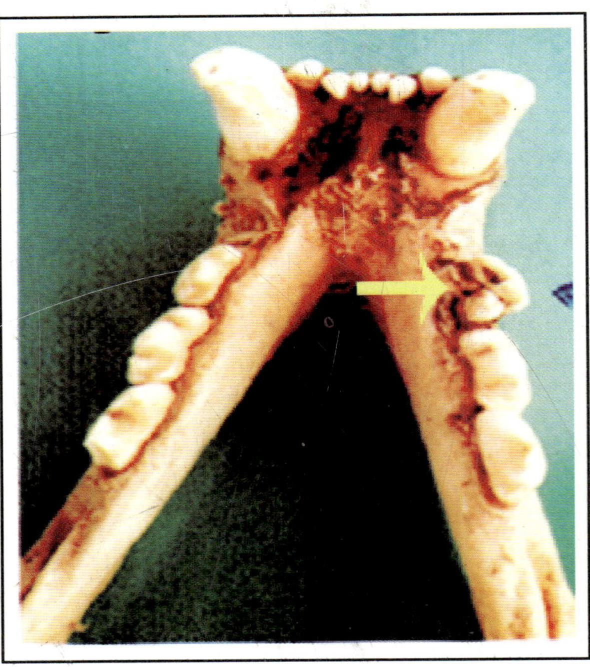

Figure 308: Mandible of leopard (*P. pardus*) showing first right premolar double in size. The incisors are not in alignment too.

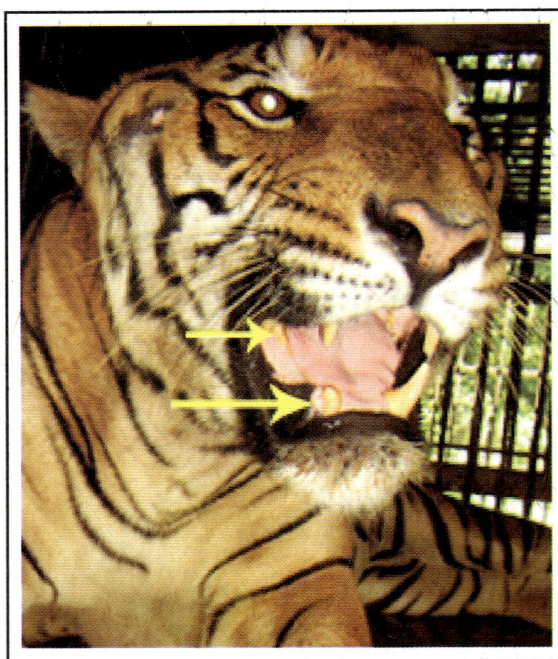

Figure 309: A tiger (*P. tigris*) belonged to Biological Park,Patna(Bihar) showing damaged right canine, mild wearing of lower incisors but extensive wear of premolars.

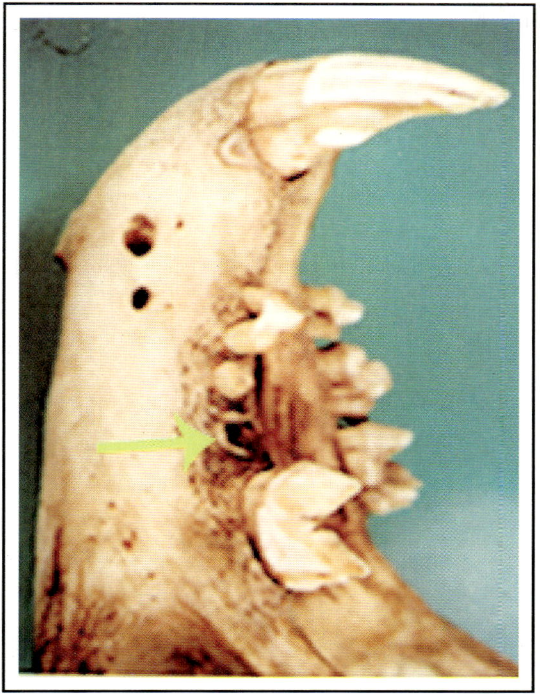

Figure 310: Photograph of mandible of young adult wild tiger (*P. tigris*) showing caries of second premolar.

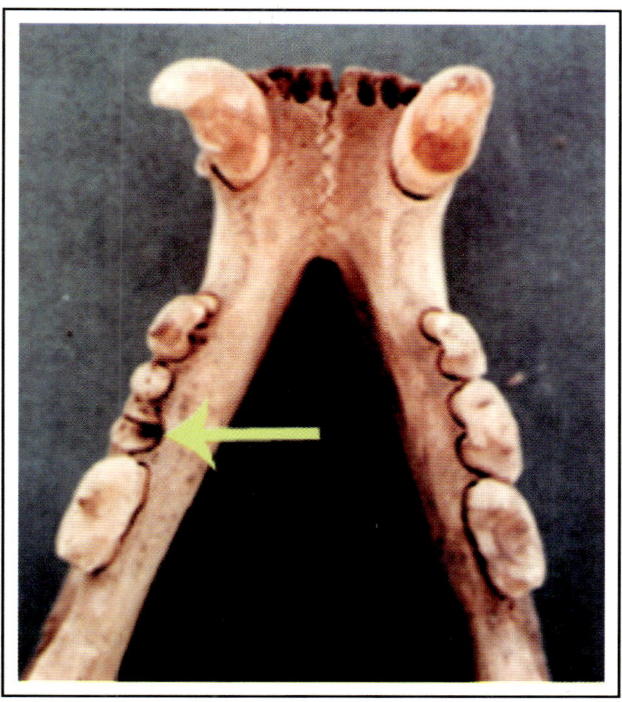

Figure 311: Photograph of mandible of wild tiger (*P. tigris*) showing caries of left second premolar tooth and wear in both canine teeth.

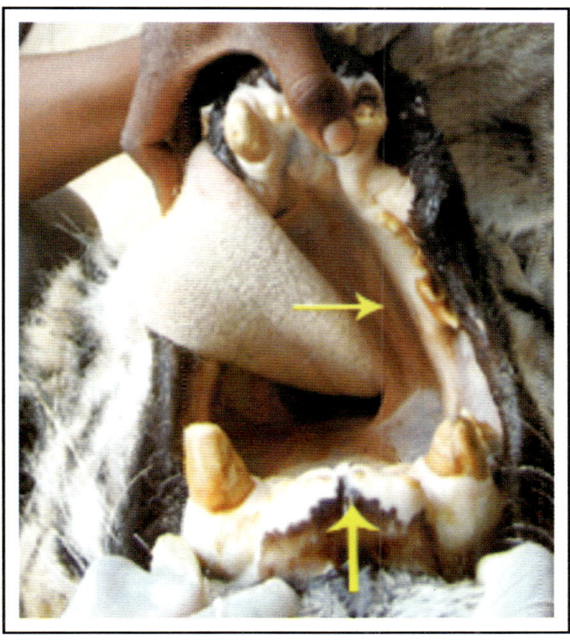

Figure 312: Loss of lower incisors and wear of canine and cheek teeth in Siberian tiger (*P. tigris altacia*).

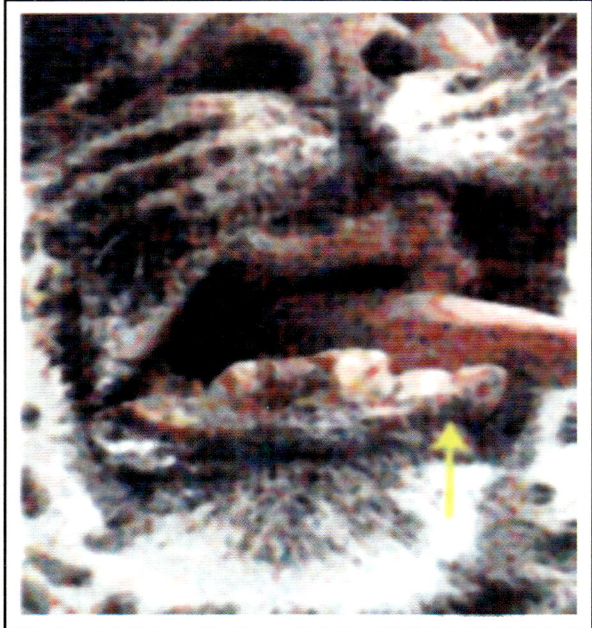

Figure 313: Decaying of incisors and canines observed in leopard (*P. pardus*).Animal had also stomatitis (Courtesy: Kishtwaria,R. S.).

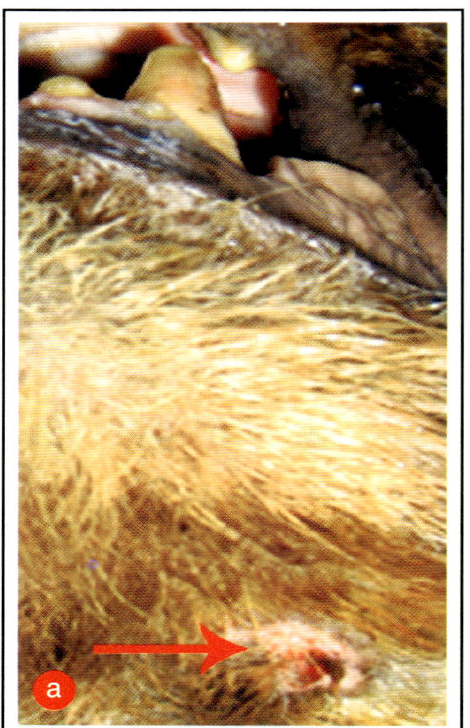

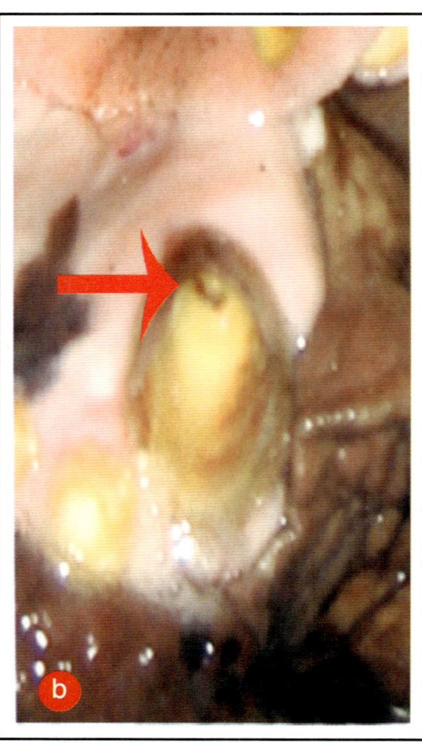

Figure 314: Photographs showing: (a) Fistula below the chin connecting to right canine tooth (b) in hybrid lioness (*P. leo*) at Biological Park,Patna (Bihar).

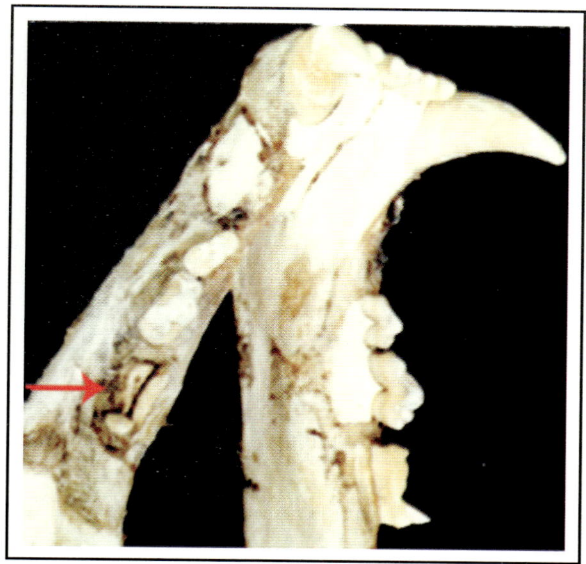

Figure 315: Photograph of mandible of captive tiger (*P. tigris*) showing damaged left carnassial tooth (M_1).

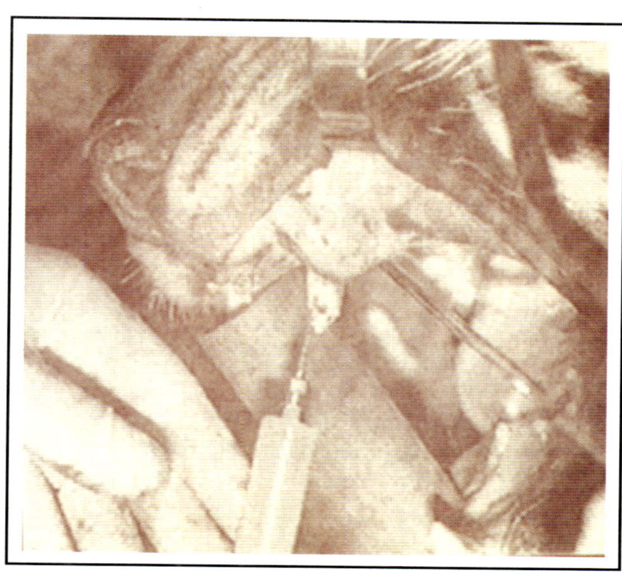

Figure 316: Photograph showing root canal treatment in tiger (*P. tigris*) at Zoological Garden, Pune (Gorhe, 1991).

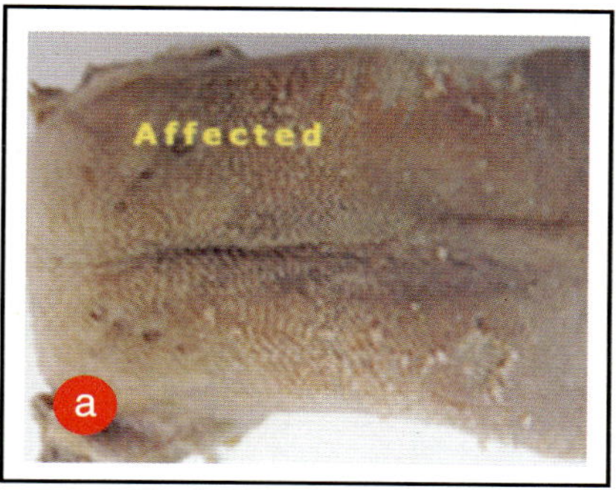

Case (i)

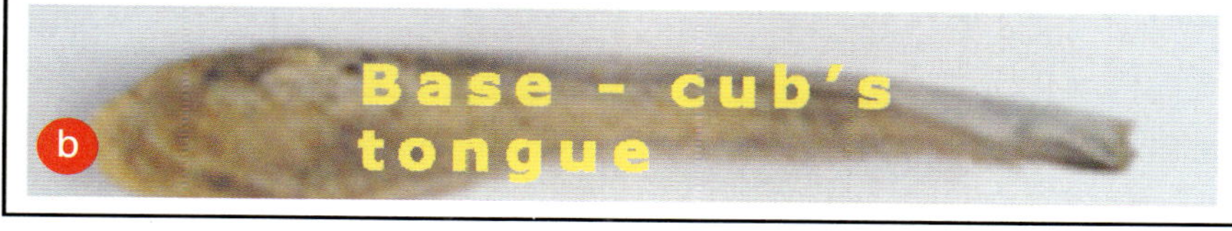

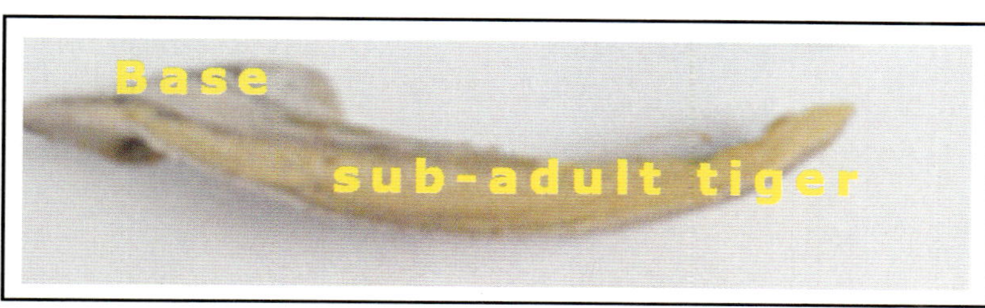

Case (ii)

Case (iii)

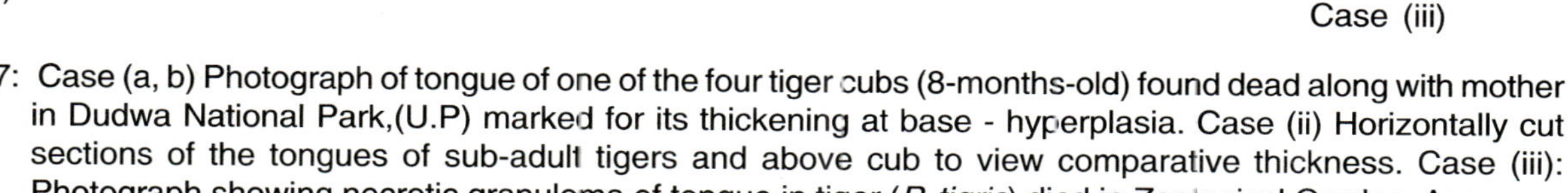

Figure 317: Case (a, b) Photograph of tongue of one of the four tiger cubs (8-months-old) found dead along with mother in Dudwa National Park,(U.P) marked for its thickening at base - hyperplasia. Case (ii) Horizontally cut sections of the tongues of sub-adult tigers and above cub to view comparative thickness. Case (iii): Photograph showing necrotic granuloma of tongue in tiger (*P. tigris*) died in Zoological Garden, Assam.

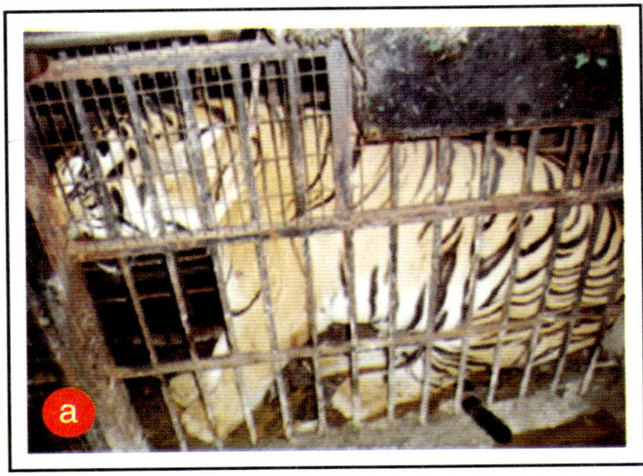

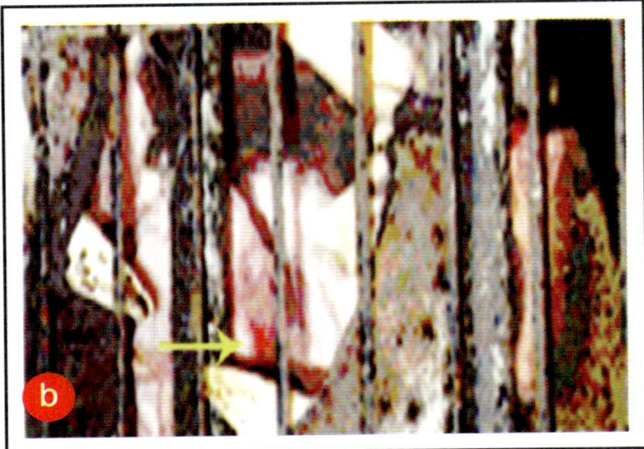

Figure 318: (a) Tiger (*P. tigris*) belonged to Tayarekoppa Wild life Sanctuary, Shimoga, (Karnataka) suffering from Calci virus infection. (b) The lesions included bleeding ulcers on tongue and hard palate. (Courtesy: Harish, B. R. & Kallappa, S.).

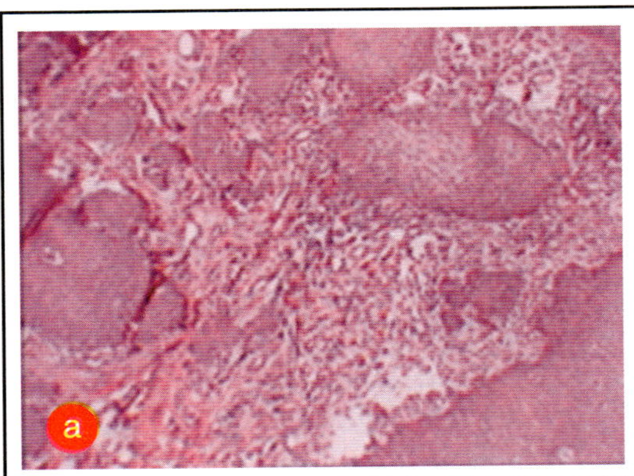

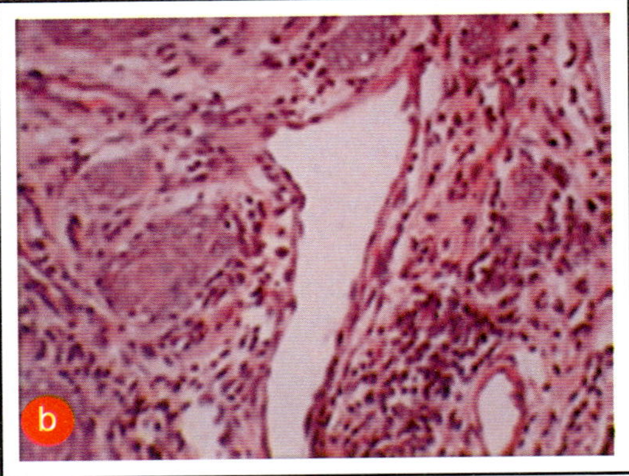

Figure 319: (a) Section of growth from oral cavity of leopard (*P. pardus*) diagnosed as fibropapilloma.H&E,x100 (b) Photomicrograph showing proliferation of epithelial cells extending deeply into the fibromatous center. H&E, x400

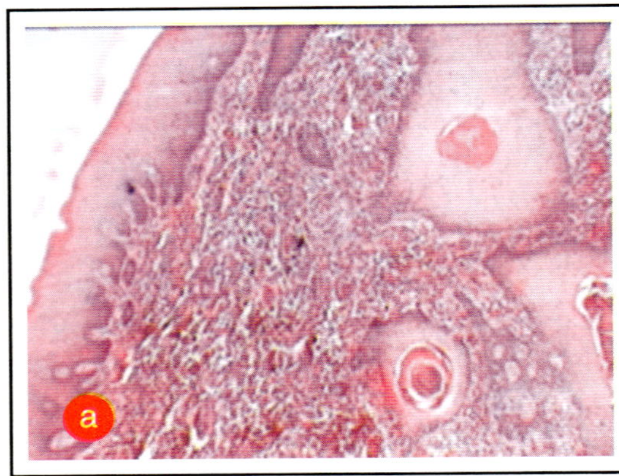

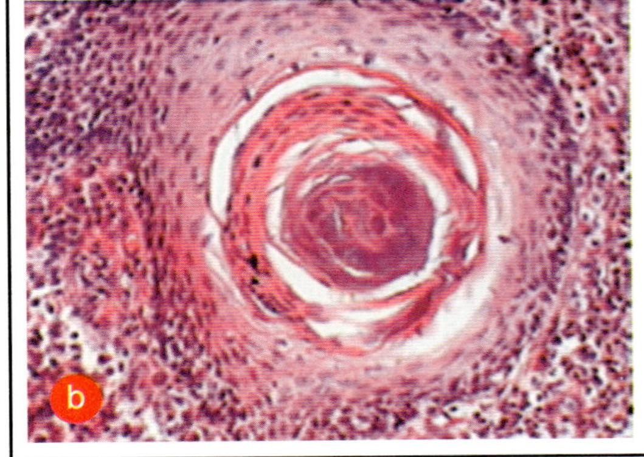

Figure 320: Photomicrograph of growth from oral cavity of tiger (*P. tigris*) died in captivity showing squamous cell carcinoma. Cells resembling normal squamous epithelium however, the pattern of growth was disorganized and formation of epithelial pearls. (a) H&E,x100(b) H&E,x400

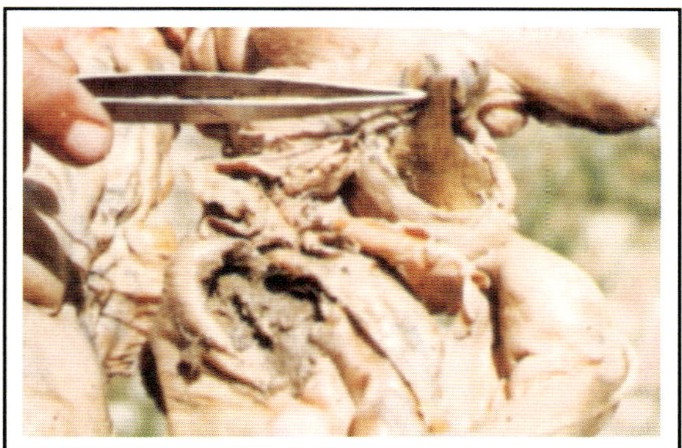

Figure 321: Perforation of intestine of Tiger (*P. tigris*) caused by bone ingested with beef.

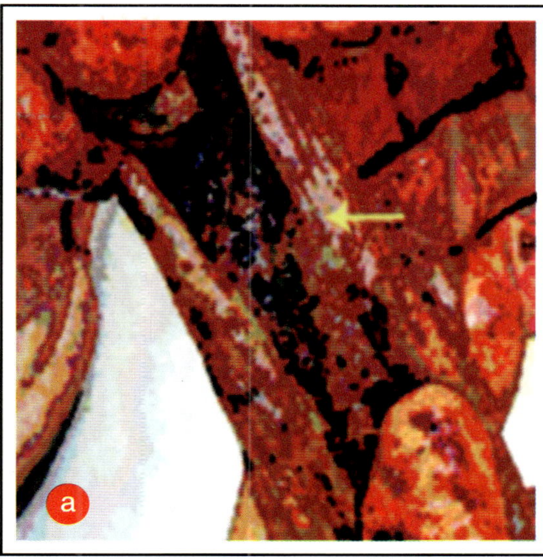

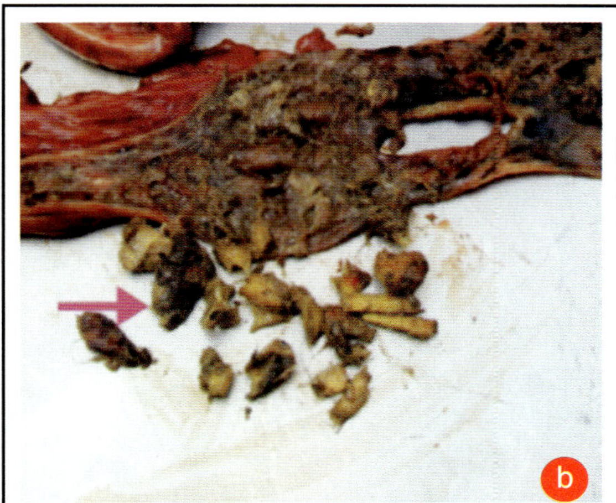

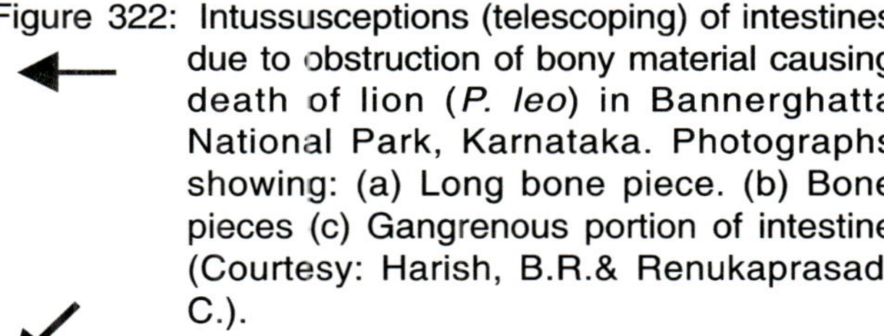

Figure 322: Intussusceptions (telescoping) of intestines due to obstruction of bony material causing death of lion (*P. leo*) in Bannerghatta National Park, Karnataka. Photographs showing: (a) Long bone piece. (b) Bone pieces (c) Gangrenous portion of intestine (Courtesy: Harish, B.R.& Renukaprasad, C.).

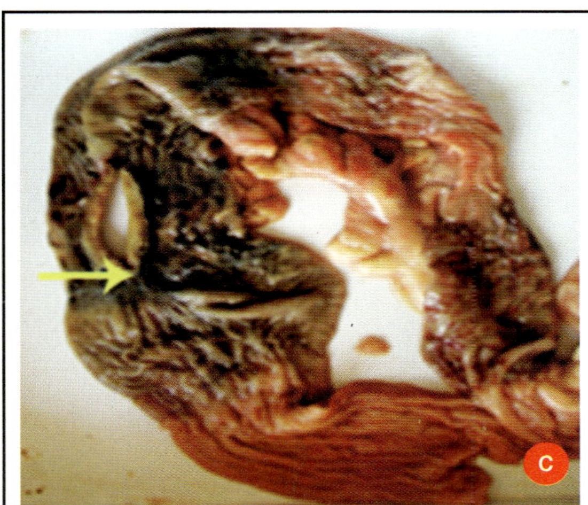

Figure323. Photograph of stomach of panther (*P. pardus*) showing mass of its own hair licked and and ingested. The animal had suppurative lesions over the surface of the body.

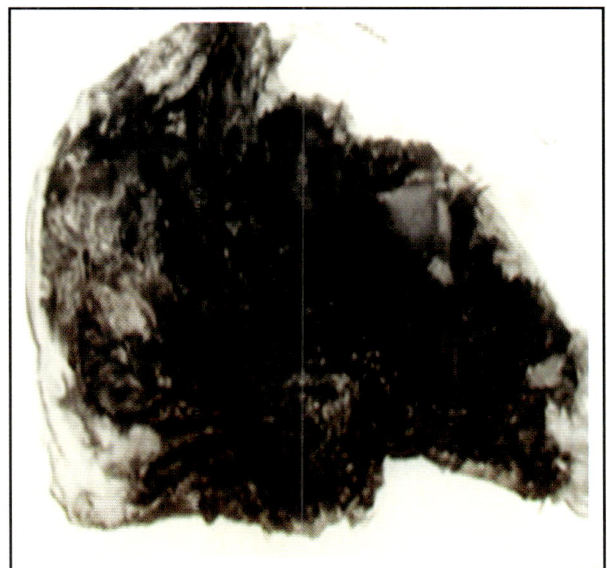

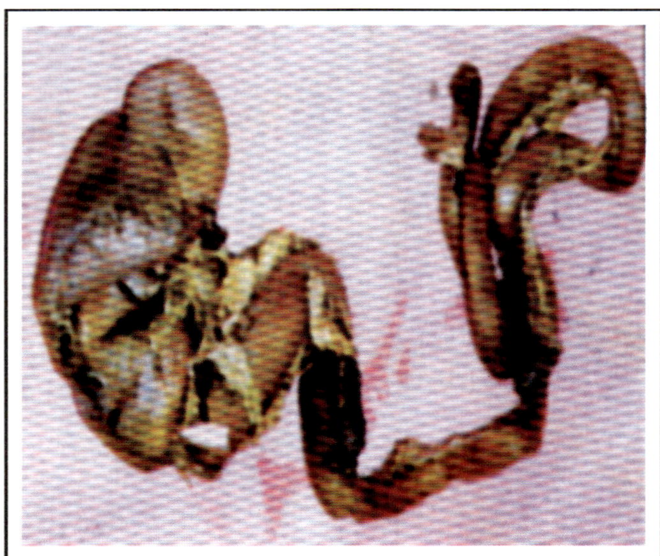

Figure 324: Photograph showing invagination of anterior segment of duodenum into pylorus in leopard (*P. pardus*) which had died in captivity (Courtesy: Srivastava, A.B.).

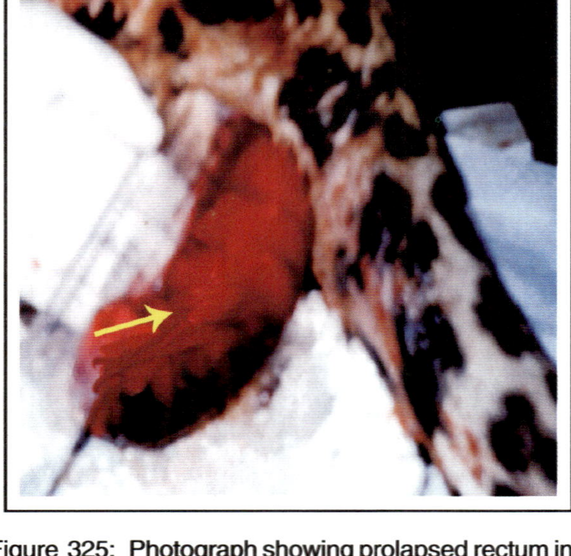

Figure 325: Photograph showing prolapsed rectum in leopard (*P. pardus*) belonging to Bannerghatta Biological Park. (Courtesy: Murthy. S.).

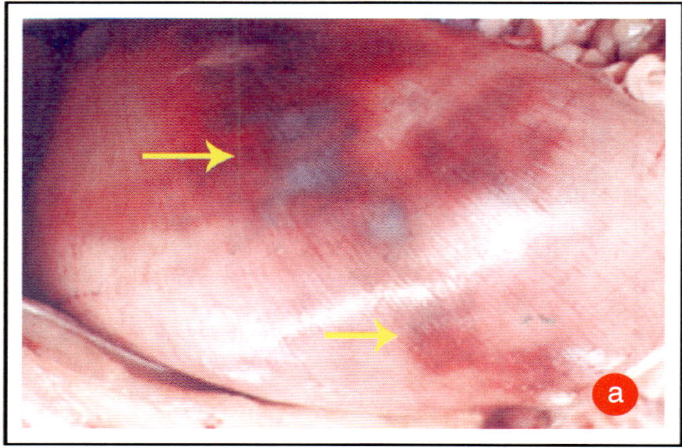

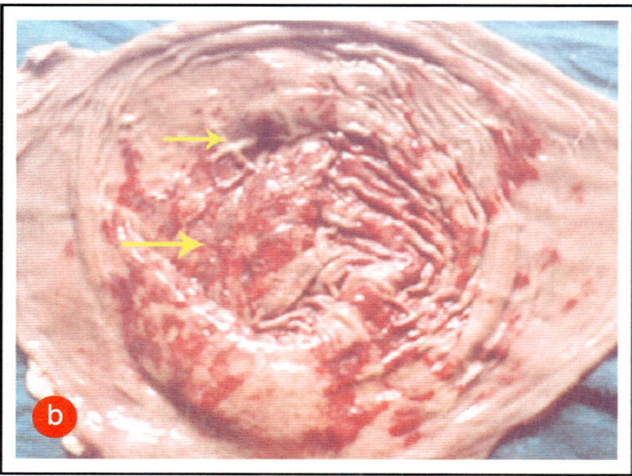

Figure 326: Carbamate poisoning in leopard (*P. pardus*). Photographs showing haemorrhagic lesions on: (a)Serosal surface of stomach. (b) Stomach mucosa (Courtesy: Suryawanshi, D.S.).

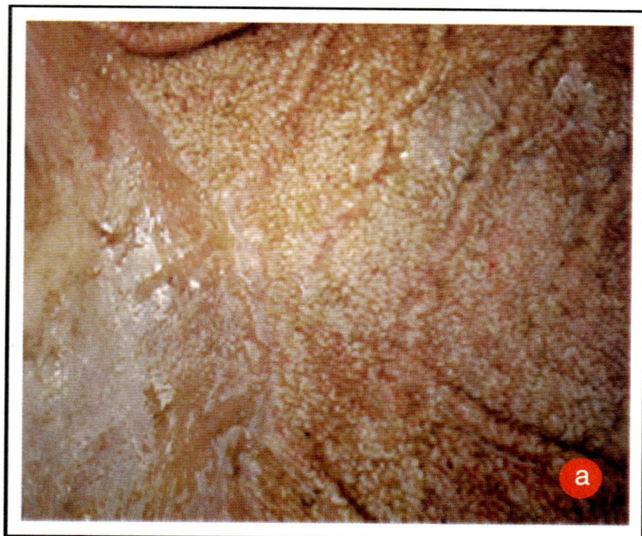

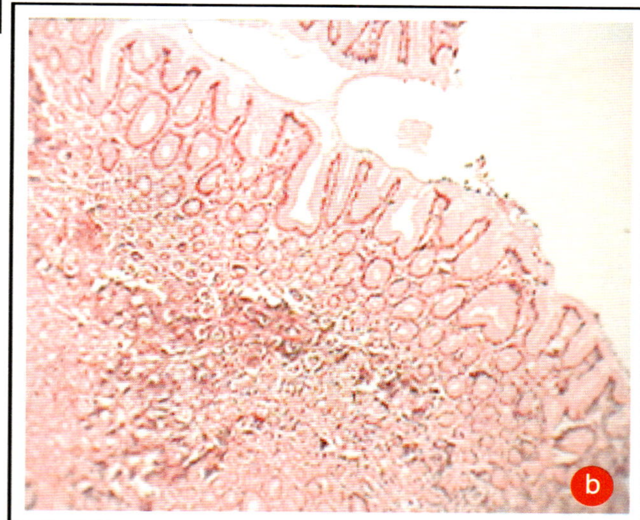

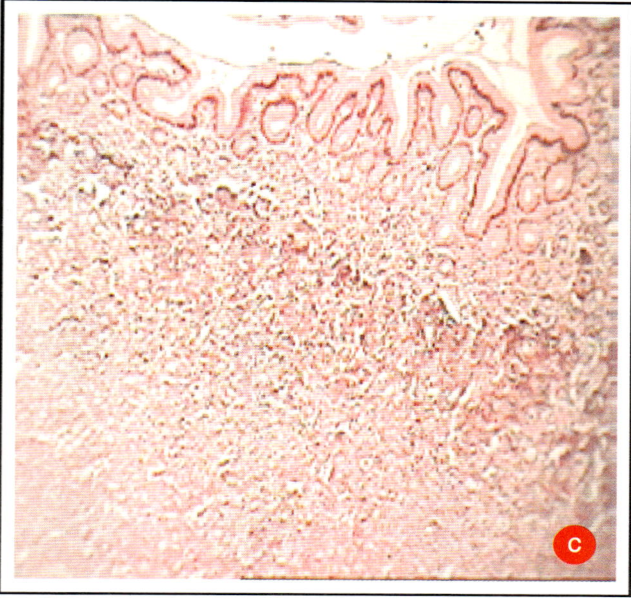

Figure 327: (a) Stomach mucosa showing congestion and focal areas of ulcerations encountered in Siberian tiger (*P. t. altacia*) died in captivity. (b, c) Photomicrographs of(a) showing mild erosions and ulcerations of gastric mucosa H & E, x 100. The condition was related to NTN component (Arun A. Sha *et al.*, 2007).

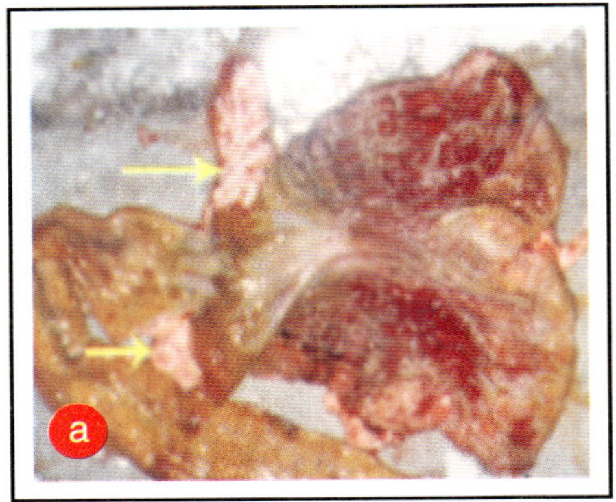

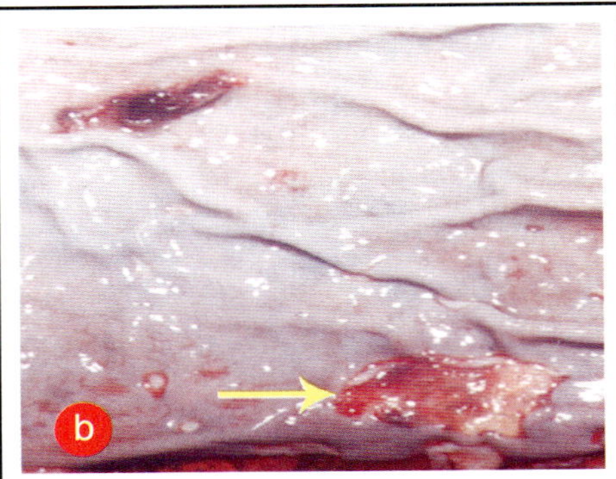

Figure 328: Photographs (a, b) showing uremic ulcers in mucosa of stomach and duodenum encountered in tiger (*P. tigris*) died in captivity (Courtesy: Suryawanshi, D.S.).

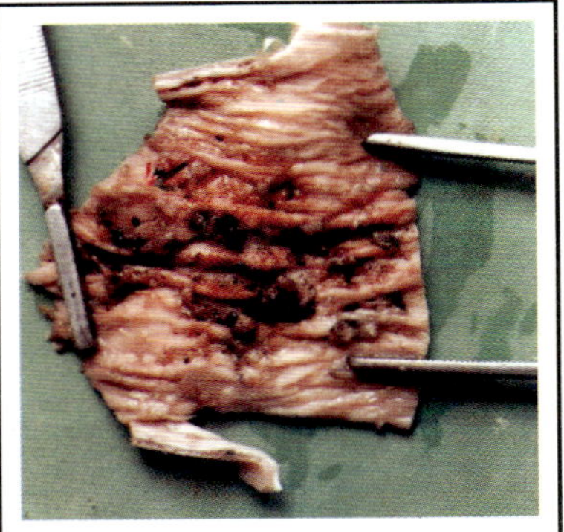

Figure 329: Ulcer in the stomach of lion (*P. leo*).

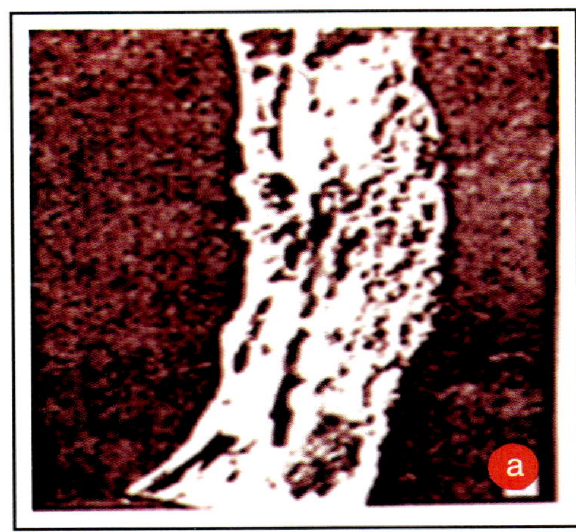

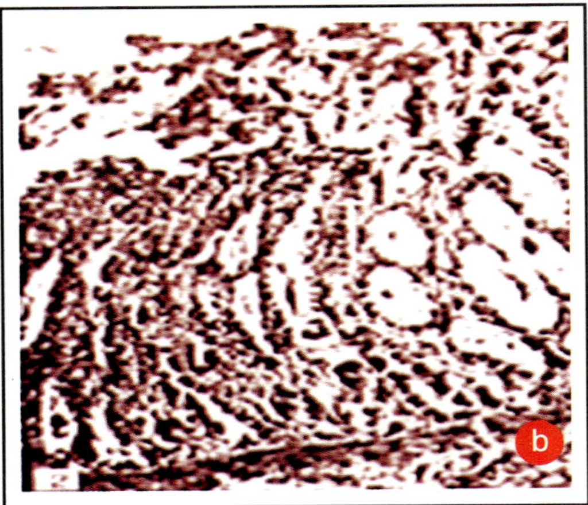

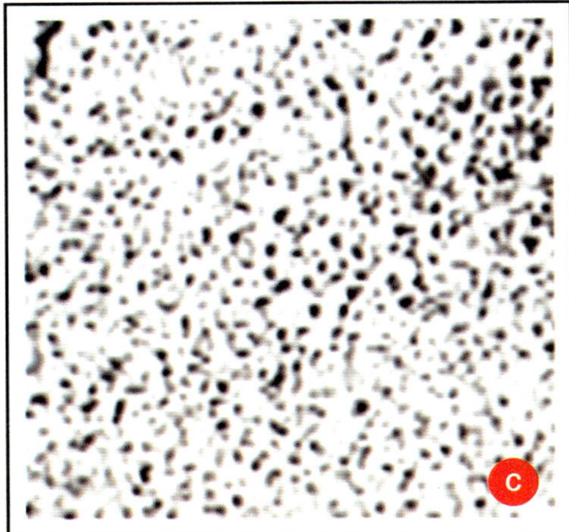

Figure 330: (a) Infectious feline enteritis in panther cub (*P. pardus*). (a) Photograph showing diphtheritic inflammation of mucosa of colon. (b) Photomicrograph showing degeneration and desquamation of intestinal epithelial lining. H&E, x100 (c) Photomicrograph showing severe necrosis and loss of cord arrangement in liver. H&E, x100 (Singh *et al*., 1983).

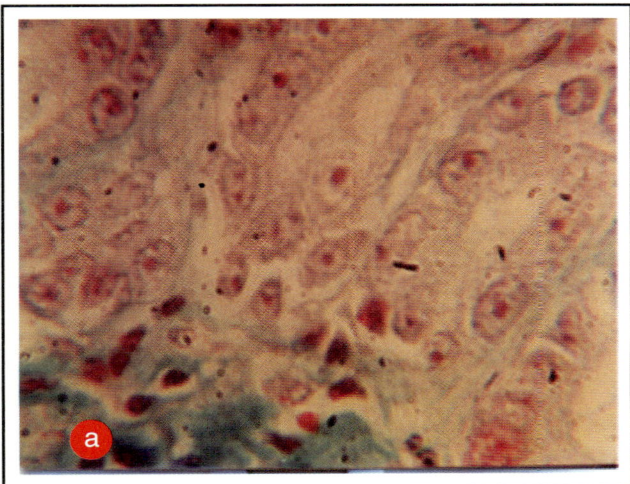

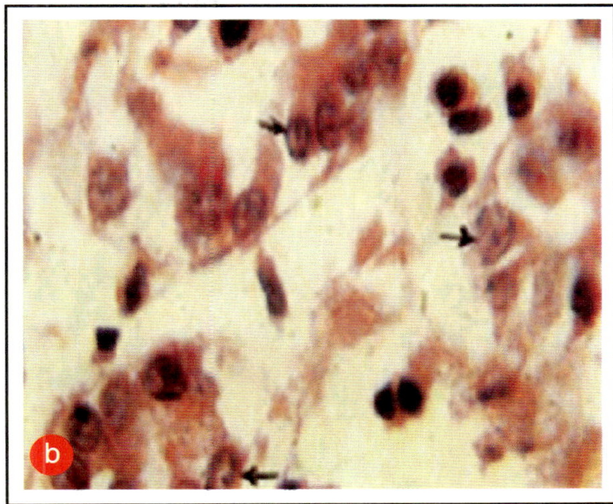

Figure 331: Feline panleucopenia in tigers (*P. tigris*) died in captivity. Photomicrographs (a, b) showing intranuclear inclusion bodies in the intestinal epithelium H & E x 1000. Courtesy: (a) Garg, U.K. (b) Srivastava, A.B.

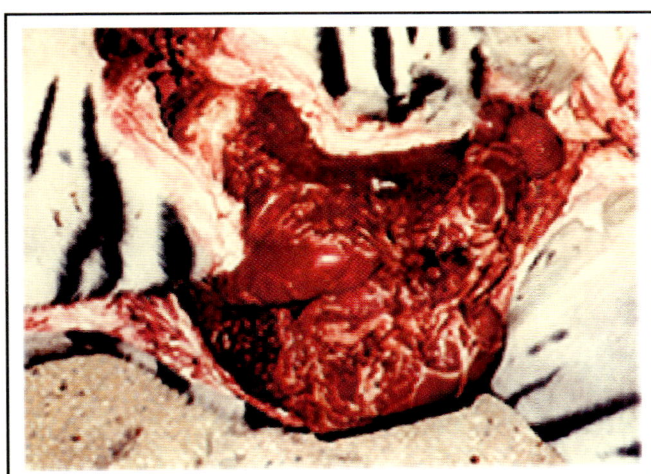

Figure 332: Photograph showing severe haemorrhagic peritonitis(specific cause remained undermined) encountered in tiger (*P. tigris*) died in National Park,Dudwa (U.P.).

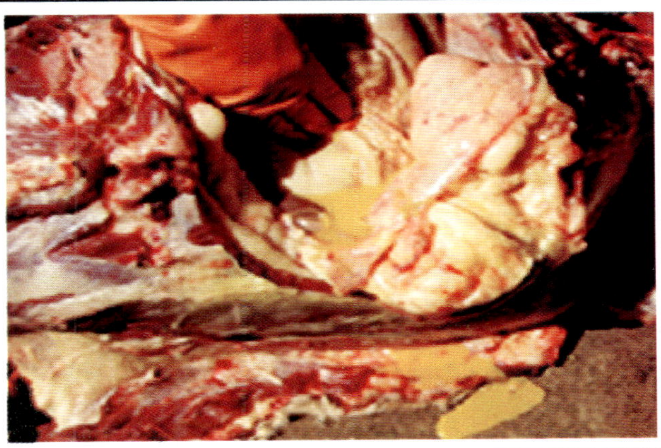

Figure 333: Photograph showing peritonitis in lion (*P. leo*) died in captivity.(Courtesy: Harish, B.R.).

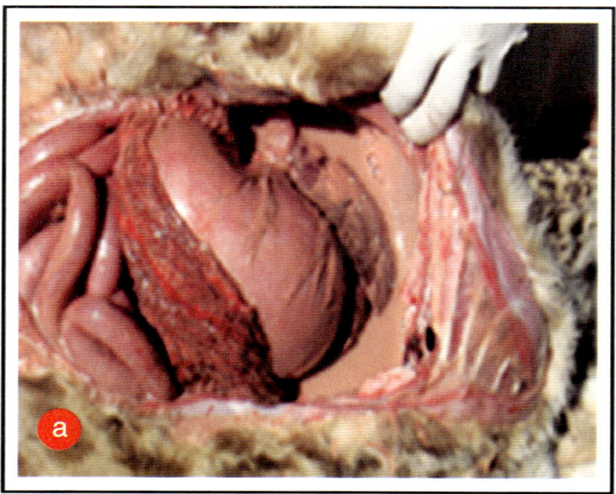

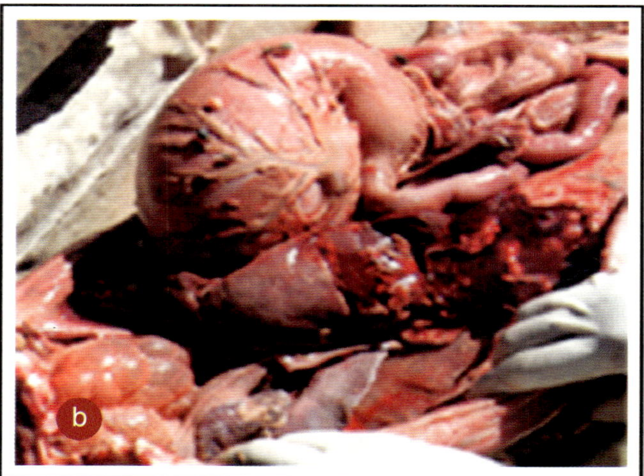

Figure 334: Photographs (a, b) showing suppurative peritonitis in wild leopard (*P. pardus*) died at Rescue Centre, Kaziranga, Assam (Courtesy: Boro, P.K).

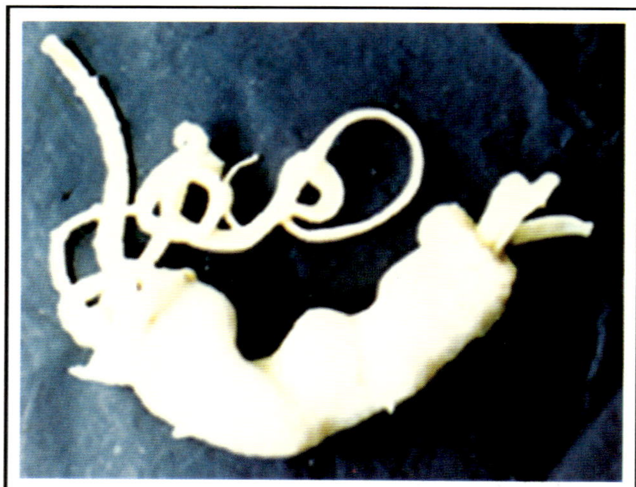

Figure 335: Photograph showing intestine of wild leopard (*P. pardus*) packed with tapeworms died in the forests of Uttarakhand.

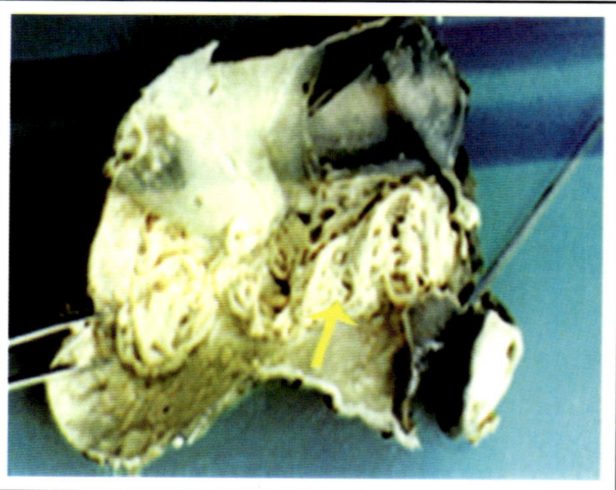

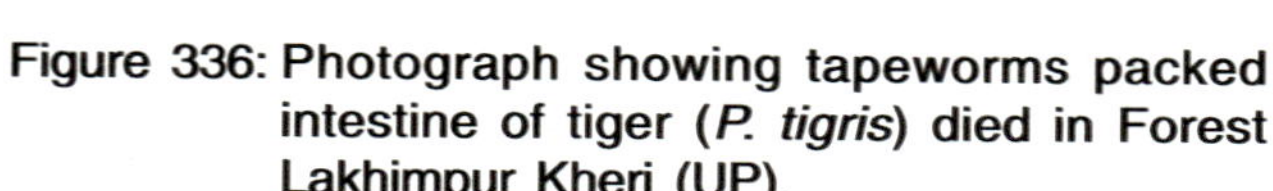

Figure 336: Photograph showing tapeworms packed intestine of tiger (*P. tigris*) died in Forest Lakhimpur Kheri (UP).

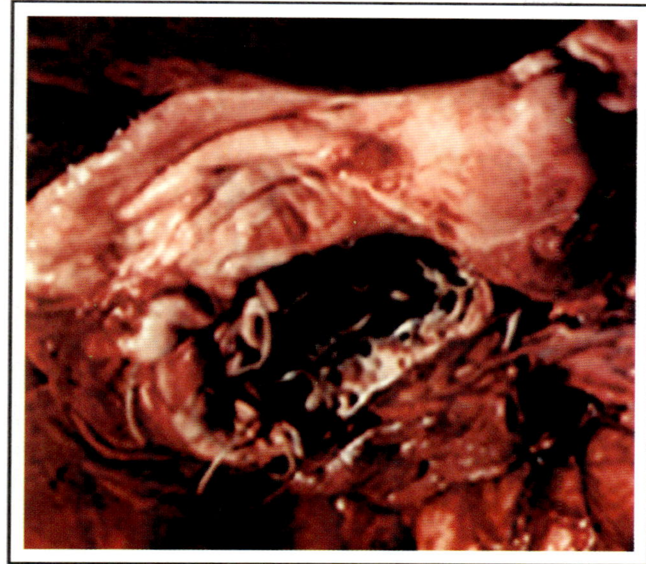

Figure 337: Photograph showing *Physaloptera* sp. and *Toxocara cati* impacting stomach of wild tigress. The case is also referred under respiratory system.

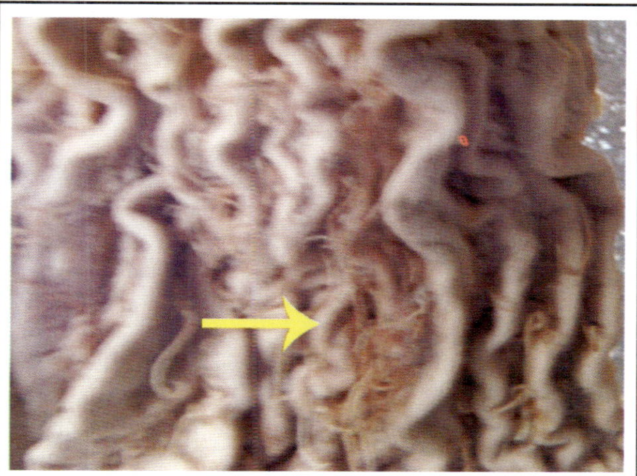

Figure 338: Intestine of lion (*P. leo*) showing round worms. (Courtesy: Dept of Pathology, CVSc, Nagpur, M.S).

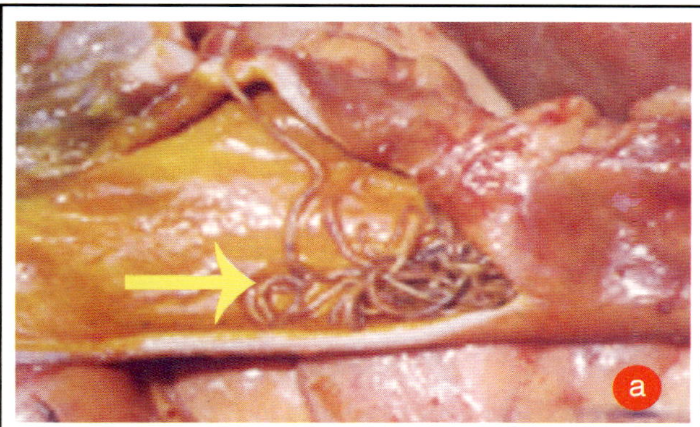

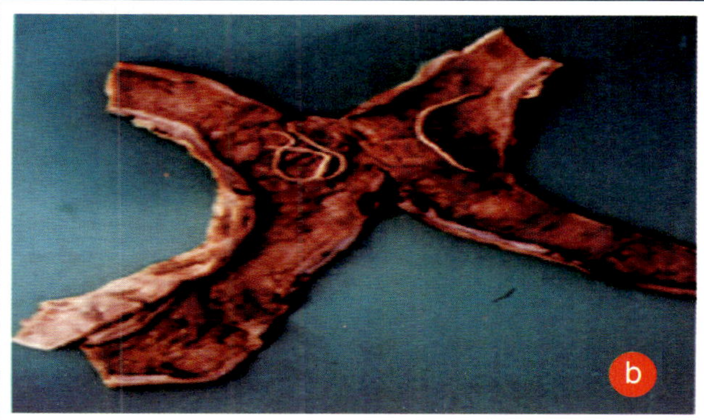

Figure 339: Photographs showing roundworms in the intestine of tigers (*P. tigris*) died in capacity (a) captivity and (b) wild.

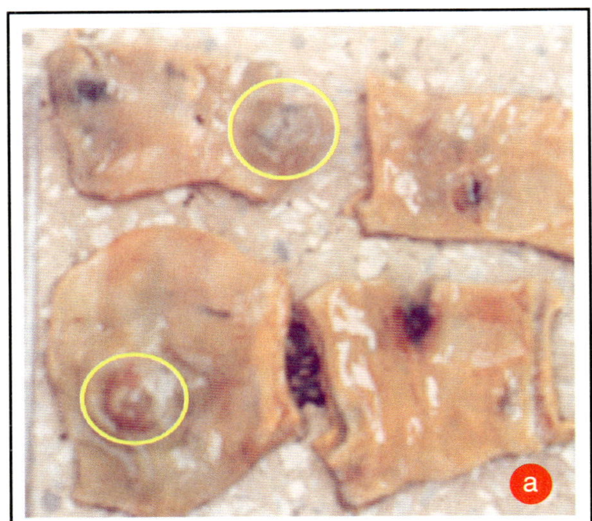

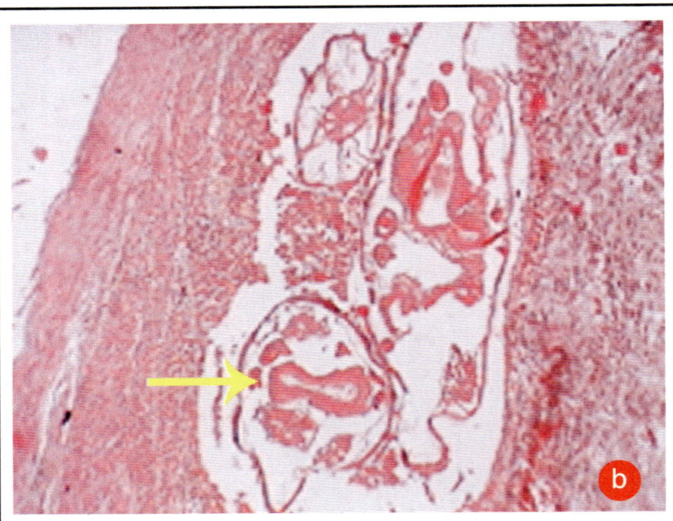

Figure 340: (a) Photograph showing *Galonocus pernisiosus* nodules in the intestine of tiger (*P. tigris*) died in captivity. (b) Photomicrograph of(a) showing cross section of *Galonocus pernisiosus* in the necrotic debris. H&E, x100.

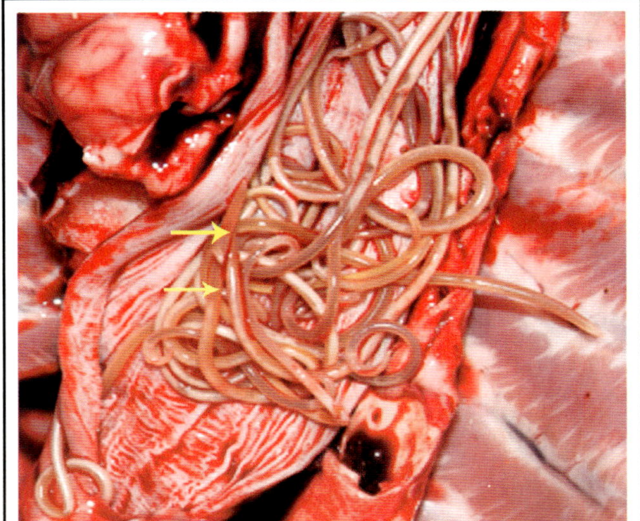

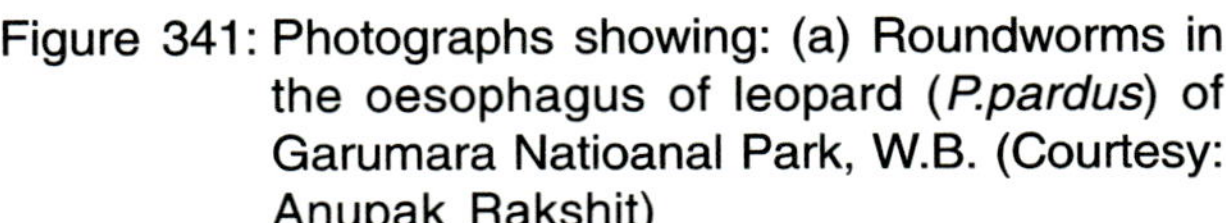

Figure 341: Photographs showing: (a) Roundworms in the oesophagus of leopard (*P.pardus*) of Garumara Natioanal Park, W.B. (Courtesy: Anupak Rakshit)

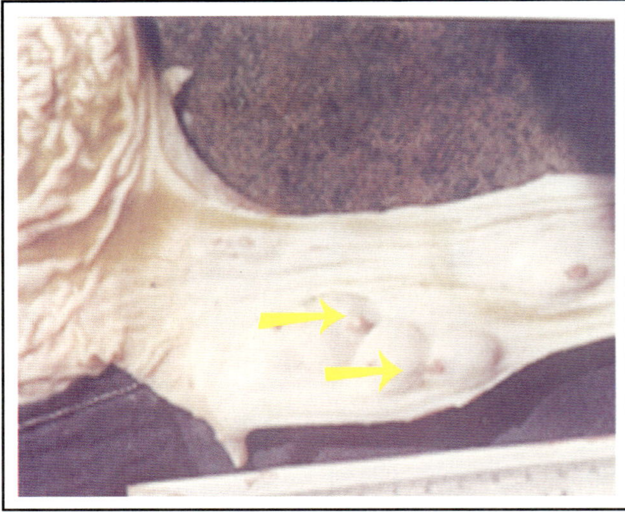

Figure 342. *Spirocercus lupi* infestation causing nodular masses in the oesophagus of leopard (*P. pardus*) of Zoological Garden, Guwahati (Assam).

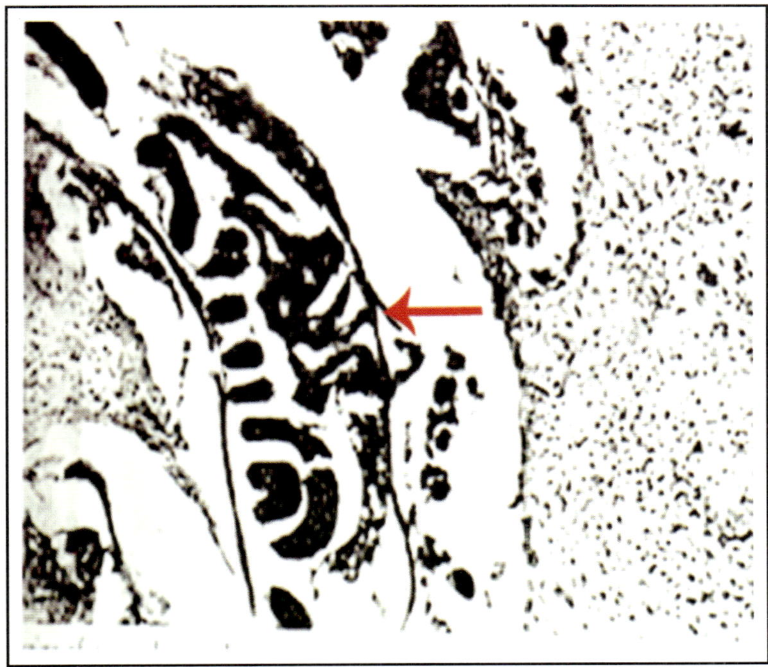

Figure 343: Photomicrograph of intestine of leopard (*P. pardus*) showing nematode sections in submucosa surrounded by a chronic inflammatory reaction. H&E, x 100 (Singh. *et al.*, 1981).

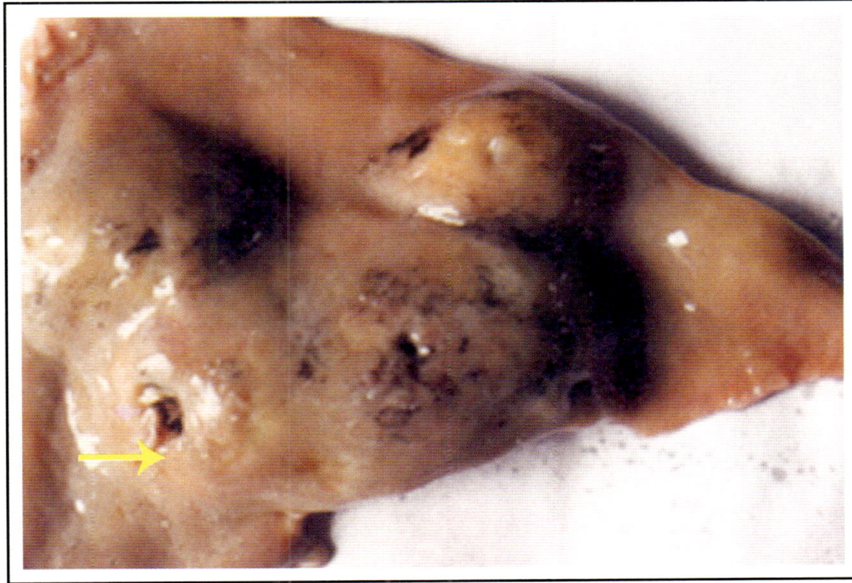

Figure 344: Photograph showing *Gnathostomum* sp. nodules in the stomach of Leopard (*P. pardus*) died in Zoological Garden, Mumbai (Courtesy: Suryawanshi, D.S.).

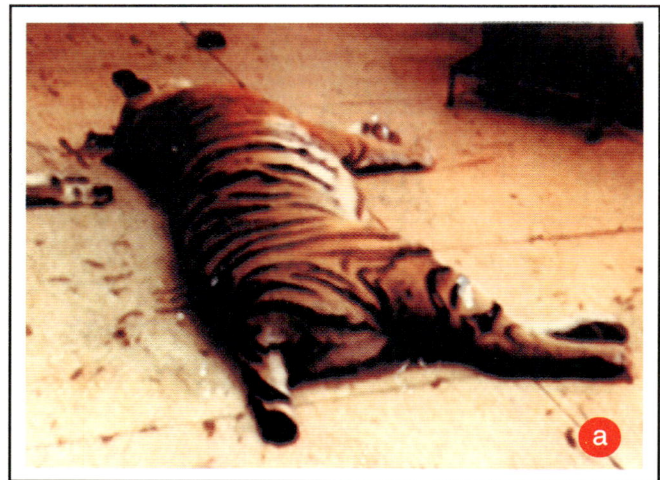

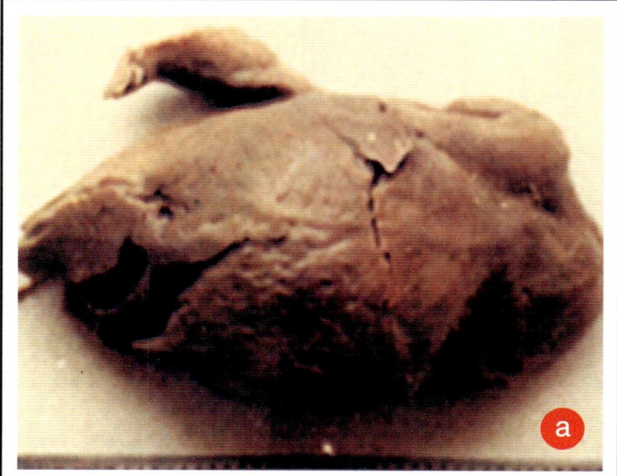

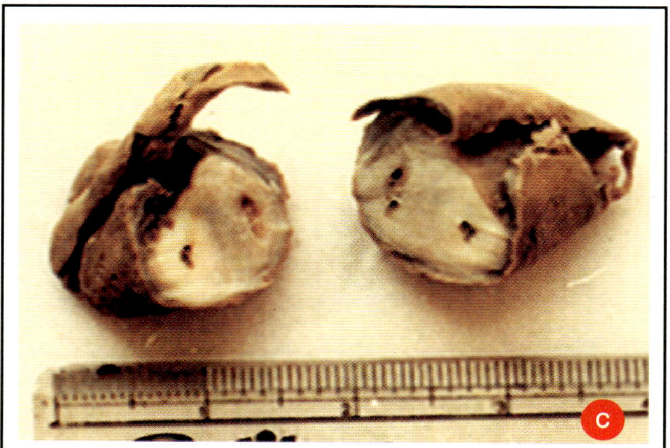

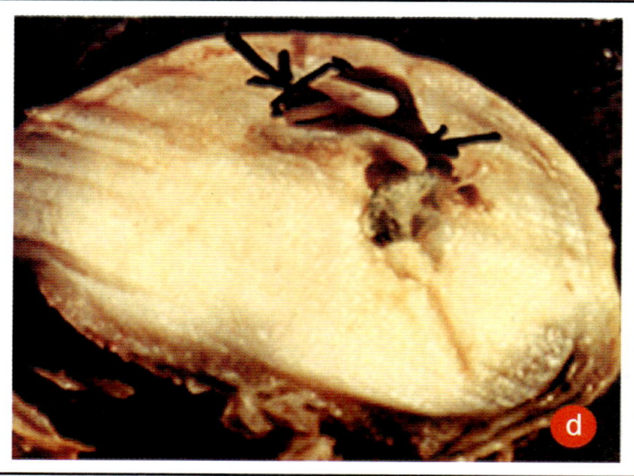

Figure 345: (a) Carcass of an adult tiger . (b) Gastric nodules encountered in (a) caused by *Gnathostomum spinigerum*. (c)Sections of (b) showing parasitic tunnels. (d) *Gnathostomum spinigerum* lying in a tunnel.

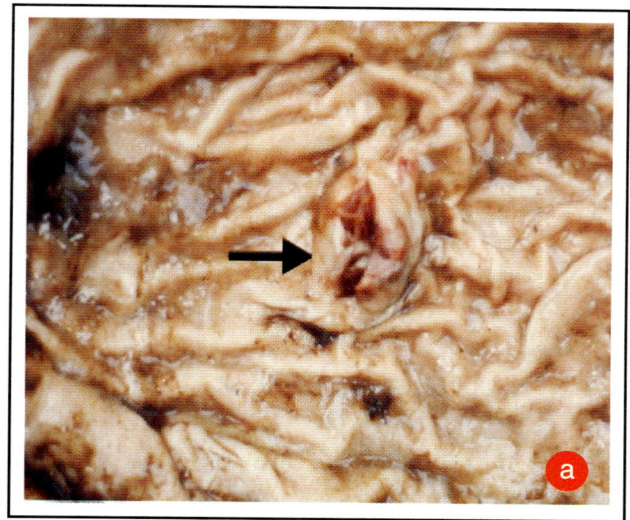

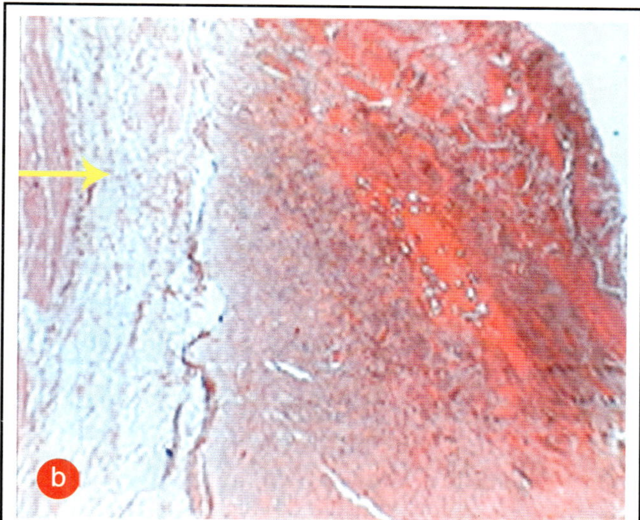

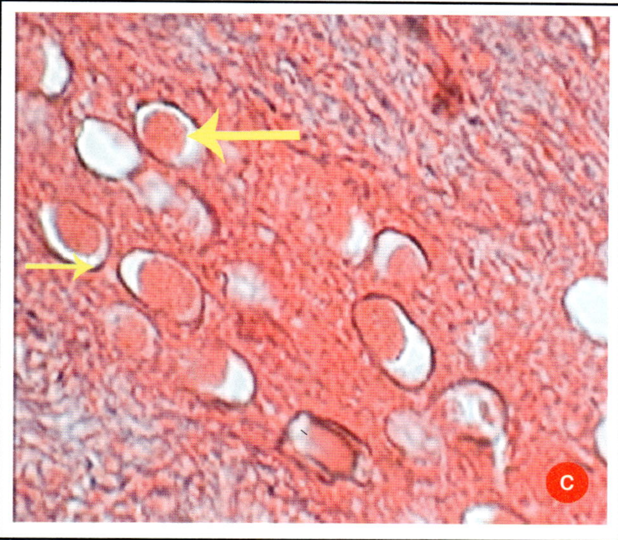

Figure 346: (a) Photograph showing nodules with *Gnasthostomum* sp. in the stomach of tigress (*P. tigris*) died in Manas Tiger Reserve, Assam. Photomicrograph of (a) showing (b) Proliferation of fibrous tissue around nodule where eggs of *Gnathostomum spinigerum* could be seen. H&E, x 40. (c) Eggs of *G. spinigerum* in the nodule. H&E, x 400.

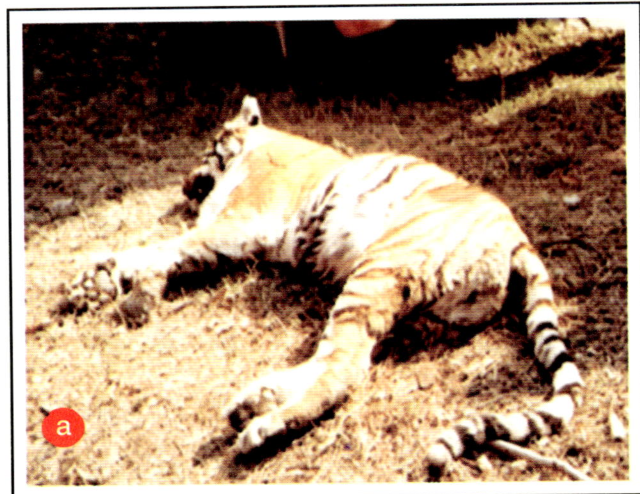

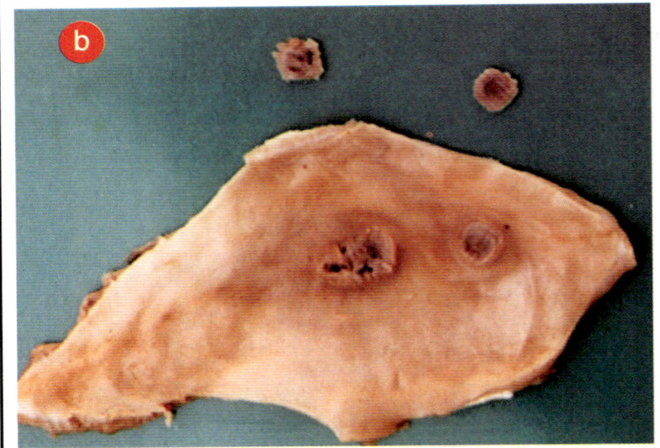

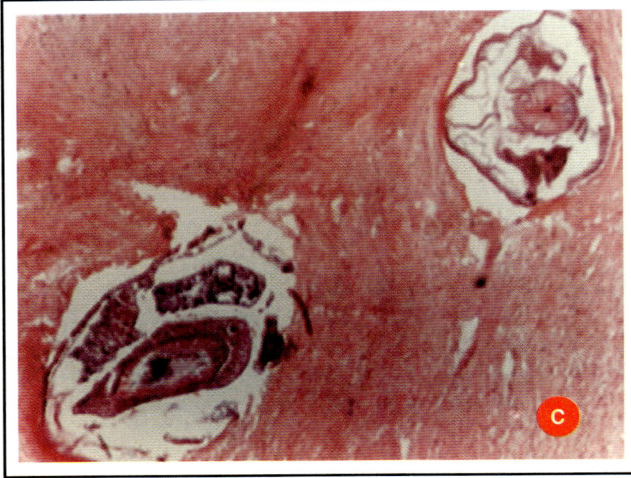

Figure 347: (a) Carcass of sub-adult tigress (25.1.2002) died in Dudwa N.P. (b) Its necropsy showed intestinal nodules and (c) histological section of the same (procesed by A.K.Sharma) revealed *Gnathostoma* sp. in the nodules encapsulated by fibrous tissue.

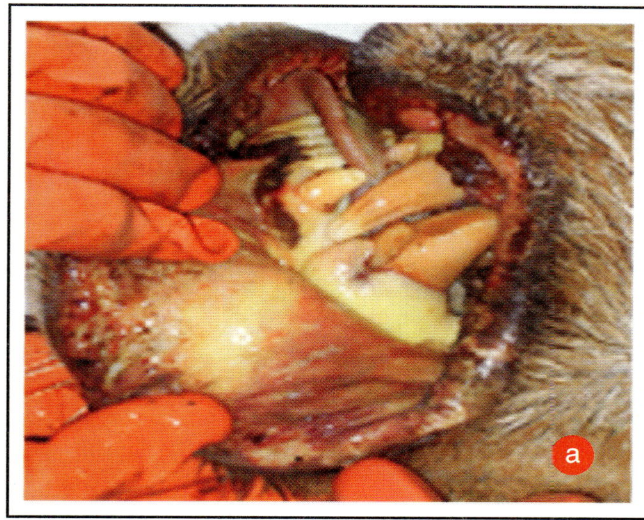

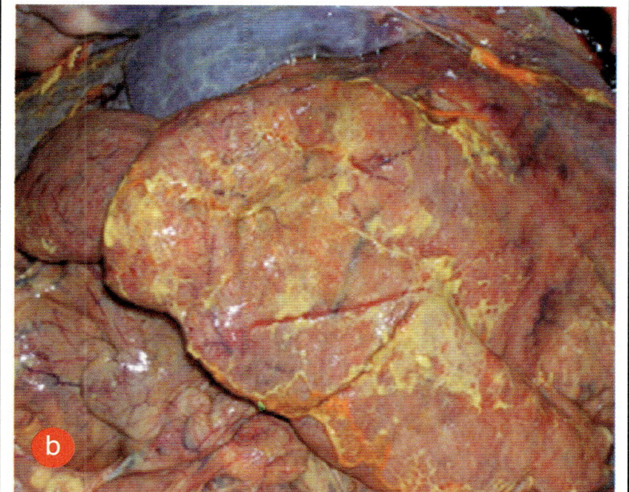

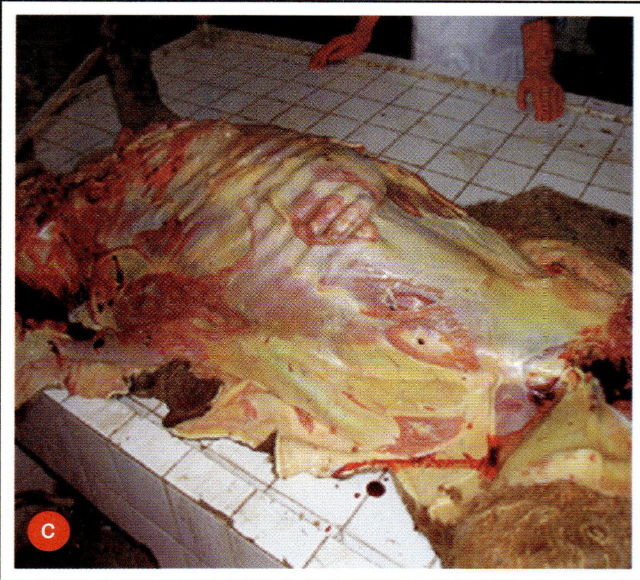

Figure 348: Jaundice diagnosed in lioness (*P. leo*) died in captivity. The gross lesions included: (a) yellowish discoloration of gums and teeth ,(b) liver (hepatitis) and (c) peritonium (peritonitis). (Courtesy: Department of Pathology, CVSc, Bangalore).

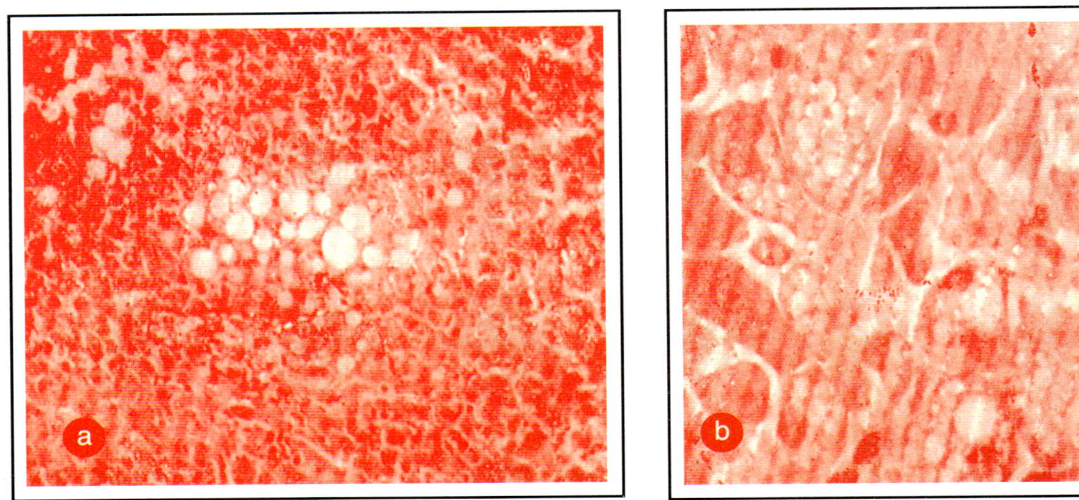

Figure 349: Photomicrographs (a, b) of liver of cheetah (*A. jubatus*) showing fatty changes including lipomatus changes. (Parihar *et al.*, 1976).

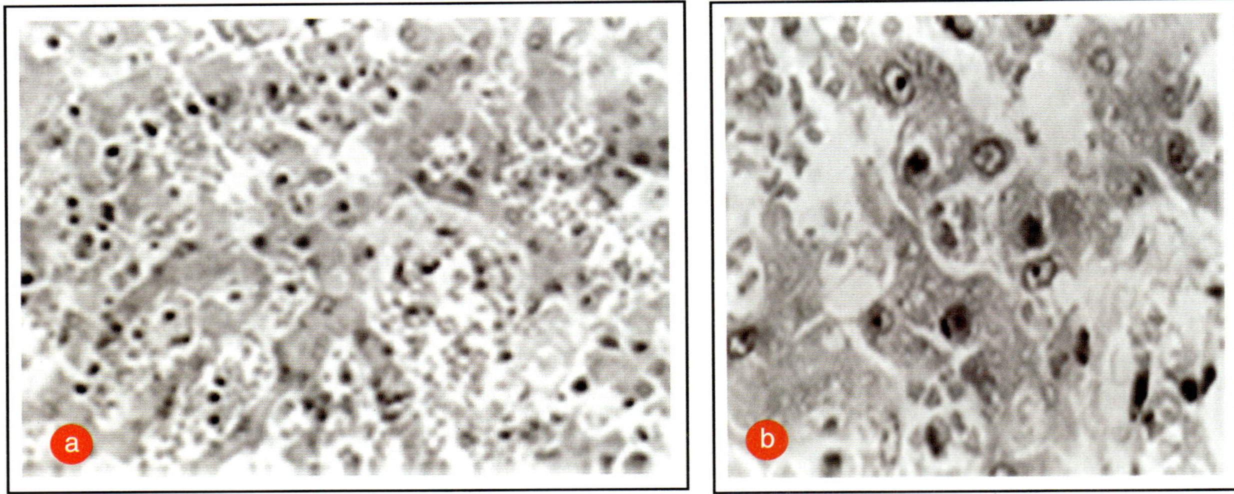

Figure 350: Photomicrographs (a.b) demonstrating intranuclear basophilic inclusions in the hepatic cells (Inclusion body hepatitis) in lion (*P. leo*). (a) H&E, x100. (b) H&E, x400. Clinically animal had showed anorexia and icterus. (Courtesy: Lal Kishan & Gupta, V.K).

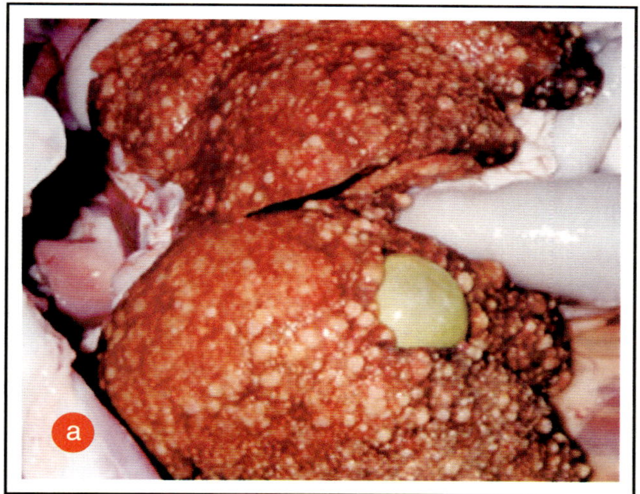

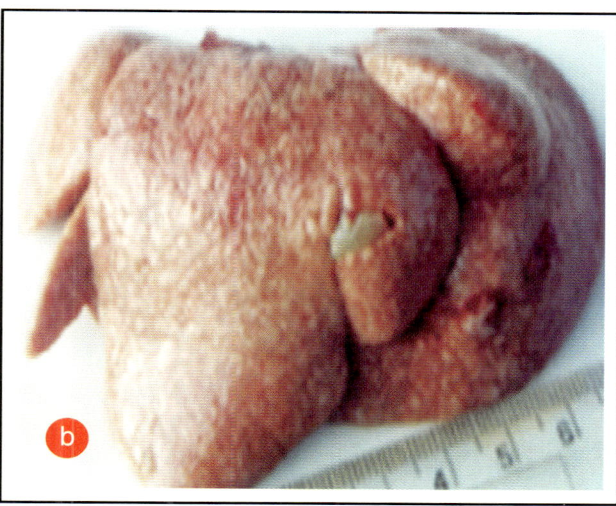

Figure 351: Photograph (a) of cirrhotic liver (Hobnail appearance) of leopard (*P. pardus*). Courtesy: Dept. Pathology, C.V.Sc., Anand,Gujarat. (b) Another case of cirrhotic liver in leopard died at Zoological Garden, Guwahati, Assam.

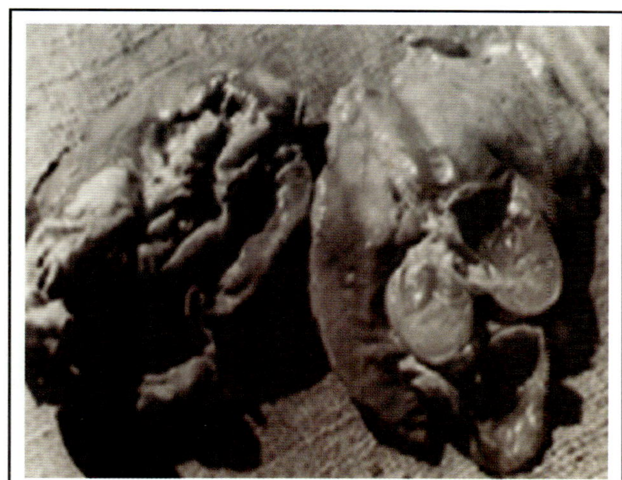

Figure 352: Photograph showing cysts of various sizes on parietal surface of liver of tiger (*P. tigris*) died in captivity.

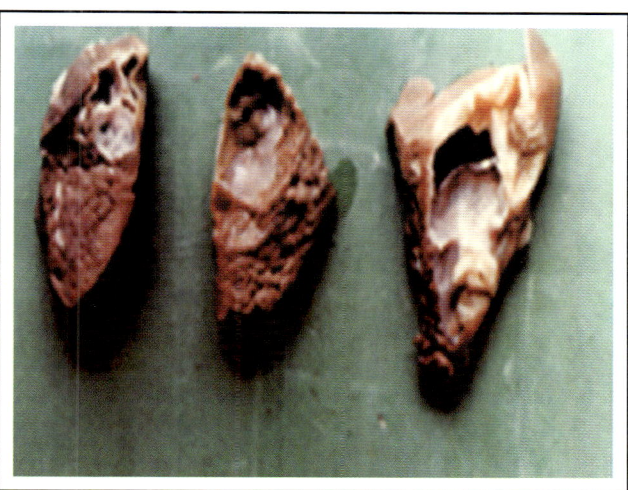

Figure 353: Photograph showing cysts of various sizes in liver of lion (*P. leo*) died in captivity.

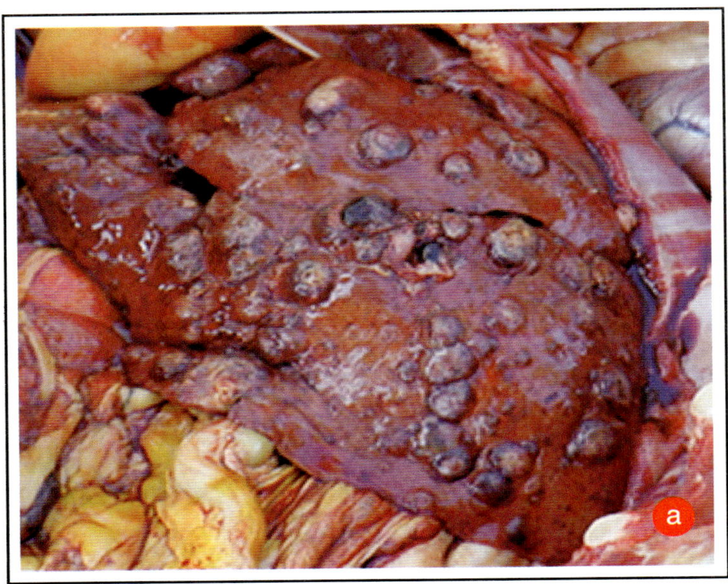

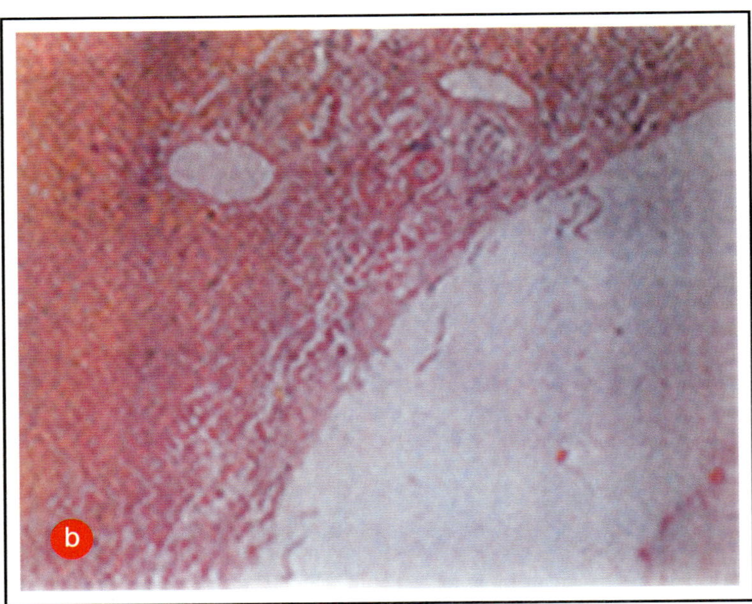

Figure 354: (a) Photograph showing multiloculated cysts (*Echinococcus multilocularis*) in the liver of lioness (*P. leo*) died at Rescue Centre, Chennai, TN. (Courtesy: Thirumurugan, R.). (b) Photomicrograph showing wall of hydatid cyst lined by cuboidal cells along with marked congestion in liver sinusoids encountered in lion (*P. leo persica*) died in captivity. H&E, x10 (Courtesy: Dept.of Wildlife Sci, C.V.Sc., Chennai).

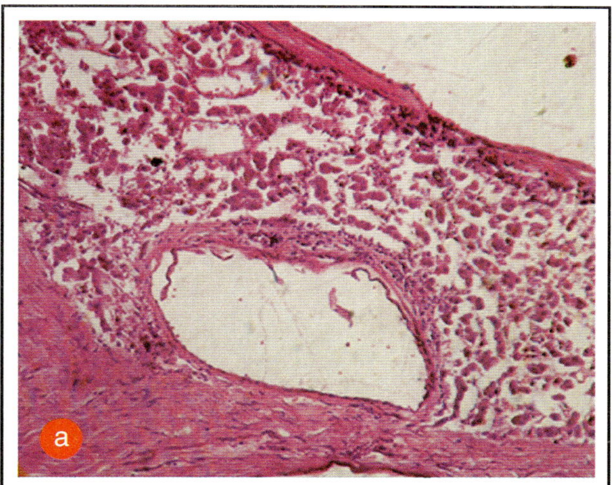

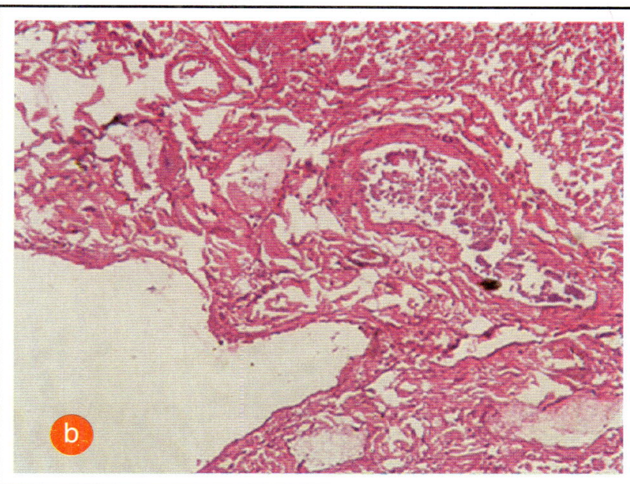

Figure 355: Photomicrographs (a,b) showing cystic liver in lion (*P. leo*) died in captivity (a) H & E, x 200 (b) H & E, x 70 (Courtesy: Dept of Pathology, C.V.Sc., Nagpur).

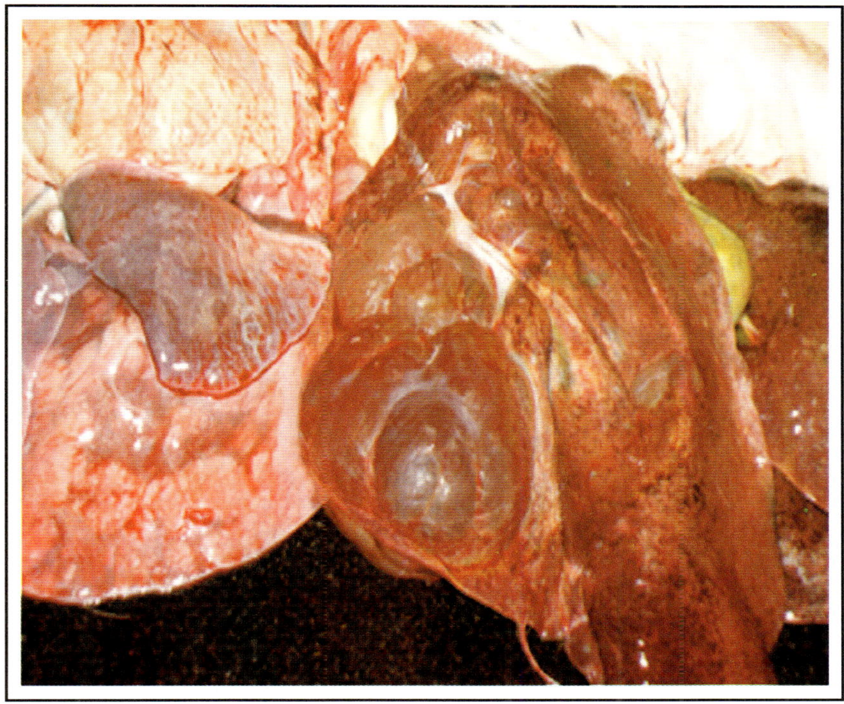

Figure 356: Photograph showing cysts in the liver of leopard (*P. pardus*) died in Zoological garden, Mysore (Courtesy: Nanjappa, K.A.).

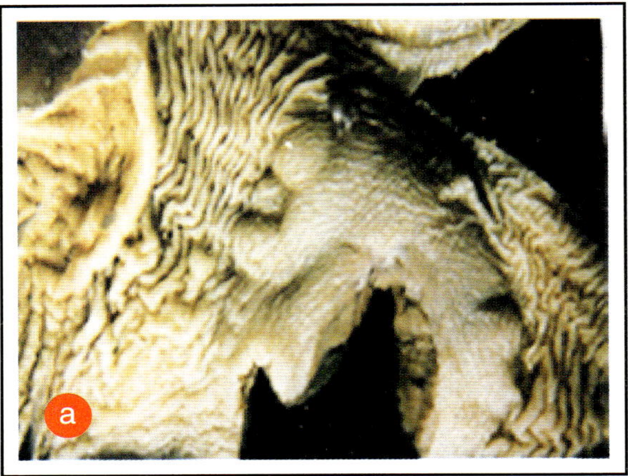

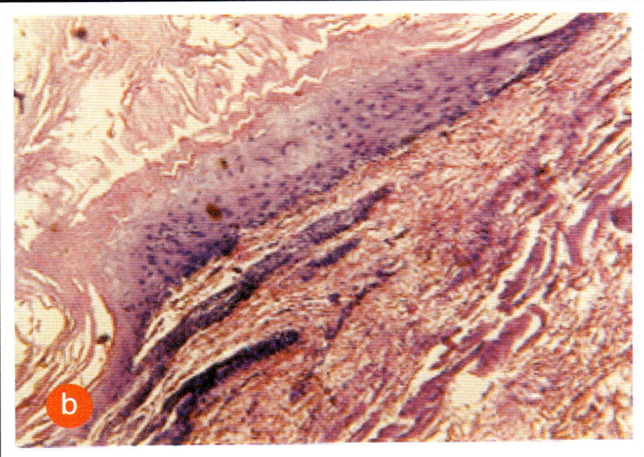

Figure 357: (a) Photograph showing growth in fundic stomach of leopard (*P. pardus*) died in captivity. (b) Photomicrograph of (a) showing changes characteristic of papilloma. H & E x 100 (Nashiruddullah *et al.*, 2007).

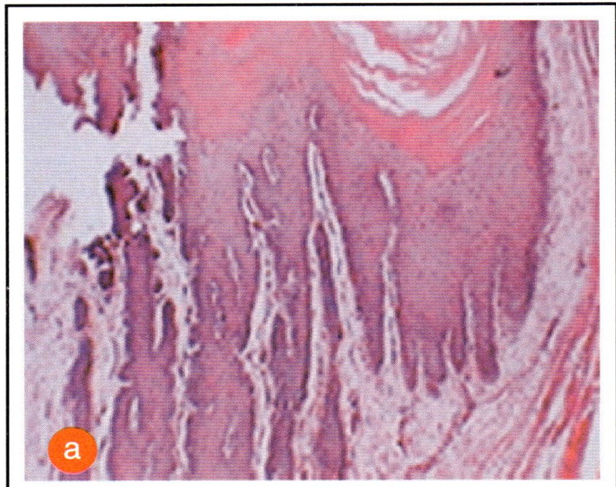

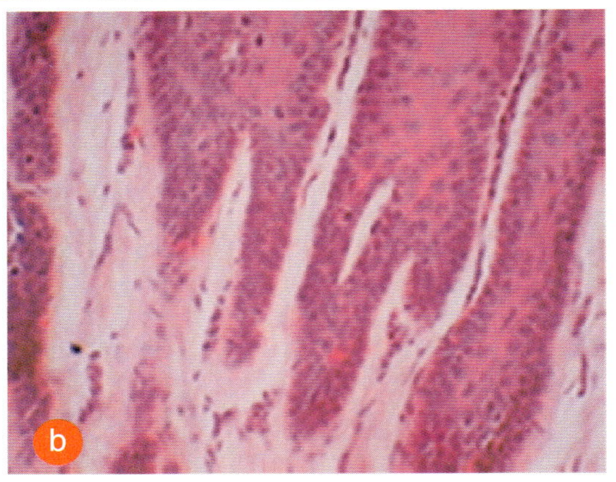

Figure 358: Photomicrograph of stomach growth from panther (*P. pardus*) diagnosed for Papilloma. (a) H&E, x 100 (b) H&E, x 400.

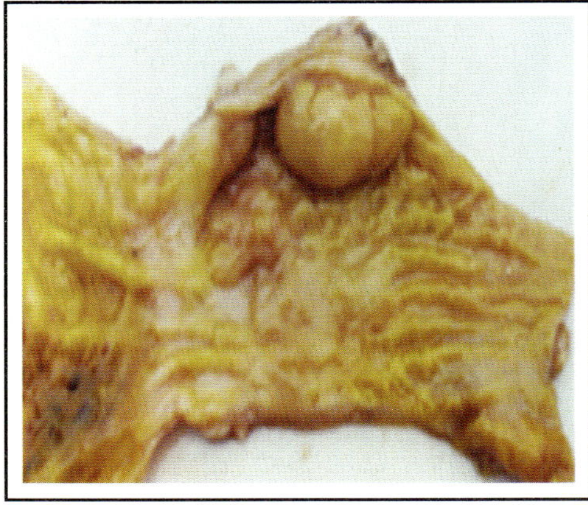

Figure 359: Photograph showing leiomyoma at the base of duodenum in leopard (*P. pardus*).

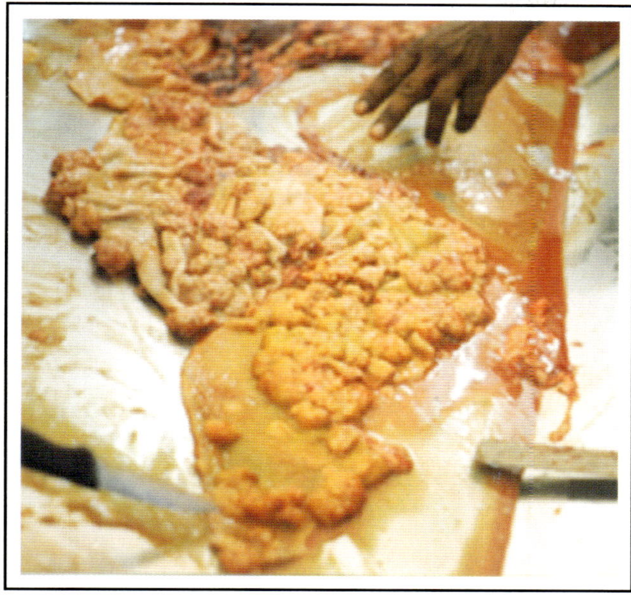

Figure 360: Cauliflower like growth of adenocarcinoma on the mucosa of intestine of lioness (*P. leo persica*) died in captivity(Courtesy: Dept.of Vet. Pathology, C.V.Sc. Tirupati, A.P).

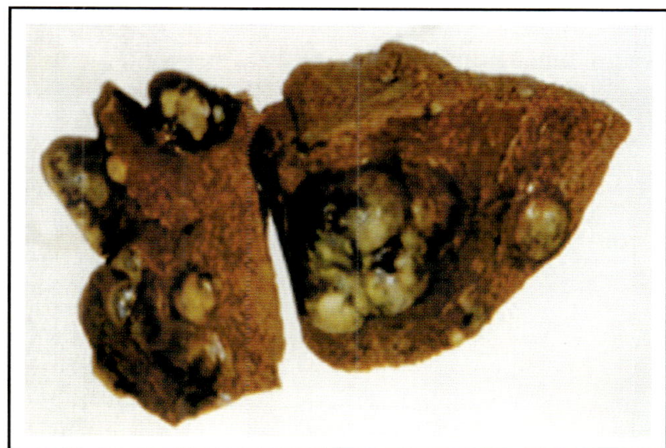

Figure 361: Photograph showing cholengiocellular carcinoma in leopard (*P. pardus*). (Courtesy: Jani, R.G.)

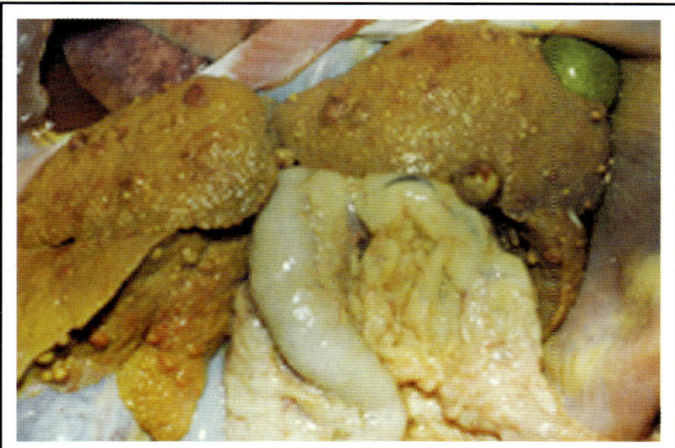

Figure 362: Photograph showing adenocarcinoma of liver in leopard (*P. pardus*) died in captivity.

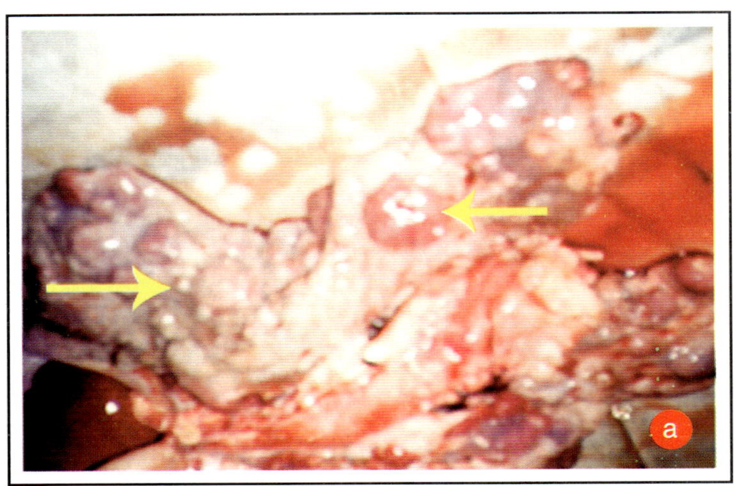

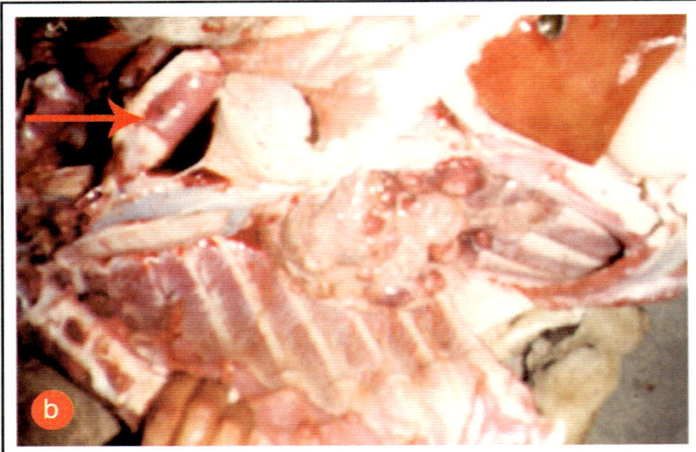

Figure 363: Photographs (a,b) showing metastasis of carcinoma in mesenteric lymph nodes (and lungs) of an Asiatic lioness (*P. leo persica*) died at Zoological Park, Chhatbir,Chandigarh.(Singh, 2004).

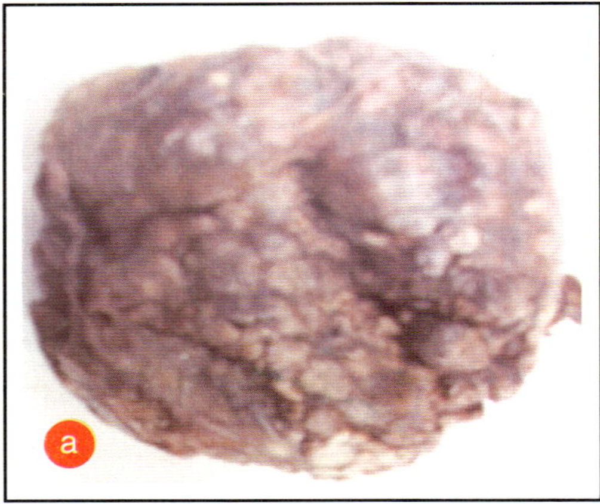

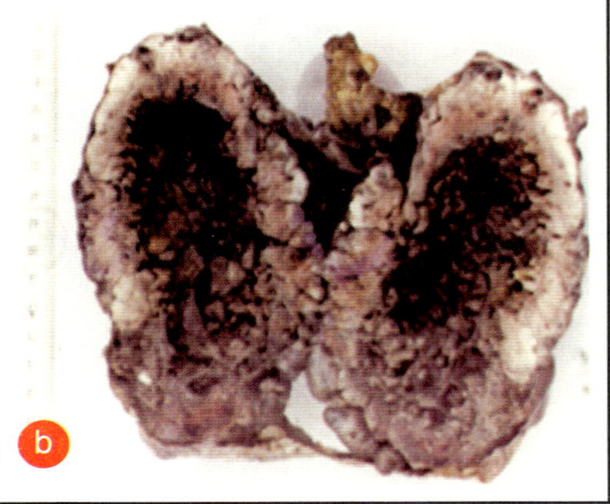

Figure 364: Photographs showing: (a) Tumorous mass from mesentery of tiger (*P. tigris*) died in National Park, Ranthambore (Rajasthan). (b) Cut opened (a) diagnosed as mesothelioma.

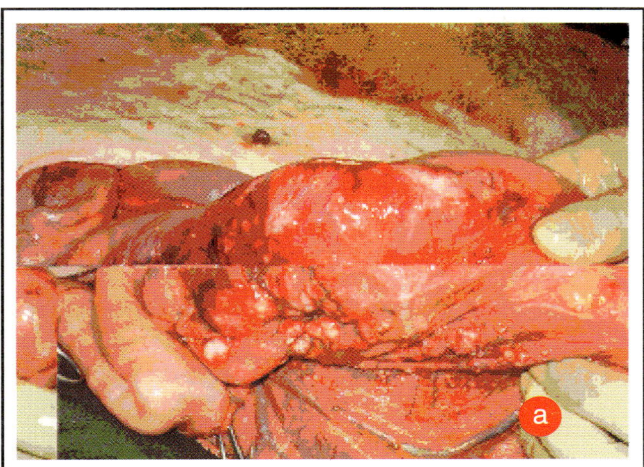

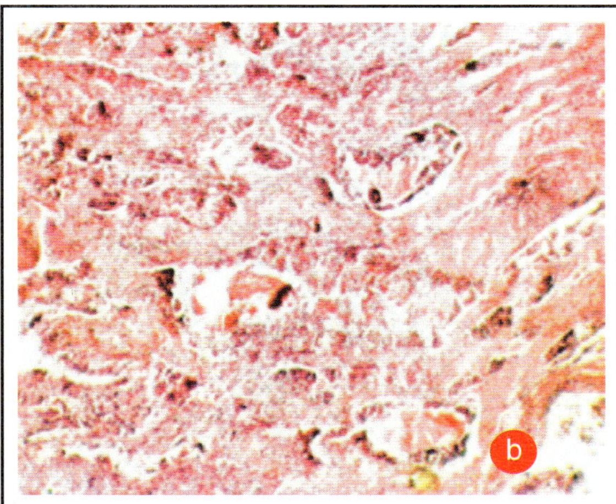

Figure 365: Haemangiosarcoma encountered in a lioness (*P. leo*) died at Biological Park, Bhubneshwar,Orissa.(a) Photograph of a growth attached to mesentery (b) Photomicrograph of (a) showing numerous neoplastic bloods vessels of varying sizes lined with poorly differentiated endothelial cells. H&E, x40 (Courtesy: Panda, S.K. & Nath, I.).

Urinary System

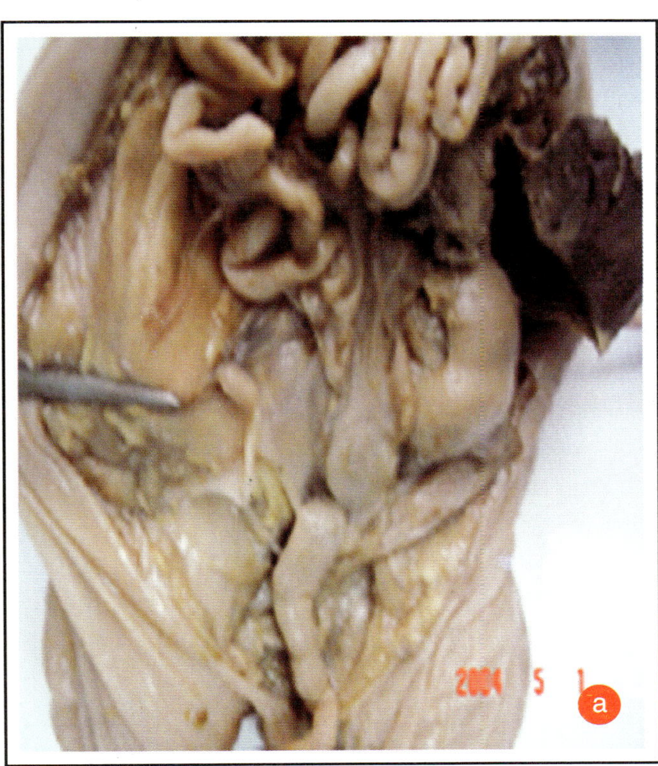

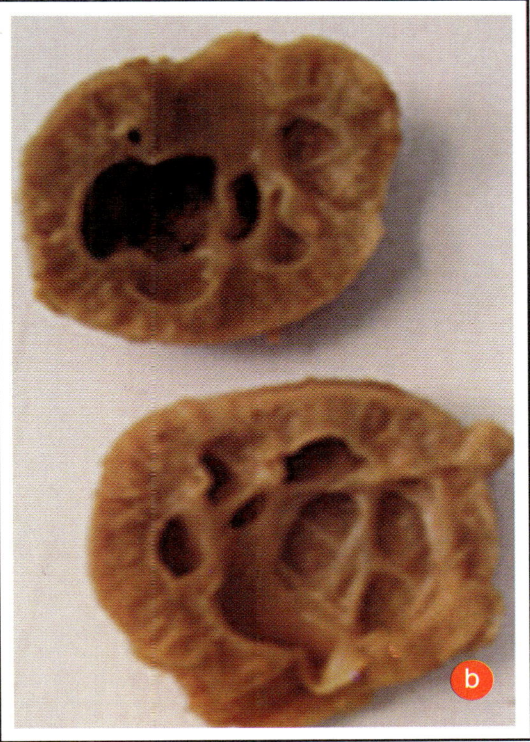

Figure 366: Photograph showing (of a) absence of right kidney in tiger (*P. tigris*) foetus aborted at about 60 days of gestation. (b) Left kidney when cut opened showed cavitations.

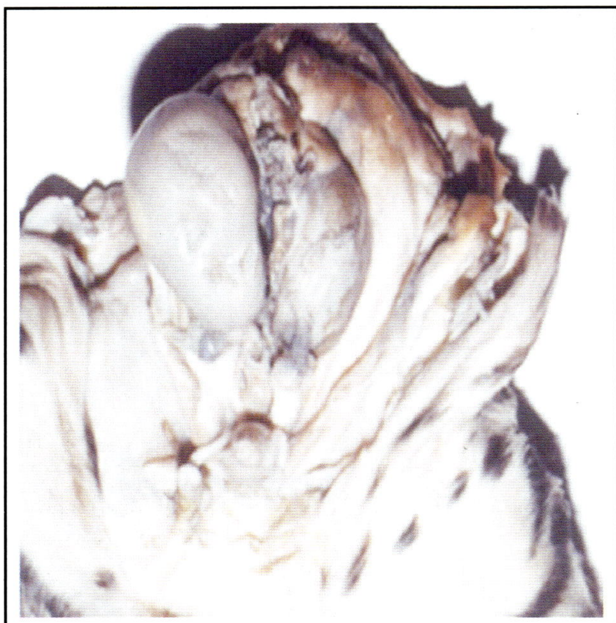

Figure 367: Photograph showing cystic kidney in tiger (*P. tigris*) cub.(Courtsey: Suryawanshi, D.S.).

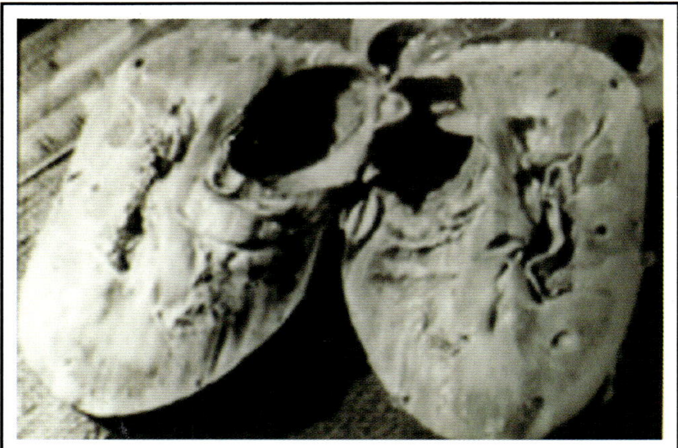

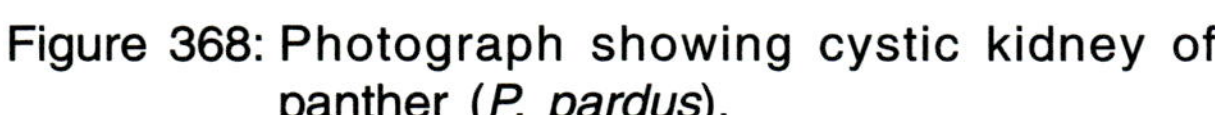

Figure 368: Photograph showing cystic kidney of panther (*P. pardus*).

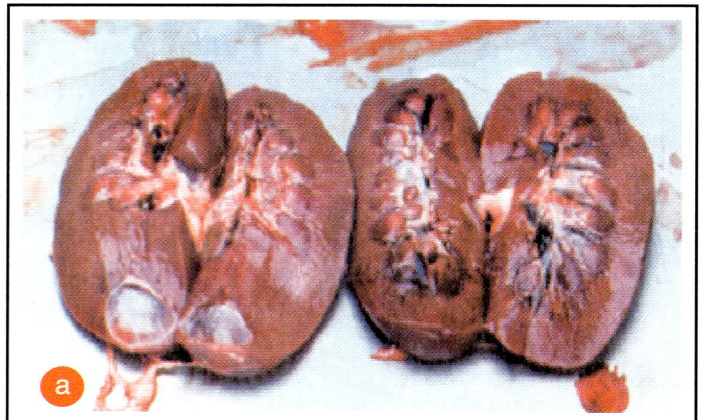

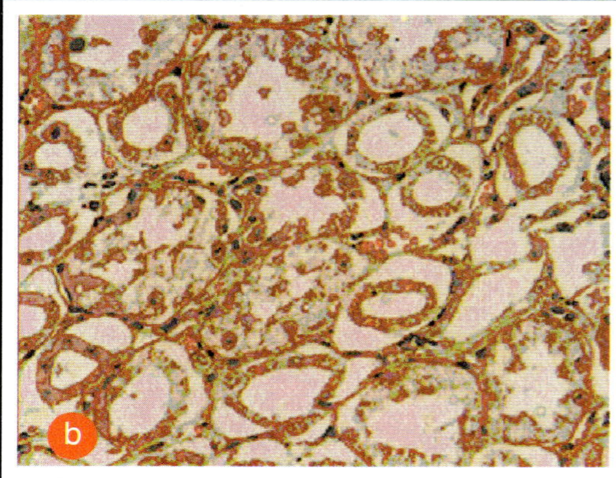

Figure 369: (a) Photograph showing polycystic kidney of tiger (*P. tigris*) died in captivity. (b) Photomicrograph of kidney of lioness (*P. leo*) showing degeneration and necrosis of tubular epithelium with cystic tubules, sclerosed vessels, interstitial tissue fibrosis and infiltration of inflammatory cells. (Courtesy: Harish, B.R.).

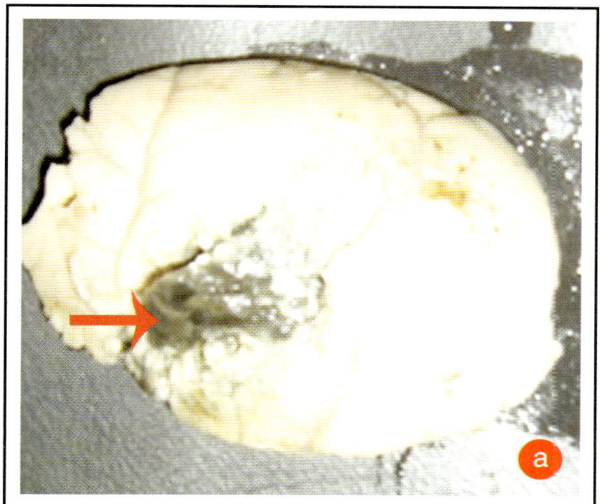

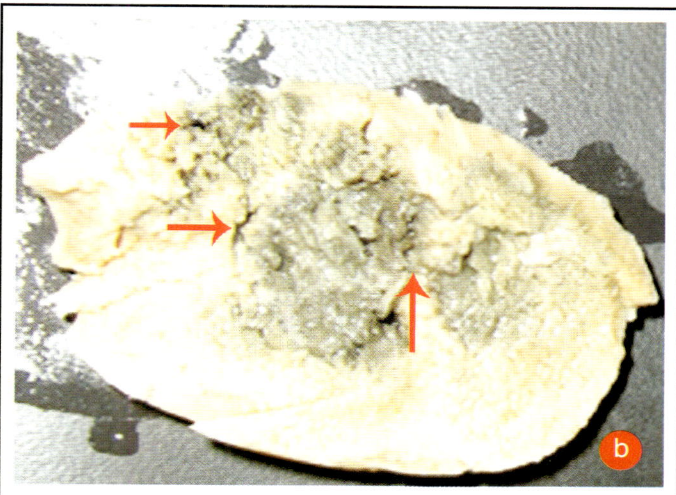

Figure 370: Photograph showing an embedded pellet in the kidney of leopard (*P. pardus*) shot dead around Delhi (Courtesy: Paneer salvam). (b) Cut section of (a) showing the extent of damage from cortex to medulla caused by the pellet.

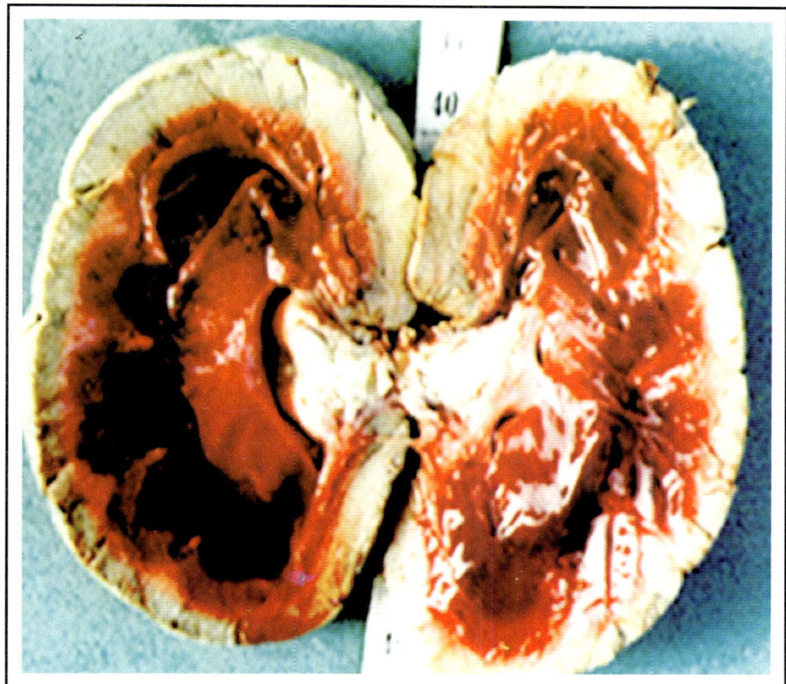

Figure 371: Photograph showing severe haemorrhagic lesions in the medulla of kidney of tiger (*P. tigris*) died in the forest of Uttar Pradesh.

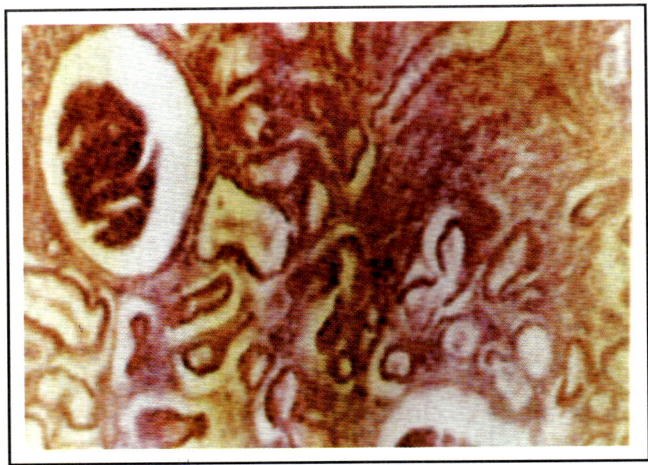

Case (i)

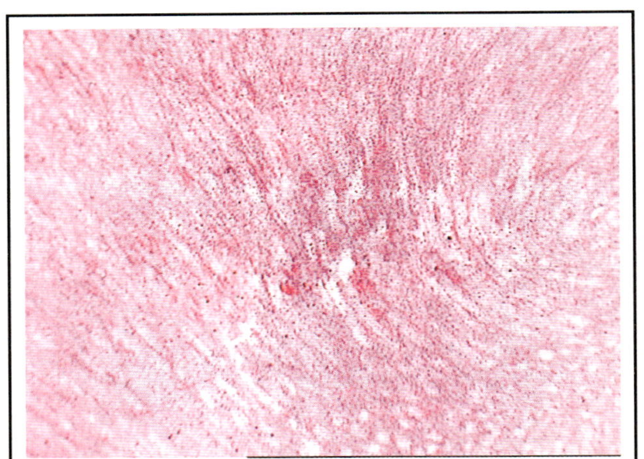

Case (iia)

Case (iib)

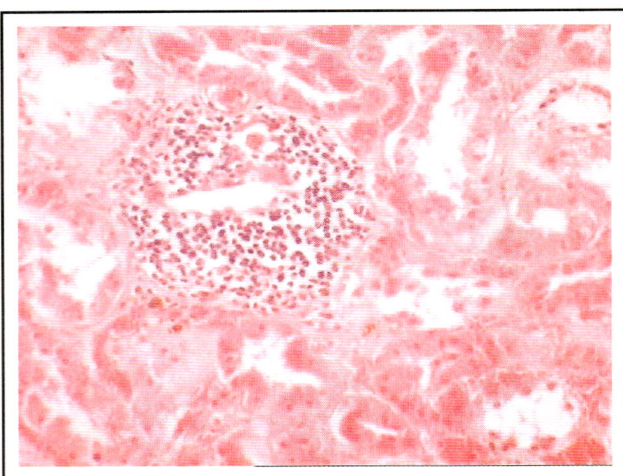

Case (iii)

Figure 372: Case (i): Hydronephrosis encountered in tiger (*P. tigris*) died in National Park Bannerghatta, Bangalore. Photomicrograph showing connective tissue between the tubules and areas of mononuclear cell infiltration blood vessels. H& E, x 100 (Gajenderagad *et al.* 2004). Case (iia): Pyelonephritis in tiger (*P. tigris*) polymopho nuclear cells are seen in the pelvis adjacent interstitial tissues of the medulla. H&E,100 Case (iib): Higher magnification of (a) showing polymorph nuclear cells in the tubular casts within tubules and interstitial spaces. H&E. x 400. Case(iii) Chronic glomerulo-nephritis encountered in tiger (*P. tigris*) showing a single glomerulus with infiltrating and sclerotic changes. H&E,x100

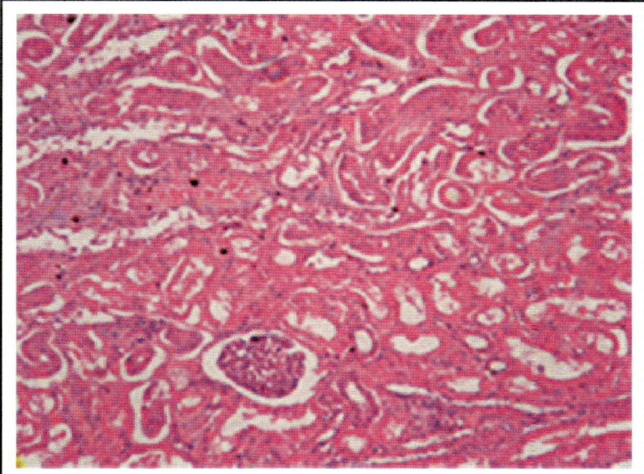

Figure 373: Photomicrograph of kidney of lion (*P. leo*) showing suppurative nephritis H & E, x 100. (Courtesy: Dept of Pathology C.V.Sc. (Nagpur, M.S.)

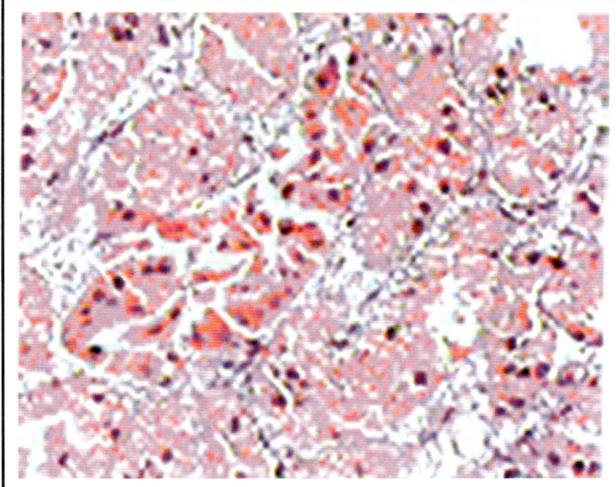

Figure 374: Photomicrograph of kidney from leopard (*P. pardus*)showing focal tubular cellular swelling. H & E, x 400.

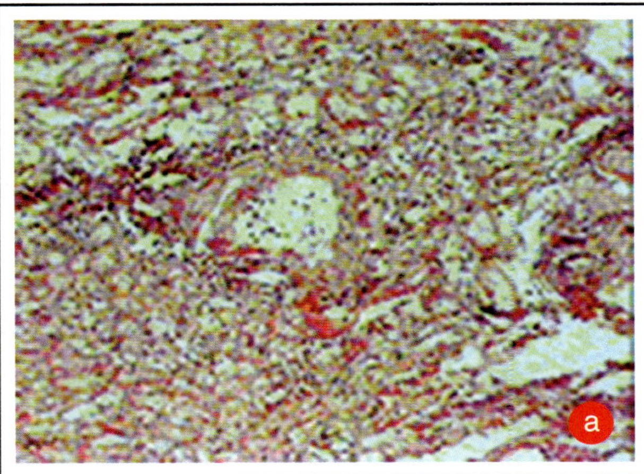

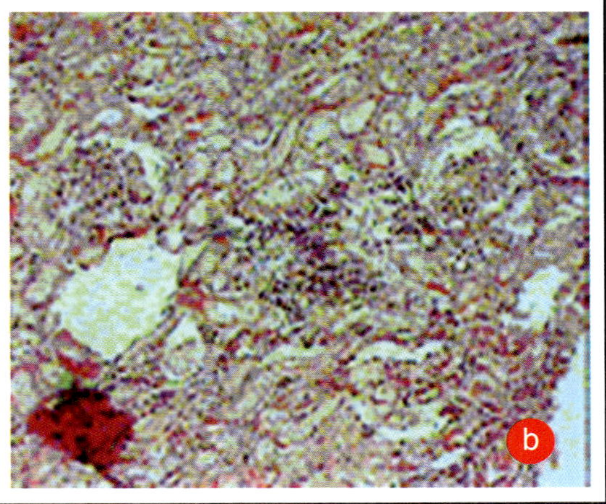

Figure 375: Interstitial nephritis in panther (*P. pardus*). Photomicrographs (a, b) showing interstitial infiltration of mononuclear cells with granular material within the glomeruli and tubular degeneration H & E x 100 (Courtesy: Dept Wildlife Science, CVSc, Chennai, TN).

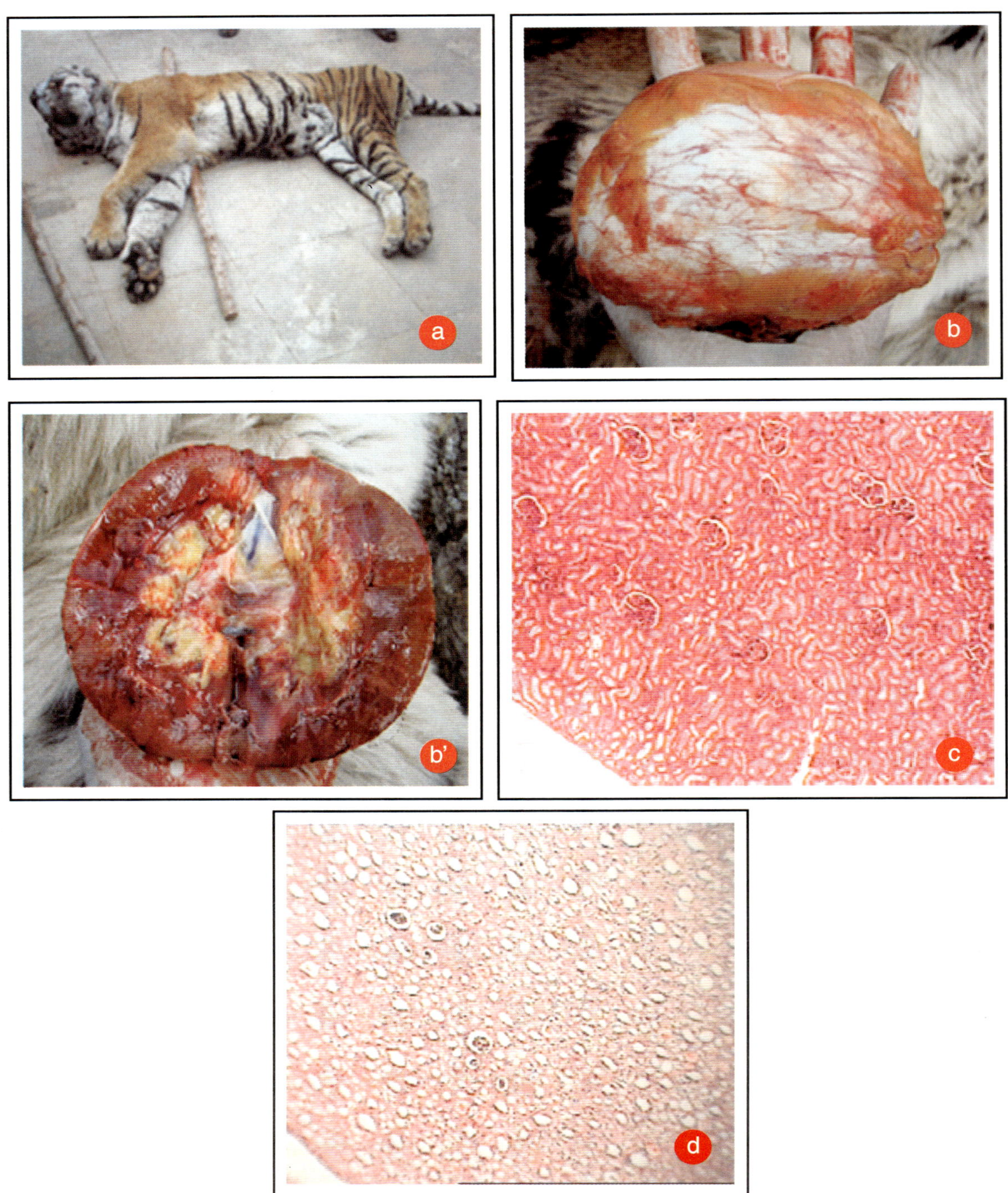

Figure 376: (a) Carcass of Siberian tiger (*P. t. altacia*). (b) Photograph of kidney of (a) surrounded by gelatinized fat. (b')Cut section of (b) showing congestion. (c) Photomicrographs of (b) showing formation of cystic spaces and abscess formation. (d) Photomicrograph showing normal architecture of kidney with intact glomeruli and tubules. H & E x 100 (Courtesy: Arun A. Sha).

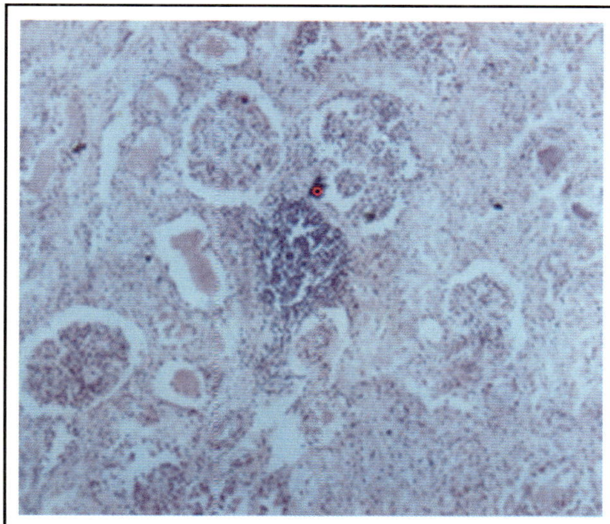

Figure 377: Photomicrograph showing chronic interstitial nephritis encountered in tiger (*P. tigris*) related to leptospiral infection. H& E, x100 (Courtesy: Suryawanshi, D. S.).

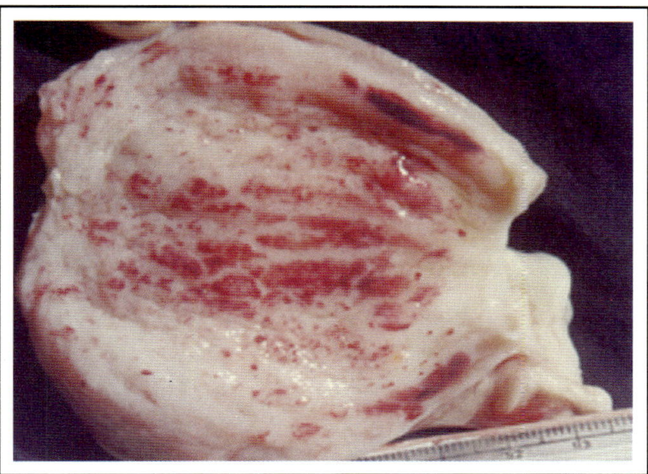

Figure 378: Photograph showing haemorrhagic lesions encountered in the urinary bladder of leopard (*P. pardus*) died in captivity.

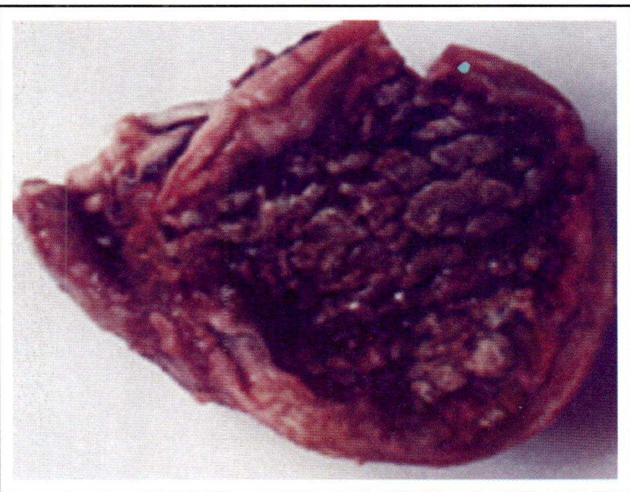

Figure 379: Photograph of urinary bladder of leopard (*P. pardus*) showing hard, thickened uneven gritty growth, which was diagnosed as granulomatous cystitis.

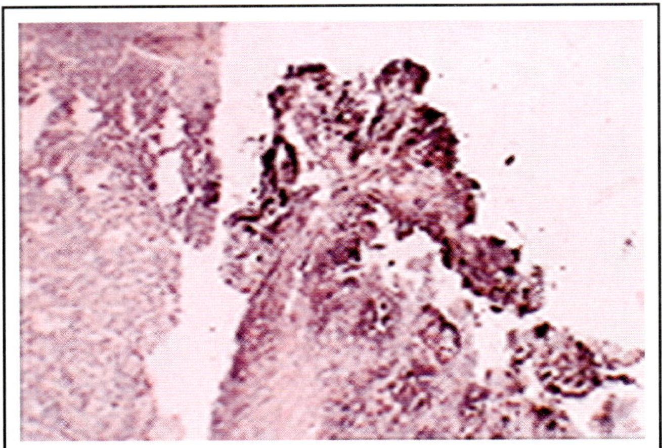

Figure 380: Cystitis in leopard (*P. pardus*) died in captivity. Photomicrograph showing necrosis and calcification in the mucosal layer of urinary bladder. H&E, x 100

Figure 381: Photomicrograph of urinary bladder of panther (*P. pardus*) showing changes characteristics of pyaemic cystitis. H&E, x 40.

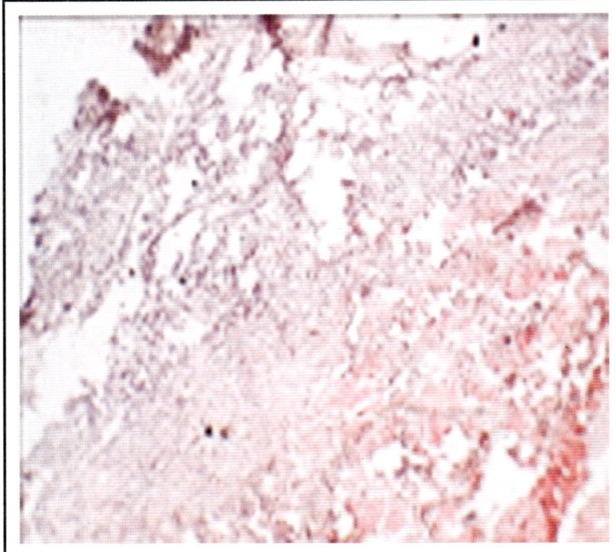

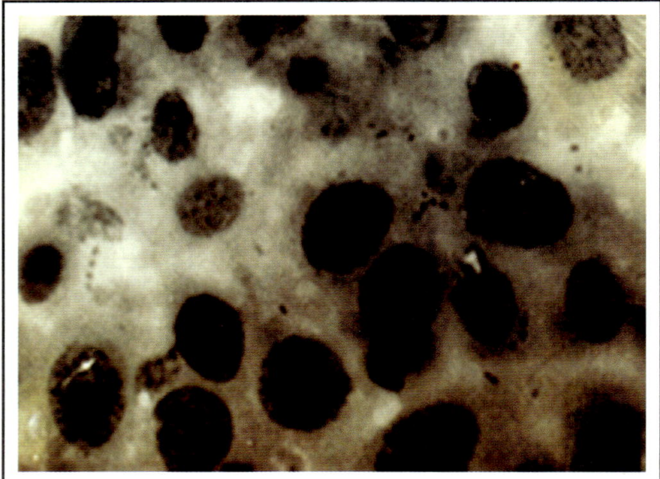

Figure 382: Gram stained impression smear from mucosa of urinary bladder of puma (*Felis concolor*, an exotic sp.) marked for pyaemic cystitis due to Streptococcus infection.

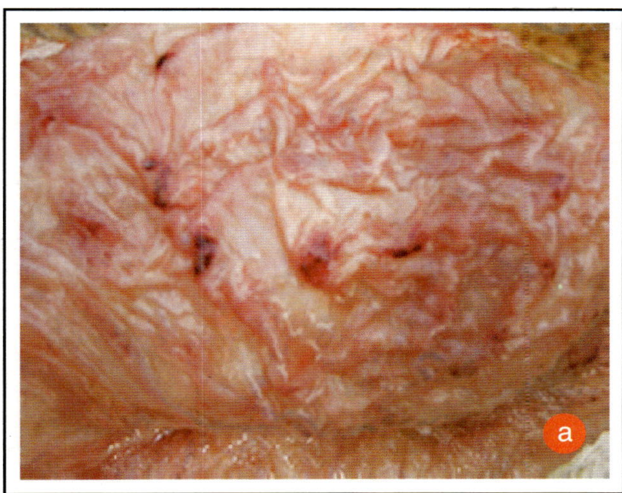

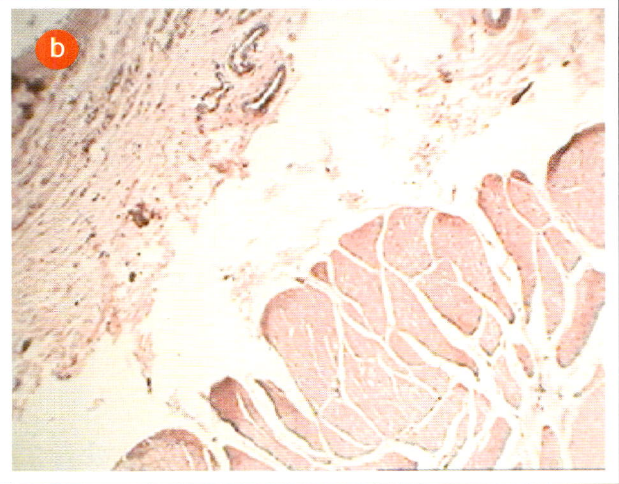

Figure 383: (a) Photograph showing congestion and mucosal erosions of urinary bladder of Siberian tiger (*P. t. altacia*). (b) Photomicrograph of (a) evidencing cystitis related to non-infectious factor. H & E, x 100. The case is also referred for nephritis.

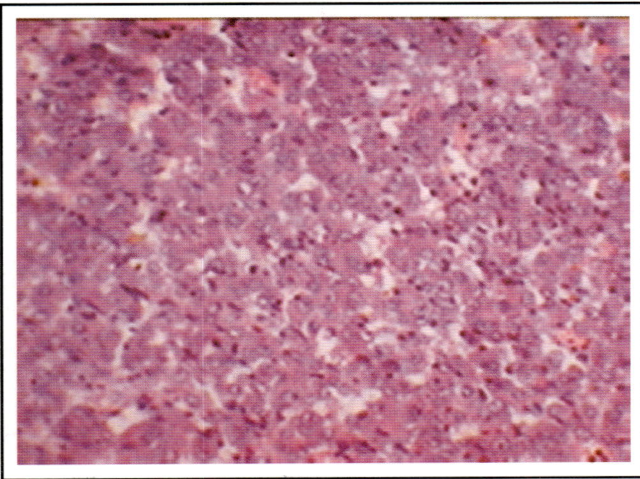

Figure 384: Adrenal cortical carcinoma in lion (*P. leo*). Photomicrograph showing pleomorphic cortical tumour cells replacing the normal cells of the gland with abundant of mitotic figures in cortex. H&E, x 400.

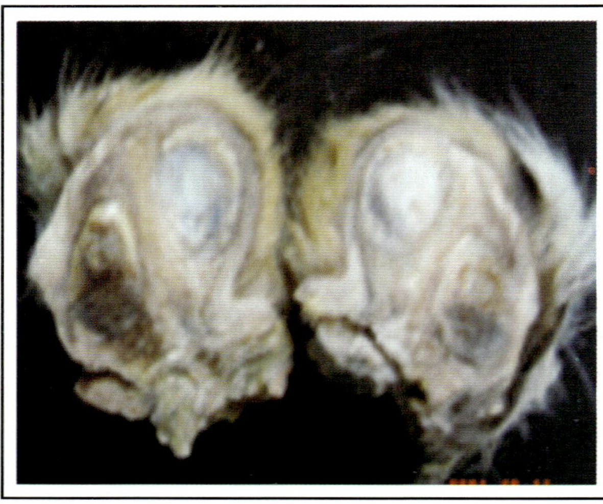

Figure 385: Photograph of testis(cut opened) of wild tiger (*P. tigris*) showing haemorrhagic clot.

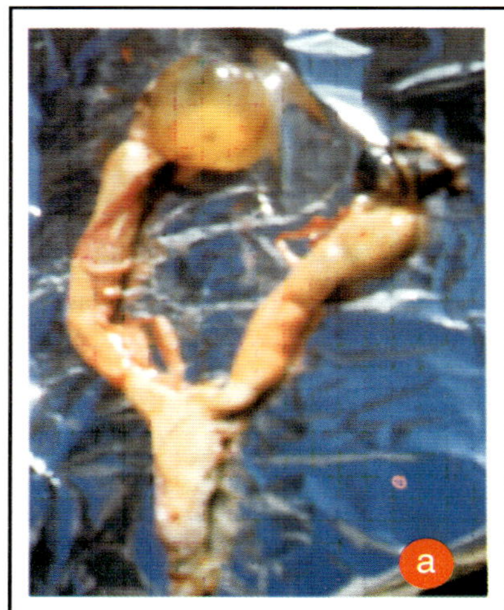

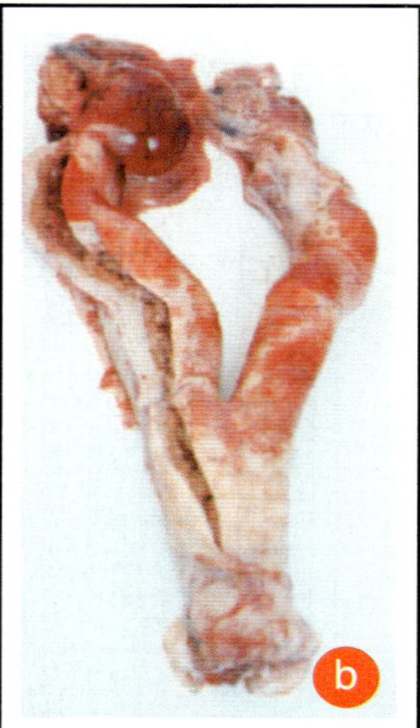

Figure 386: (a) Follicular cyst encountered in hybrid lioness (*P. leo*) died in captivity. (b) Cut open follicular cyst and uterine horn showing acute endometritis (Courtesy: Harish, B.R.).

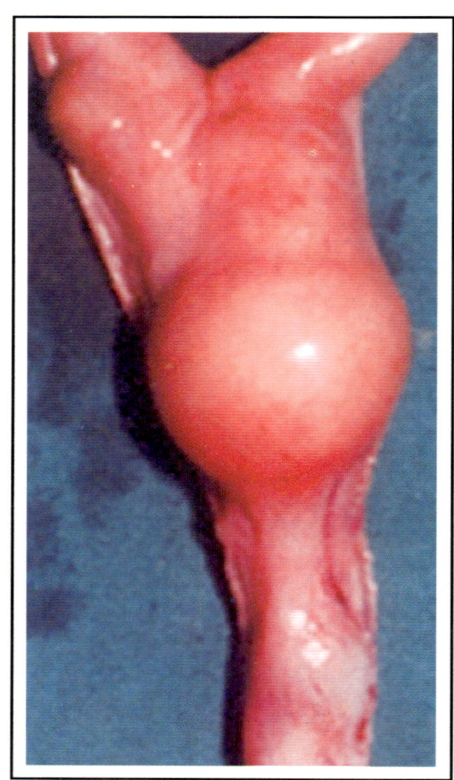

Figure 387: Photograph showing cystic endometriosis encountered in tigress (*P. tigris*) died in captivity.

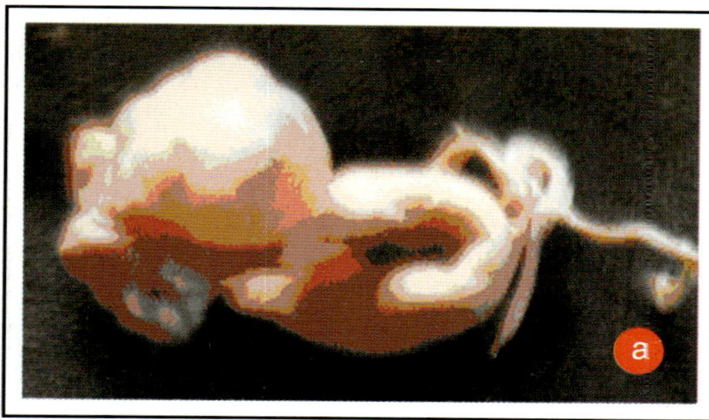

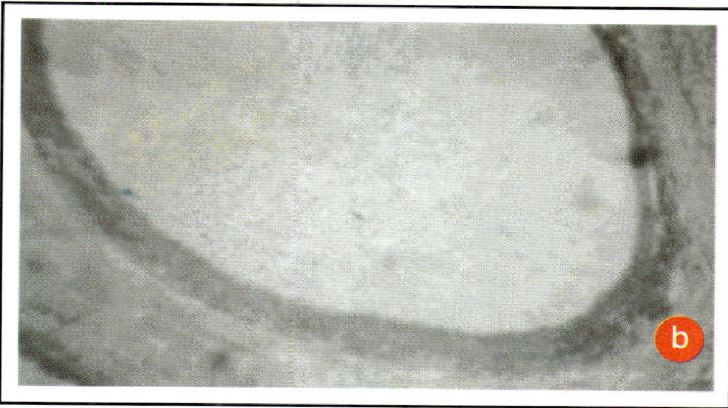

Figure 388: Photograph showing follicular cyst measuring 2 to 2.5 cm encountered in both ovaries of tigress (*P. tigris*) died in captivity. (b) Photomicrograph of (a) showing cyst filled with clear serous fluid and thin walled granulosa cell (Courtesy: Garg, U.K).

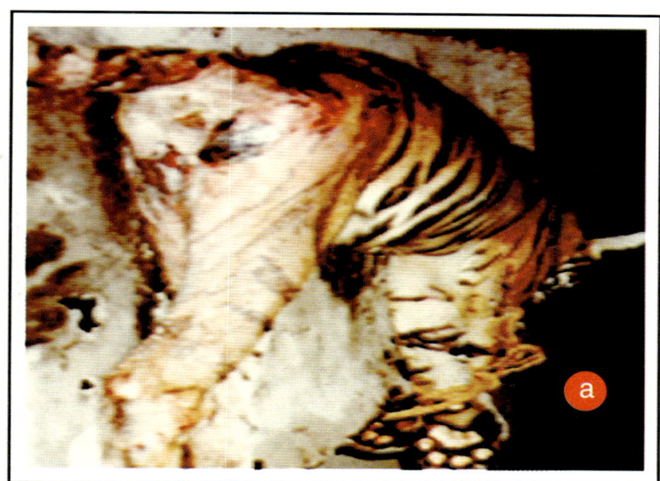

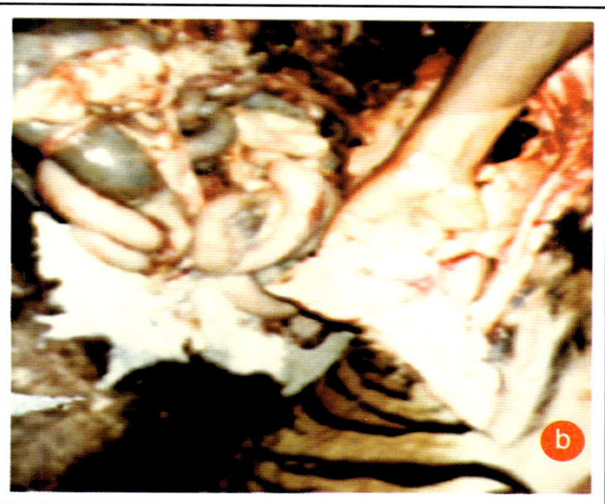

Figure 389: (a) Dead tigress (*P. tigris*) at National Zoological Park, New Delhi showing suppurative lesions extending from vagina to vulva. (b)Necropsy of (a) showing Pyometra.

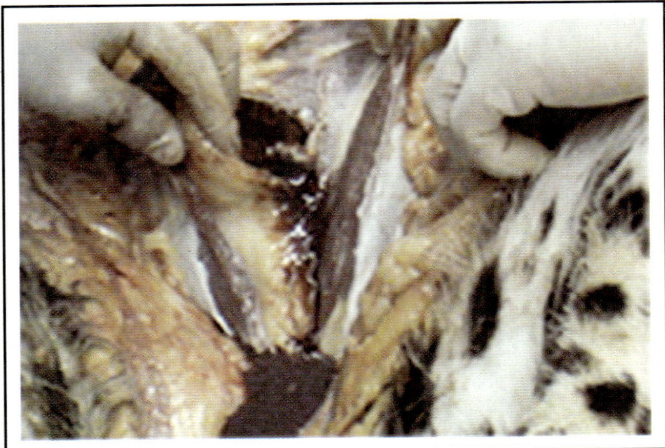

Figure 390: Photograph showing lacerated vagina of leopard (*P. pardus*) that died of dystocia. Note presence of blood clots.

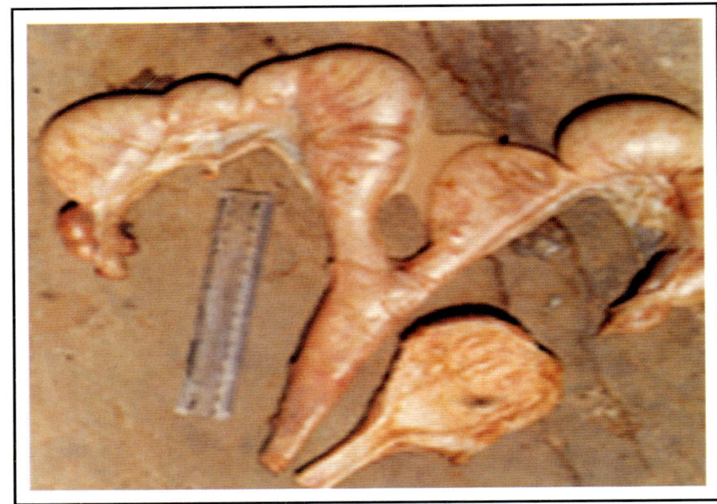

Figure 391: Pyometra in tigress (*P. tigris*). Note copious pus in uterus. Mucosa of urinary bladder also showed necrotic foci. The case is also referred under urinary system.

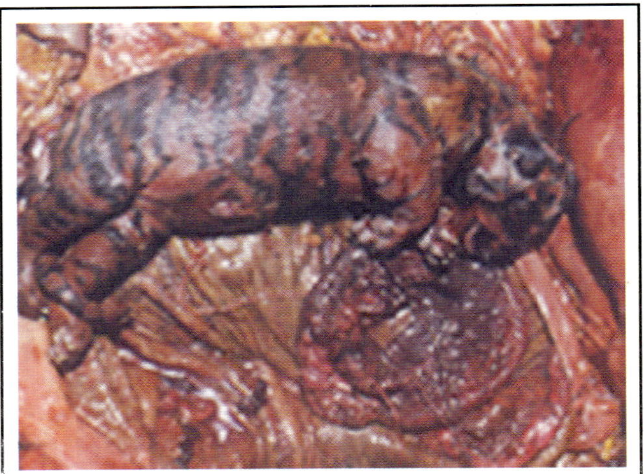

Figure 392: Photograph of oedematous and putrefied fully developed foetus of tigress (*P. tigris*), which had died due to dystocia at Zoological Garden, Guwahati, Assam.

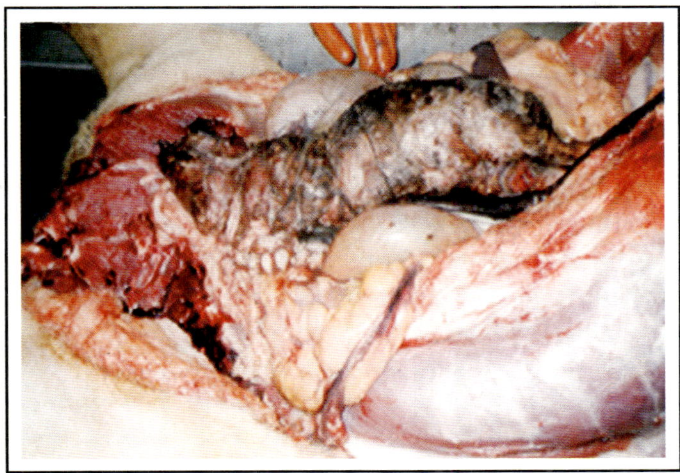

Figure 393: Macerated foetus in uterus of lioness (*P. leo persica*). (Courtesy: R.G.Jani)

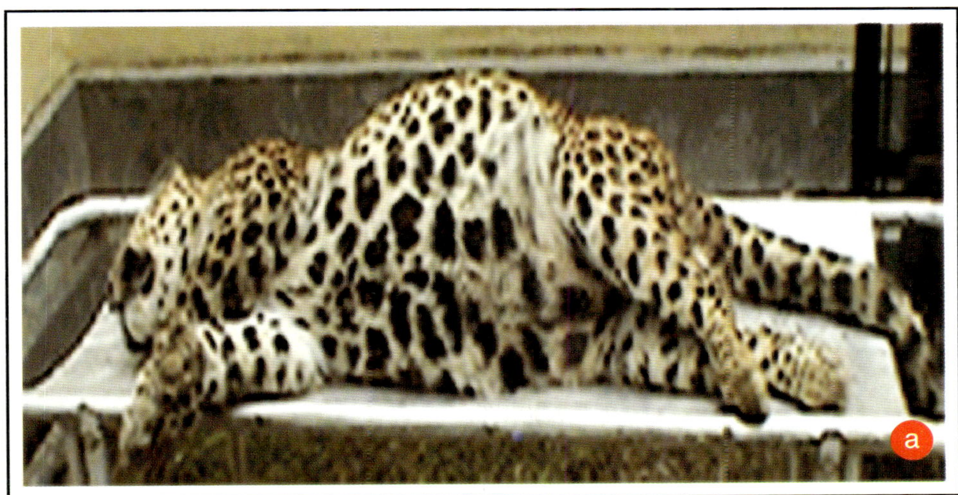

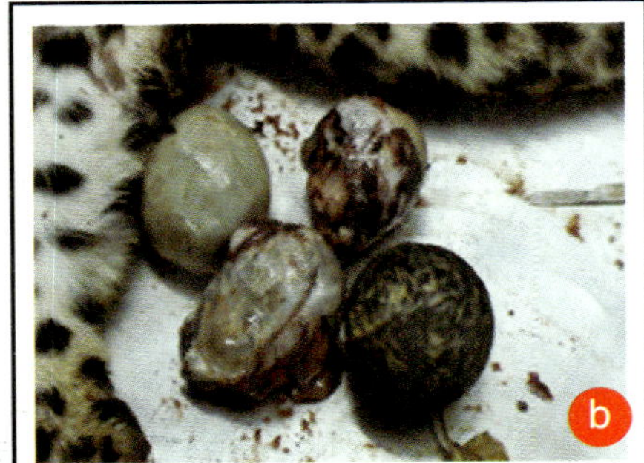

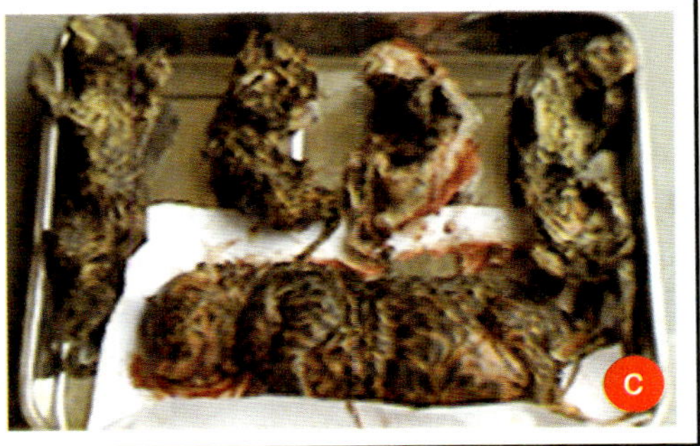

Figure 394: A swollen carcass (postmortem Bloat) of leopardess (*P.pardus*) belonging to Himalayan Zoological Park, Bulbulay, Gangtok, Sikkim. (b) Ball shaped four of the five foetuses recovered during necropsy of (a). (c) Autoysed deformed foetuses unrolled (b) and the fifth one of full sized. (Courtesy: Shankar, K.S.M.).

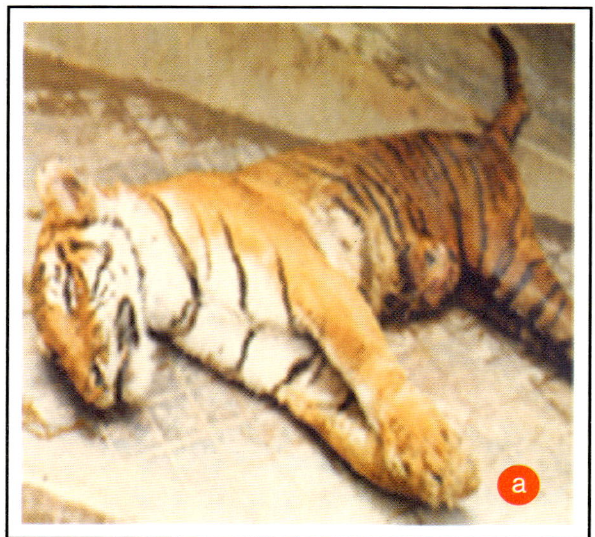

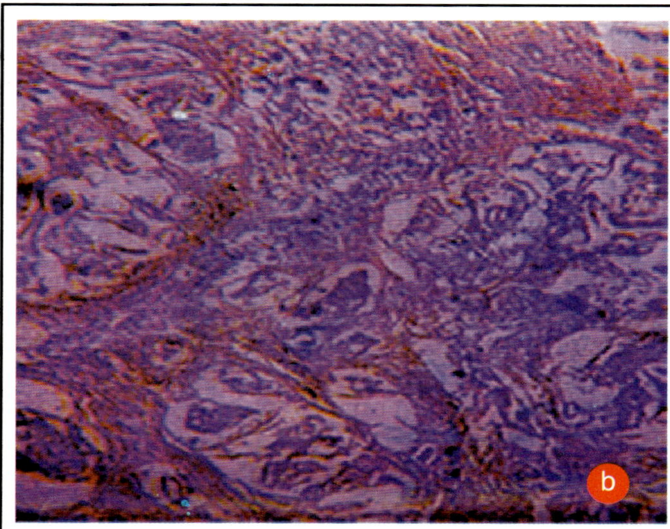

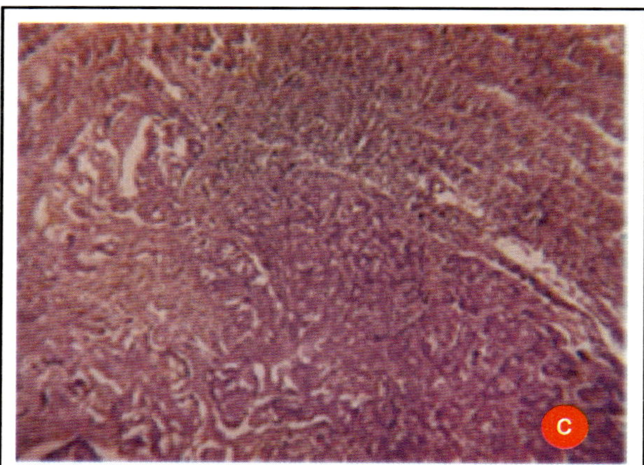

Figure 395: (a) Carcass of adult tigress (*P. tigris*) showing tumorous growth,involving mammary gland. (b) Photomicrograph of (a) showing changes characteristic of mammary gland adenocarcinoma. H&E, x100. (c) Metastasis of (b) to lymph node. H&E, x 70.

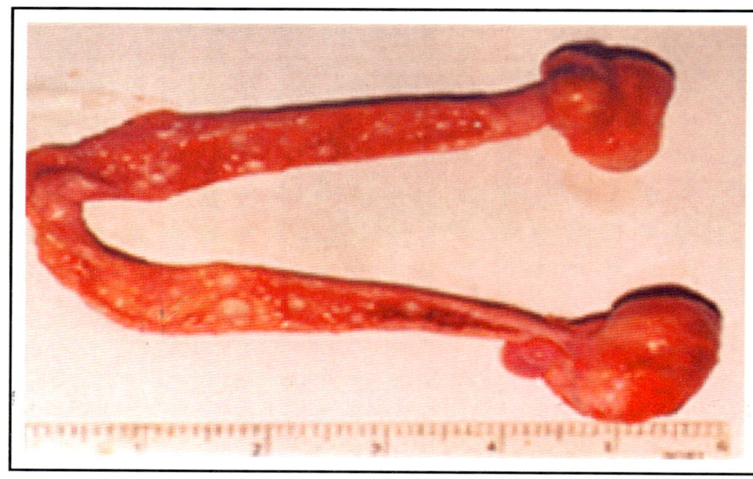

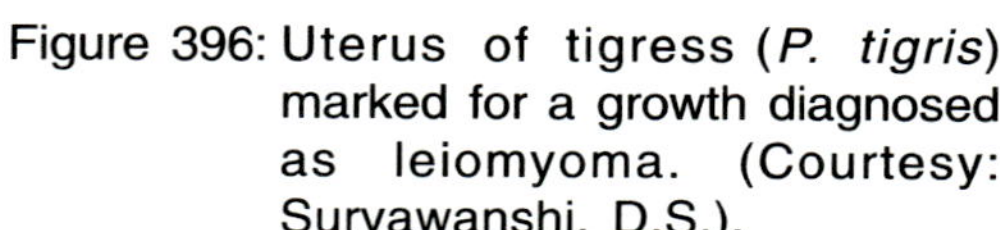

Figure 396: Uterus of tigress (*P. tigris*) marked for a growth diagnosed as leiomyoma. (Courtesy: Suryawanshi, D.S.).

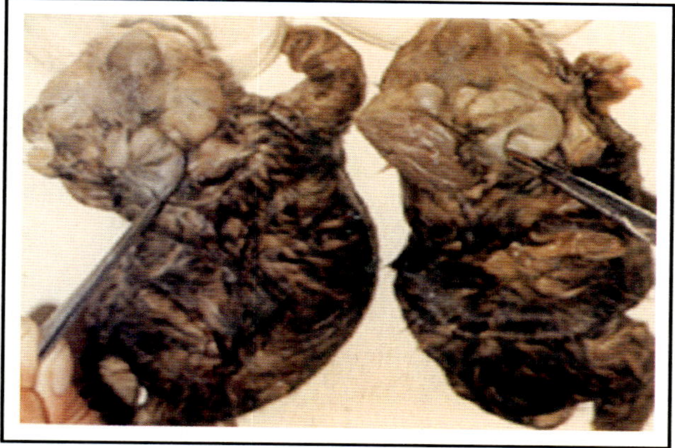

Case (ia)

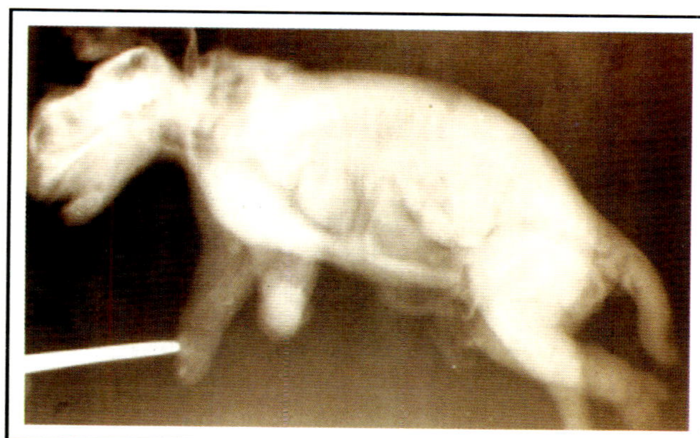

Case (ib)

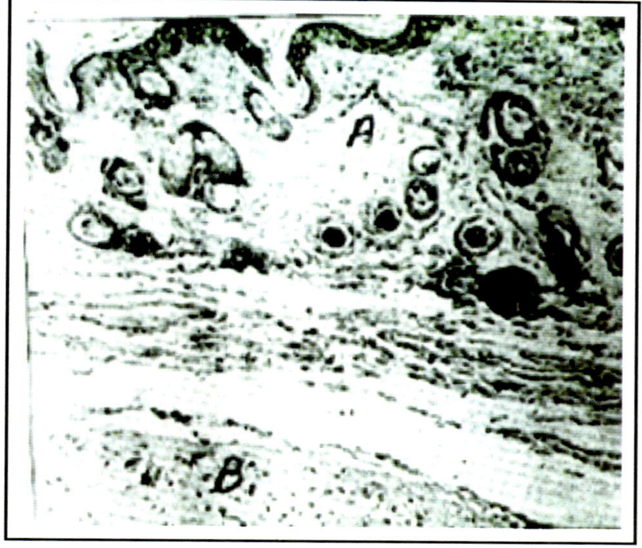

Case (ii)

Figure 397: Case1. (a) Photograph showing two stillborn panther cubs born (of wild parents were brought to Zoological Park, Kanpur) with meningoencephalocele. (b) Radiograph of one of the cubs showing imperfect development of scalp. Case 2. Exencephaly in still born panther (*P. pardus*) at Zoological Park, Bhubneshwar, Orissa (Rao and Acharjyo, 1993). Photo with permission.

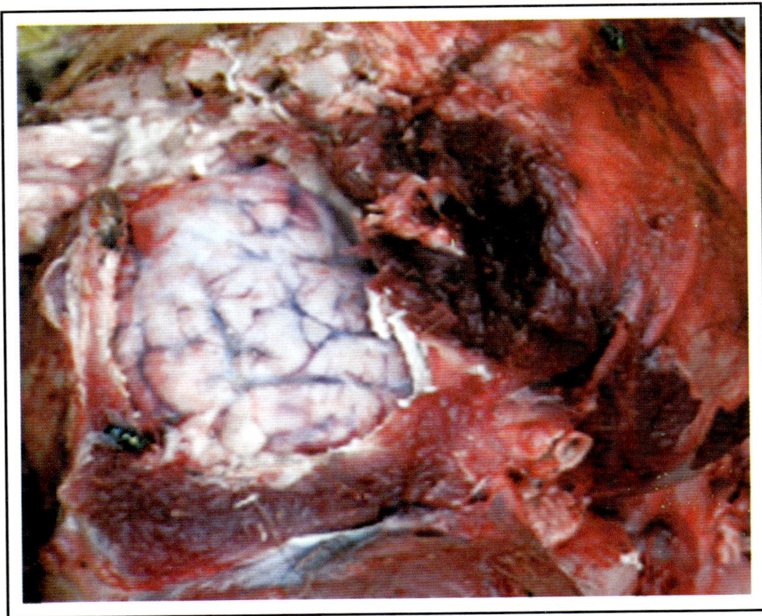

Figure 398 : Photograph showing congestion of brain of wild leopard (*P. pardus*) associated with severe traumatic impact on its scalp belonged to Corbett Tiger Reserve, Ramnagar (Courtesy: Choudhury, B.).

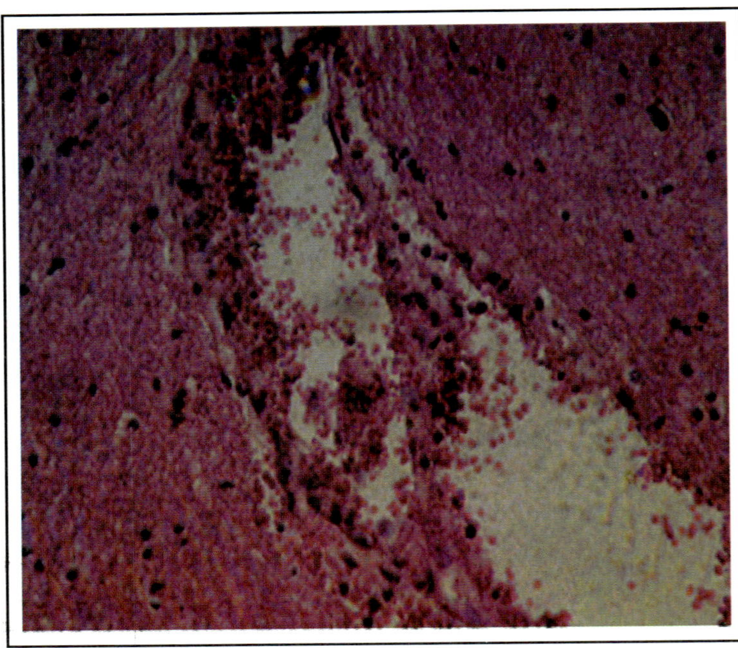

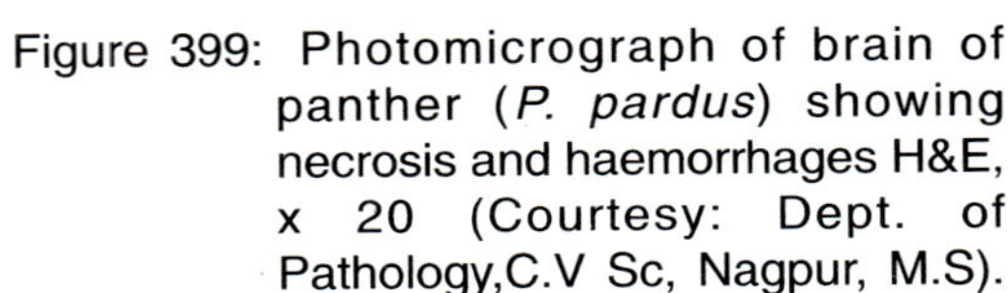

Figure 399: Photomicrograph of brain of panther (*P. pardus*) showing necrosis and haemorrhages H&E, x 20 (Courtesy: Dept. of Pathology,C.V Sc, Nagpur, M.S).

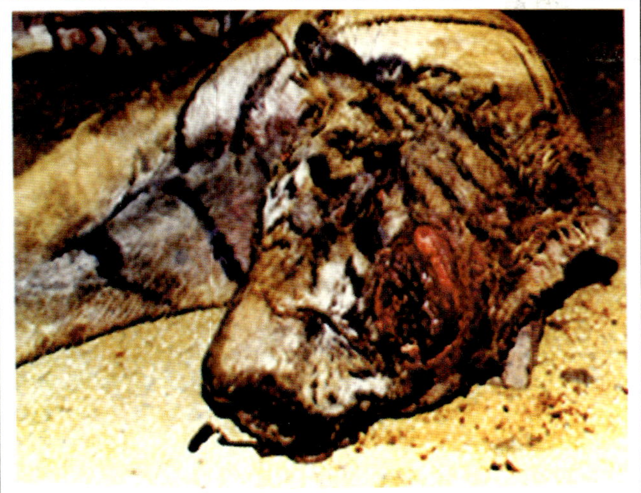

Figure 400: Left Eye of wild tiger (*P. tigris*) completely damaged due to some traumatic insult.

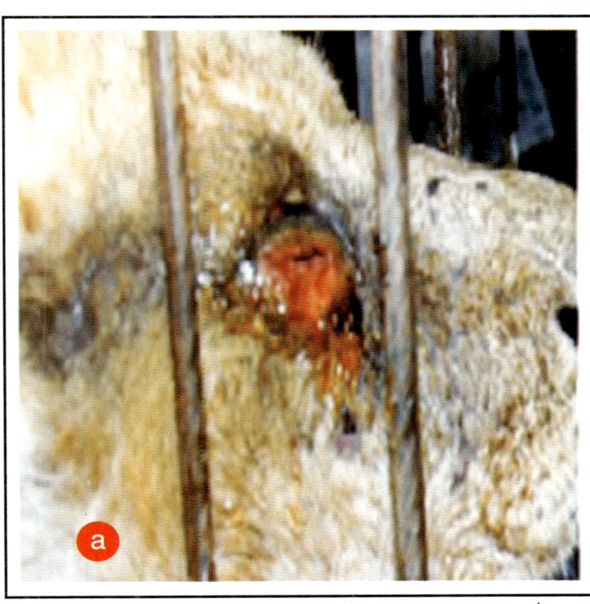

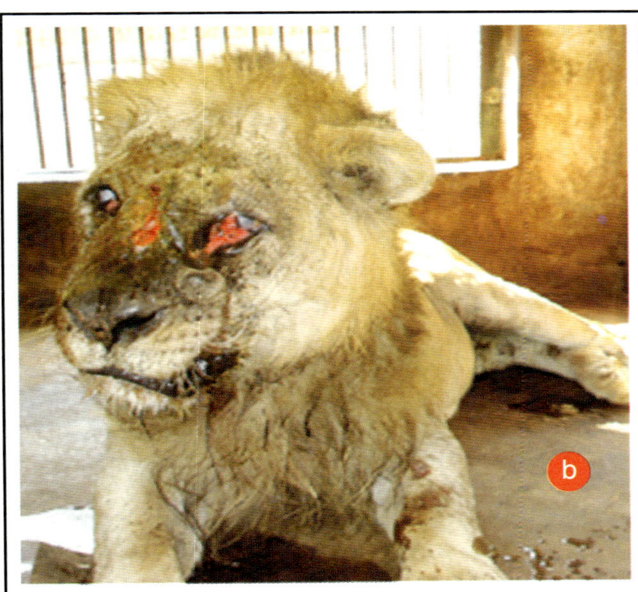

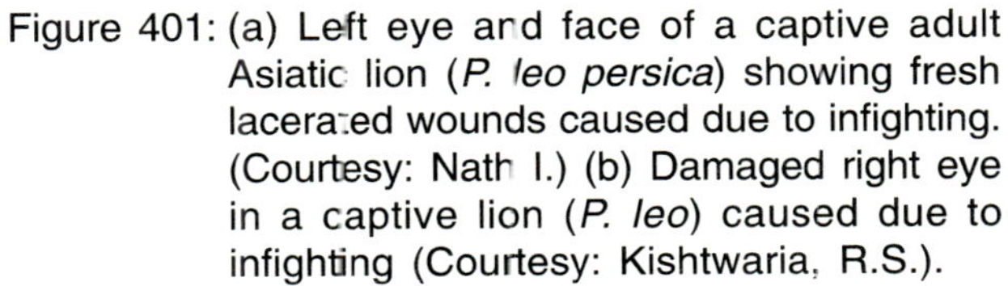

Figure 401: (a) Left eye and face of a captive adult Asiatic lion (*P. leo persica*) showing fresh lacerated wounds caused due to infighting. (Courtesy: Nath I.) (b) Damaged right eye in a captive lion (*P. leo*) caused due to infighting (Courtesy: Kishtwaria, R.S.).

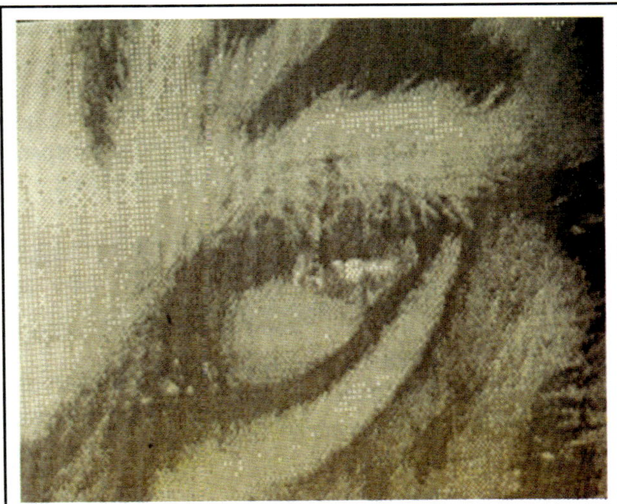

Figure 402: Photograph showing luxation of lens in the anterior chamber of left eye of tiger (*P. tigris*) belonged to a captive facility (Bhardwaj & Chandra, 1991).

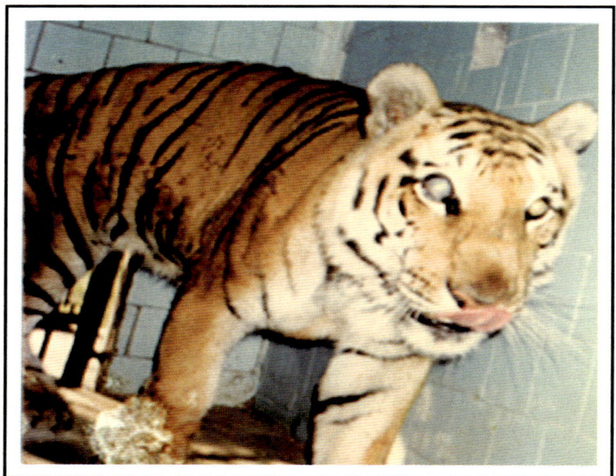

Figure 403: Young adult tiger (*P. tigris*) suffering from corneal opacity in right eye.

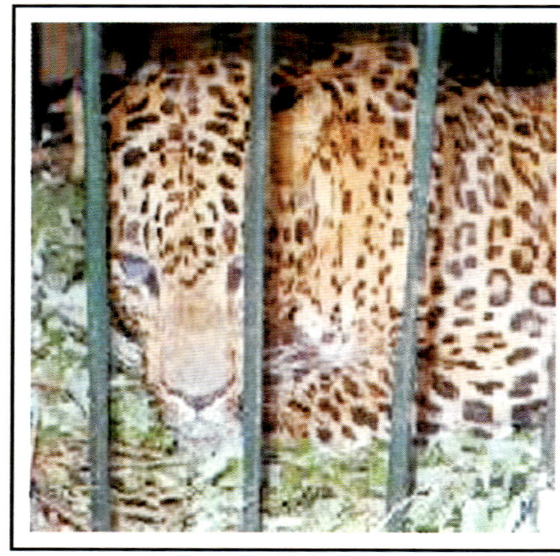

Figure 404: Young adult leopard (*P. pardus*) suffering from corneal opacity in right eye (Courtesy: Kishtwaria, R.S.).

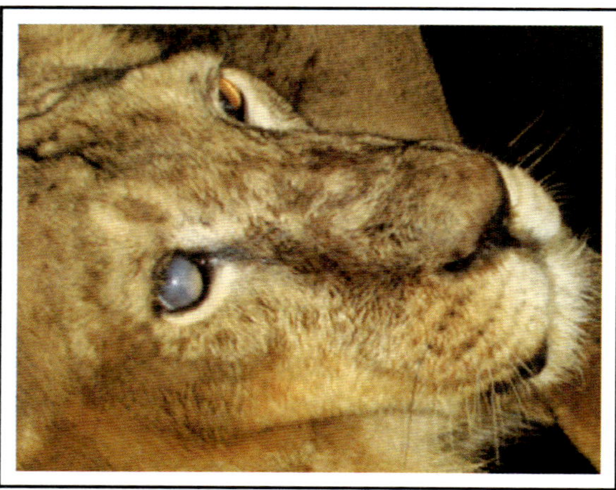

Figure 405: Asiatic lioness (*P. leo persica*) suffering from cataract in right eye at National Zoological Park, New Delhi.

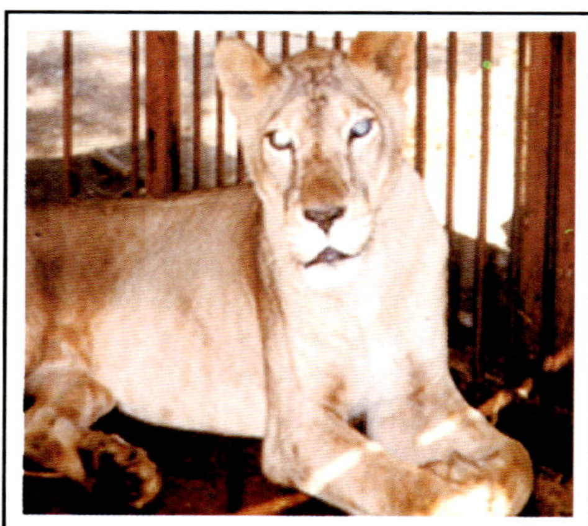

Figure 406: Hybrid lioness (*P. leo*) rescued from circus and housed at Zoological Garden, Kanpur (U.P.) with corneal opacity in both eyes.

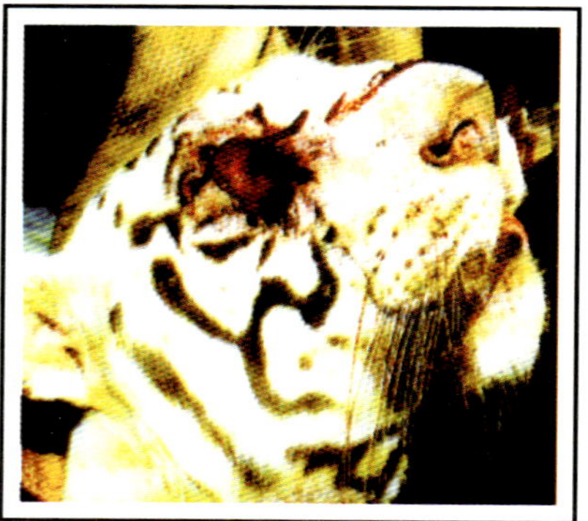

Figure 407: Epidermoid carcinoma of eye lid encountered in tiger belonged to Biological Park, Bhubneshwar (Photo: Bose, V.S.C. cited by Rao, A. T. & Achrjyo, 2002).

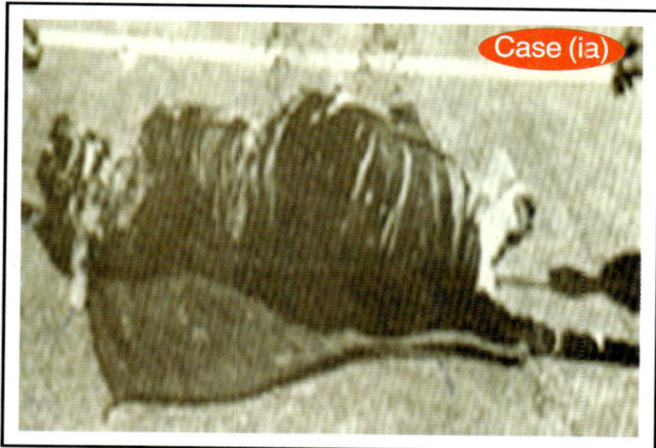

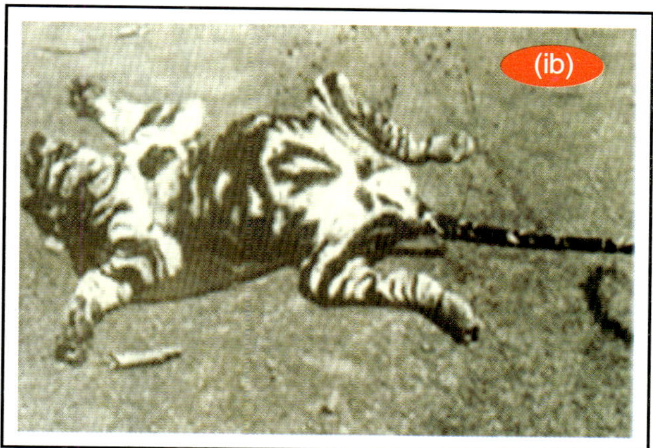

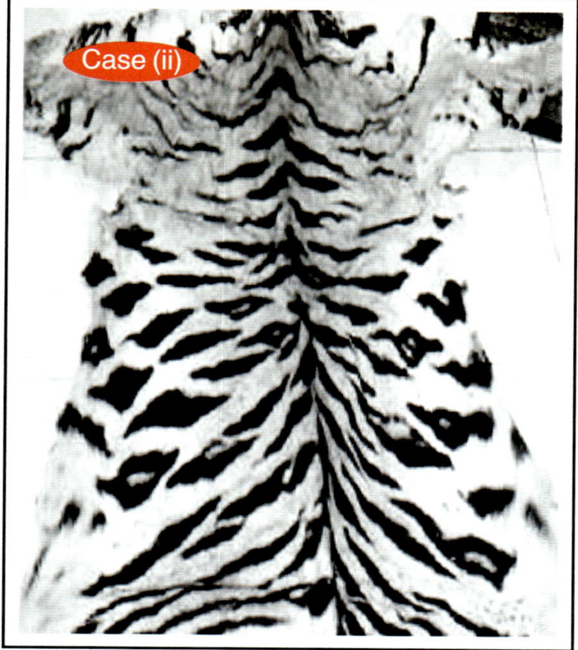

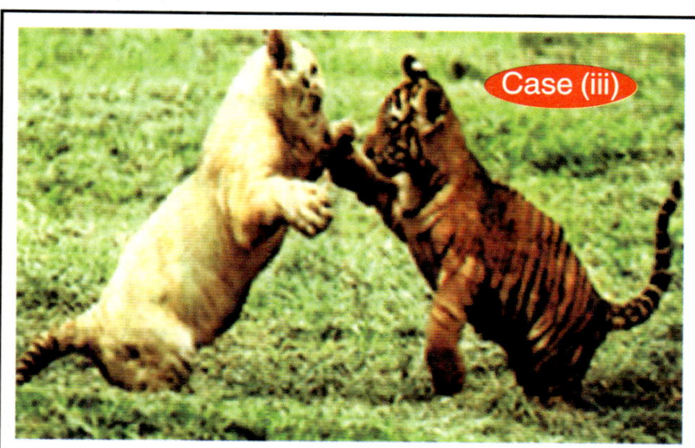

Figure 408: Case (i)Tiger (*P. tigris*) skin showing stripes of different shape and pattern from Orissa (a) dorsal view and (b) ventral view of the same. Case (ii)Tiger (*P. tigris*) skin from Karnataka showing stripes of different shape and pattern (Courtesy: Ashok Kumar). Case (iii). Bengal tiger cubs playing at the zoo in Guadalajara, Mexico (Times of India New Delhi, July 7, 2007). Note white among two cubs carrying stripes only on the tail.

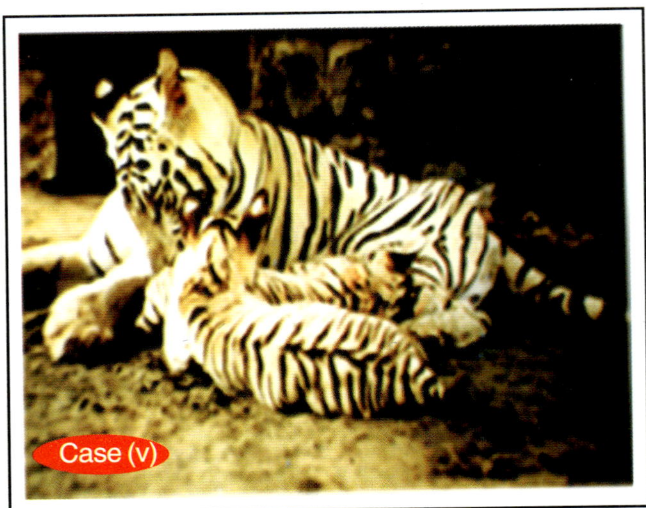

Case (iv) White tigress (*P. tigris*) with her white cubs having stripes of normal pattern.

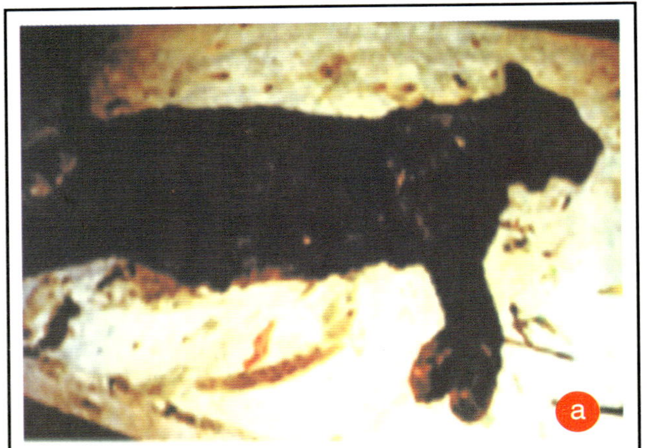

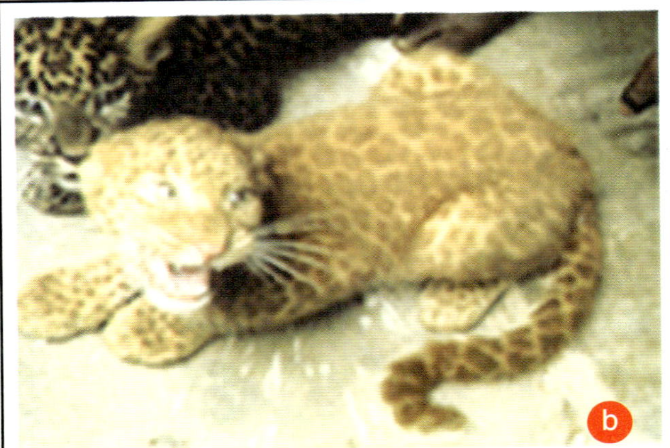

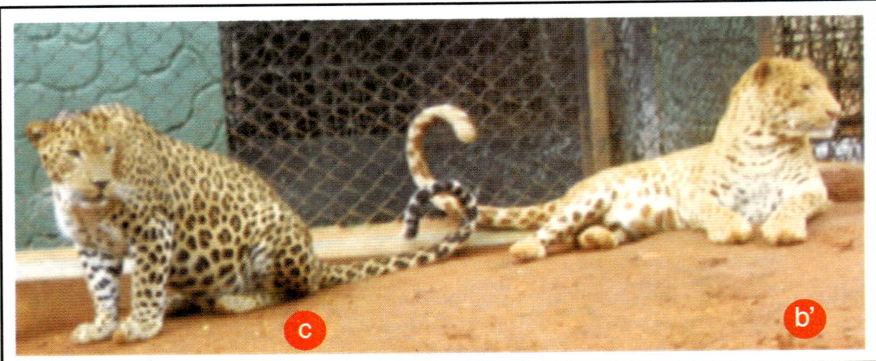

Figure 409: Leopard (*P. pardus*). (a) Black. (b) One of the two cubs rescued from wild and lodged at Zoological Garden Mysore (Karnataka) with light yellowish-white fur coat due to rosettes lacking black color. (b') The same at about 6-year of age along with normal colour partner (c).

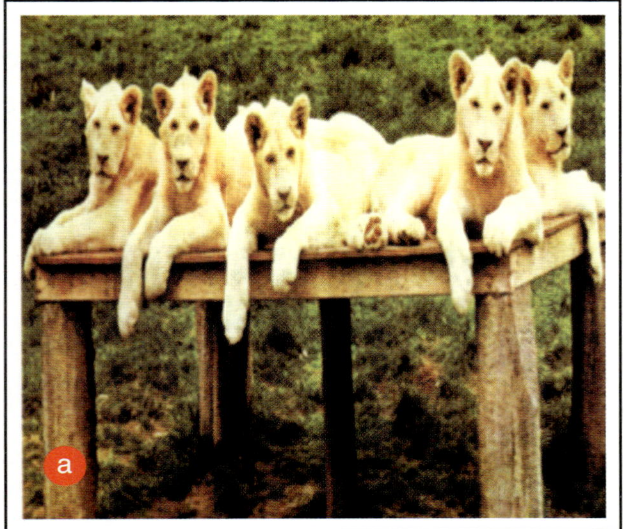

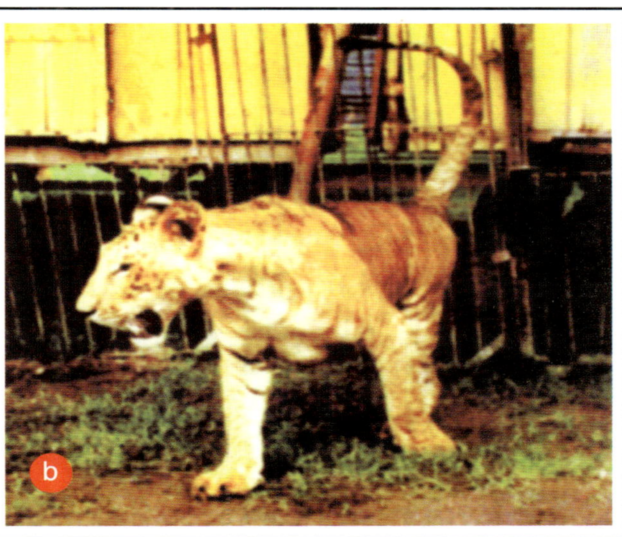

Figure 410: (a) A litter of five male white lion cubs at Zoo near Sydney, Austraila. (Times of India New Delhi, November 9, 2007).(b) Hybrid of TigerX Lioness with faint stripes in a circus of Bareilly (U.P.).

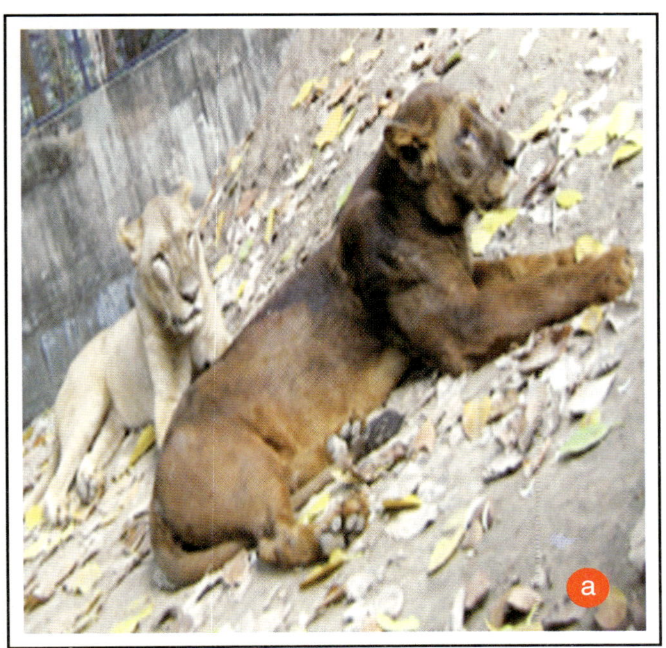

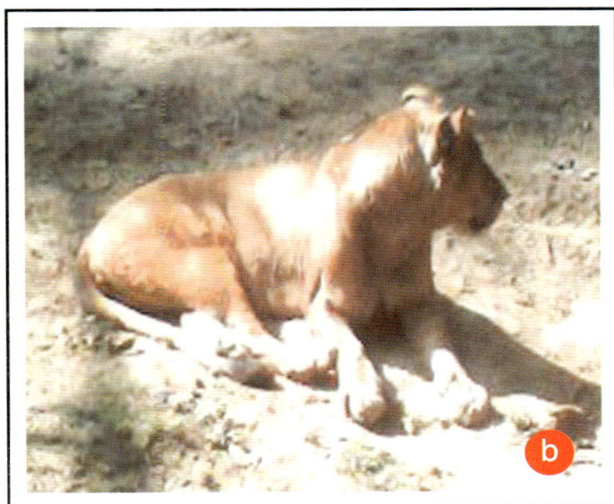

Figure 411: (a) Blackish brown fur in about 6- year-old hybrid lioness (*P. leo*) belonging to Biological Park, Patna (Bihar). As per history her body coat colour changed when she was under treatment for dental fistula and ecto-parasitic infestation(with Butox -Deltamethrin washing). (b) But after about four months when lioness suffered from urinary infection and treated with Norfloxacin, her coat colour reverted almost to its normal colour. (Ajay, S.K. Personal Comm.).

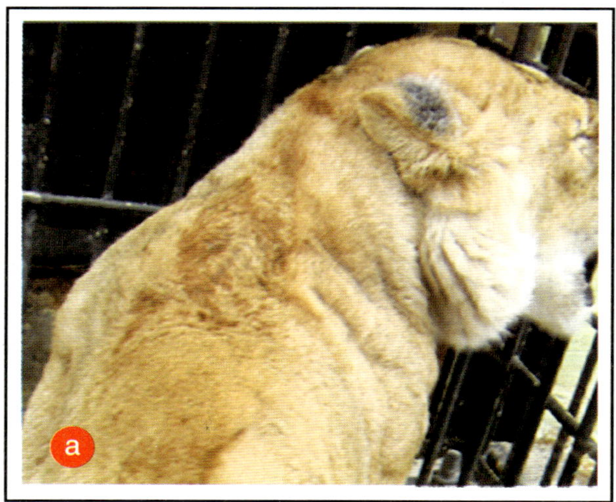

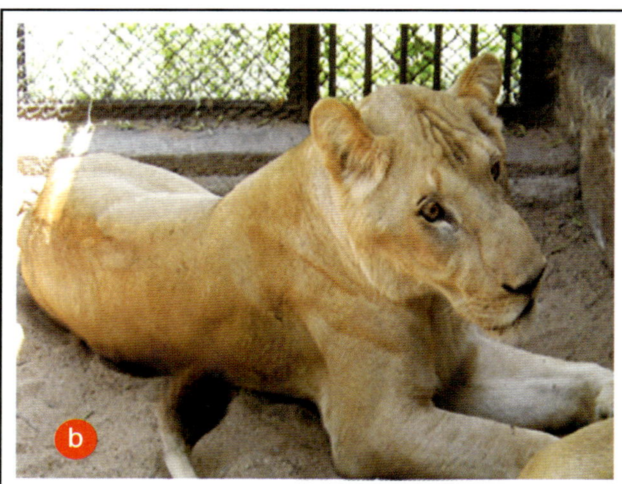

Figure 412: Male hybrid lions (*P. leo*) without mane (generally castration follows disappearance of mane) stationed at Rehabilitation Center of: (a) Bannerghatta National Park,Bangalore, Karnataka .(b) Zoological Park,Chennai, Tamil Nadu.

Figure 413: One of the leopard cubs had second to fifth toes syndactyly. The other cub too had syndactyly in some of the digits but its paws were partly cannibalized by mother.

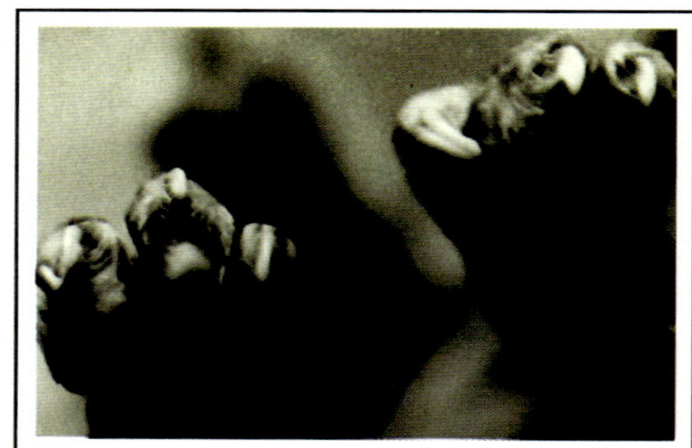

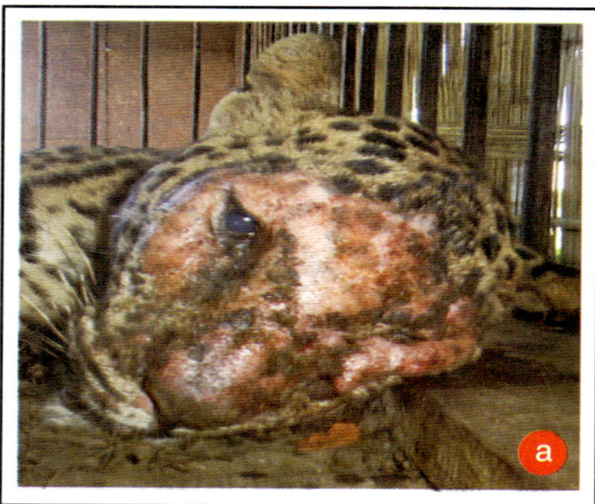

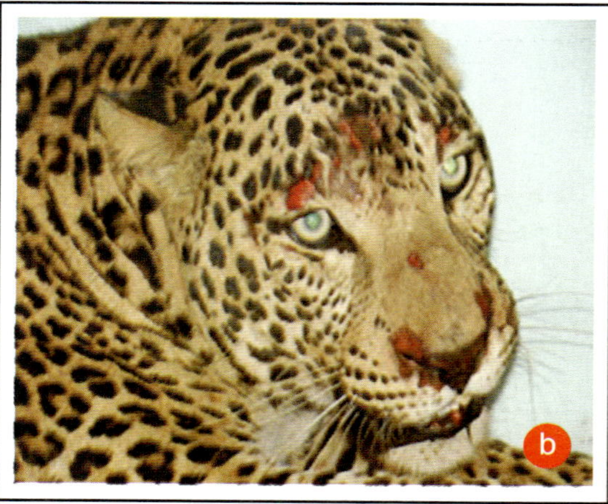

Figure 414: Photographs showing injuries occurred during trapping of man- eating leopards on their face. Courtesy: (a) Talukdar, A. and Choudhury, B. (b) on head (Courtesy: Joshi, H.C.).

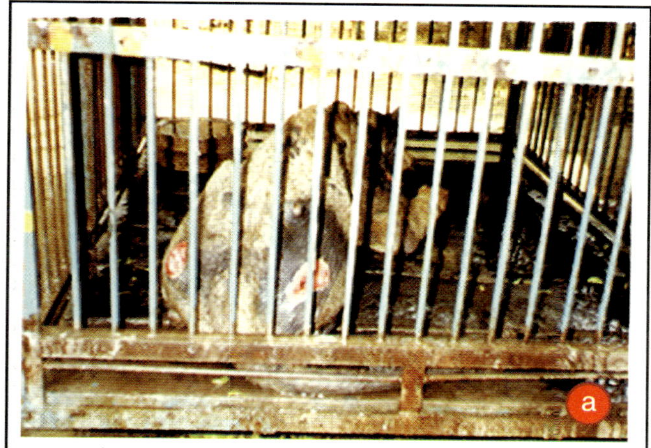

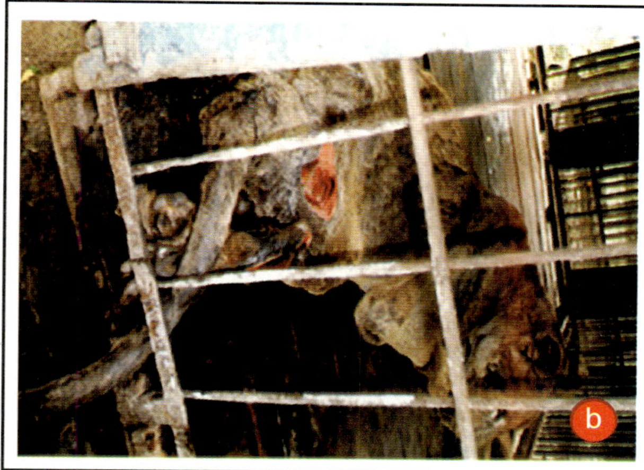

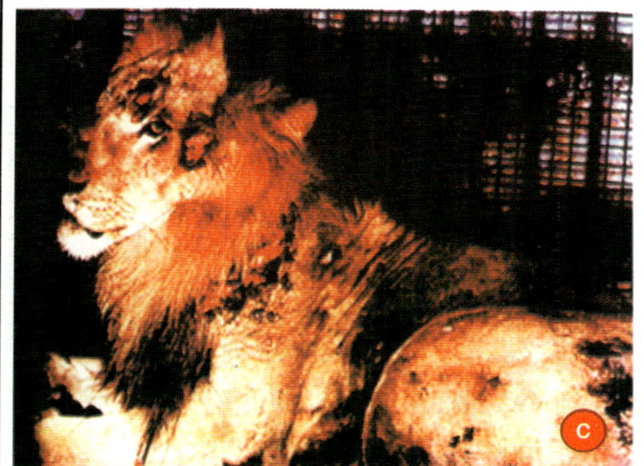

Figure 415: (a-c) During restraint operations traumatic wounds and abrasions are often encountered on face and quarters in large cats.

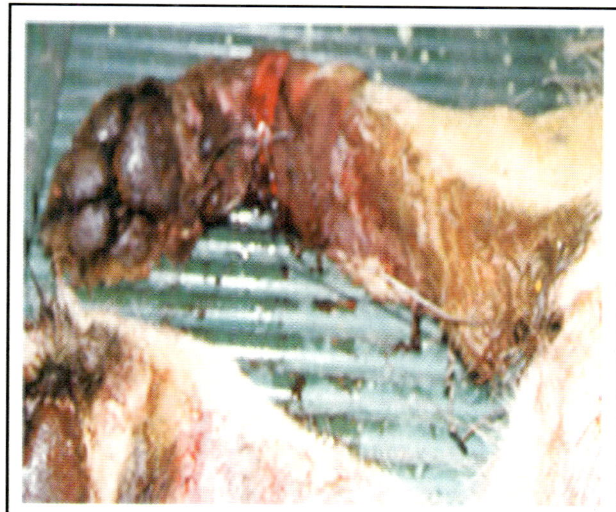

Figure 416: Photograph showing left fore foot of lion when trapped in snare trap (*P. leo persica*).

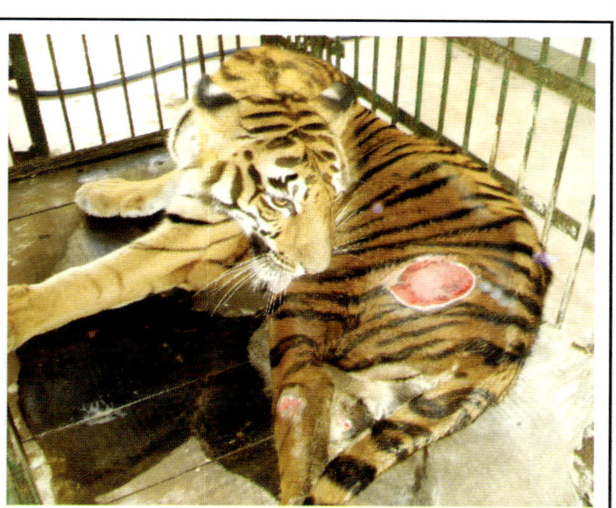

Figure 417: Bed sore developed in captivity in the upper thigh region of wild rescued tiger(Courtesy: Nath, I.)

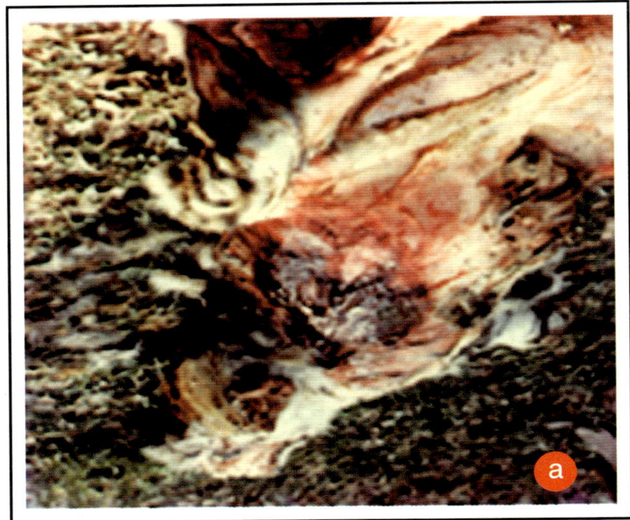

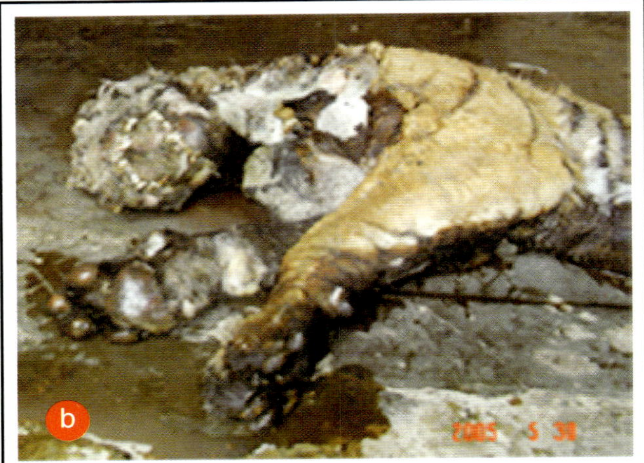

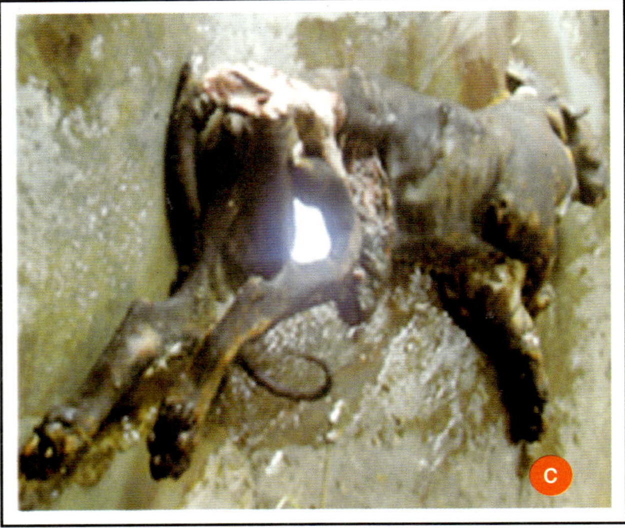

Figure 418: Photographs showing : (a) Charred right hind limb of wild tiger (*P. tigris*). (b, c) Charred body of another tiger (*P. tigris*). Both the cases belonged to Dudhwa National Park, Uttar Pradesh.

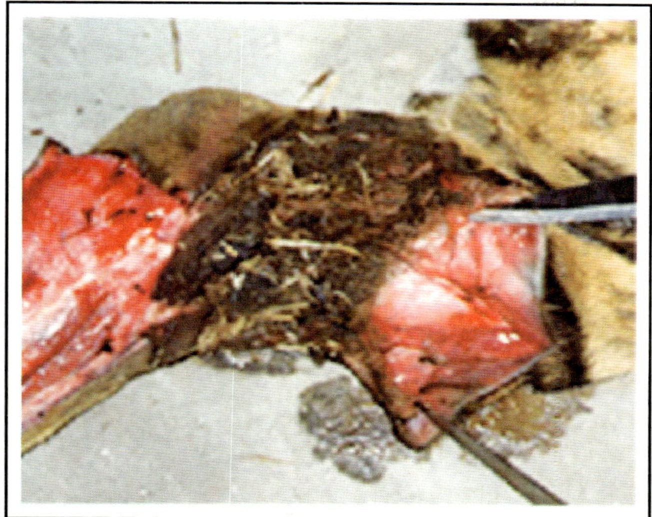

Figure 419: Charred (electrocuted) skin and muscles with haemorrhagic areas just above the hock joint in tigers(*P. tigris*) electrocuted in the forests of Madhya Pradesh (Courtesy: Srivastava, A.B.).

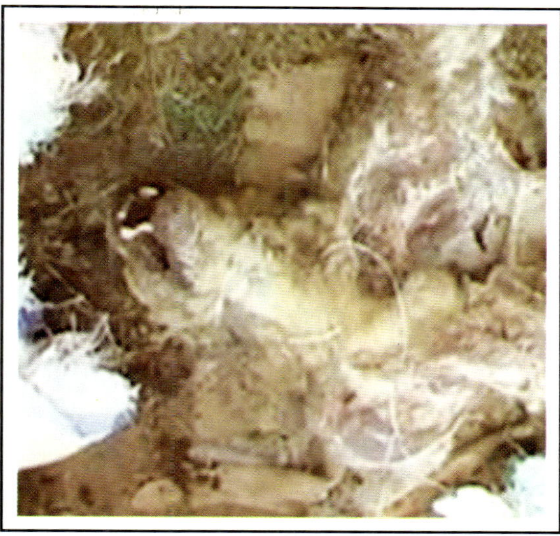

Figure 420: Carcass of one of the five lions (*P. leo persica*) found electrocuted on 19th October, 2007 in the Prempara village of district Amrelinear in Gujarat (Courtesy: Kishore bhai Kotecha).

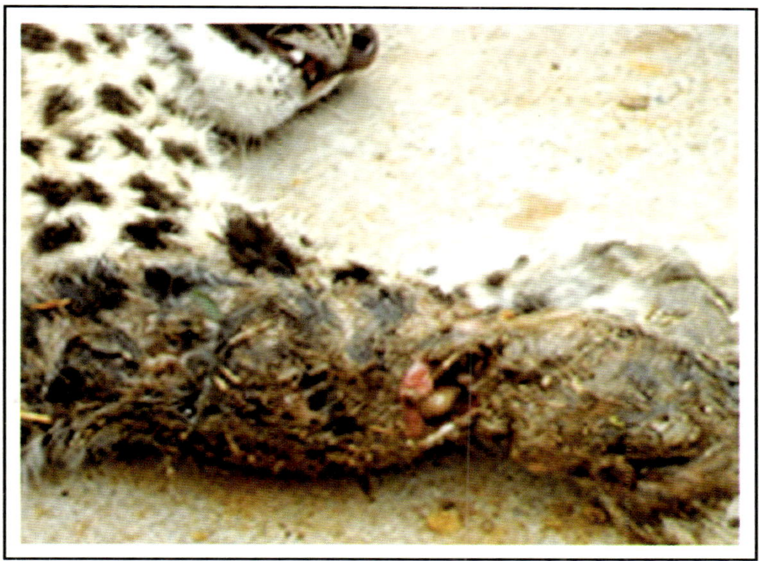

Figure 421: Leopard (*P. pardus*) victim of forest fire. Photograph showing 3rd degree burn injuries on skin of fore limbs, body and footpads,and wounds infested with maggots (Courtesy: Kishtwaria, R.S.).

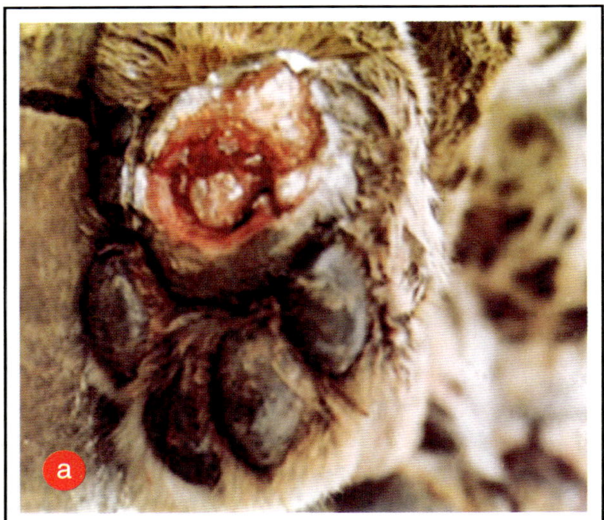

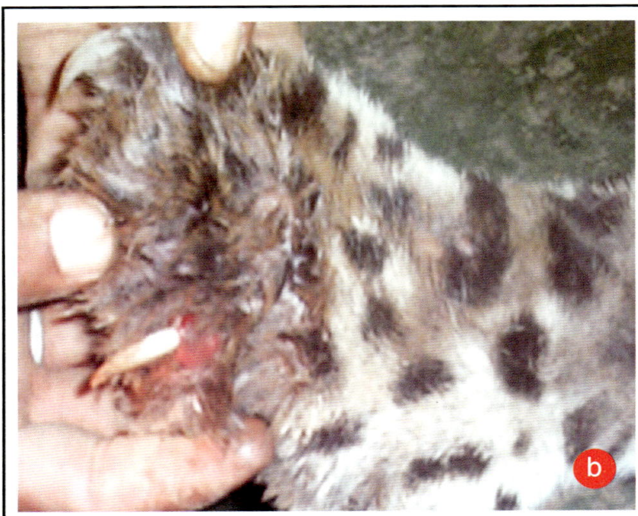

Figure 422: Man-eating leopards (*P. pardus*) sustained severely lacerated wounds in fore paws. (a) Leopard with injured fore paw foot pad belonging to Forest Div., Uttarakhand (Courtesy: Joshi, H.C.). (b) Wild leopard with injured fore foot toes belonging to Forest of Himachal Pradesh (Courtesy: Kishtwaria,R.S.).

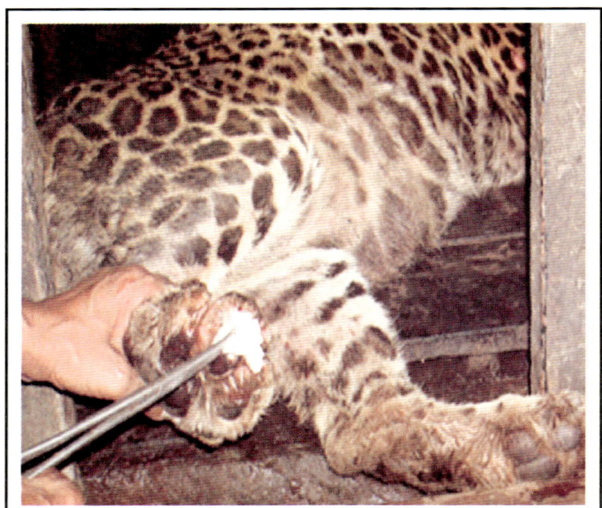

Figure 423: Photograph showing severe lacerated wound in the right hind foot pad of adult female leopard (*P. pardus*) at Biological Park, Patna. (Courtesy: Ajay, S.K.)

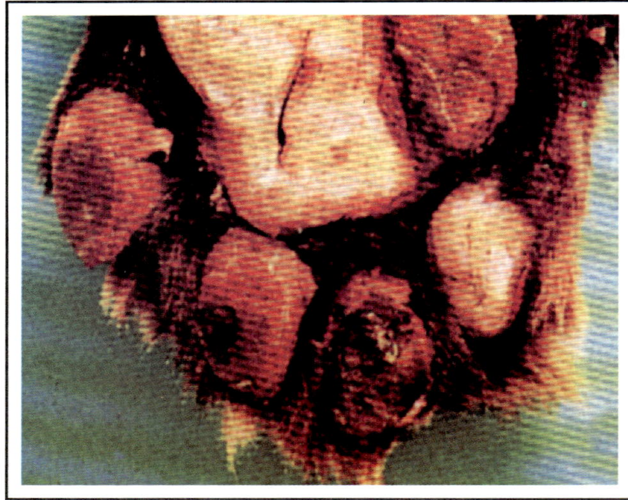

Figure 424: Lacerated wounds on left foot with necrotic lesions in toes encountered in wild tiger (*P. tigris*). Also note a sharp cut on the footpad.

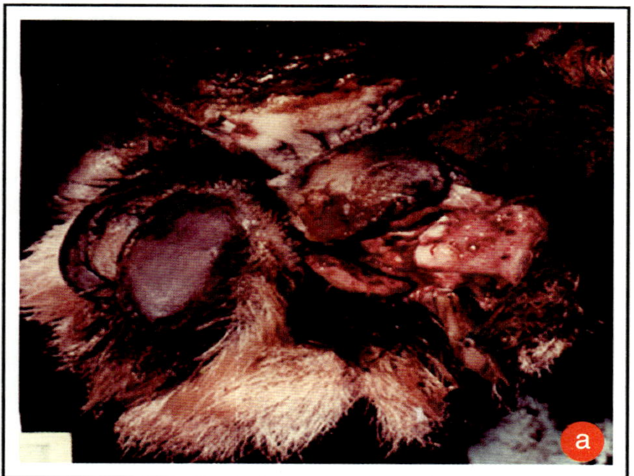

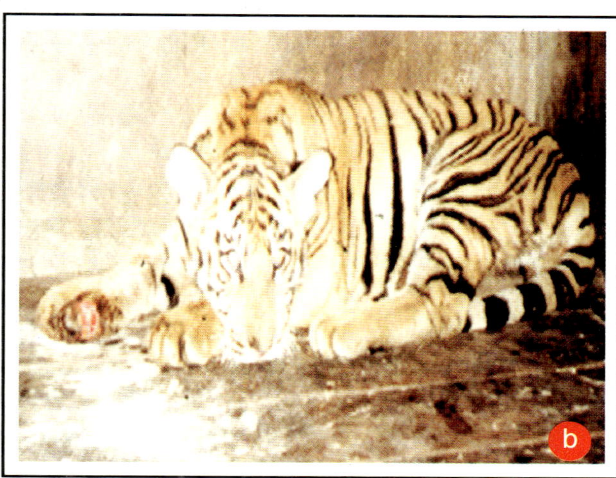

Figure 425: (a)Lacerated wounds in the footpad and toes of captive adult tiger (*P. tigris*).(b) Tiger (*P. tigris*) cub in Zoological Park, Chhatbir (Chandigarh) with lacerated wound in footpad of its right paw.

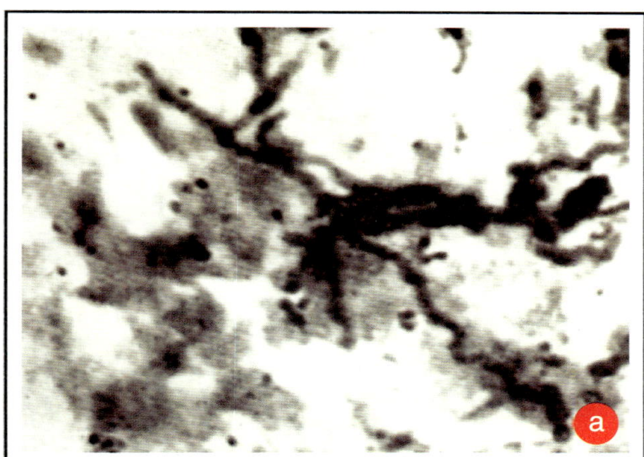

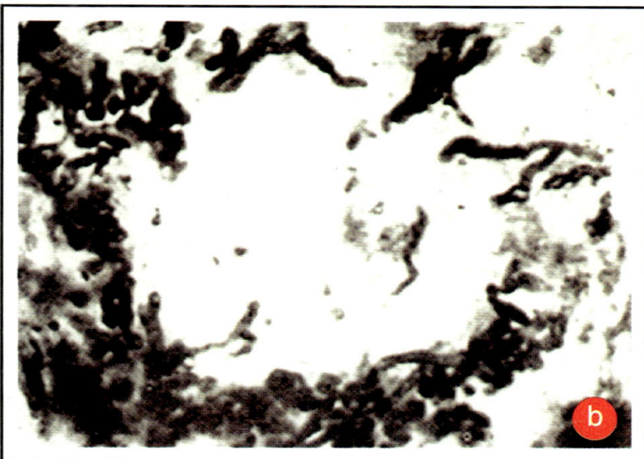

Figure 426: *Candida tropicalis* cultured from generalized cutaneous lesions in a hybrid lion (*P. leo*) cub died in National Zoological Park, New Delhi (a) Filamentous form of the organism in the lesion. PAS, x 440. (b) Filamentous and yeast form of organisms in the dermis. PAS, x 440 (Verma *et al.*, 1983).

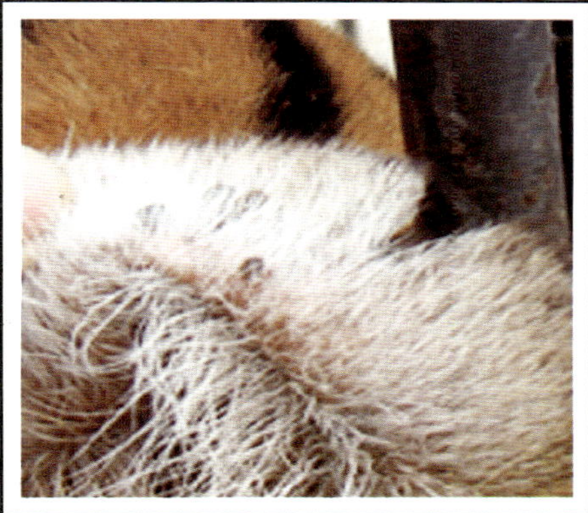

Figure 427: Soft tick infestation of ear in tiger (*P. tigris*) at Tiger Safari, Bannerghatta, Bangalore.

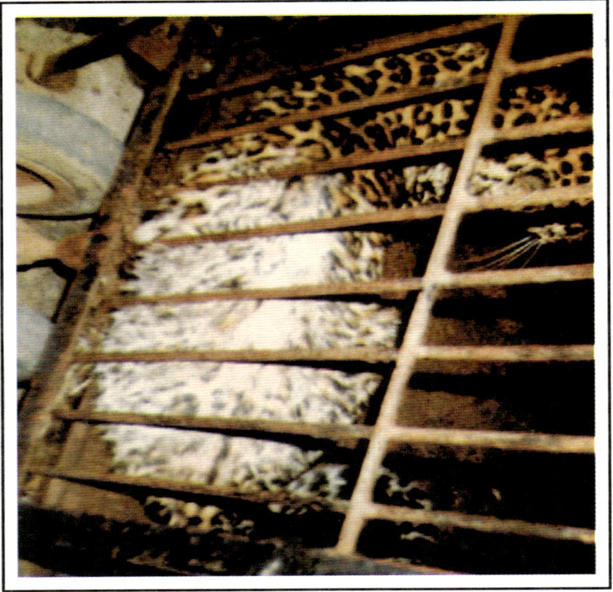

Figure 428: Photograph showing ectoparastic dermatitis in leopard (*P. pardus*) at Zoological Park,Kanpur (U.P.).

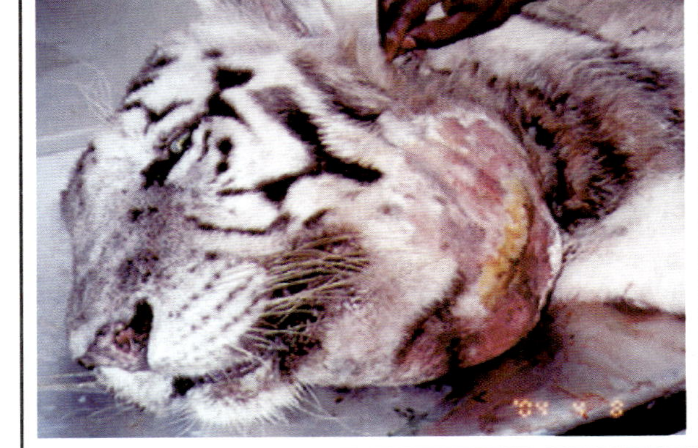

Figure 429: Swelling of left side of the face in tiger (*P. tigris*) caused due to melanoma (Courtesy: Dept. of Pathology, CVSc., Anand, Gujarat).

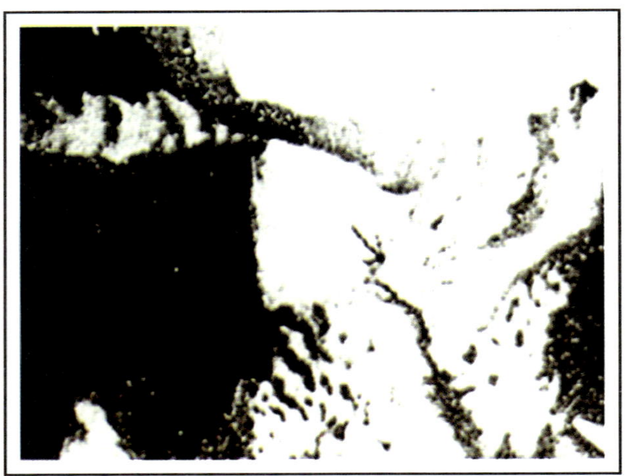

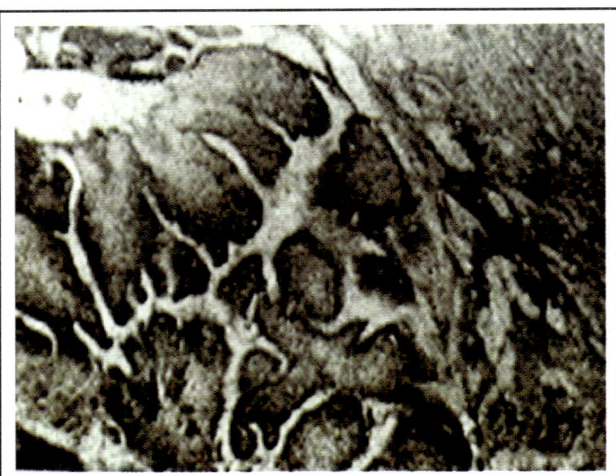

Figure 430: (a) Growth of squamous cell carcinoma around the tail of jaguar (*Panthra onca,* an exotic sp.) housed in Zoological Garden, Kolkata. (b)Photomicrograph showing well-differentiated tumour cells withabundant eosinophilic cytoplasm, intercellular bridges, concentric laminated masses of keratin, central aggregates of keratin cells. H & E x 100 (Paul *et al.*, 2002).

Musculo-Skeleton System

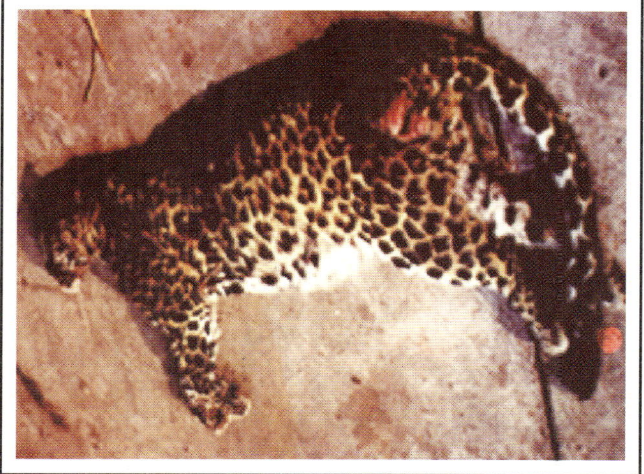

Figure 431: A leopard (*P. pardus*) carcass from wild having (inflicted) wound in its left thigh region.

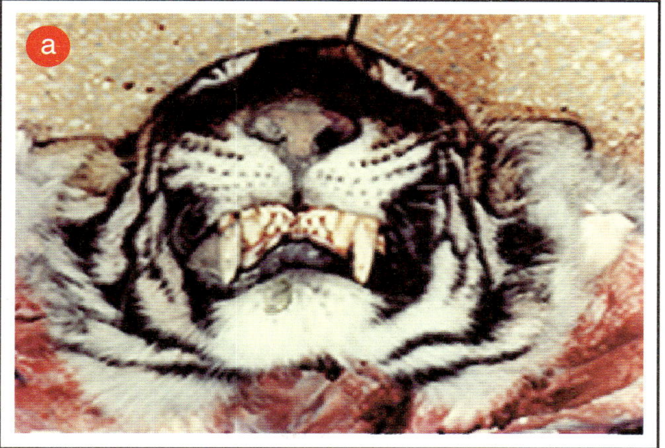

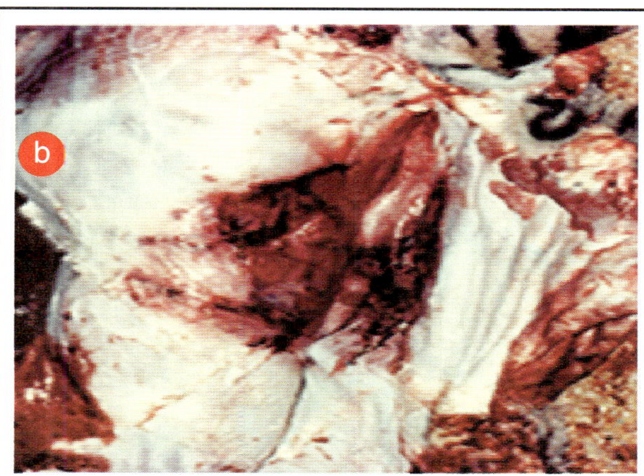

Figure 432: Carcass of tiger (*P. tigris*) shot dead in the forests of Pilibhit (U.P) showing agony of traumatic insult by clenched jaws (a) and muscular haemorrhages (b).

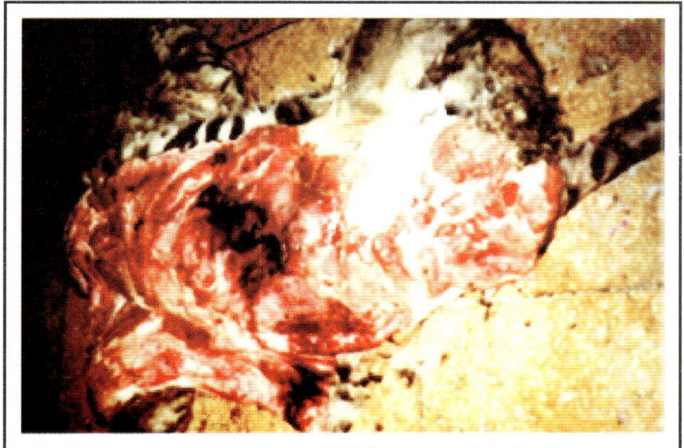

Figure 433: Photograph showing traumatic injury in wild leopard (*P. pardus*) alleged to infighting.

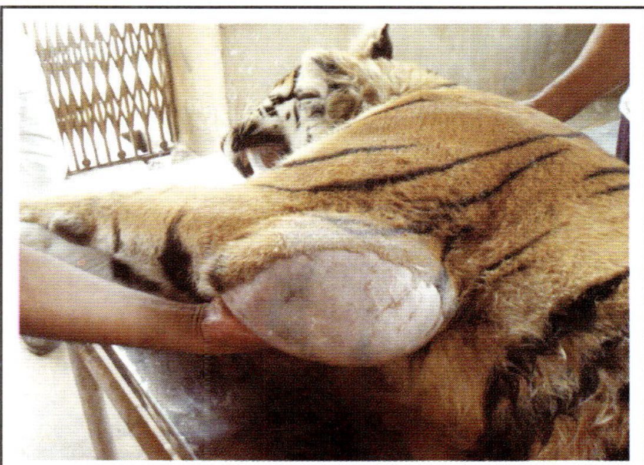

Figure 434: Hygroma at elbow in a tiger (*P. tigris*) in captivity (Courtesy: Nath, I.).

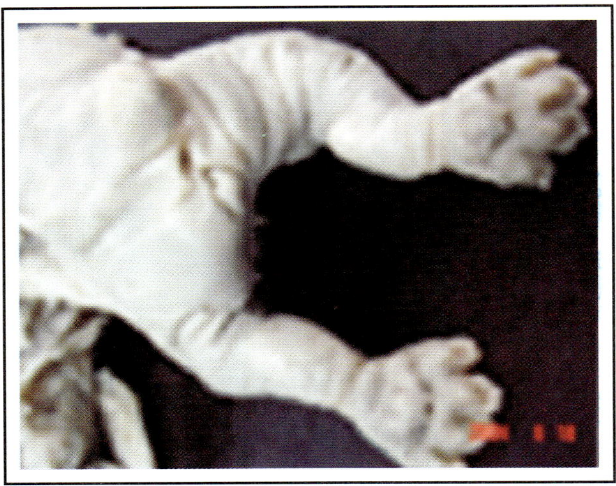

Figure 435: Stump tail encountered in an aborted leopard (*P.pardus*) foetus belonging to National Zoological Park, New Delhi.

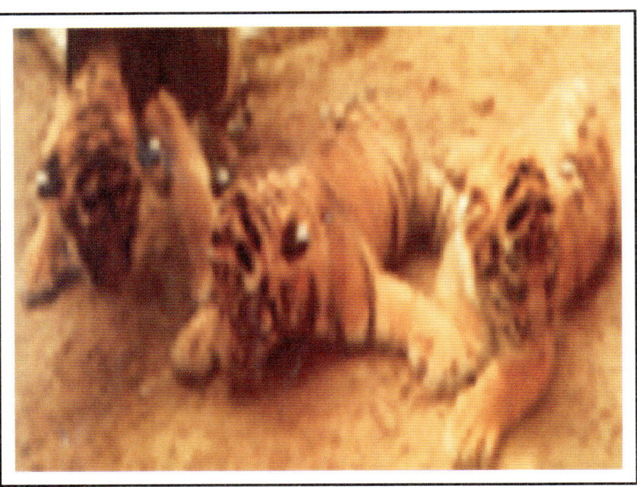

Figure 436: Photograph showing 3 tiger cubs (born in a litter) belonged to a circus suffering from congenital rickets. All the cubs had died within six months despite medical help.

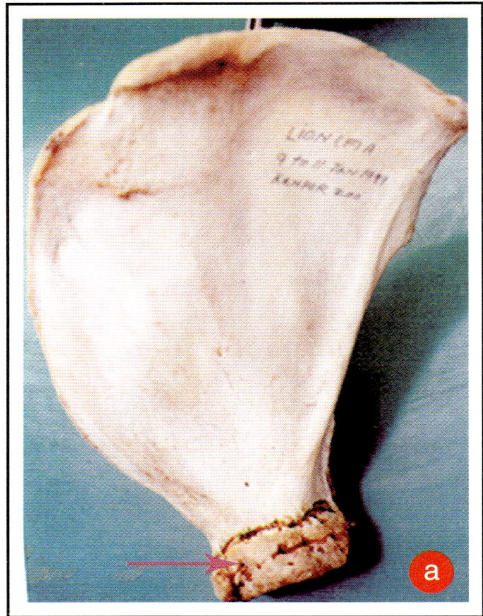

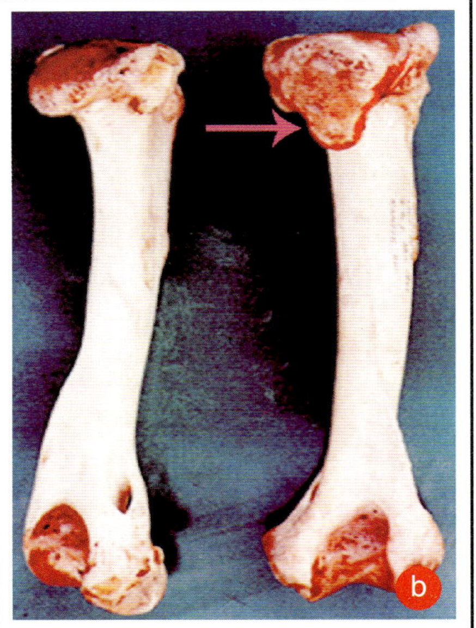

Figure 437: Photographs showing hyperostoitic growths: (a) Around the brim of scapula glenoid cavity. (b)Head of humerous encountered in an asiatic lion (*P. leo persica*) died in captivity.

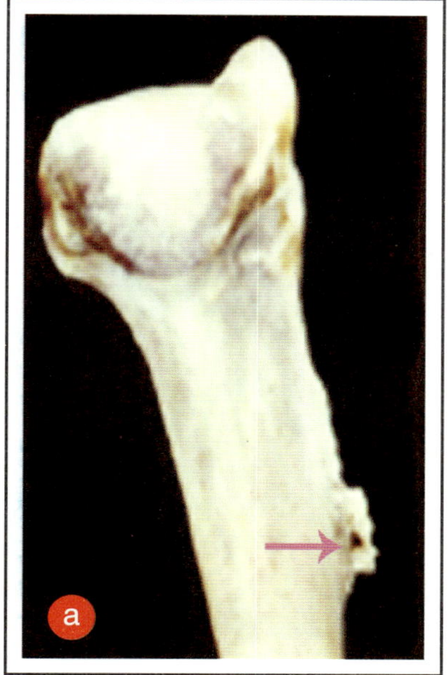

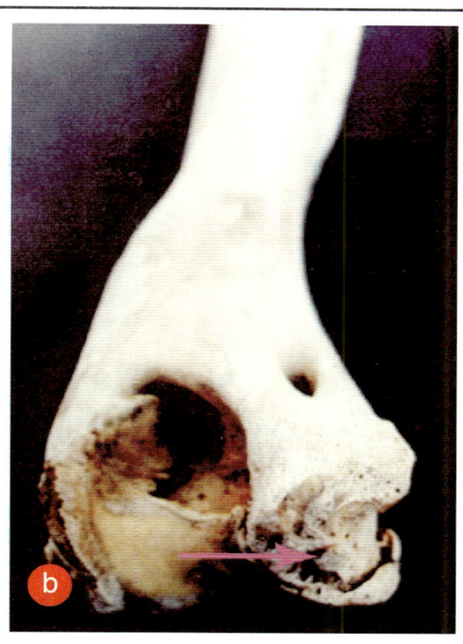

Figure 438: Photographs of humerous of wild tiger (*P. tigris*) showing: (a) Epiphytic growth on the medio-lateral aspect in the proximal third length of the shaft. (b) Formation of excrescences around the epicondyles. Note condyle damaged due to abcessation.

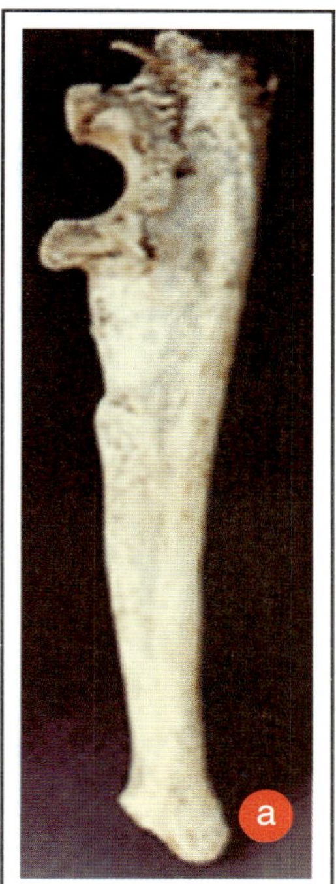

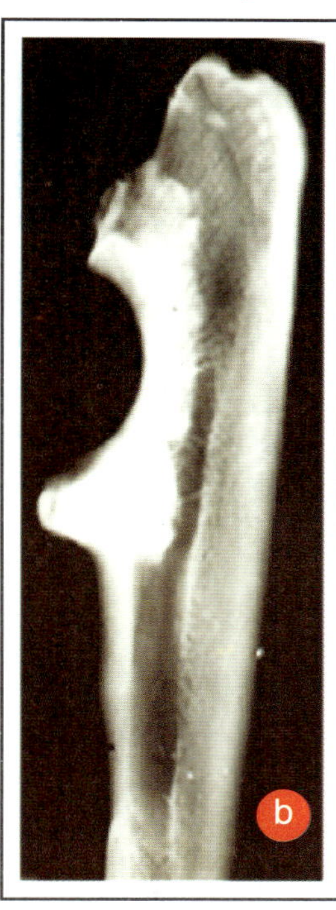

Figure 439: (a) Right ulna of wild tiger (*P. tigris*) showing excrescences in its proximal extremity and heavy excrescences along side the semi lunar notch. (b) Radiograph of (a).

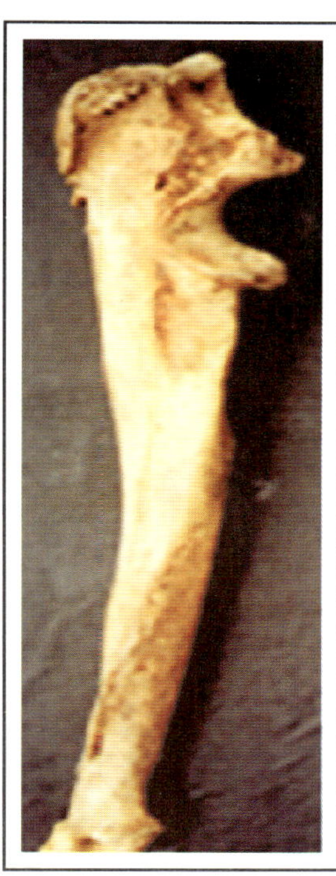

Figure 440: Left ulna of wild tiger (*P. tigris*) showing excrescences on medial aspect of olecranon and around trochlear notch.

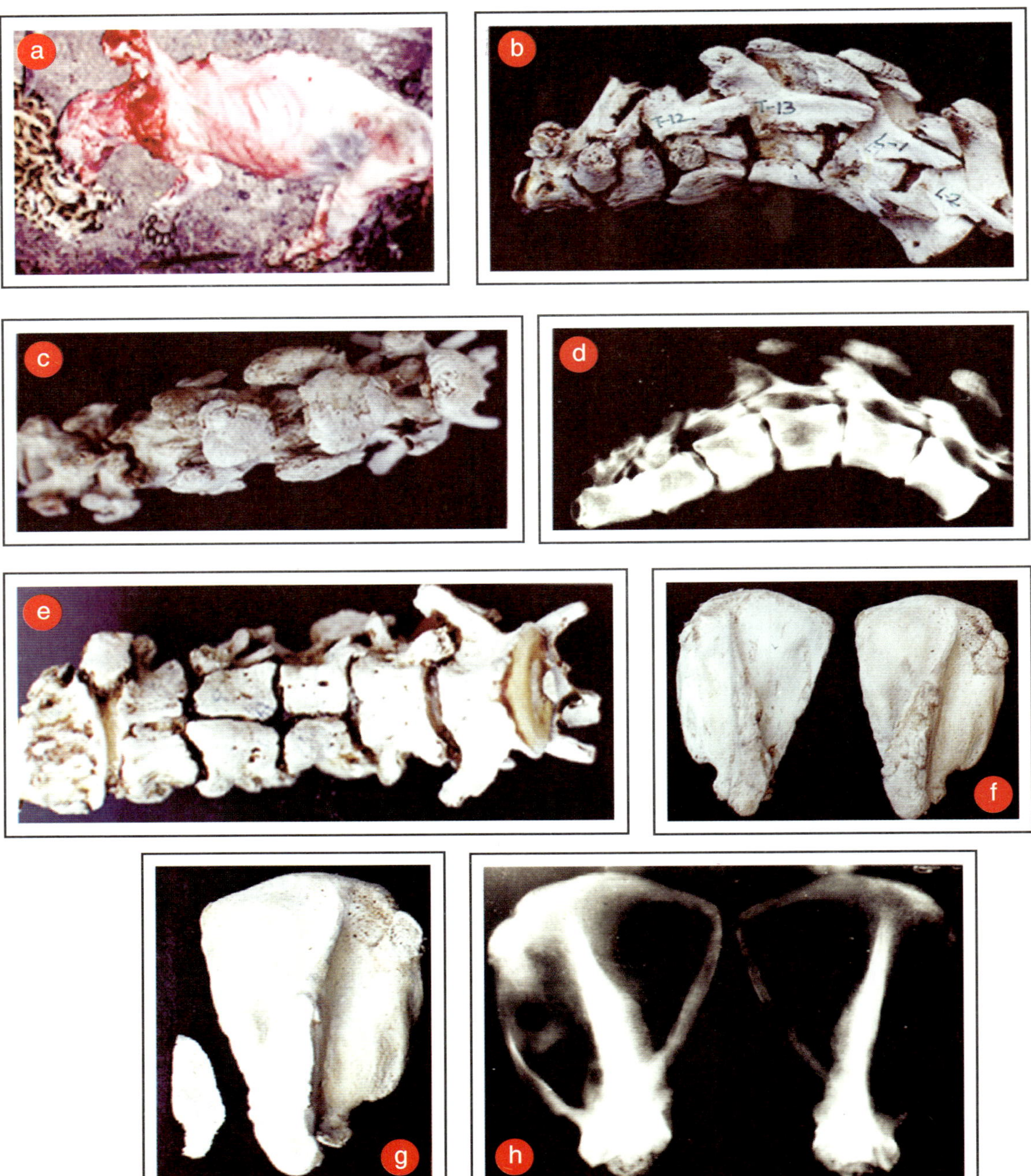

Figure 441: Osteomalacia in jaguar (*P. onca*, an exotic sp), which had died at Zoological Park, Kanpur (U.P.). Necropsy findings included: Photographs (a-c) showing: Kyphosis of thoracic vertebral region- 11th thoracic to 2nd lumbar vertebrae and exostoses of ends of spinal and transverse processes. (d) Radiograph of (b) showing lateral view of the same. (e) The ventral aspect of 3 vertebrae of (b) showing a longitudinal crack. (f, g) Thin pliable scapulae. (h) Radiograph of (f) showing depletion of bony substance in supra and infra spinatous fossae.

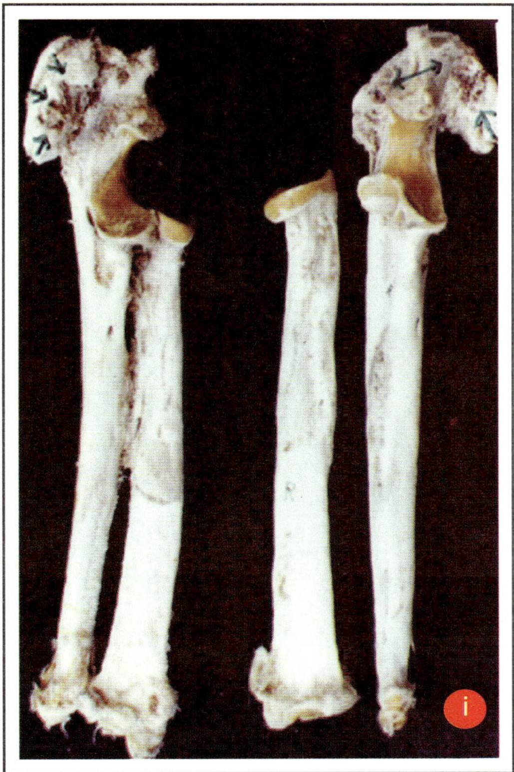

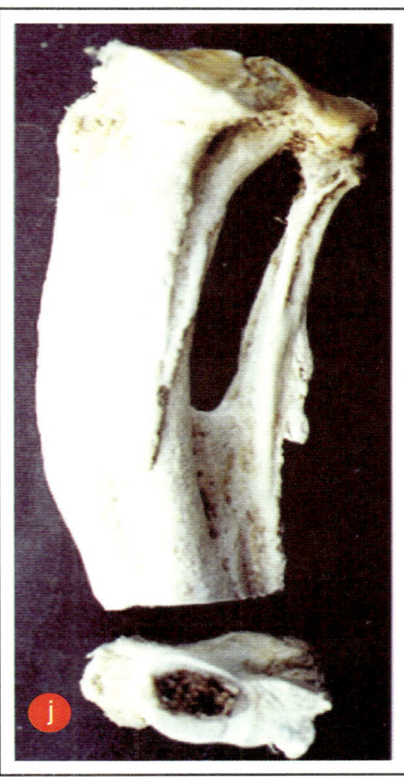

Figure 441: (i) Exostoses at Proximal extremity of each ulna (j) Fibula in its lower half joined by a thin osseous tissue with tibia. Note thickened cortex of tibia.

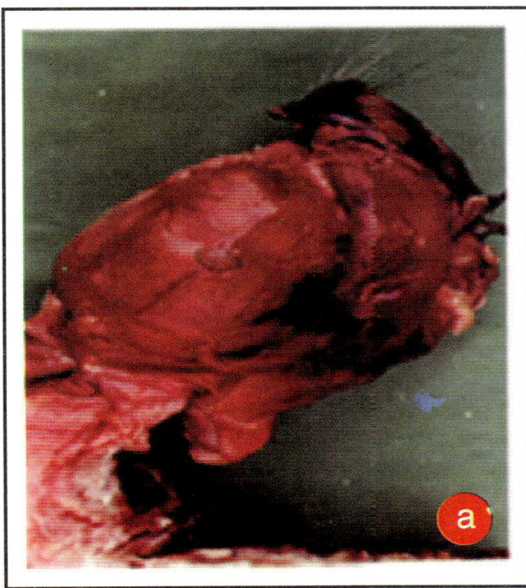

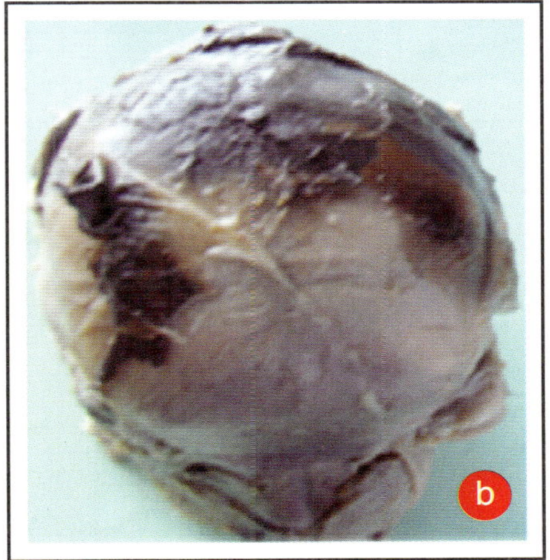

Figure 442: Photographs of de-skinned skulls of large cats showing congestion and haemorrhages. (a) 25-day-old female tiger (*P. tigris*) cub belonging to Corbett N. P. (b) Lion (*P. leo*) cub belonging to National Zoological Park, New Delhi. This could be due to stressed mother seizing firmly her offspring with the head to shift them in the face of some threat.

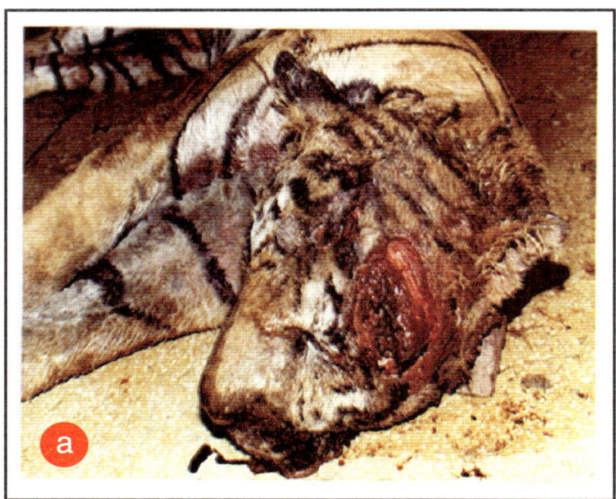

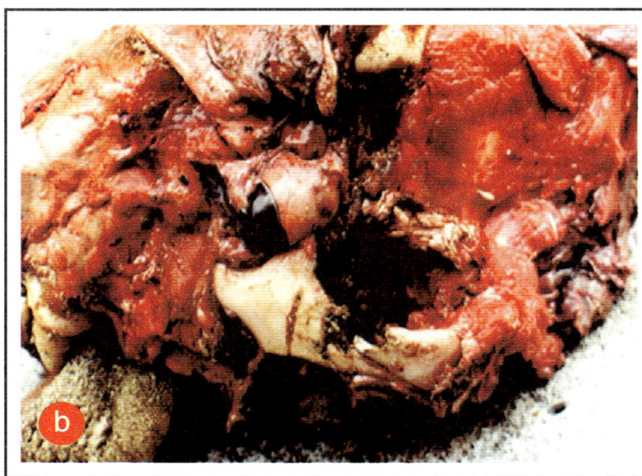

Figure 443: (a) Carcass of an adult male tiger (*P. tigris*) from Corbett National Park, Ramnagar. (b) Skull of (a) showing fracture of left zygomatic arch causing damage of its eyeball. The case is also referred for appendicular skeleton anomaly and under sense organs.

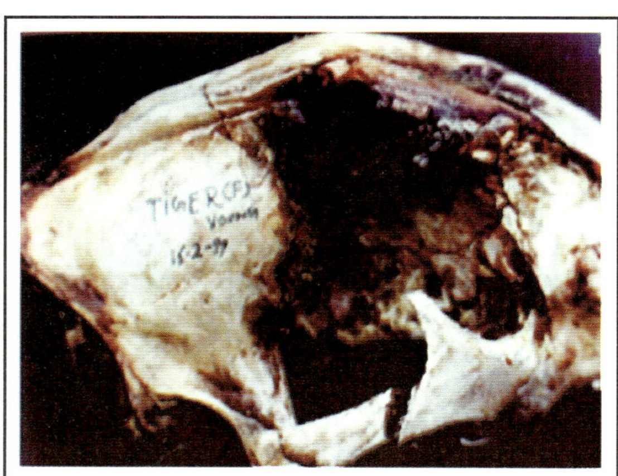

Figure 444: Young wild tiger (*P. tigris*) killed in retaliation in Haldwani forest division. Note fracture of right zygomatic arch.

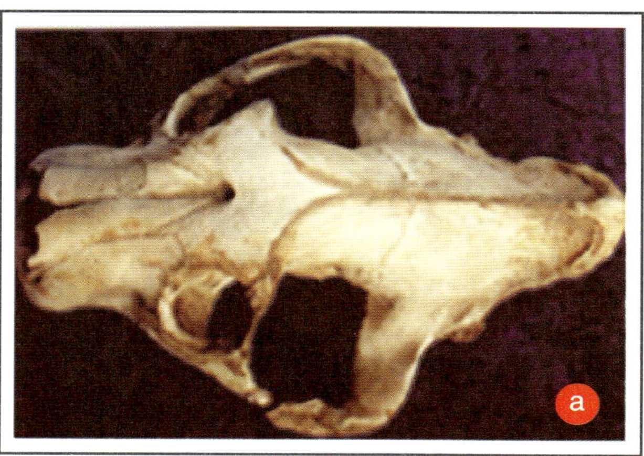

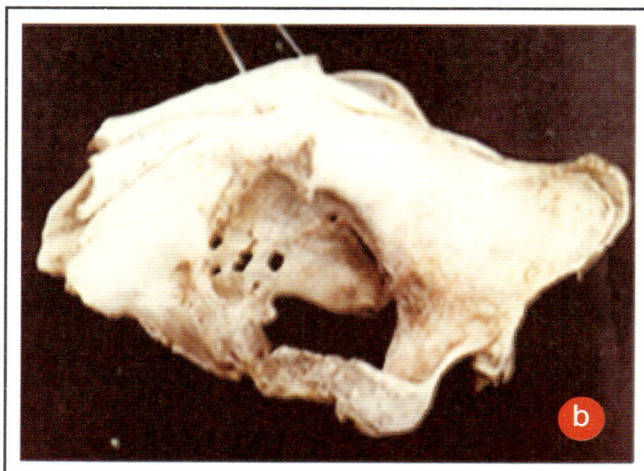

Figure 445: Photographs of tiger (*P. tigris*) skulls (a,b) from Dudwa National Park of Uttar Pradesh showing antemortem-traumatized left zygomatic arches.

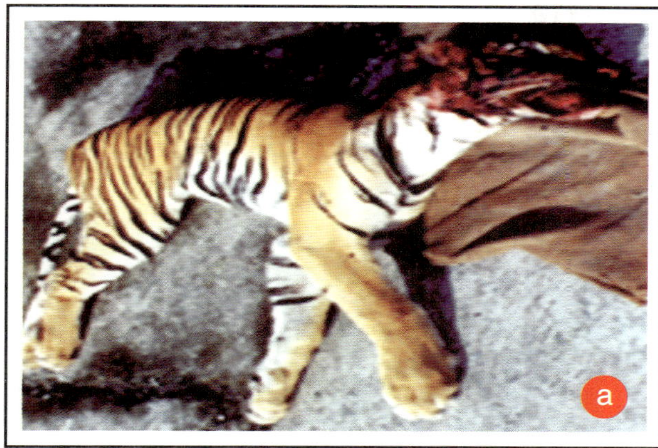

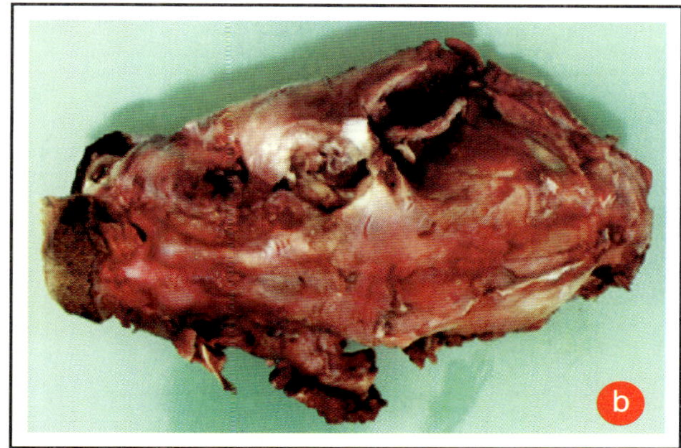

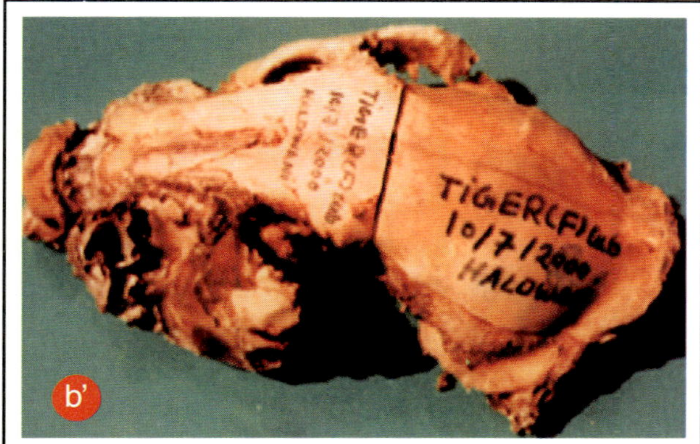

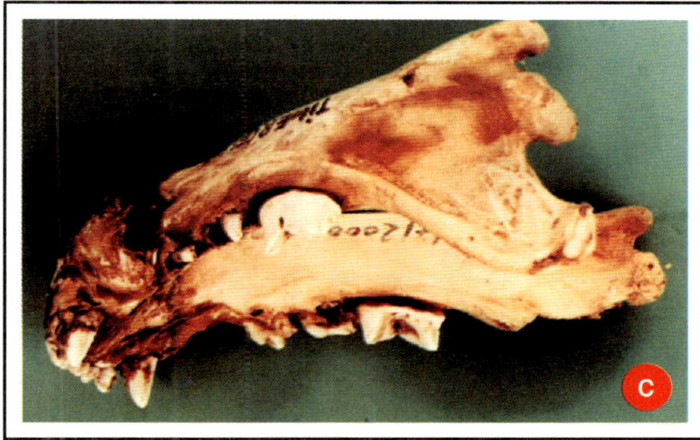

Figure 446: Photographs showing: (a) Carcass of Sub adult tigress (*P. tigris*), which entered into hut of a villager, attacked family members and in protection she was struck with an iron rod and succumbed of traumatic shock. Note spilling of blood in the head region. Necropsy showed fractures in skull (b, b') and mandible(c) of the tigress.

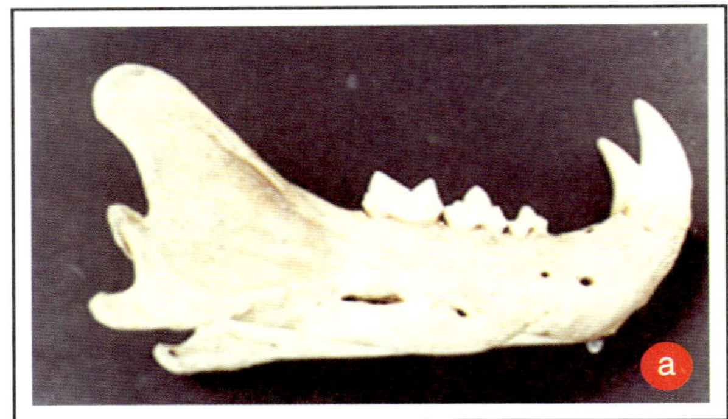

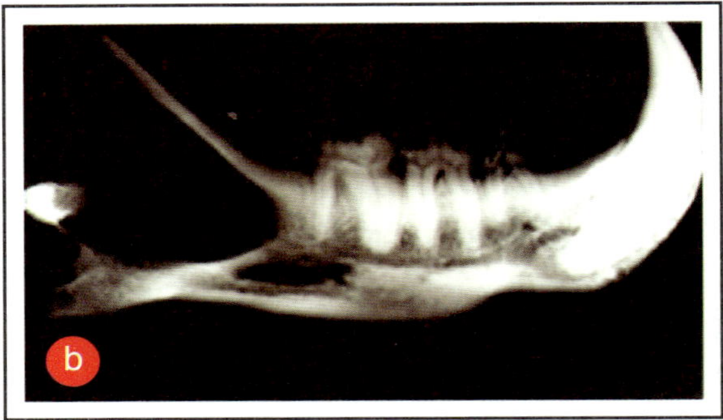

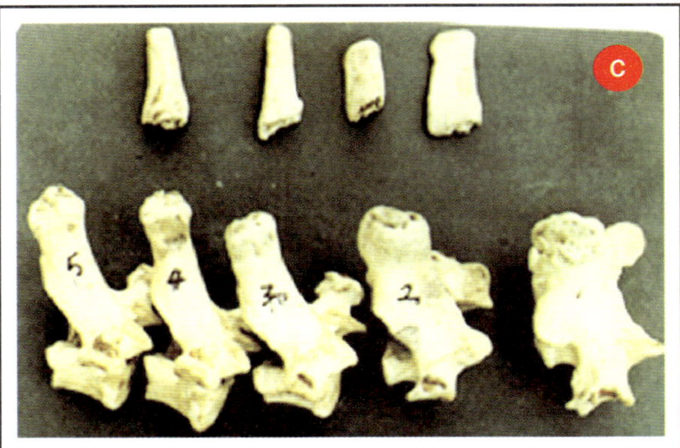

Figure 447: Photograph of right horizontal ramus of mandible of wild tiger (*P. tigris*) showing: (a) Healed fracture. (b) Radiograph of (a) showing small unresolved space. (c) Photograph showing chronic fractures of spinal processes of first to fifth thoracic vertebrae of (a).

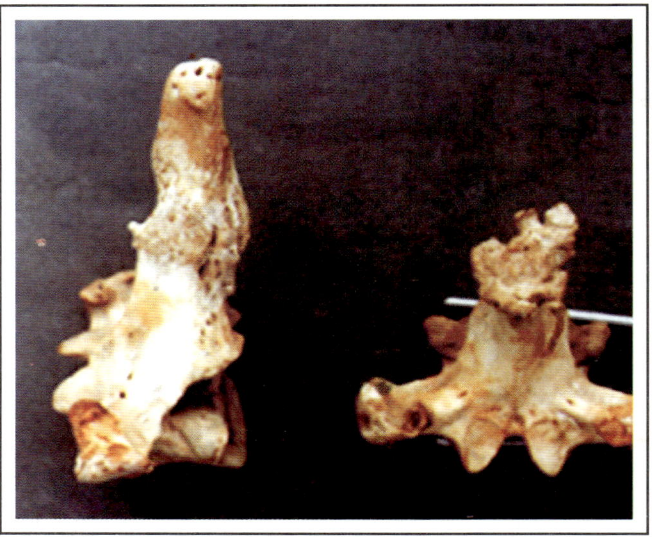

Figure 448: Photograph showing faulty healed spinal process of 4th thoracic vertebra and broken spinal process of 8th thoracic vertebra encountered in wild tiger (*P. tigris*).

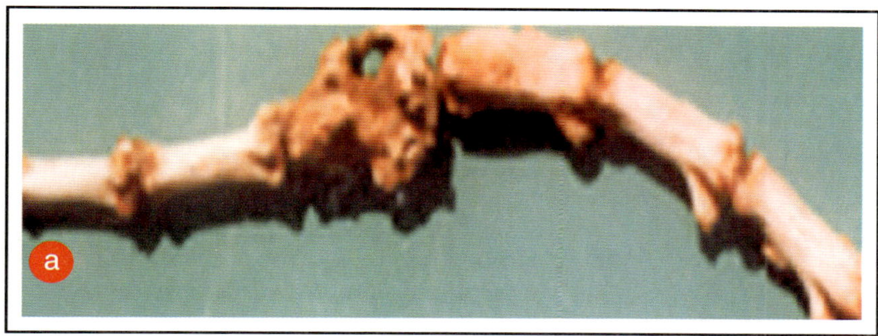

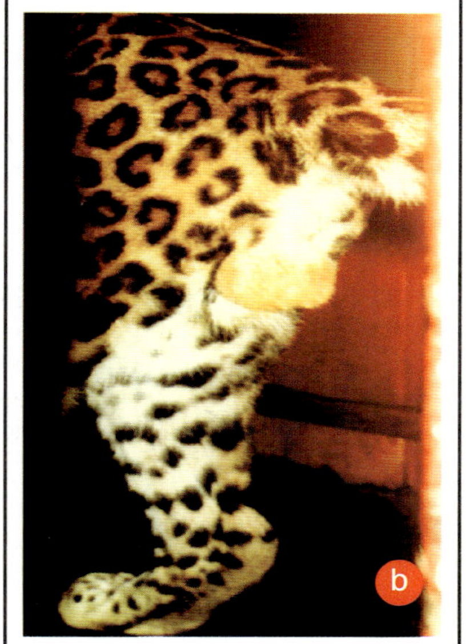

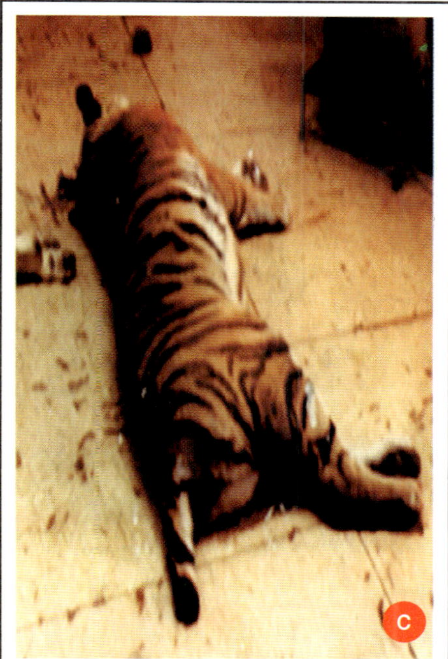

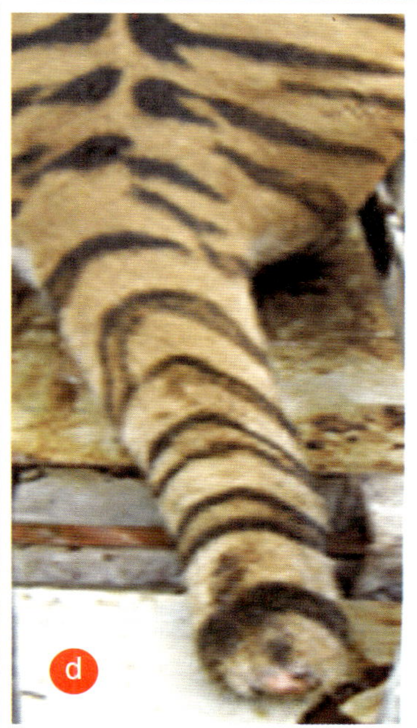

Figure 449: Tail anomalies observed in adult large cats include: (a) Uneven callus formation of fracture of 12 th coccygeal vertebra encountered in tiger (*P. tigris*) died in National Park, Dudwa (U.P). Missing of tail in: (b) leopard (*P. pardus*) from base onwards. (c, d) Loss of tail more than half of the total length wild and captive tigers (*P. tigris*).

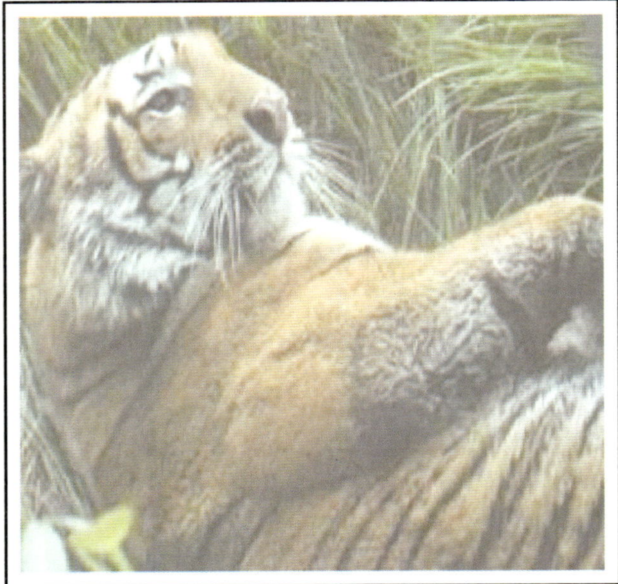

Figure 450: An adult tiger (*P. tigris*) in forest was hit in its posterior part of the body (lumbar region) by a speedy vehicle and unable to stand and bear weight on hindquarter (Courtesy: Pande, R.). Note: Animal was rescued and shifted to Zoological Garden, Lucknow, however it succumbed soon after arrival.

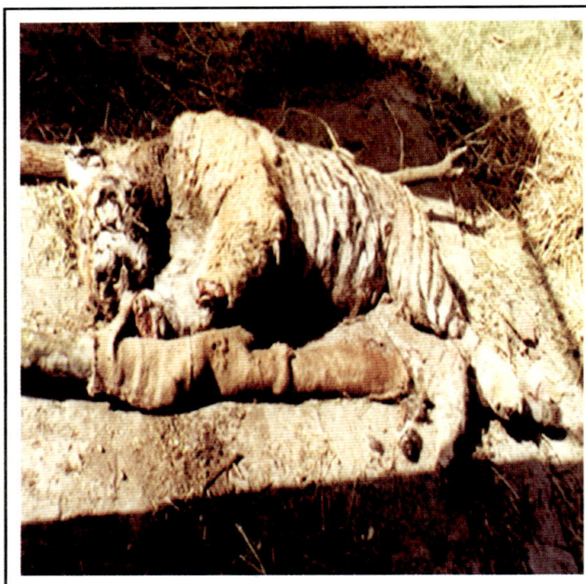

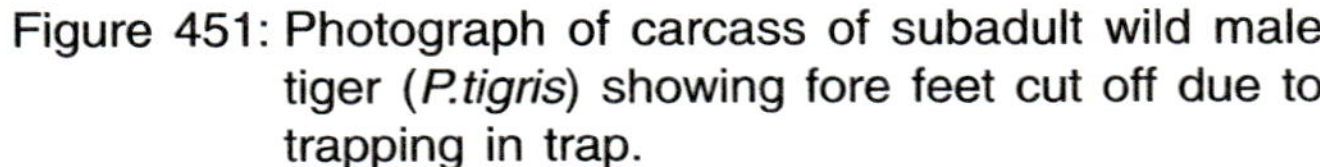

Figure 451: Photograph of carcass of subadult wild male tiger (*P.tigris*) showing fore feet cut off due to trapping in trap.

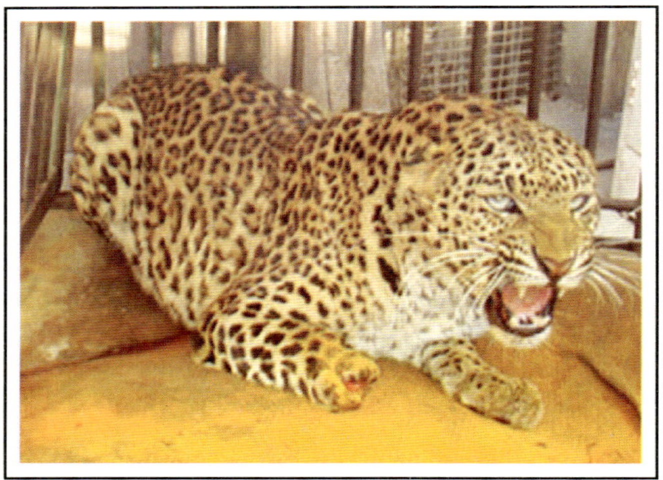

Figure 452: Fore feet cut off in a subadult leopard (*P. pardus*) due to trapping in trap and was housed in a captive facility at Shimla (HP).

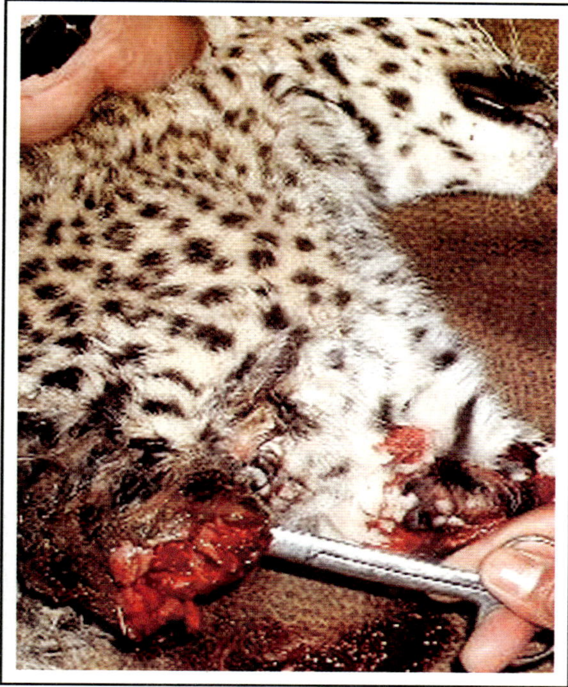

Figure 453: Amputed lower half of the right limb of a leopard (*P. pardus*) cub, which had complicated burn wound. The case is also referred under integumemtary system. (Courtesy: Kanwar, M.S.).

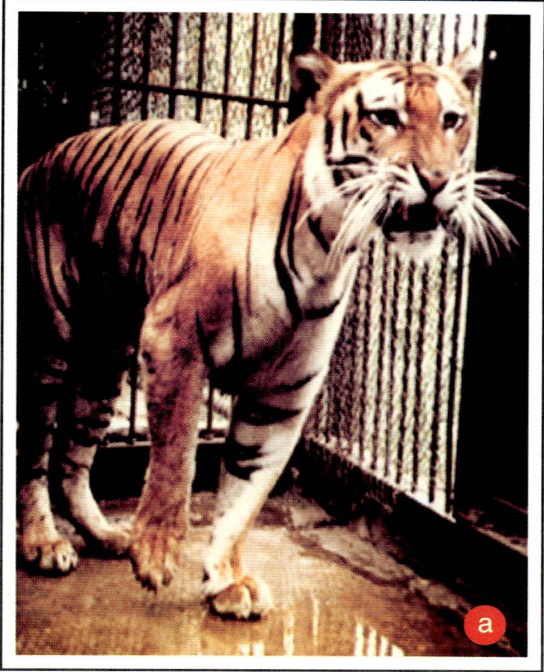

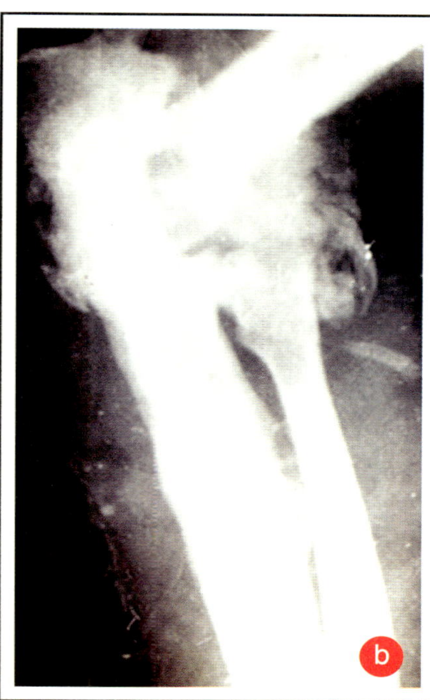

Figure 454: Photographs (a) showing gun shot injury at right elbow joint of tigress (*P. tigris*) belonging to Dudwa National Park (U.P). The bullet lodged in the elbow joint was extracted. Despite treatment the wound got infected. (b) Radiograph of traumatized joint showing osteomyelitis and ankylosis.

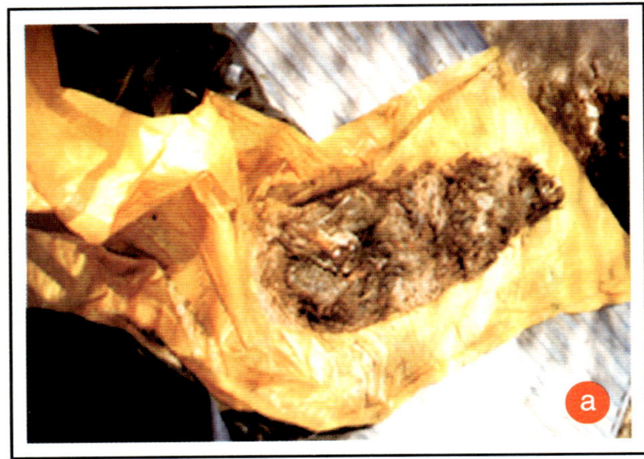

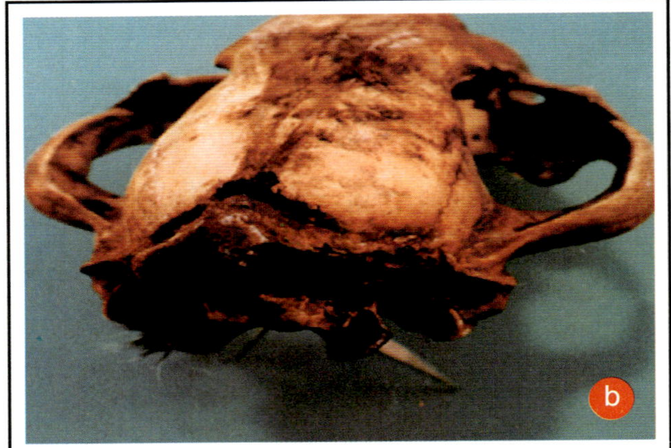

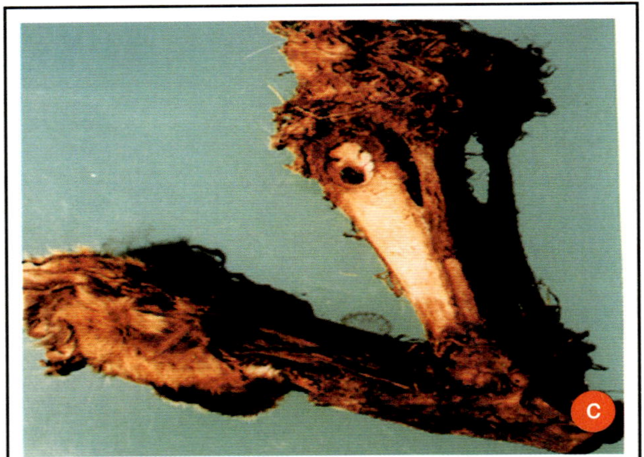

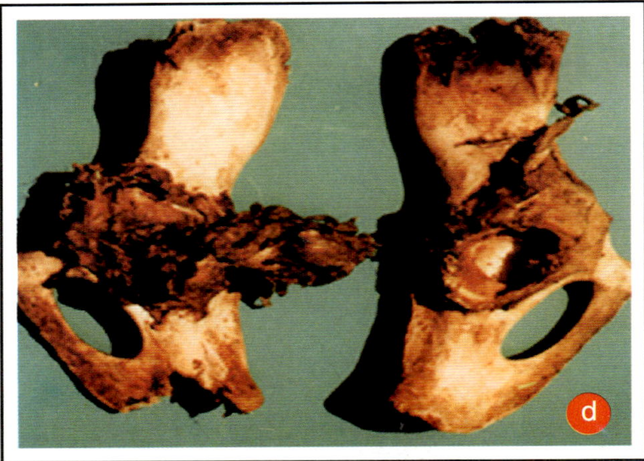

Figure 455: (a) Decomposed carcass of about one-year old wild tiger (*P. tigris*). Skeleton elements of (a) showing: (b) Deep lacerated marks in the occipital region of skull. (c) A canine mark on tibia and (d) damaged pelvic bones. A predator might have killed the cub. Male tiger may attack the cub accompanying the mother tigress in heat.

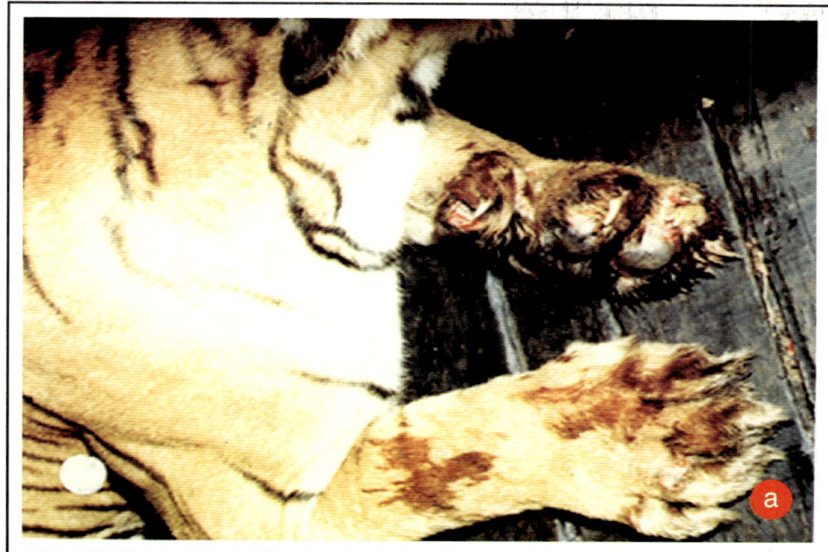

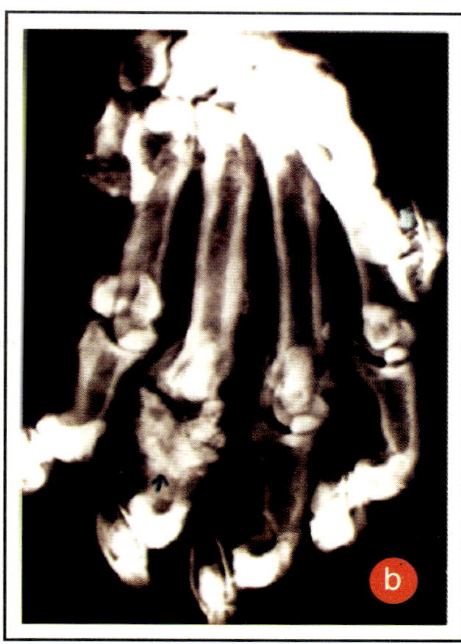

Figure 456: (a) Carcass of an adult tiger (*P. tigris*) belonging to Corbett National Park (Uttarakhand) showing chronic wound extending from footpads to metacarpal bones of both fore paws. (b) Radiograph of (a) showing healing of fractures in 1st phalanges of 3rd and 5th metacarpals of left side.

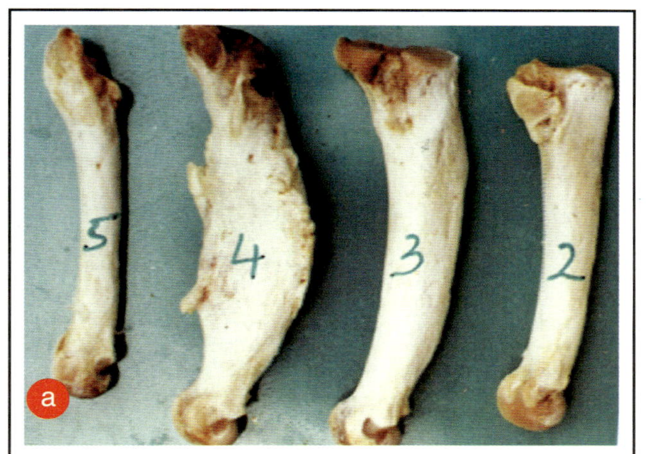

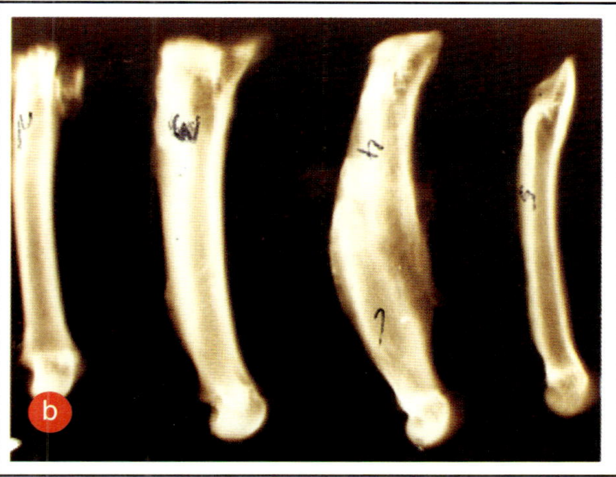

Figure 457: Photograph (a) of left metatarsals of tigress (*P. tigris*) died in Dudhwa National Park (U.P) showing: Periosteal irregular growths on 4th metatarsal and its radiograph (b) uneven healed fracture without uniting medullar canal.The left 3rd metatarsal also showed periosteal thickening. The affected 4th metatarsal scaled 44.40g, and measured 7.2 cm in girth.The corresponding figures of right metatarsal were, 27g and 4.6 cm respectively. The proximal and middle phalanges of 4th metatarsal were also affected except in their distal extremity (not shown in photo). The first phalanx weighed 27 g and measured 9.1 cm in girth. The corresponding figures of right side were; 13.95g and 4.4cm, respectively.

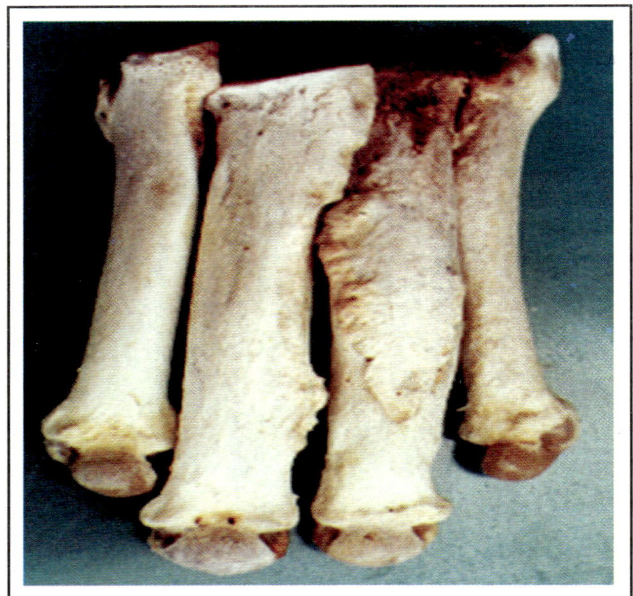

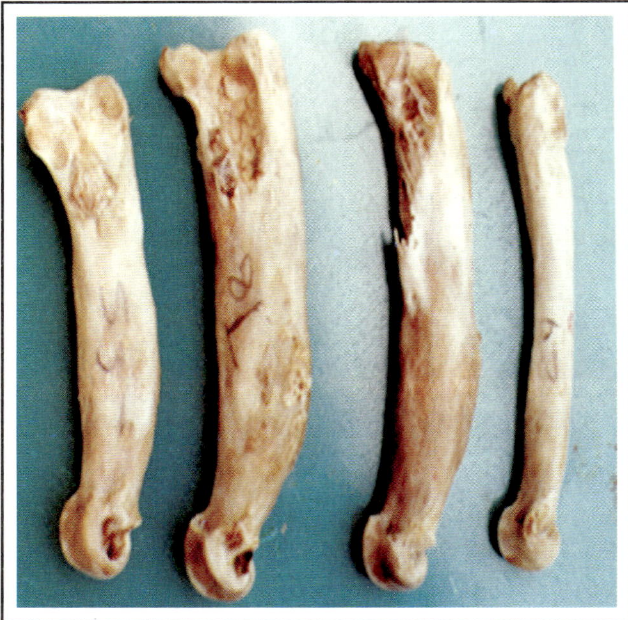

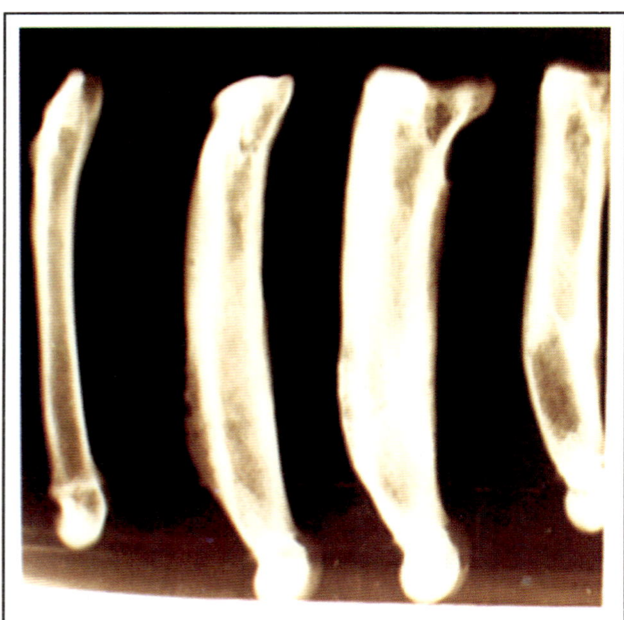

Figure 458: Necropsy of a wild male tiger (*P. tigris*) showed 2nd to 4th right metatarsal bones increased in thickness. Third metatarsal was enlarged more than alies. At the middle of palmer aspect of 4th metarsal had interrupted periosteal reaction. The radiograph showed increased thickness of the cortices but presence of medullary canal in all. Metatarsals R/L weighed(g): 1st = 55.0/35.0 ; 2nd= 78.0/60.0; 3rd= 56.0/42.0; 4th= 29.0/29.0. The above findings clearly evidenced that animal had metatarsal bones affected.

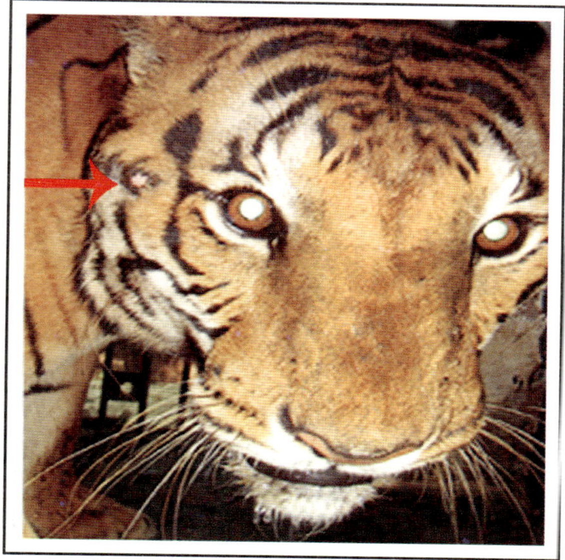

Figure 459: An adult male tiger (*P. tigris*) at Biological Park, Patna (Bihar) showing both sides of its head swollen due to either some chronic osteopathy or tumorous growth.

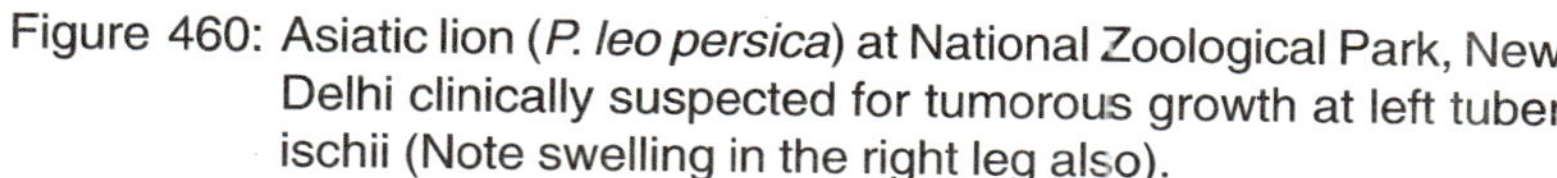

Figure 460: Asiatic lion (*P. leo persica*) at National Zoological Park, New Delhi clinically suspected for tumorous growth at left tuber ischii (Note swelling in the right leg also).

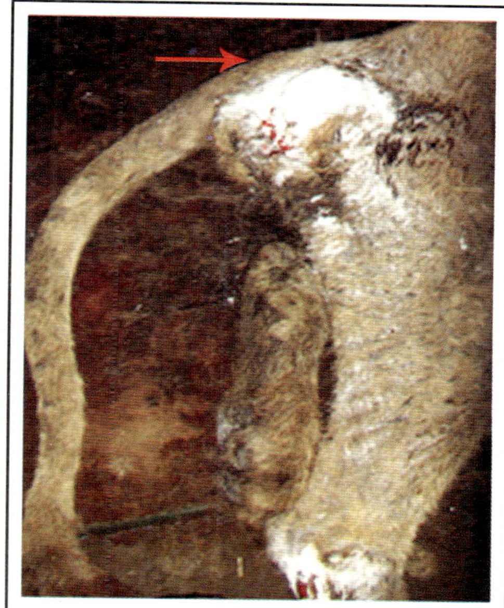

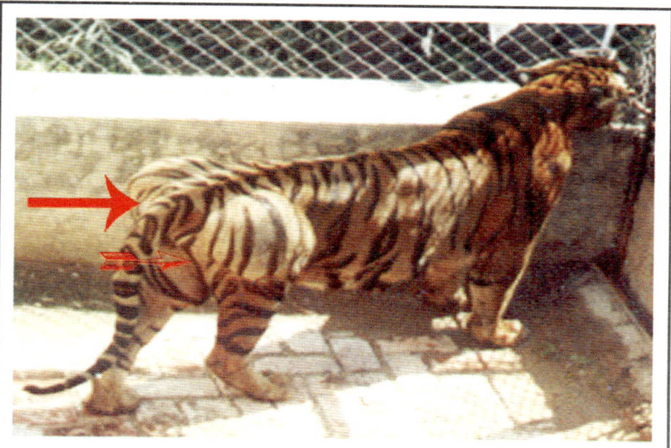

Figure 461: Adult male tiger (*P. tigris*) at Zoological Garden, Lucknow (U.P)suffering from hyperostosis. Note development of round large hard nodular masses on ribs and hip joints.

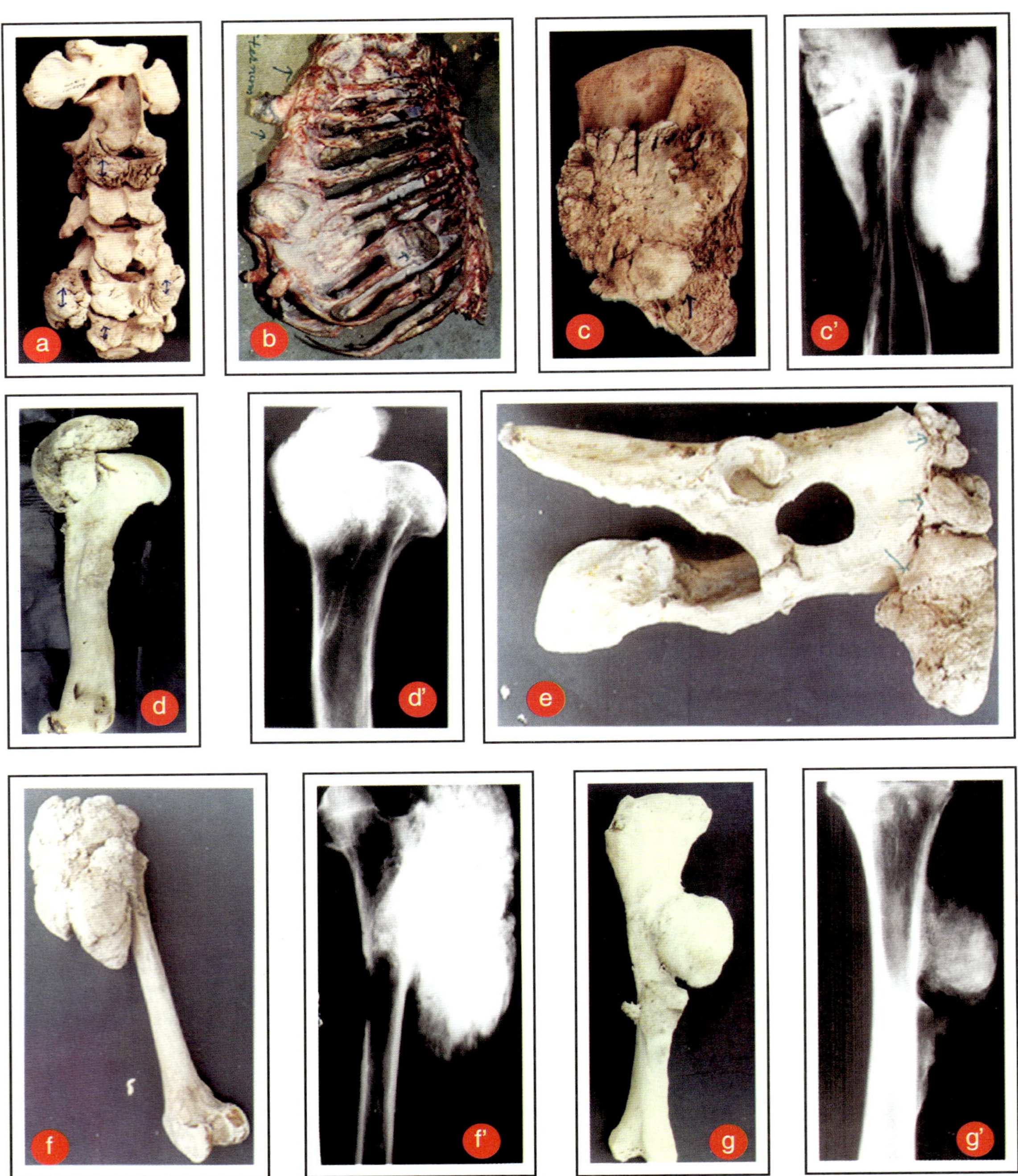

Figure 462: Multiple hyperostotic growths of different shape and size and magnitude in various bones encountered in a tiger (*P. tigris*) died at Zoological Park, Kanpur. (a) Cervical vertebrae-Transverse processes. (b) Sternum disfigured due to different sized growths and nodular growths on certain ribs, (c, c') 2/3 of the lateral aspect of scapula (d, d') Head of humerous. (e) Schiatic arch and ischiatic tuberosity of pelvis. (f, f') Greater trochanter of femur (gross and radiograph). (g, g') Tibia- involving shaft (diaphysis).

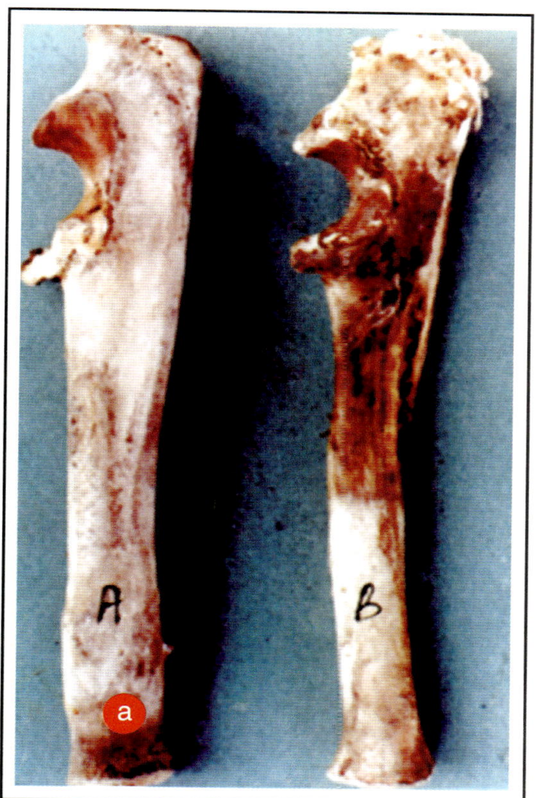

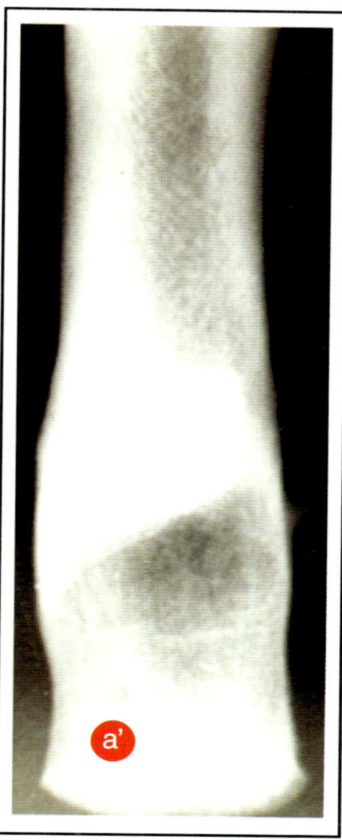

Figure 463: Photographs of ulnas of sub-adult tigress (*P. tigris*) died in Haldwani Forest Division (Uttarakhand) showing: (a) Increased dimension but mainly in its distal third. (a') Radiograph evidencing increased density due to thickening of the cortex extending focally in the distal third and proxima third. Oeteolytic changes are also discerned.

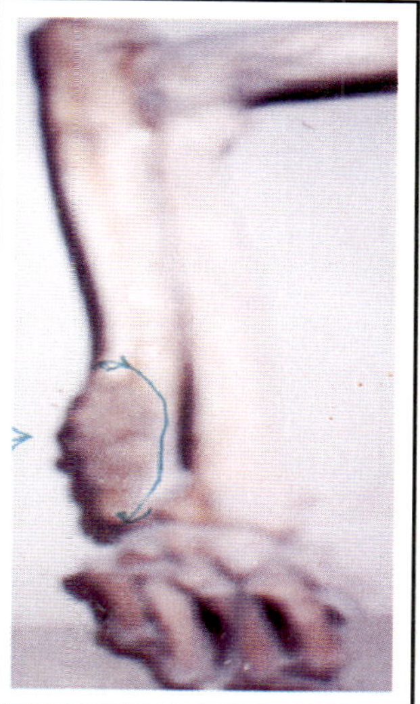

Figure 464: Photograph of left ulna and radius belonged to skeleton of an adult wild tiger (*P. tigris*) of Museum of Corbett National Park, Ramnagar (Uttarakhand) showing hard irregular brownish colored periosteal growth on the distal third of the ulna.

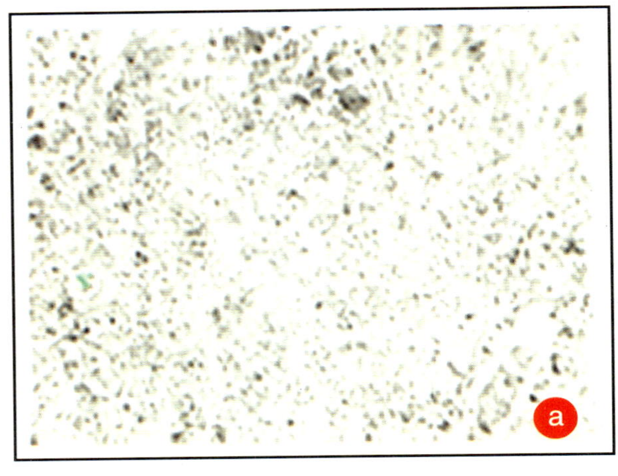

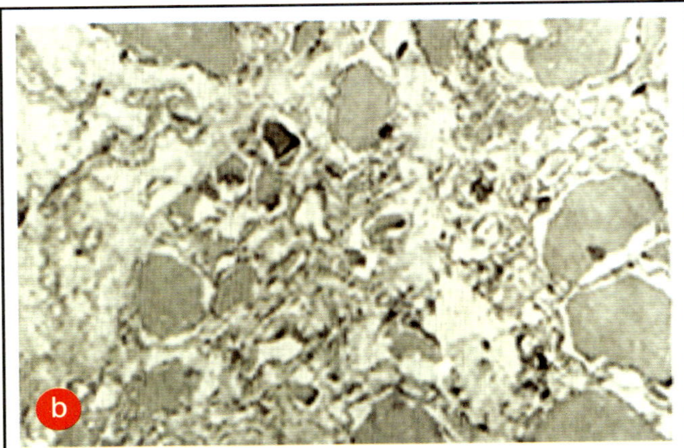

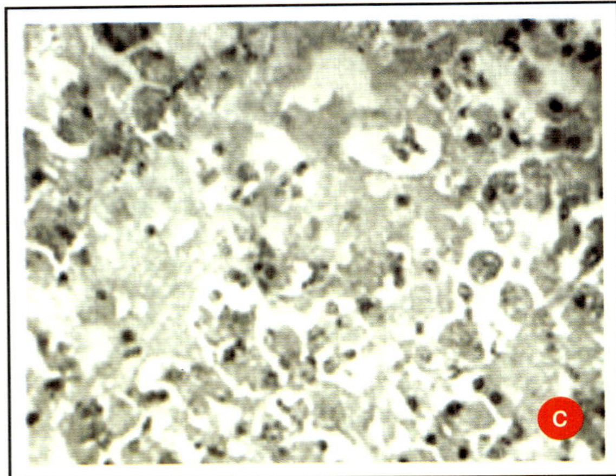

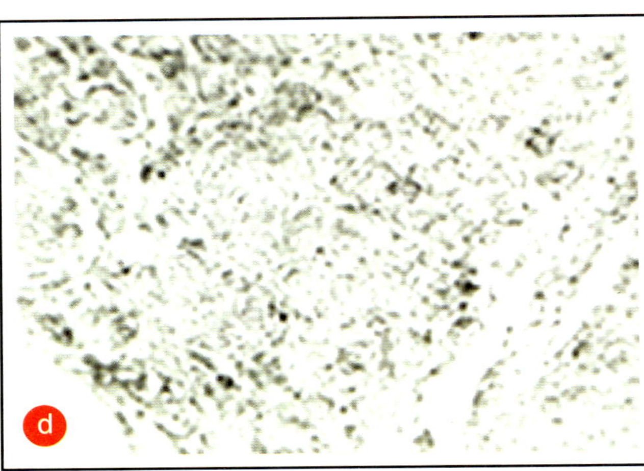

Figure 465: Senility in lion (*P. leo*). Photomicrographs showing: (a)Pituitary degeneration of acidophiles and hyalinization, H&E, x 200. (b) Hyalinization of acidophiles and stroma. Absence of granulation in acidophiles, H&E, x 200. (c) Thyroid-varying sized follicles, stromal fibrosis and hyalinization is also evident (d) Adrenal-Multiple extra capsular accessory cortical nodules. H&E, x200 (Rajan *et al.*, 1979).

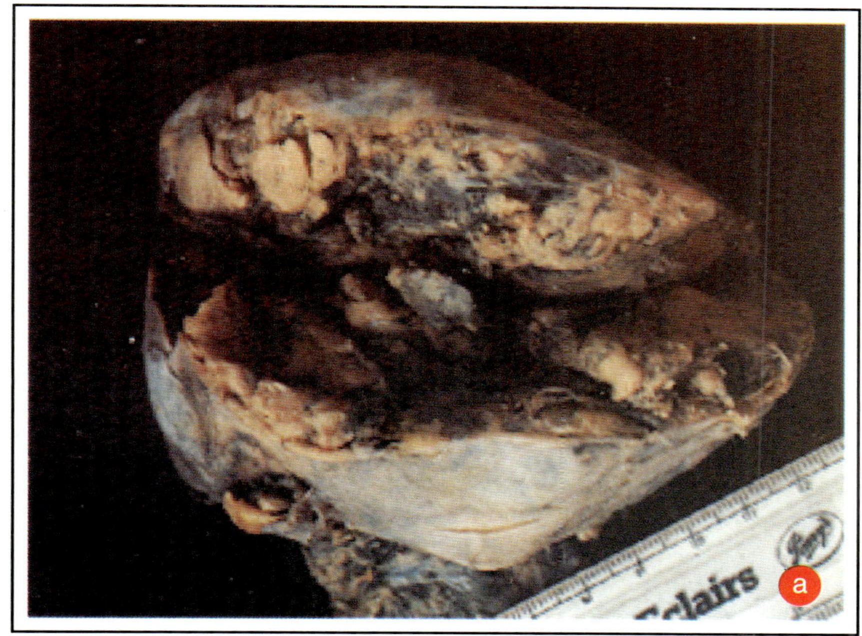

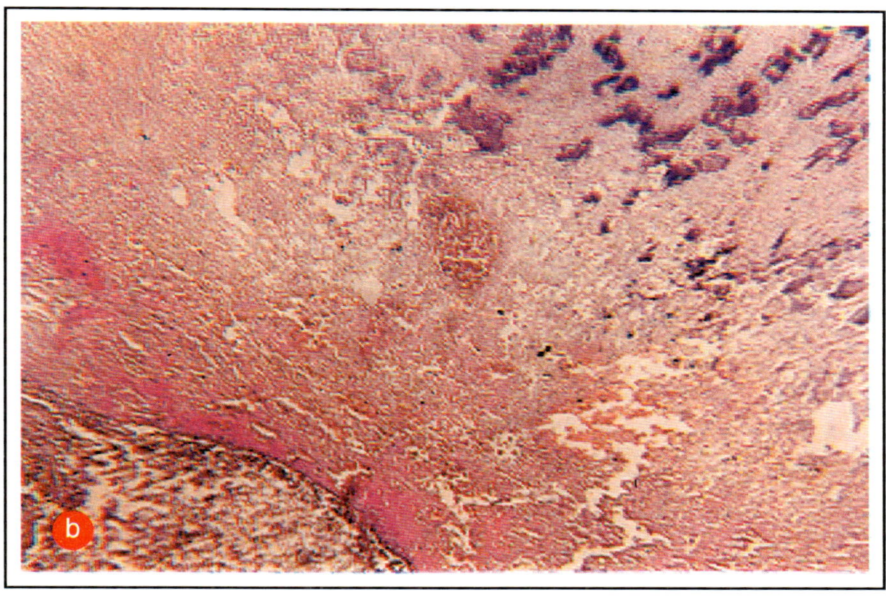

Figure 466: (a) Photograph showing a growth from adrenal of lion (*P. leo*) died at Zoological Garden, Guwahati, Assam. Note caseation on cut surface (b) Photomicrograph of (a) showing characteristic changes of adrenocortical carcinoma with caseation and mineralization. H & E, x 100 (Nashiruddullah *et al.*, 2007).

(b) Small Cats & Civets

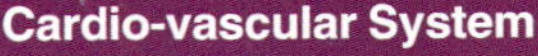

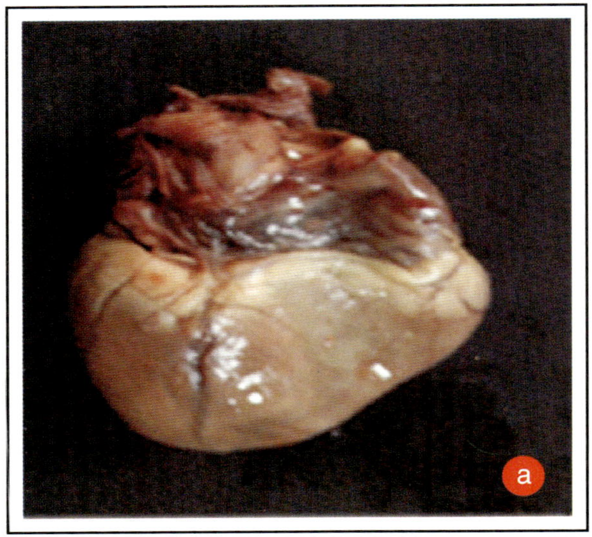

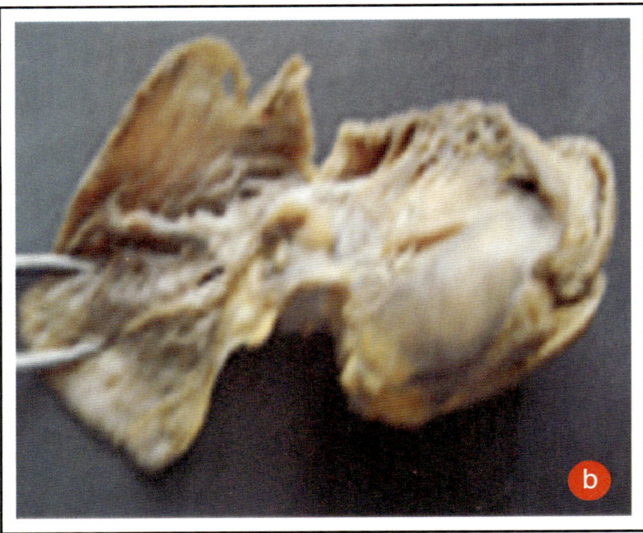

Figure 467: Photographs (a,b) showing hypertrophy of right ventricle in adult female leopard cat (*P. bengalensis*)

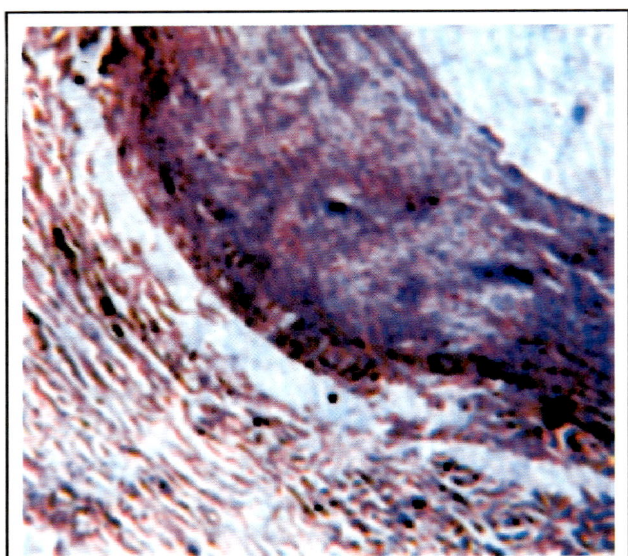

Figure 468: Photomicrograph showing atheroma of aorta in leopard cat (*P. bengalensis*) died in captivity. H& E, x 40 (Nashiruddullah and Chakaraborty, 2006)

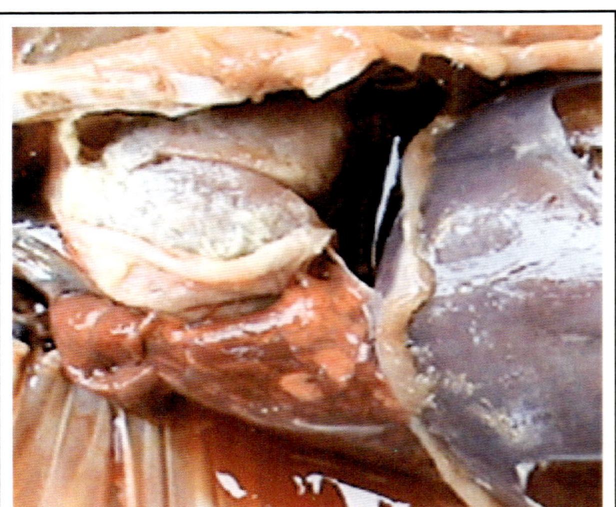

Figure 469: Photograph showing fibrinous pericarditis and fibrinous perihepatitis in small Indian civet cat (*Viverricula indica*). The condition was associated to chronic bacterial infection.

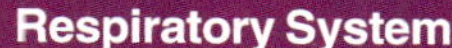

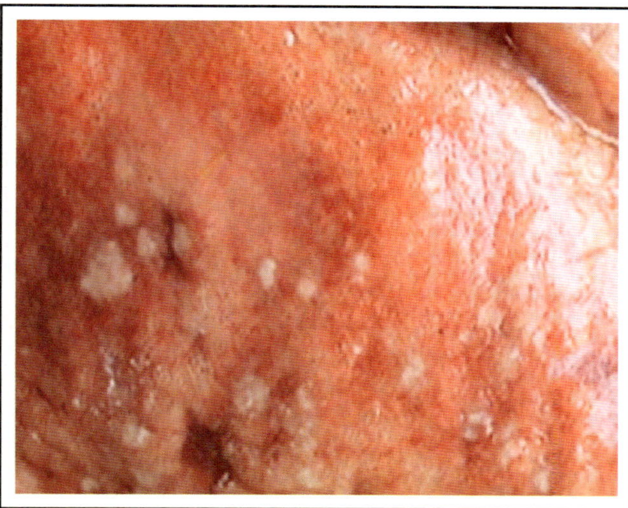

Figure 470: Photograph showing emphysema and necrotic foci in lung of leopard cat (*P.bengalensis*) died at Zoological Garden,Guwahati, Assam.

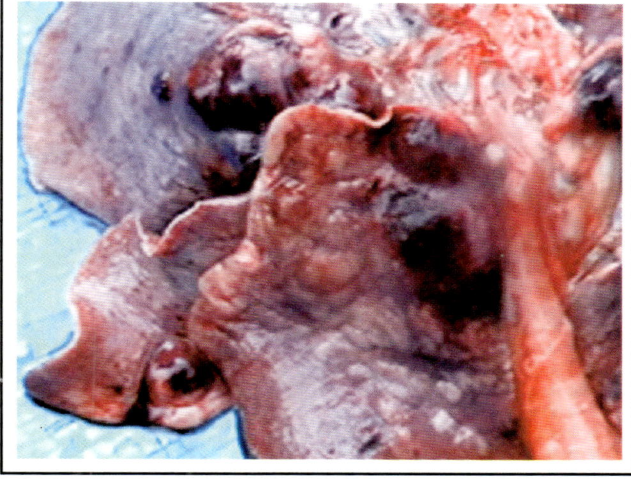

Figure 471: Photograph showing lung emphysema in Golden cat (*C. temmincki*) died at Zoological Garden, Guwahati, Assam.

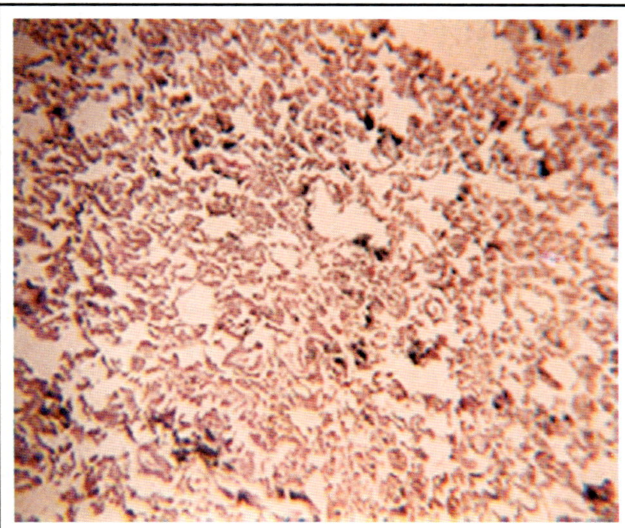

Figure 472: Photomicrograph showing pneumoconiosis in hog badger (*Arctonyx collaris*) died at Zoological Garden, Guwahati, Assam. H & E, x 100

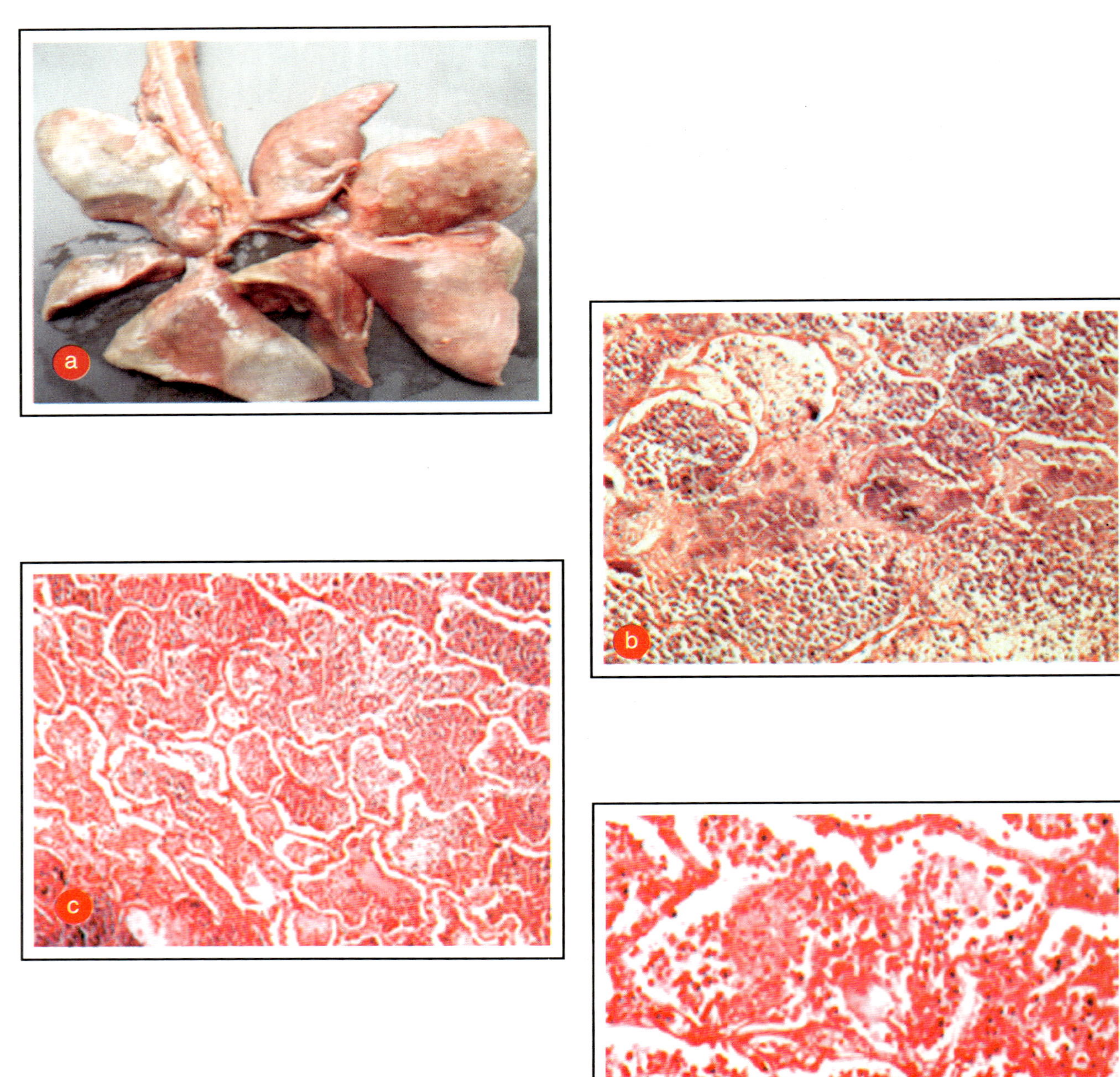

Figure 473: (a) Photograph of lung of leopard cat (*P. bengalensis*).Photomicrographs of (a) showing: (b)Necrotic foci surrounded by inflammatory cells. H& E, x160 (c) Fibrinous bronchopneumonia with mononuclear cells and fibrinous exudate in the alveoli. H & E, x 80 (d) Higher magnification,H & E,x 250 of (c).

Figure 474: Photomicrograph showing *Toxoplasma* schizont in the lung of common civet (*Paradoxurus* sp.)

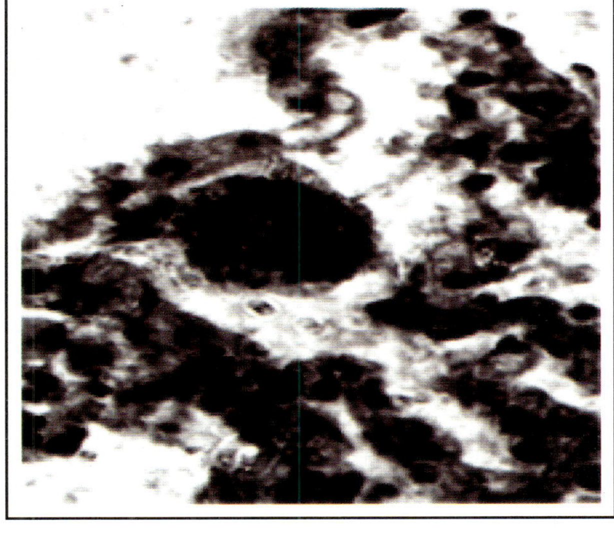

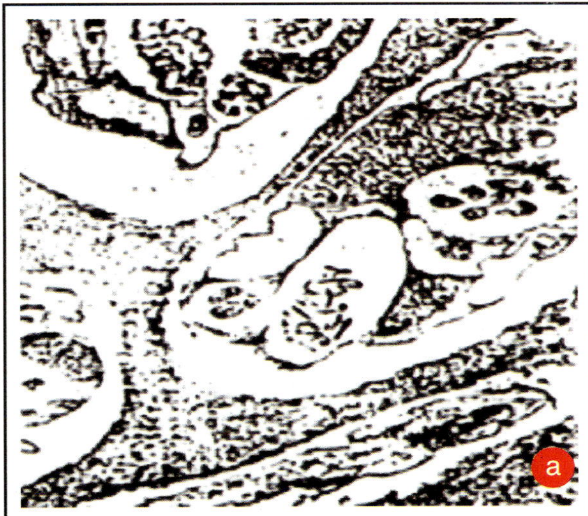

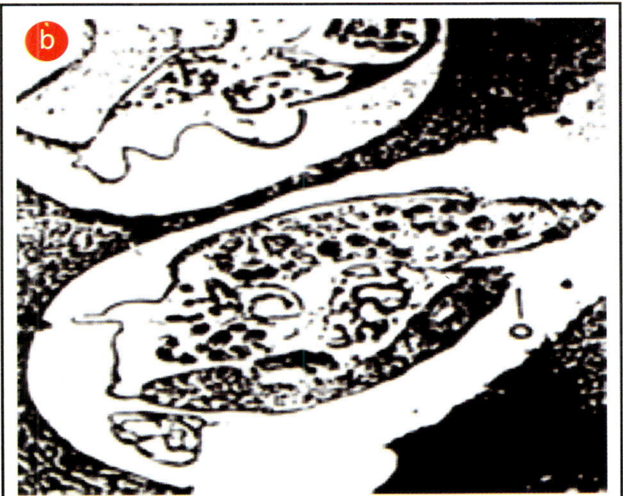

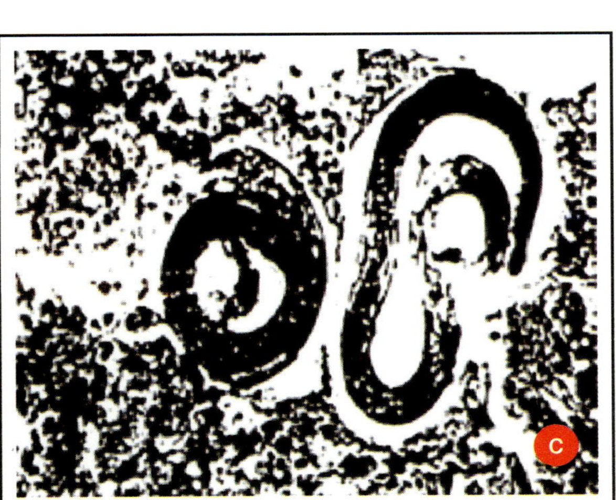

Figure 475 : Photomicrographs of pulmonary nodule caused due to *Filaroides osleri* encountered in a leopard cat (*Prionailurus bengalensis*) died in captivity showing: (a) Portions of gravid female worms.X90 (b) Vulvar opening in the posterior end of the worm (c) 'S' shaped parasite in the lung parenchyma.(Rao *et al.*, 1971).

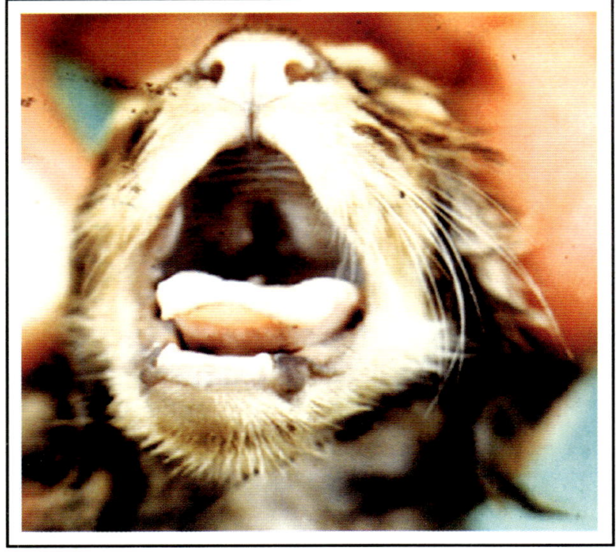

Figure 476: Photograph showing cleft palate in leopard cat (*P.bengalensis*) kitten.

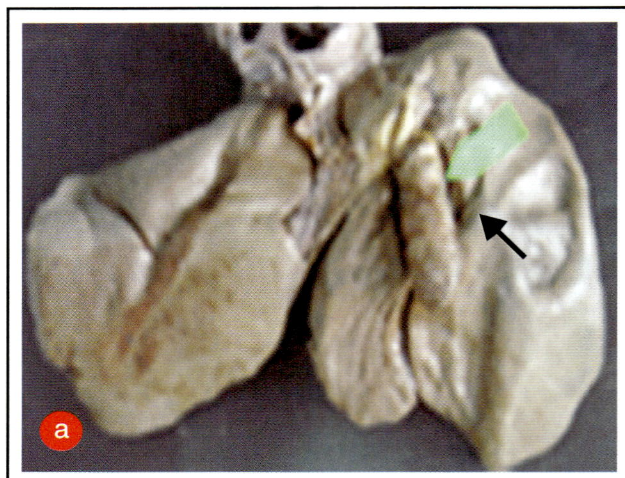

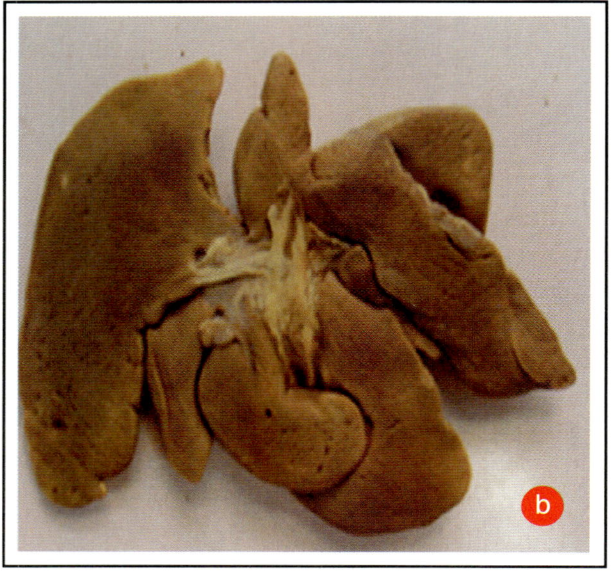

Figure 477: Photographs showing: (a) Presence of gallbladder on the parietal surface of liver (formalized specimen) of fishing cat (*P. viverrinus*) (b) Absence of gall bladder in liver encountered in common civet (*Paradoxurus* sp.).

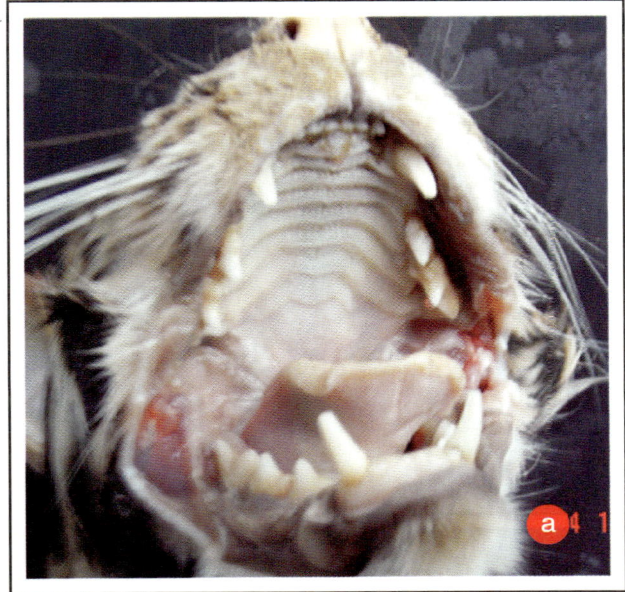

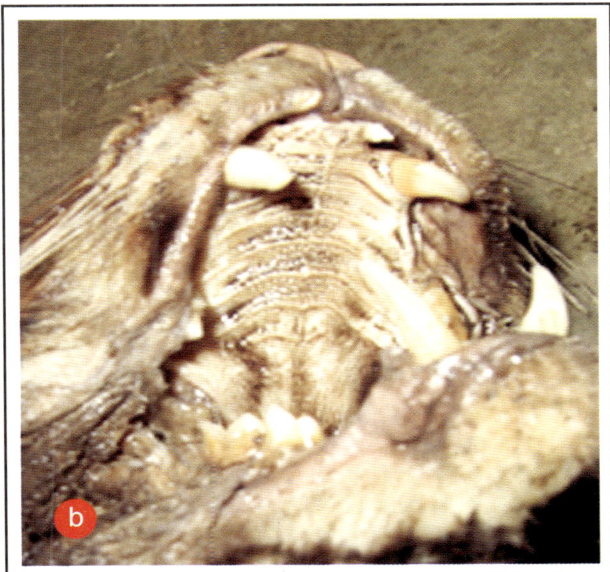

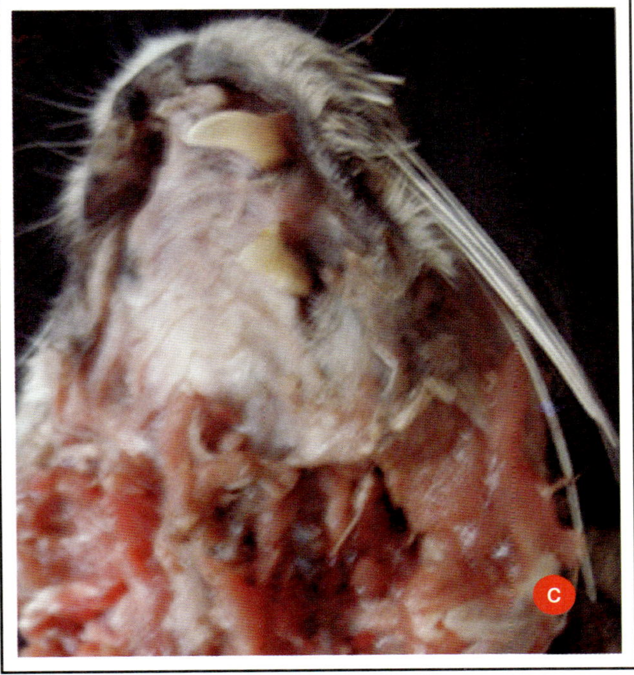

Figure 478: Photographs showing wearing of teeth in 3 leopard cats (*P. bengalensis*). (a). Complete wearing of upper and lower incisors. (b) Complete wearing of upper and lower incisors and upper premolars and molars. (c) Loss of right canine tooth.

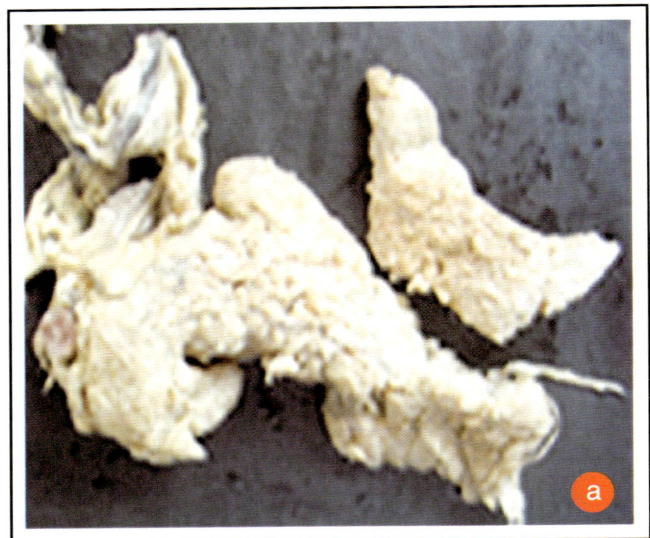

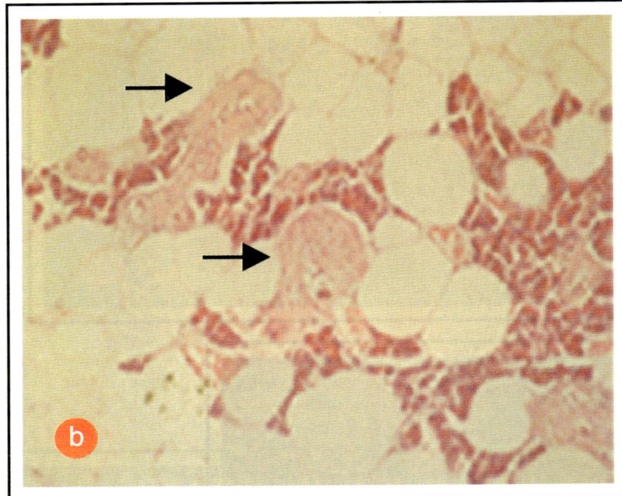

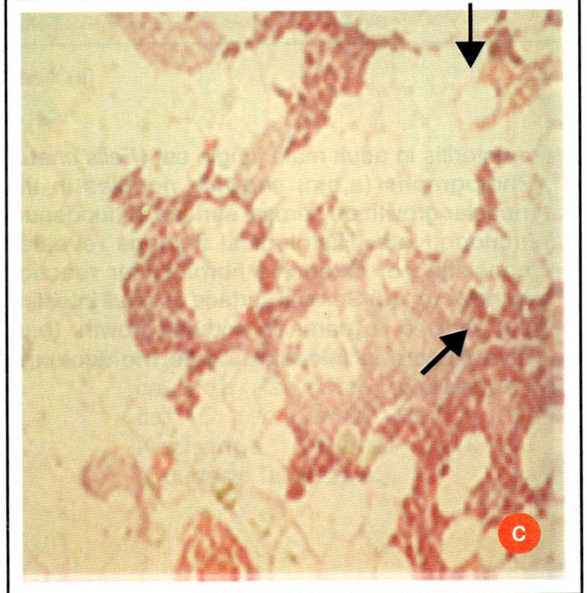

Figure 486: (a) Pancreas from large civet (*V. z. zibetha*) cut opened, showing fatty cheesy mass diffusely present. (b) Photomicrograph of (a) evidencing infiltration with adipose tissue and occasional focal necrosis H&E, x 100 (c) Pancreatic islets amyloidosis(arrow) Secretary acini showing atrophy (arrow) with deposition of amorphous eosinophilic mass (amyloid). H&E, x 200. (Singh *et al.*, 2004).

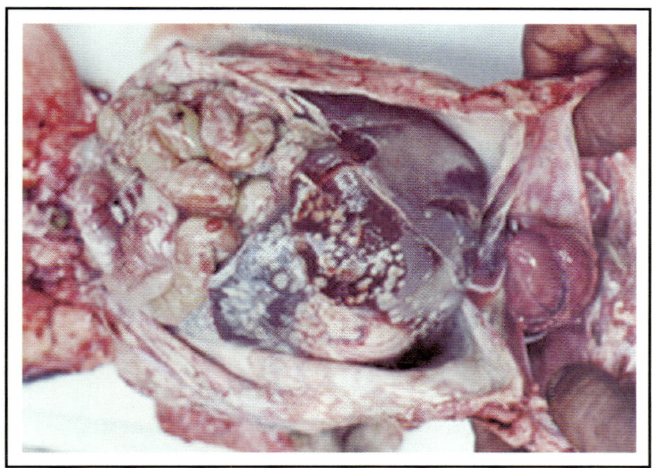

Figure 487: Photograph showing multiple raised pyogenic foci in the liver, spleen and mesentery leading to peritonitis due to *E. coli* infection in small Indian civet (*V. indica*).

Figure 488: Photograph showing suppurative hepatits in an adult male common civet (*Paradoxurus* sp.).

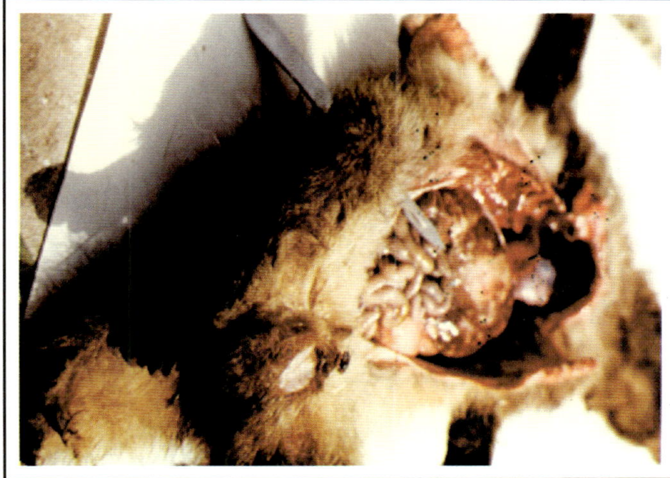

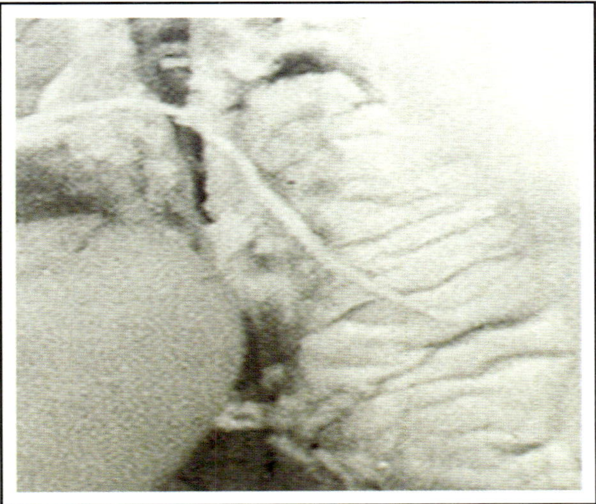

Figure 489: Photograph of pancreas of hog badger (*Arctonyx collaris*)showing *Acheilostoma collaris* nematode within the pancreatic duct.

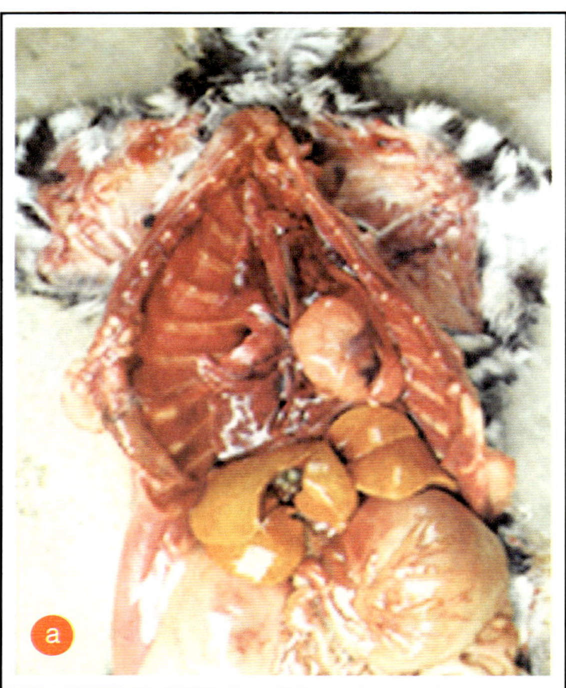

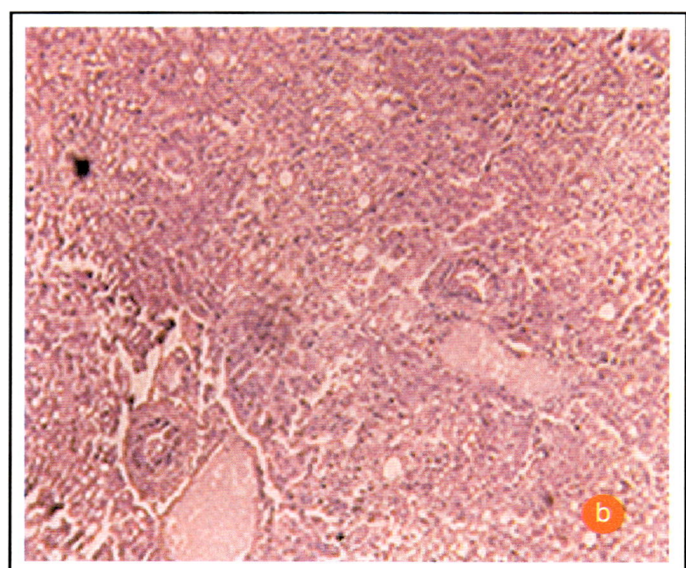

Figure 490: Photograph of leopard cat (*P. bengalensis*) showing (a) Massive perirenal and pericardial fat along with yellowish appearance of liver. (b) Photomicrograph of (a) showing acute fatty changes of the hepatocytes. H & E, x 100.

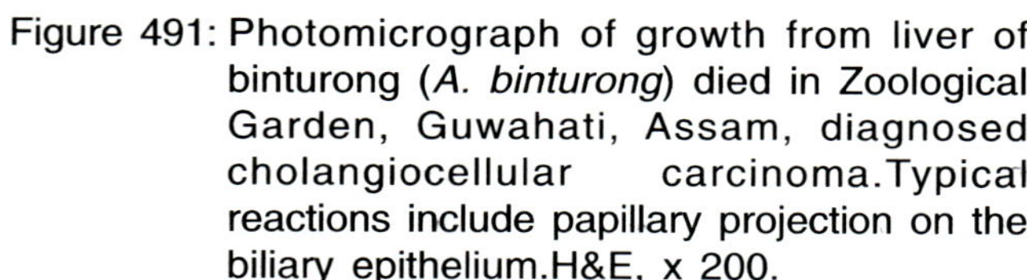

Figure 491: Photomicrograph of growth from liver of binturong (*A. binturong*) died in Zoological Garden, Guwahati, Assam, diagnosed cholangiocellular carcinoma.Typical reactions include papillary projection on the biliary epithelium.H&E, x 200.

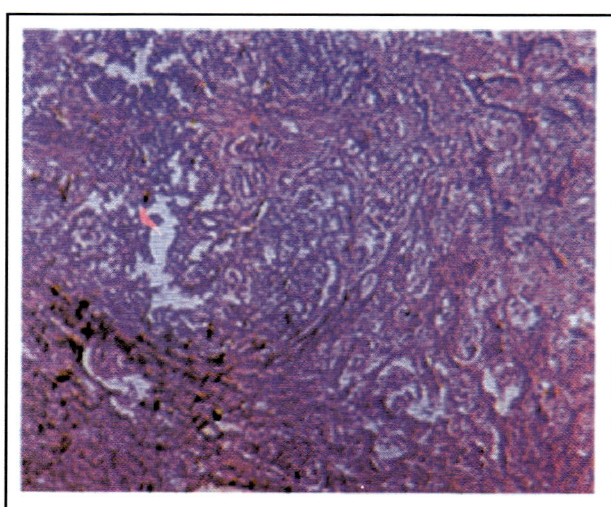

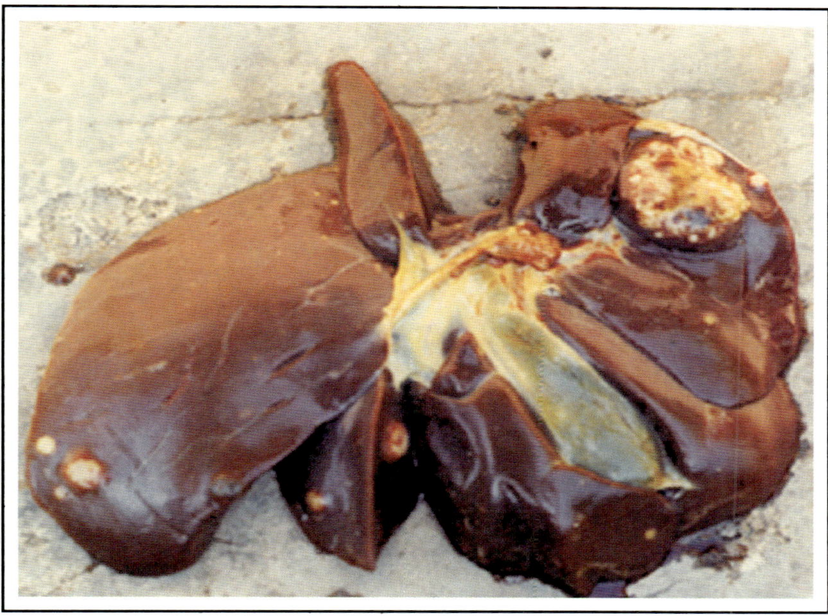

Figure 492: Photograph showing tumorous growth in the liver of binturong (*Arctictis binturong*). Histopathologically the growth was diagnosed as hepatocellular carcinoma.

Figure 493. Photograph of spleen of binturong (*A. binturong*) died at Zoological Garden, Guwahati (Assam) showing metastatic lesion of cholangiocellular carcinoma.

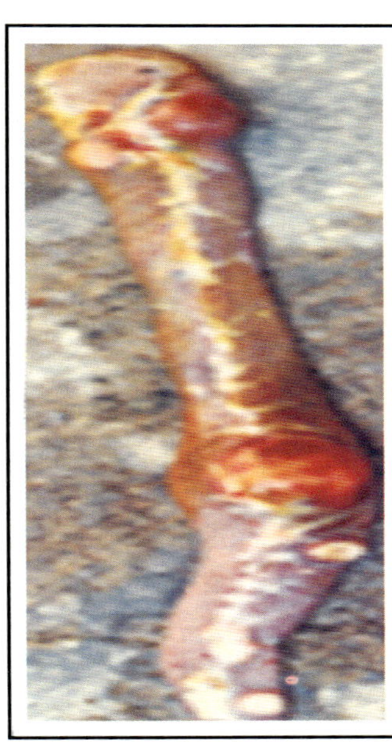

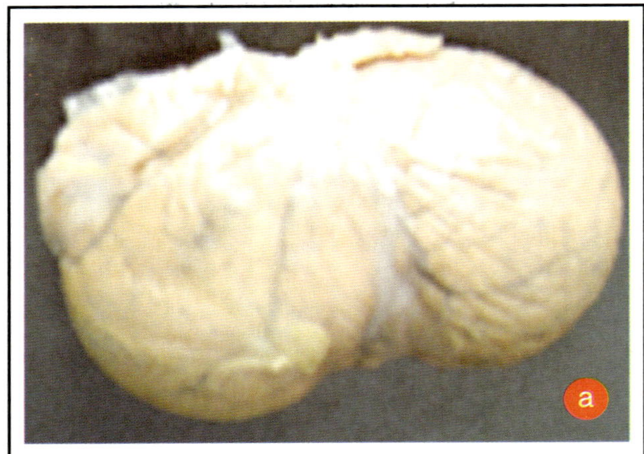

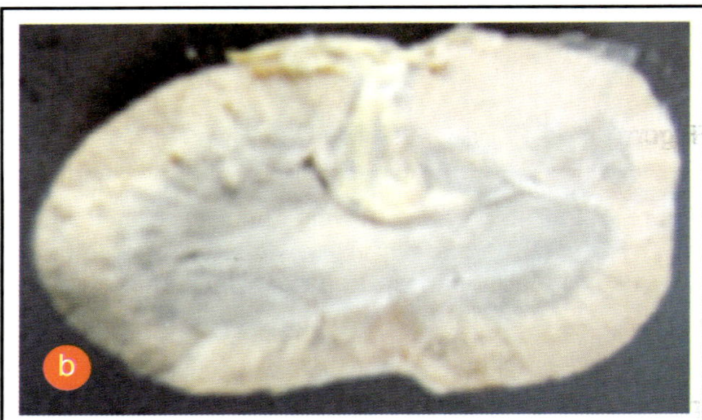

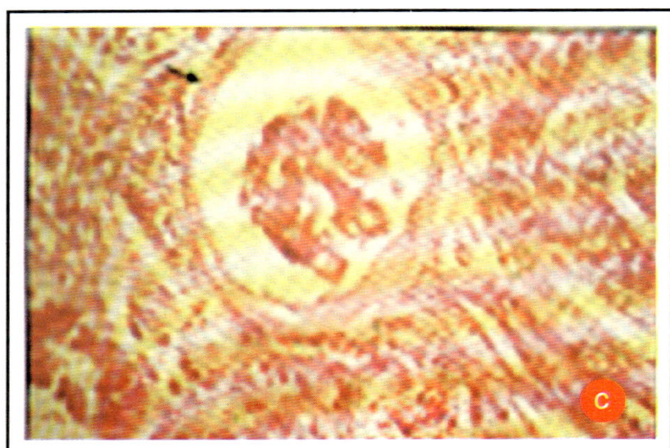

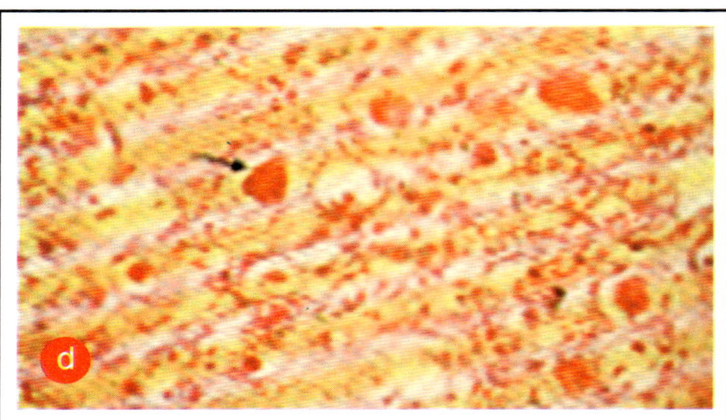

Figure 494: (a) Photograph of right kidney of large civet (*V. z. zibetha*) died in captivity showing focal constriction nearly in middle transversely. (b) Cut section of (a) showing variably thickened cortex. Photomicrographs showing: (c) Moderate thickening of parietal layer of Bowman's capsule (arrow) and proximal tubular degeneration. H&E, x400. (d) Tubules ending in pelvic region filled with homogenous fluid mass. H&E, x100. The case is also referred under digestive system.

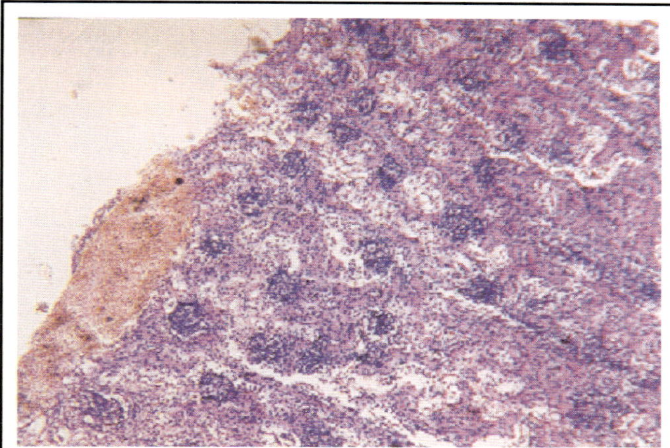

Figure 495: Photomicrograph showing pyelonephritis in Jungle cat (*F. chaus*) died in Zoological Garden, Guwahati, Assam. Note polymorphonuclear cells infiltration in the cortical areas, H & E, x 100.

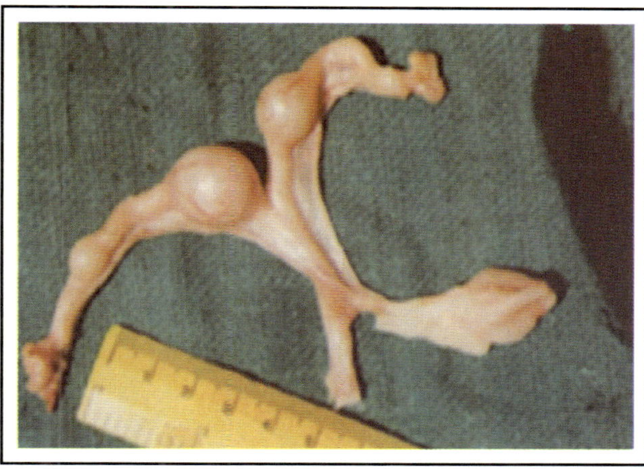

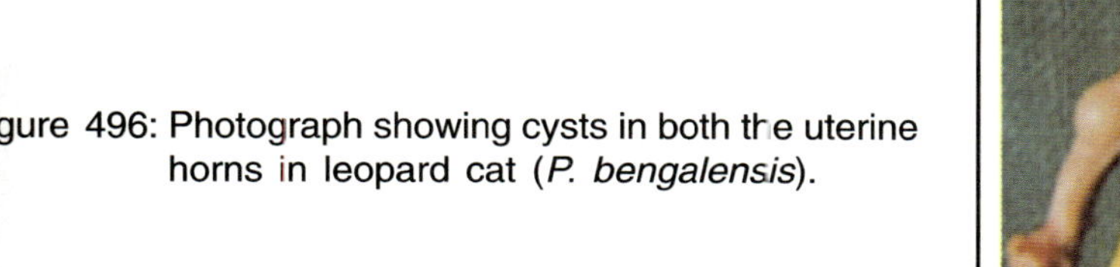

Figure 496: Photograph showing cysts in both the uterine horns in leopard cat (*P. bengalensis*).

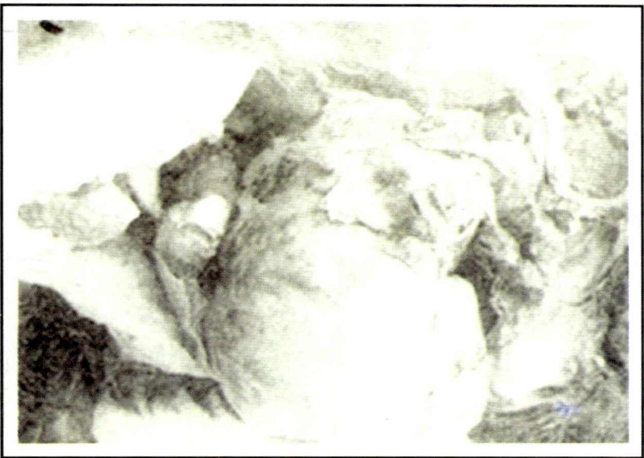

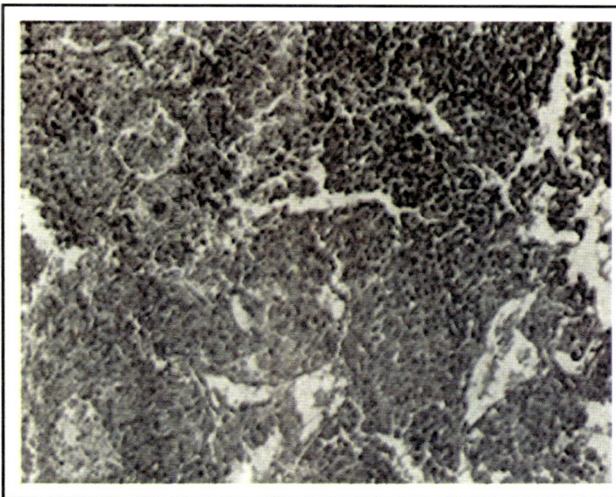

Figure 497: Granulosa cell tumour of ovary in civet (*V. indica*). (a)Photograph showing a huge mass of growth filling the abdominal cavity. (b) Photomicrograph showing sheets of neoplastic cells amidst dilated blood vessels. H&E,x 400(Valsala *et al.*,1995).

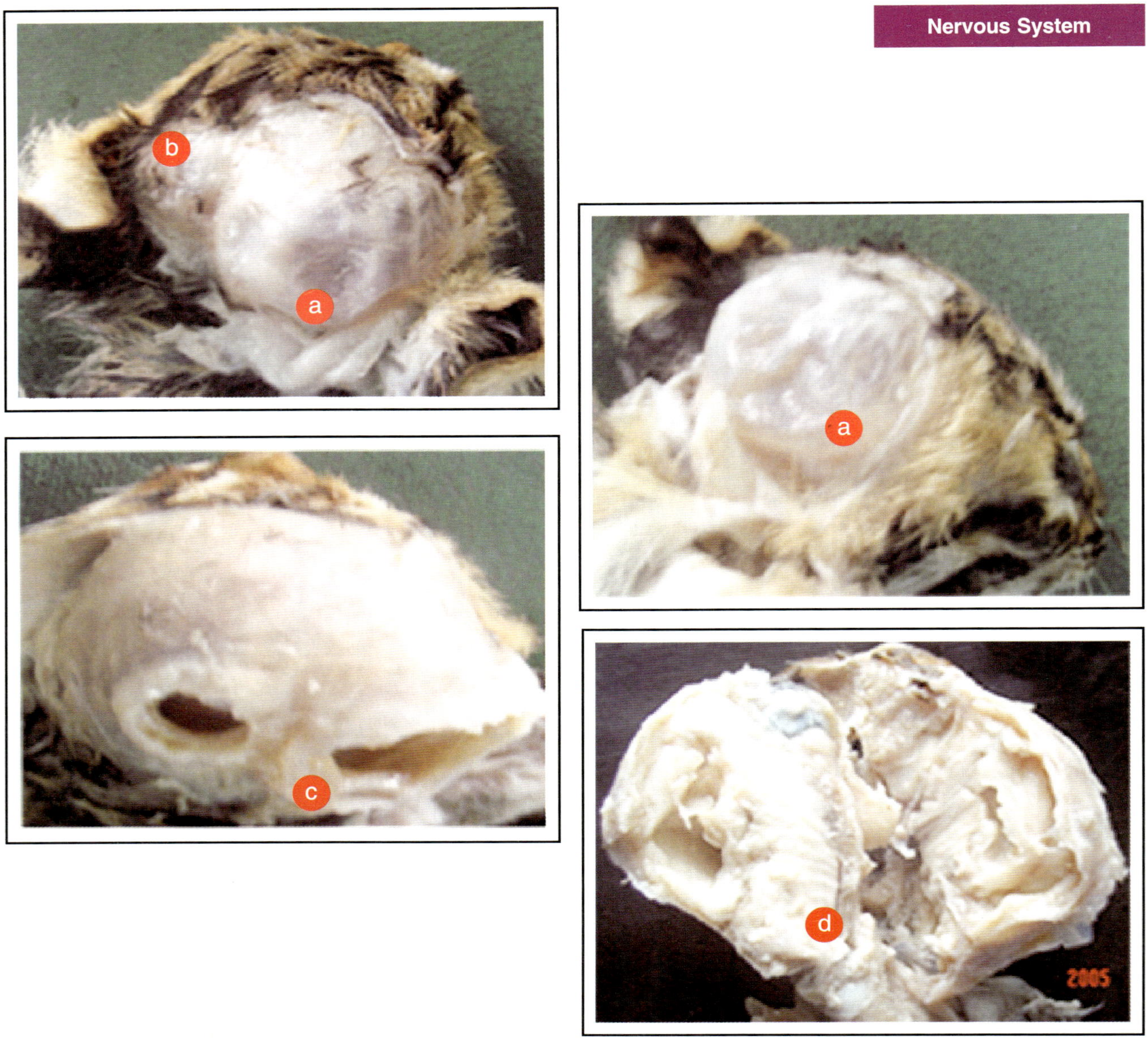

Figue 498: Meningoencephalocele diagnosed in 75-day-old leopard cat (*P. bengalensis*) kitten died at Biological Park,Patna (Bihar).Photographs (a,b) showing: (a) A large cystic protuberance(8.0 cm) on right side and also nearby a small protuberance (4.5cm) at left side of parietal bones of the skull. (c,d) Their dissection showed absence of development of parietal bones. The growths were filled with straw colored fluid.

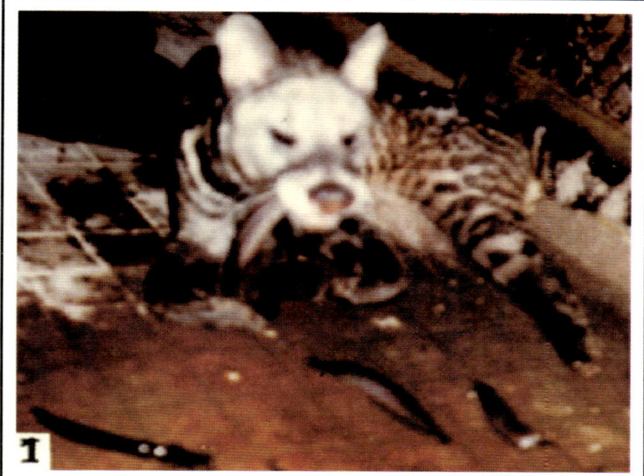

Figure 499: Large Indian civet (*V. z. zibetha*) showing the cured limbs those had paralysis. Feeding of live fish and administration of Vitamin B_1 had cured the condition.

Integumentary System

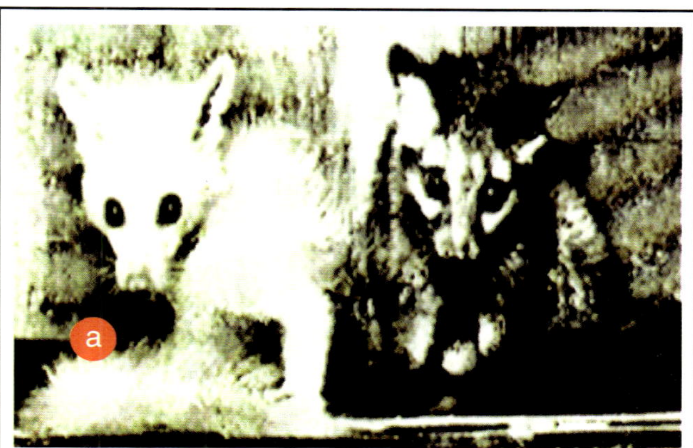

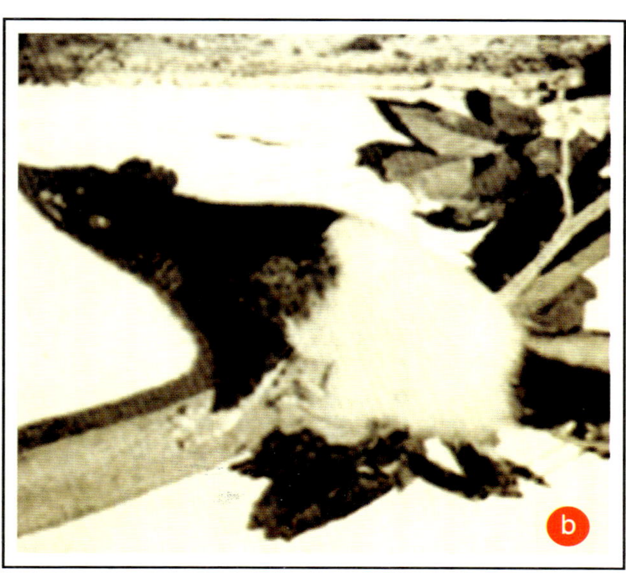

Figure 500: (a) An albino common palm civet (*Paradoxurus hermaphroditus*) with its normal cousin in Zoologica Garden, Ahmedabad, Gujarat. (b) semi-albino palm civet (*P.hermaphroditus*) at Zoological Garden, Coimbatore (Ashraf, 1992).

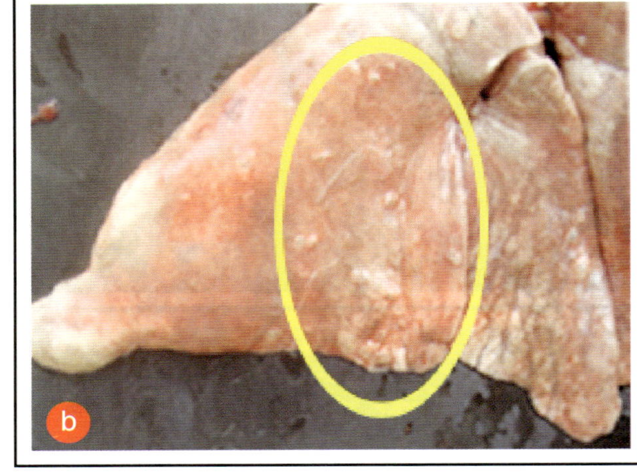

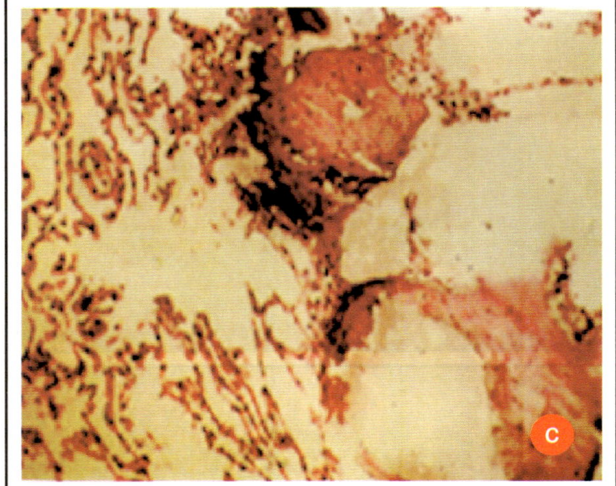

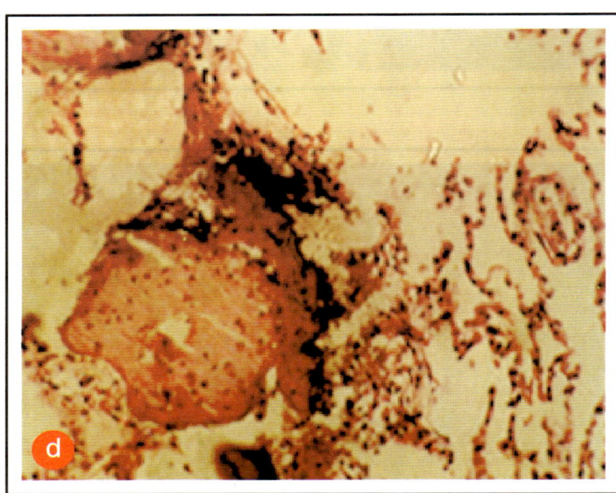

Figure 509: Photographs (a,b) of lungs from wolf (*C. lupus*) showing white -yellowish hard pin head sized nodules. Photomicrographs (c, d) showing ossification and calcification within pulmonary tissue. H &E, x100 (H.P. aid by Division of Pathology, IVRI, Izatnagar).

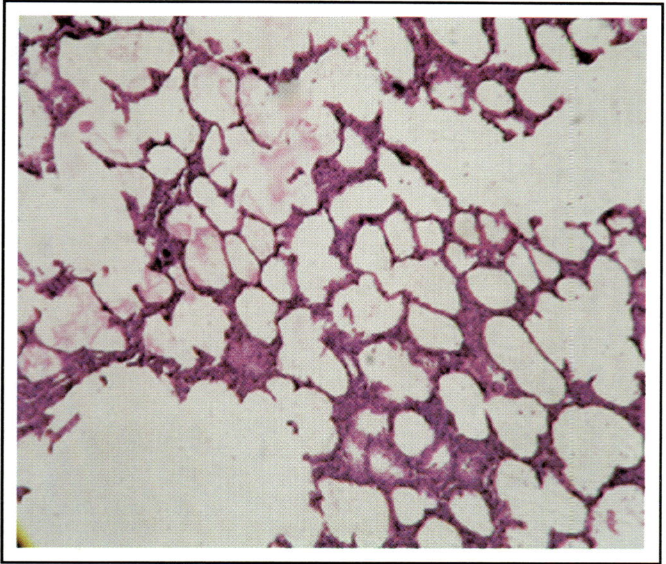

Figure 510: Photomicrograph showing pulmonary emphysema in Jackal (*C. aureus*). H & E, x 100 (Courtesy: Dept.of Pathlogy, C.V.Sc., Nagpur, M.S.).

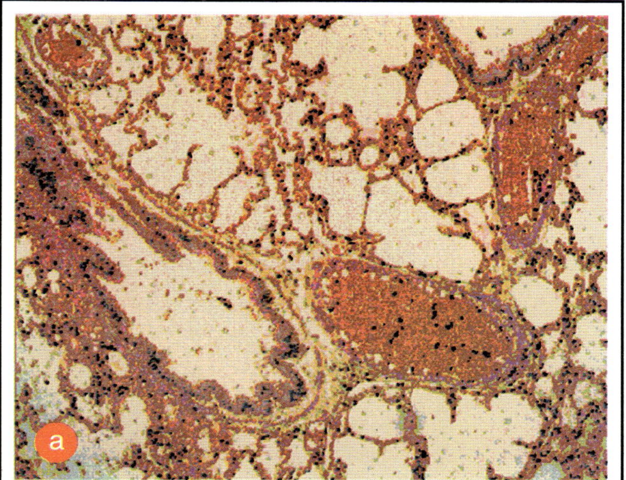

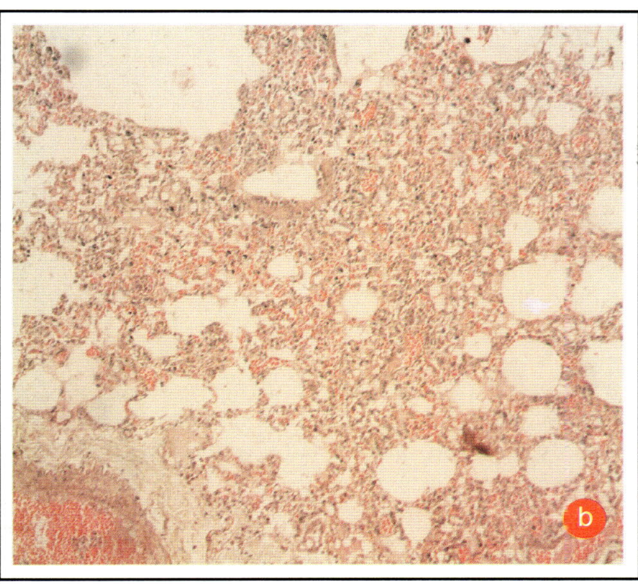

Figure 511: Pneumonia in jackal (*C. aureus*). Photomicrographs showing: (a) Enlarged and ruptured alveoli,alveolar emphysema and most of the alveoli atelectased. Peribronchiolar area filled with oedema fluid and infiltration of inflammatory cells. All the arterioles and vessels engorged with RBCs. (b)Deciliation in bronchial epithelium was also noticed. Few areas of parenchyma showed carbon/dust particles. H & E x 100 (Courtesy: Harish, B.R. & Shiva Shanker)

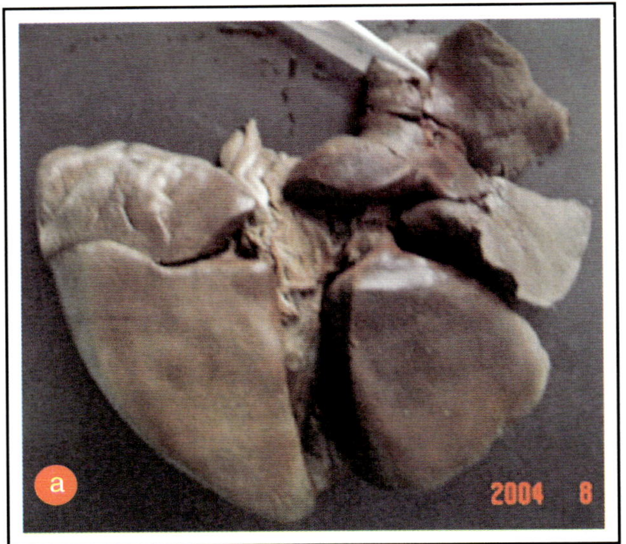

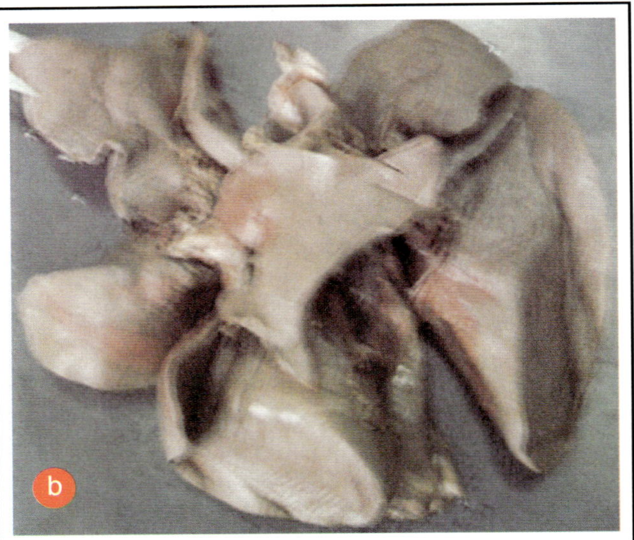

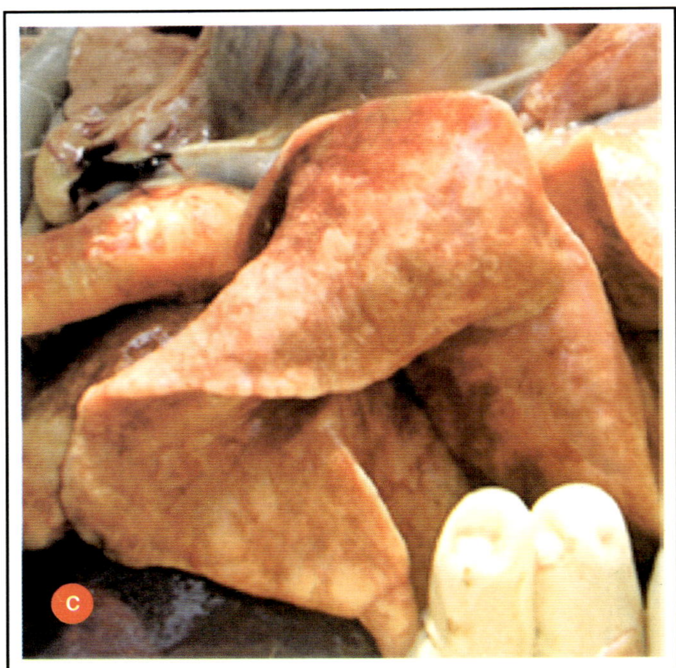

Figure 512: Photograph of lungs of jackal (*C. aureus*) died in National Zoological Park, New Delhi showing: (a) Grey hepatisation of all the lobes resembling liver. (b) Medial view of the same (a). (c) Photograph of lungs of Jackal (*C. aureus*) showing congestion. Animal died of Trypanosomiasis. (Courtesy:Kallappa, S.) Note: case is also referred under Urinary system.

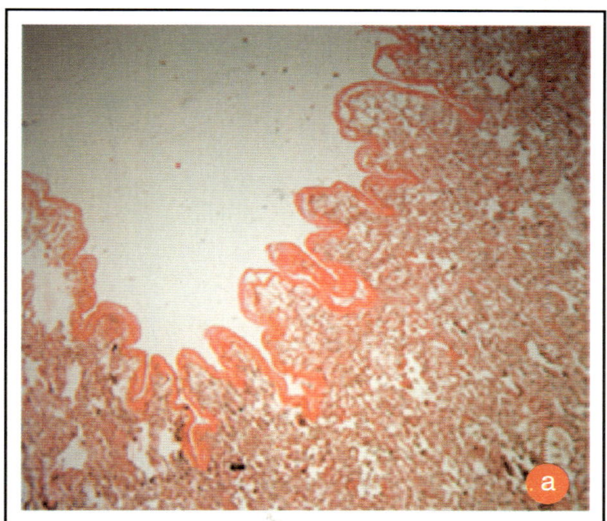

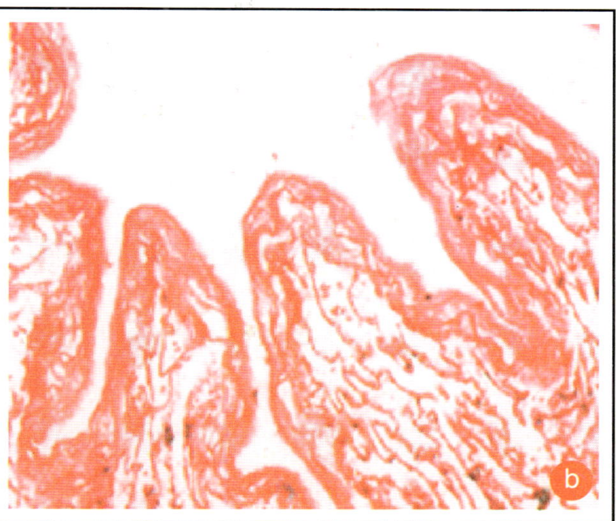

Figure 513: Photomicrographs of lung of jackal (*C. aureus*) showing cross section of parasite with disrupted cuticle. H&E,(a) x 50; (b) x 160 .

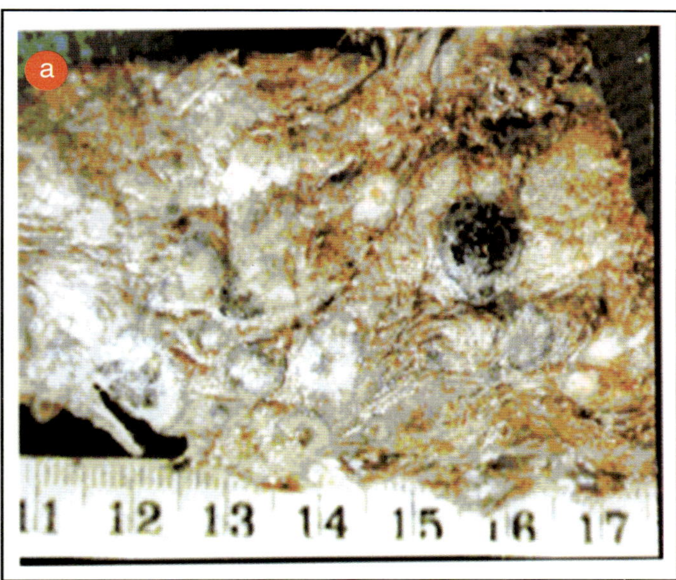

Figure 514: Photograph of melanosarcoma of lung encountered in hyena (*H. hyaena*) died in captivity showing blackish tan coloured circumscribed raised nodules. (b) Photomicrograph of (a) showing pulmonary tissue infiltrated with melanoblastic cells. H& E, x100

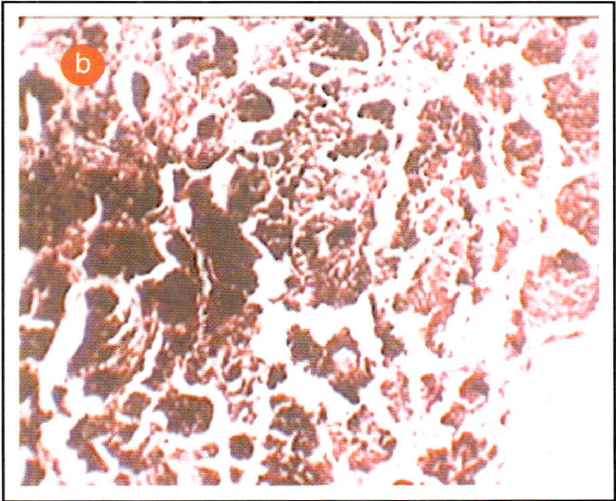

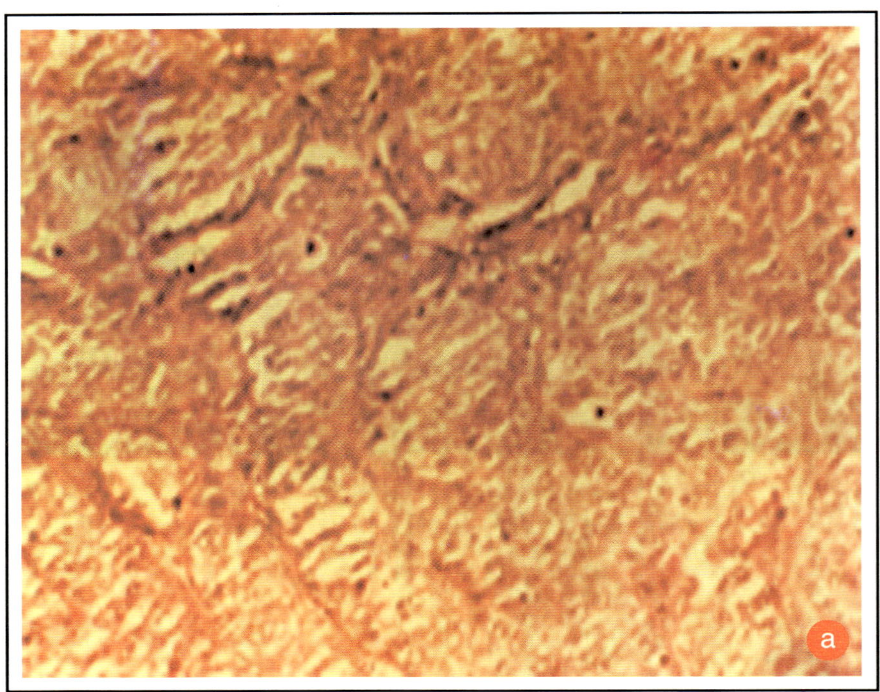

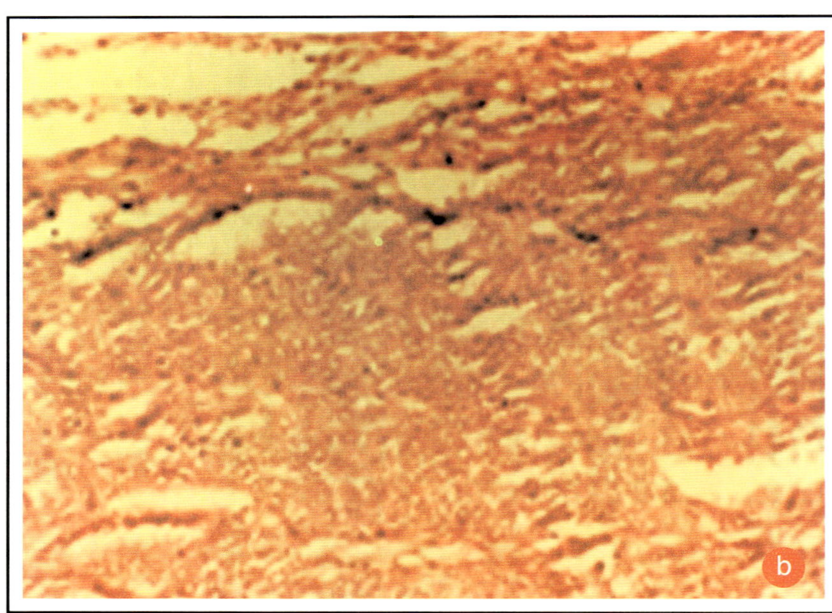

Figure 515: Photomicrographs showing: (a) Alveolar cell carcinoma in wolf (*C. lupus*) died at Zoological Garden, Lucknow (U.P).(b) Same as of (a).Pulmonary tissue filled with neoplastic masses. H & E x 100. (Histologic aid Div. of Pathology, I.V.R.I., Izatnagar)

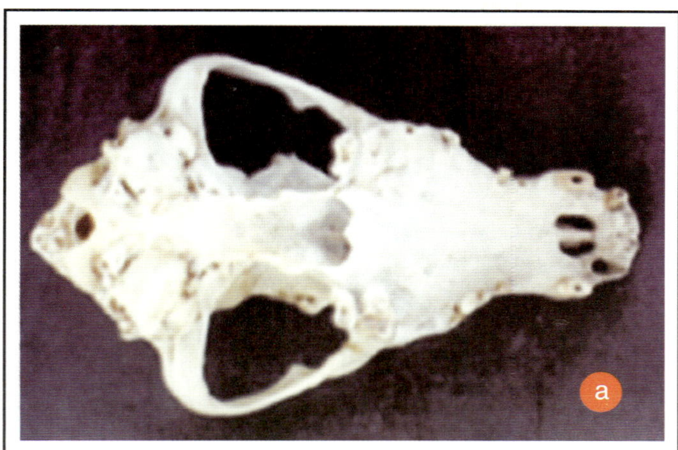

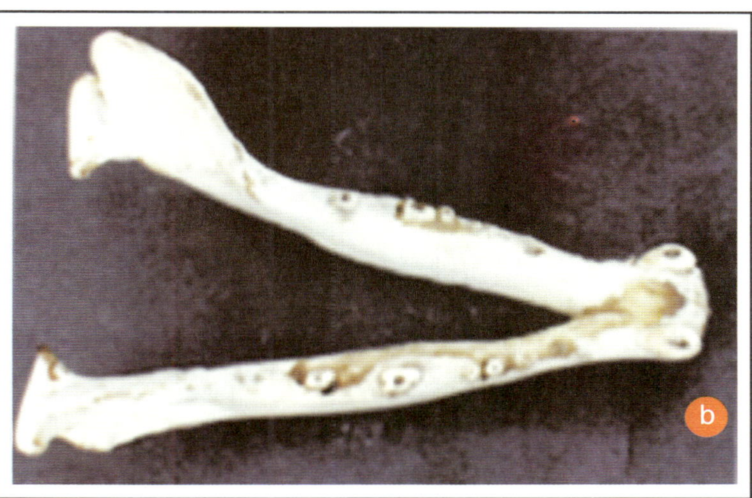

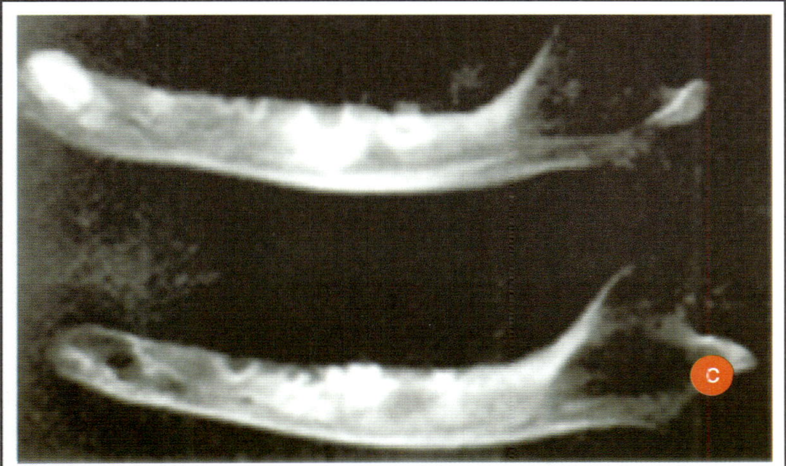

Figure 516: Photographs of upper (a) and lower(b) jaws of wolf (*C. lupus*) showing worn out teeth.(c) Radiograph of (b) showing resolved alveoli of premolars and molars.

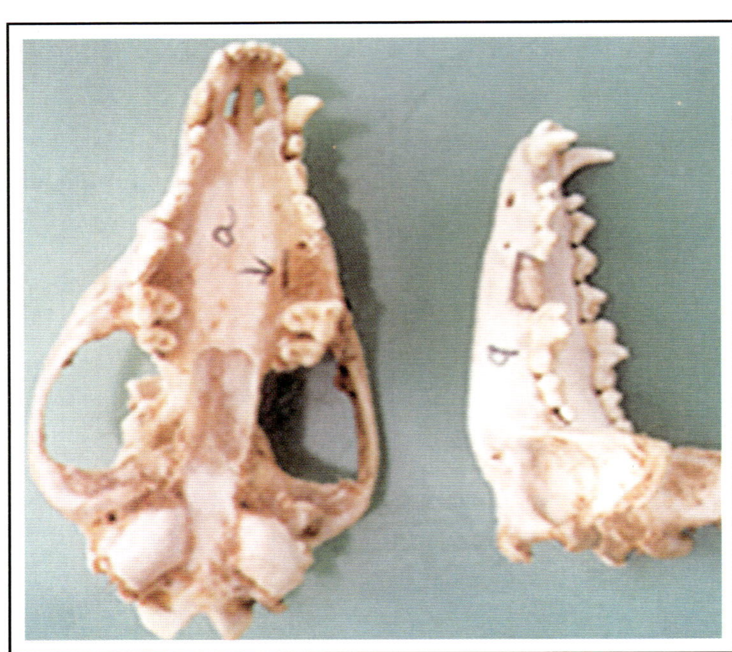

Figure 517: Photograph of skull and mandible of jackal (*C. aureus*) showing loss of upper PM4 and (b) lower 2nd premolar tooth and thier alveoli resolved.

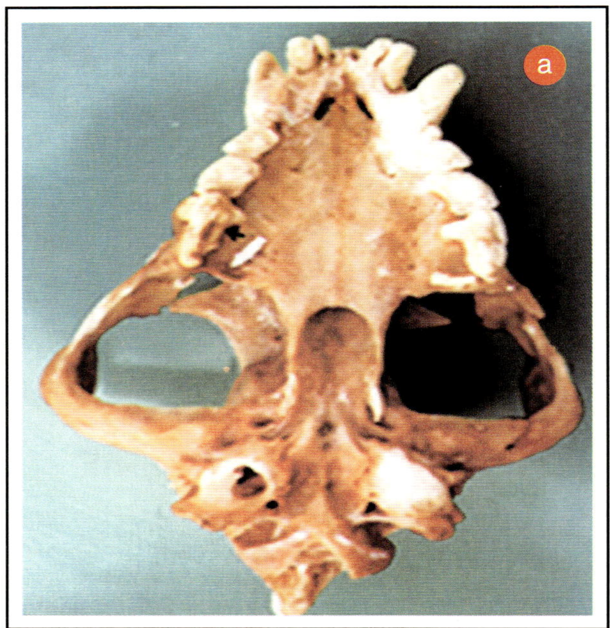

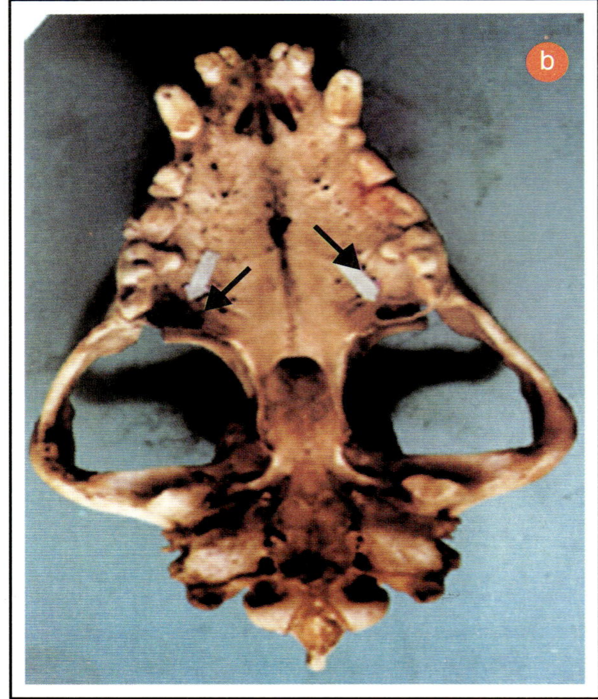

Figure 518: Photograph of hyena (*H.hyaena*) skulls showing: (a) Loss of right last molar and its alveolus completely resolved (arrows).(b) Loss of central pair of incisors and last molars. Note cusps of cheek teeth and tip of canines are blunt rounded because of their heavily use in bone crushing and chewing.

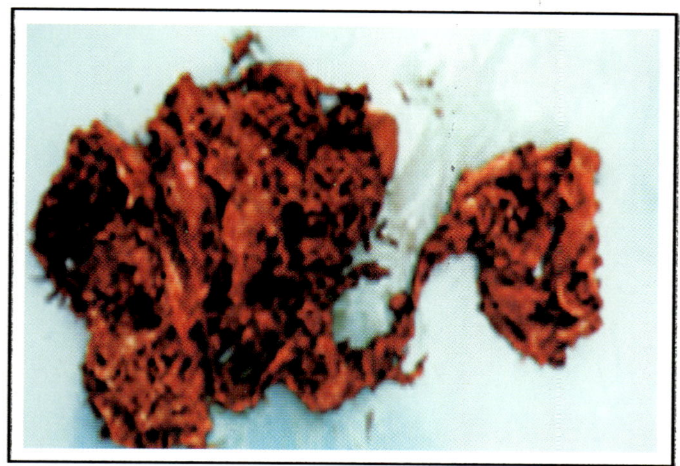

Figure 519: Photograph of stomach of wild jackal (*C. aureus*) packed mainly with insects and mucosal folds flattened.

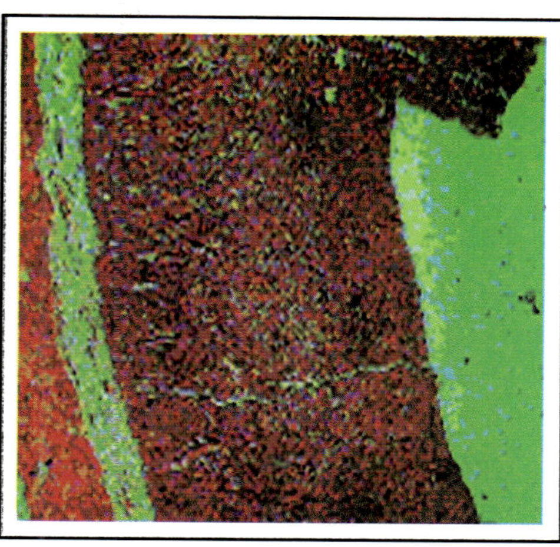

Figure 520: Photomicrograph showing enteritis in wild dog (*C. alpinus*) died in Zoological Park,Chennai. H & E x 100 (Courtesy: Dept. of Wildlife Sciences, C.V.Sc., Chennai, Tamil Nadu).

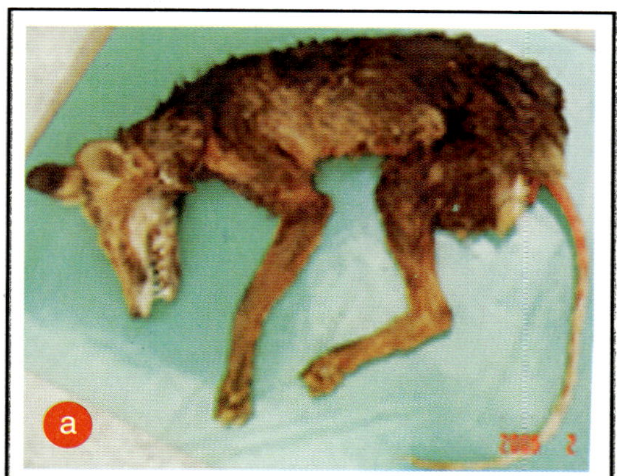

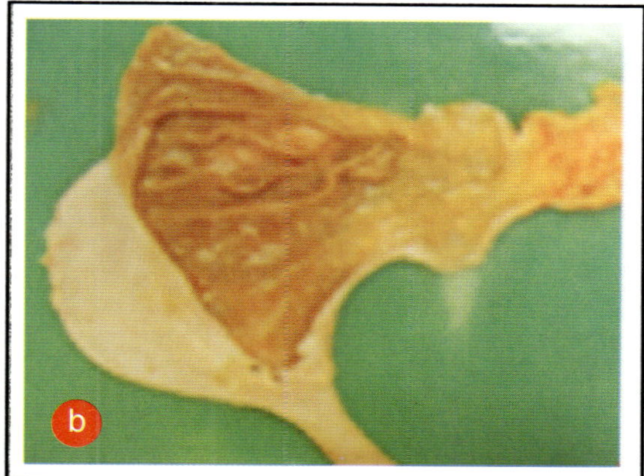

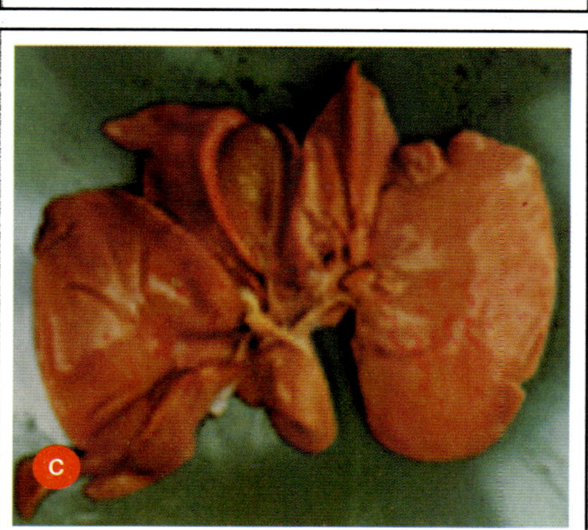

Figure 521: (a) Carcass of cachoectic Himalayan red fox (*V.v.montana*). Necropsy of (a) showed: (b) stomach and intestine mucosa extensively stained with bile pigment. (c) Yellowish liver. The condition was attributed to jaundice.

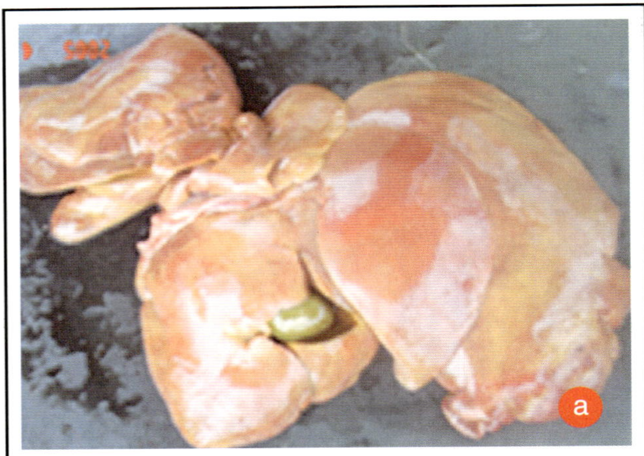

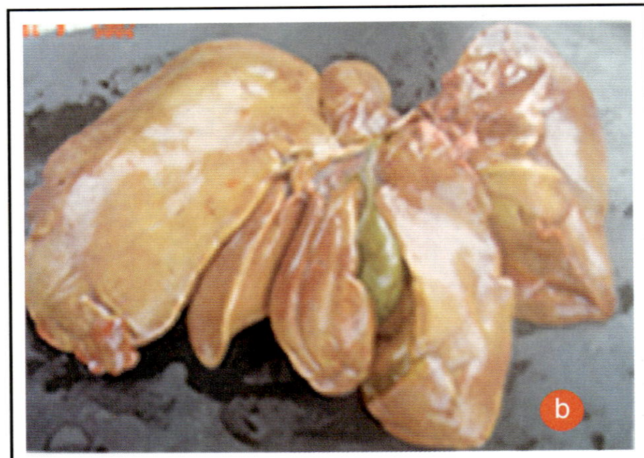

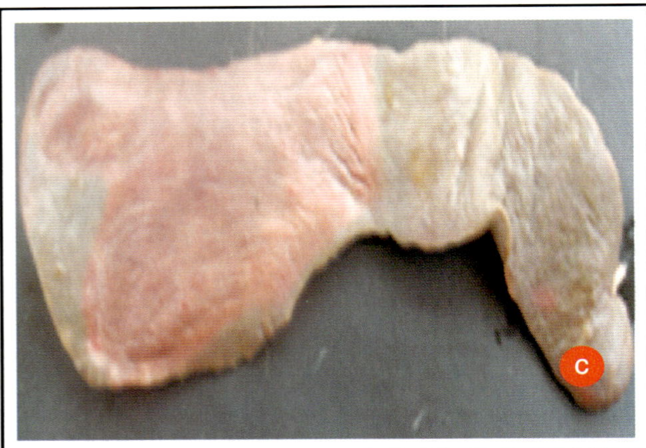

Figure 522 : Photograph of anemic liver from an adult female wolf (*C. lupus*) died in Zoological Garden, Lucknow of Uttar Pradesh(a) Parietal surface view (b) visceral surface view. (c) Spleen of the animal was discolored and flabby. The case is also referred under respiratory system .

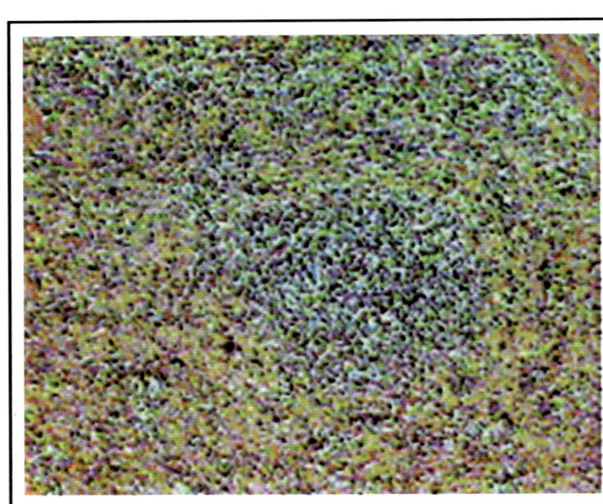

Figure 523: Photomicrograph of spleen from wild dog (*C. alpinus*) died in Zoological Park,Chennai (TN) showing lymphoid depletion. (Courtesy: Dept. of Wildlife Science,C.V.Sc.,Chennai,T.N).

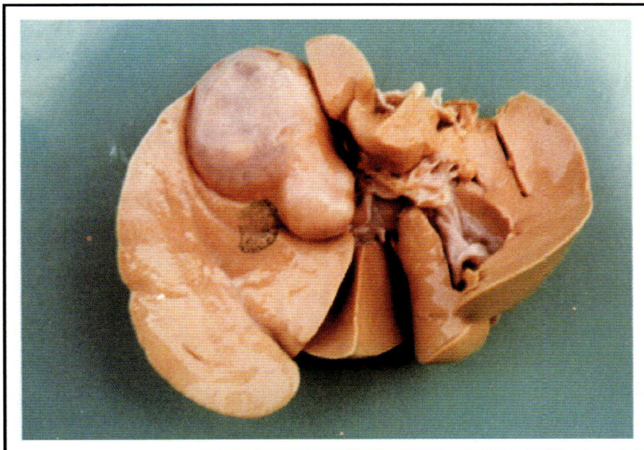

Figure 524: Photograph showing a large abscess in left lateral lobe of the liver of common fox (*V.v.bengalensis*) died at National Zoological Park, New Delhi.

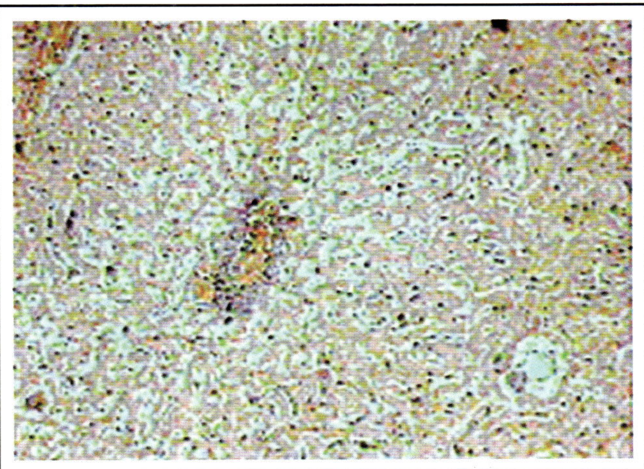

Figure 525: Photomicrograph of liver of wild dog (*C. alpinus*) showing infiltration of mononuclear cells in perivascular area, sinusoidal distension and congestion. H & E, x 100 (Courtesy: Dept. of Wild life Sci, CVSc, Chennai)

Uro-Genital System

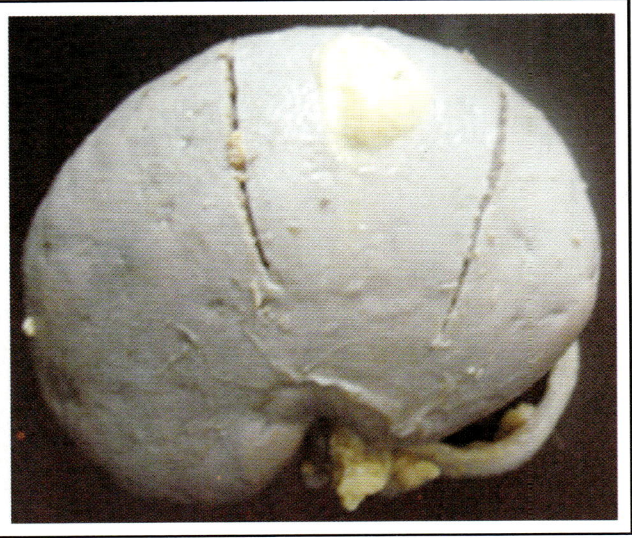

Figure 526: Kidney from jackal (*C. aureus*) showing abscess on its surface.

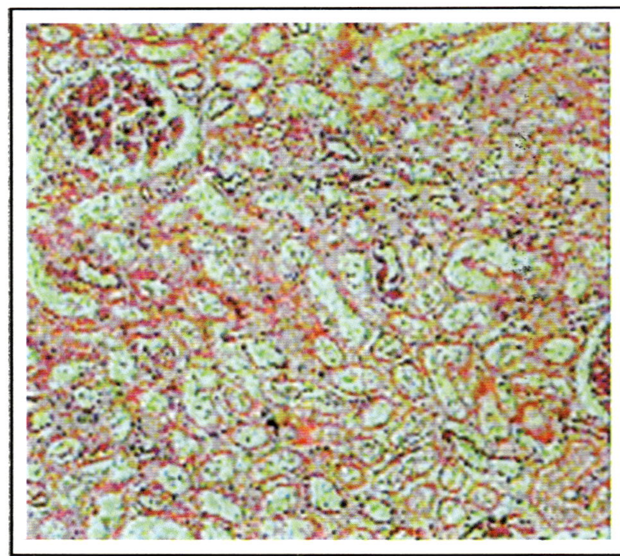

Figure 527: Photomicrograph showing tubular degeneration and necrosis of kidney of wild dog (*C. alpinus*) died at Zoological Park, Chennai, H & E x 100 (Courtesy: Dept of Wildlife Science, C.V.Sc., Chennai, T.N).

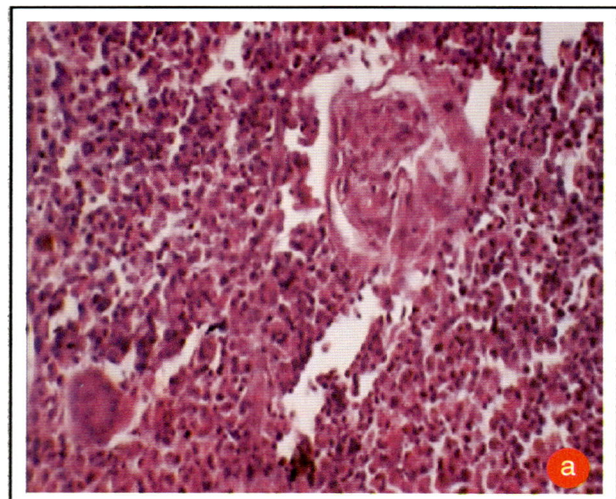

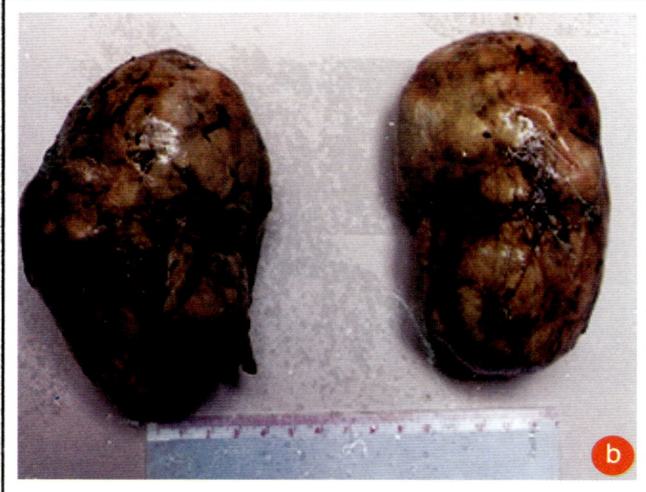

Figure 528: (a) Kidneys of hyena (*H. hyaena*) died in Zoological Garden, Guwahati (Assam) showing nodular elevations on the surfaces.(b) Photomicrograph of (a) showing sheets of lymphoid tumour cells replacing the cortical tubules of the kidney. H & E, x 200. The condition is diagnosed as lymphosarcoma. (Nashiruddullah *et al.*, 2007)

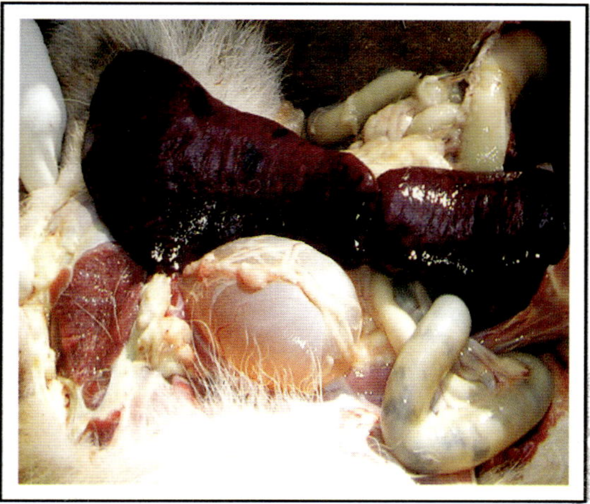

Figure 529: Photograph showing retension of urine in jackal (*C. aureus*) reported to have died of trypanosomiasis.

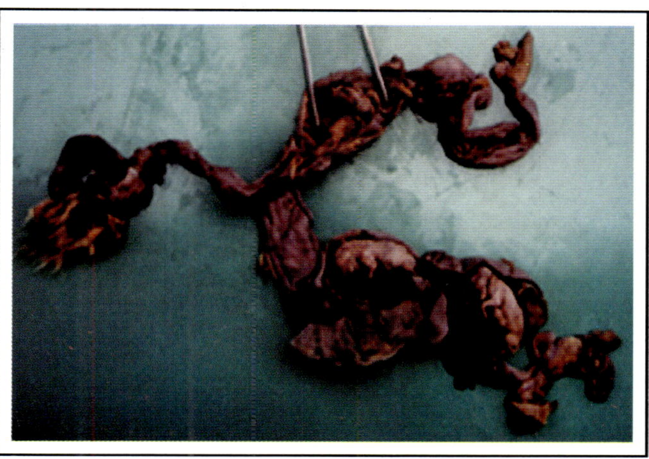

Figure 530: Photograph showing mutilated foetuses in the uterine horns of jackal (*C. aureus*), crushed by a speedy vehicle while crossing the highway.

Nervous Sytem(Brain) & Sense Organs (Eye)

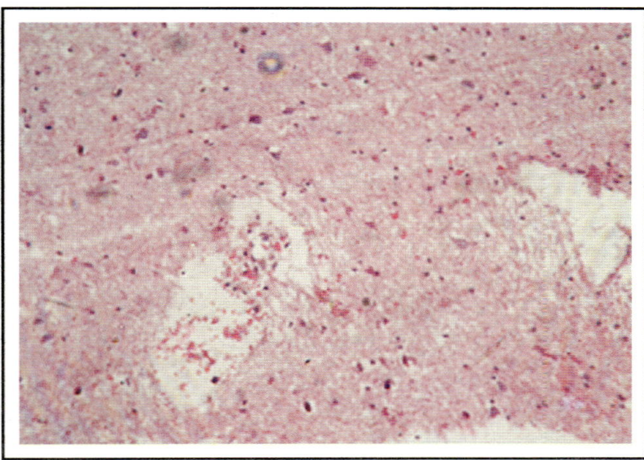

Figure 531: Histopathologic section of brain from jackal (*C. aureus*) showing haemorrhages H & E x 100 (Courtesy Dept. of Pathology C.V.Sc., Nagpur, M.S).

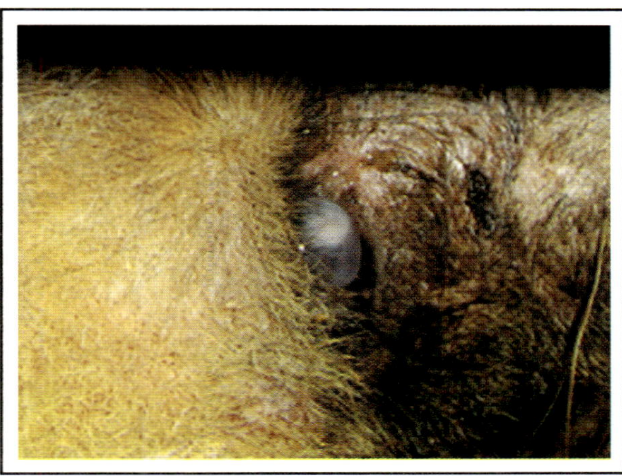

Figure 532: Photograph showing corneal opacity in right eye in hyena (*H.hyaena*) belonging to National Zoological Park, New Delhi.

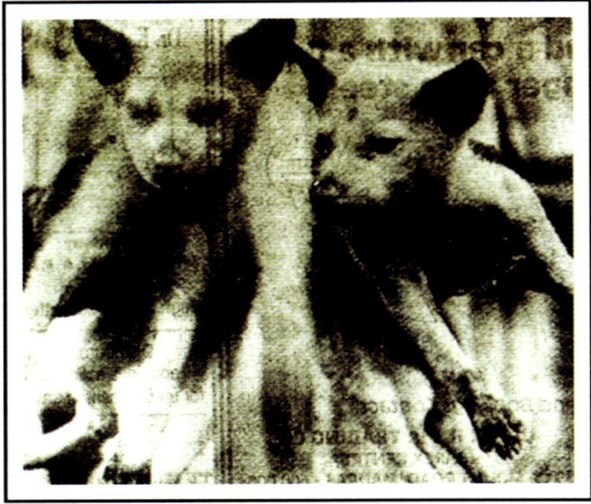

Figure 533: Albino jackals (*C. aureus*) collected from wild and kept in Zoological Garden, Kolkata (Hindu Newspaper, Delhi Ed. 5-4-1991).

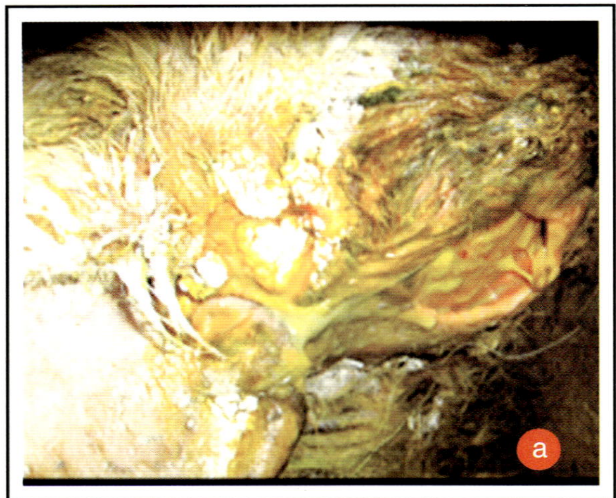

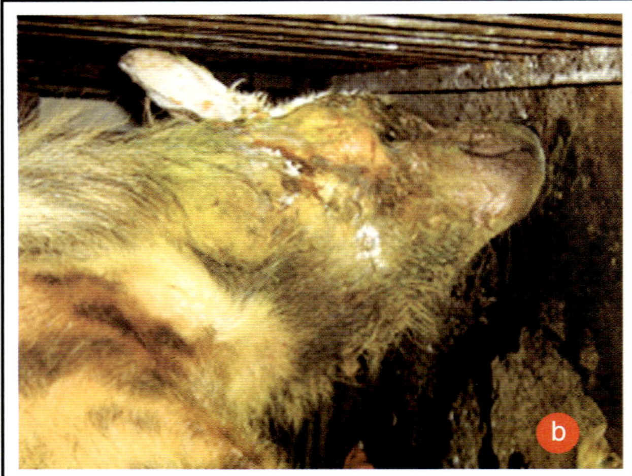

Figure 534: Photograph (a,b) showing suppurative dermatitis on right side of the face, involving mandible in hyena (*H. hyaena*) belonging to National Zoological Park, New Delhi.

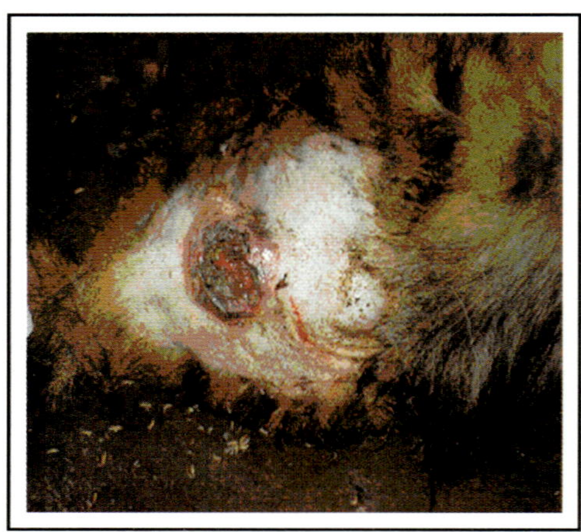

Figure 535: Photograph showing maggot infested fistula on the left thigh and on rump region in captive hyena (*H. hyaena*). (Courtesy: Nanjappa, K.A.)

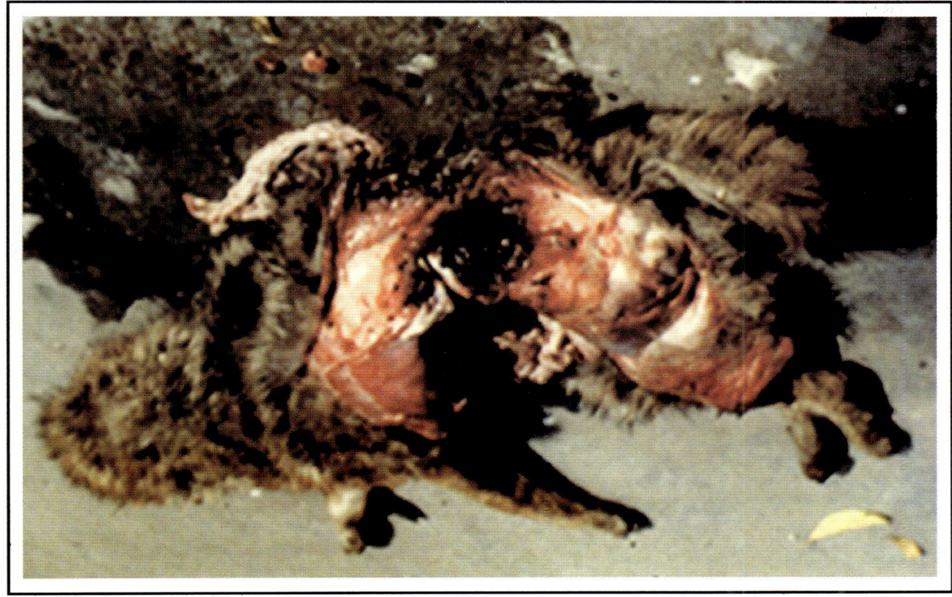

Figure 536: Photograph showing deep muscular wounds on the left dorso lateral aspect of body of jackal (*C. aureus*) sustained during infighting in captivity.

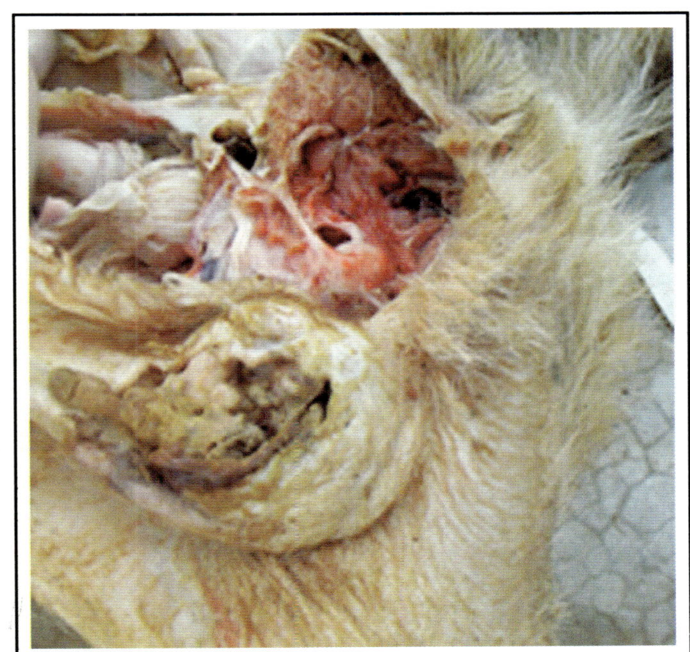

Figure 537: Photograph showing tumorous growth on the lower abdomen of the wolf (*C. lupus*) died in Zoological Garden, Lucknow (U.P).

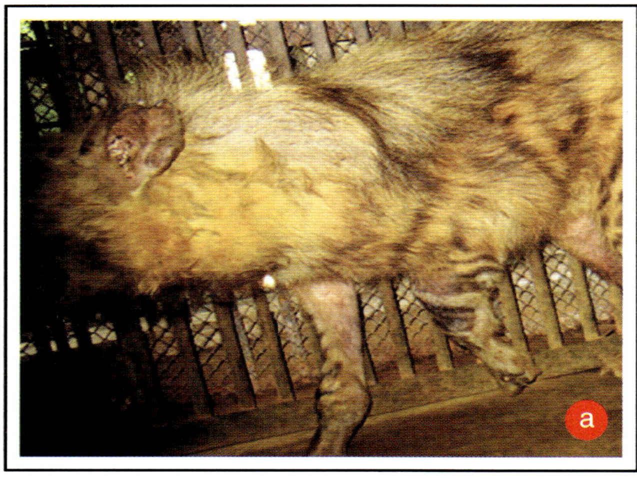

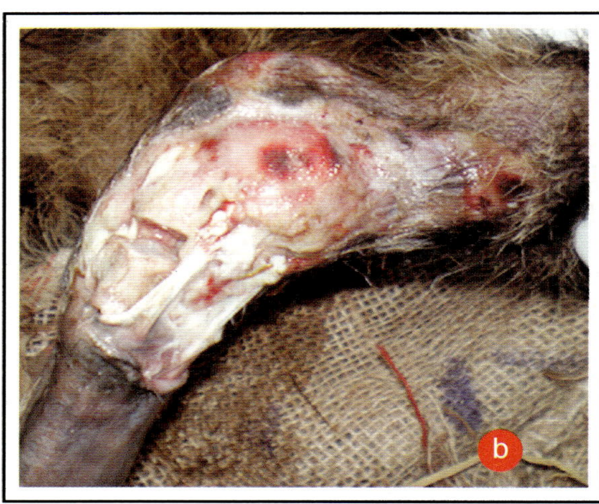

Figure 538: (a) Hyena (*H.hyaena*) having fracture in its left fore limb under treatment at Zoo hospital, Chennai (b) Hyena having fracture of right hind limb under treatment at Z.G. Pune (MS).

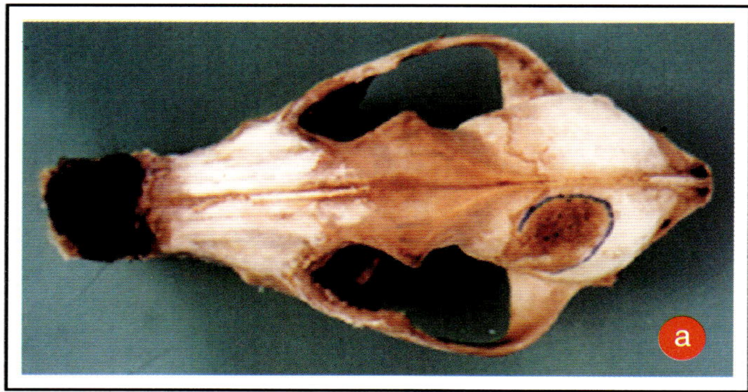

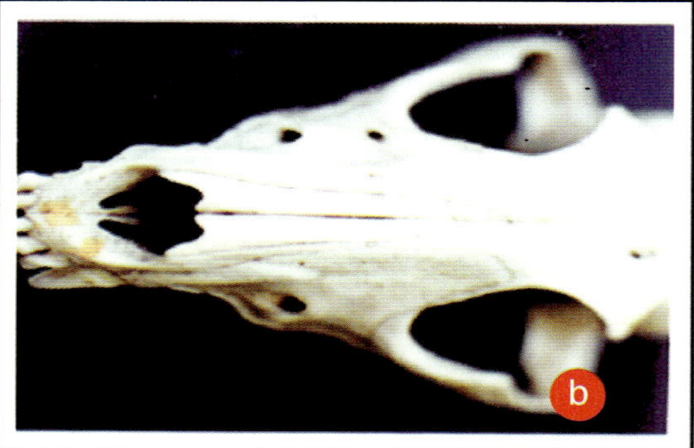

Figure 539 (a) Fresh deskinned skull of jackal (*C. aureus*) showing periosteal thickening of left parietal. (b): Fresh deskinned skull of jackal (*C. aureus*) showing two holes in right maxilla and one hole in the left maxilla. Also an elongated hole present in left frontal bone.

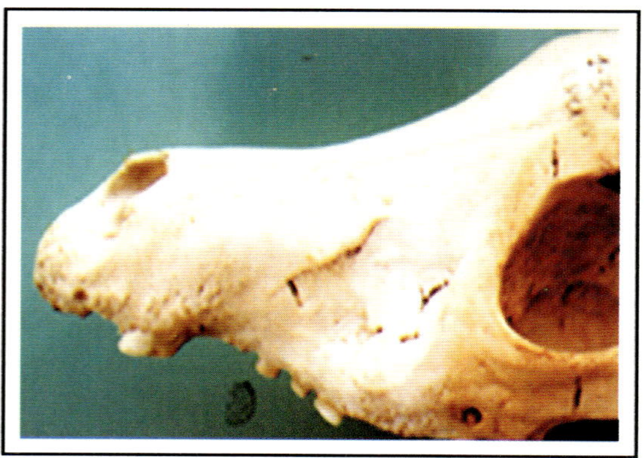

Figure 540: Photograph showing fracture on left maxilla encountered in necropsy of wolf (*Canis lupus*). Also infra orbital foramen not discerned.

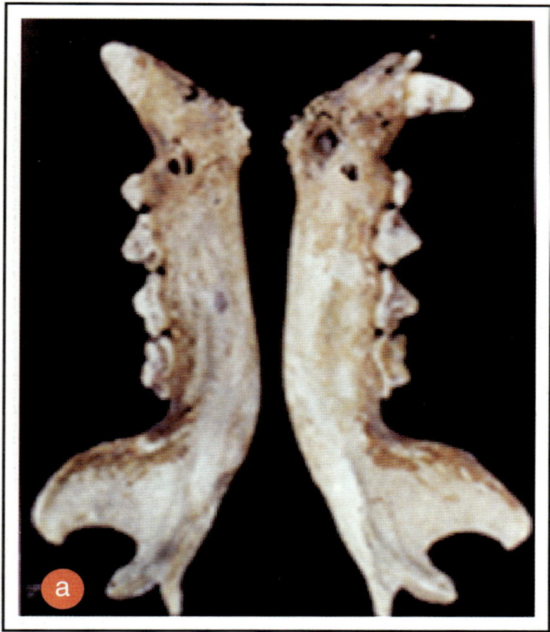

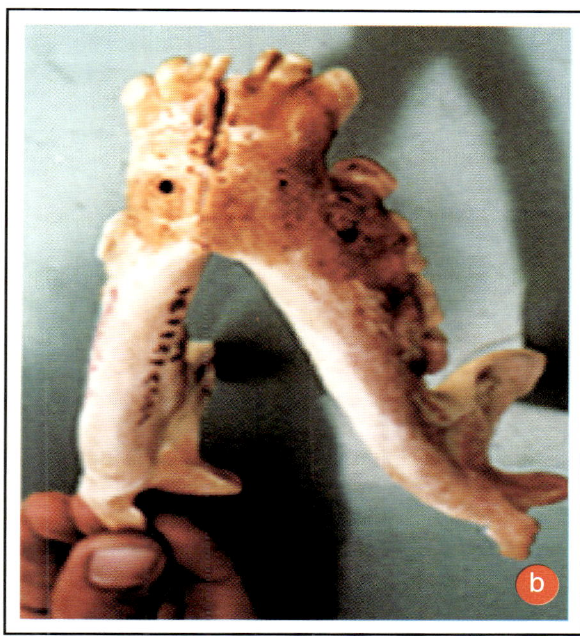

Figure 541: Hyena (*H. hyaena*) mandible showing a pin head sized hole on the ventral surface of the left ramus at the level of body of symphysis and at the lateral aspect of right ramus at the level between first and second premolars.(b) Lingual surface of the rami showing holes at the level of diastema in other case.

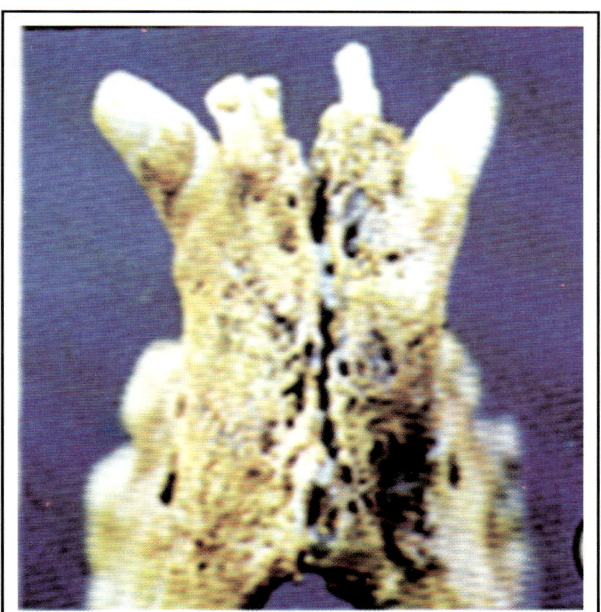

Figure 542: Photograph of mandible of hyena (*H. hyaena*) showing osteoporotic lesions extending from the level of symphysis to the base of molars teeth.

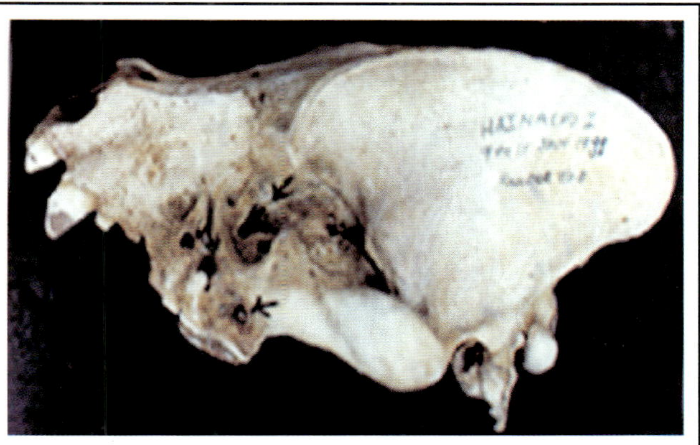

Figure 543: Photograph showing necrotic lesion of left maxilla in hyena (*H. hyaena*) died in captivity.

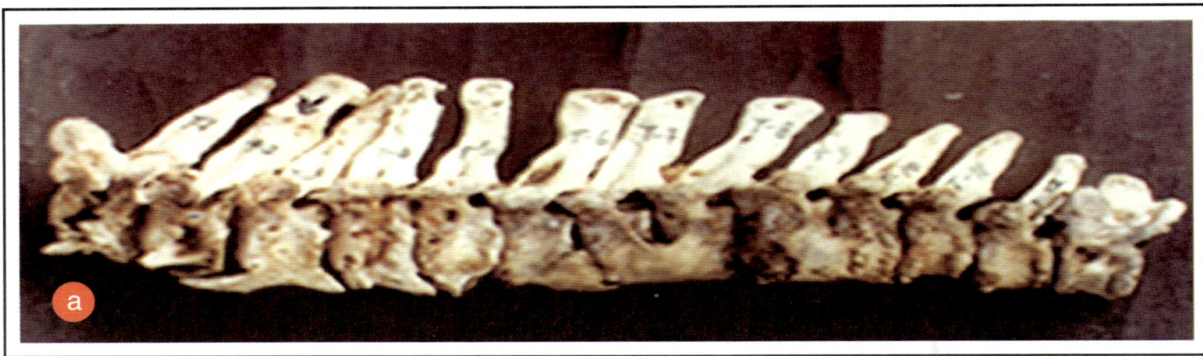

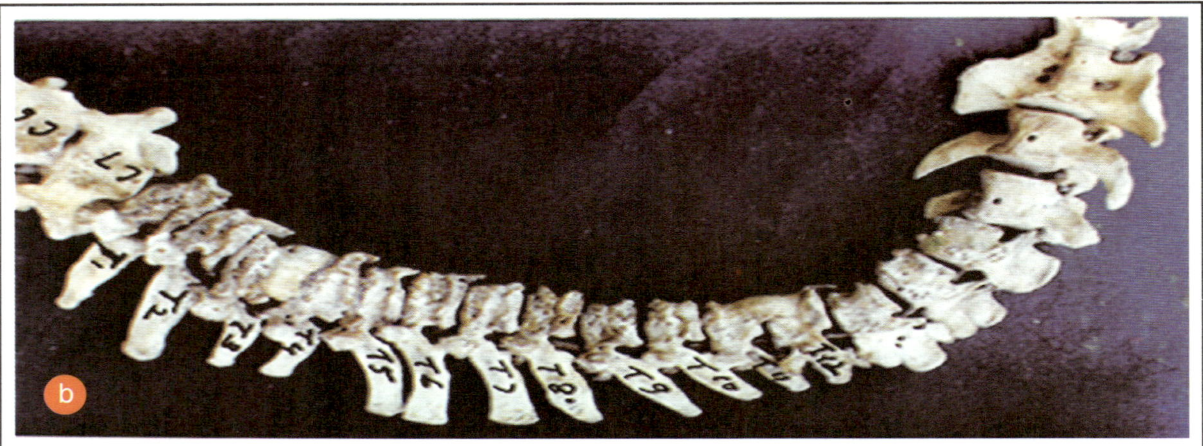

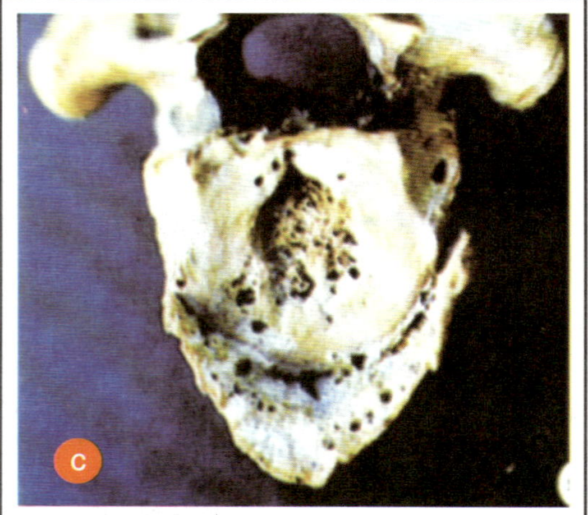

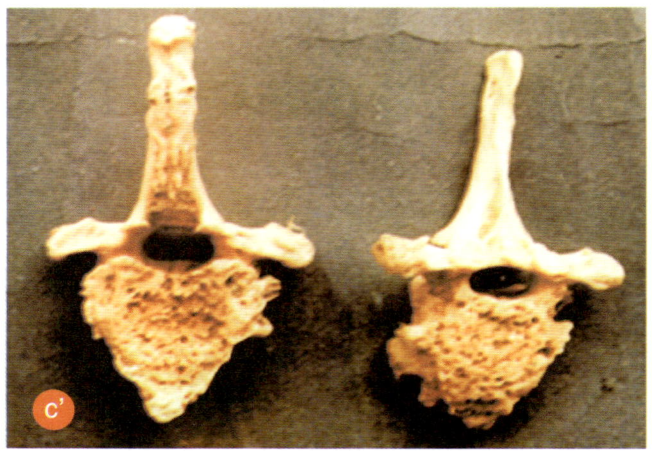

Figure 544: Spondyloarthopathy in hyena (*H. hyaena*) died in captivity. Photographs showing latero-ventral (a) and ventro-lateral (b) views of the vertebral bodies and their marginal ends with osteophytic growths. Growths at the ventral aspect of body are lipping over the adjacent vertebra. Note: Some of the last thoracic vertebrae not shown . The important features included: (c, c') Osteophytic growths.

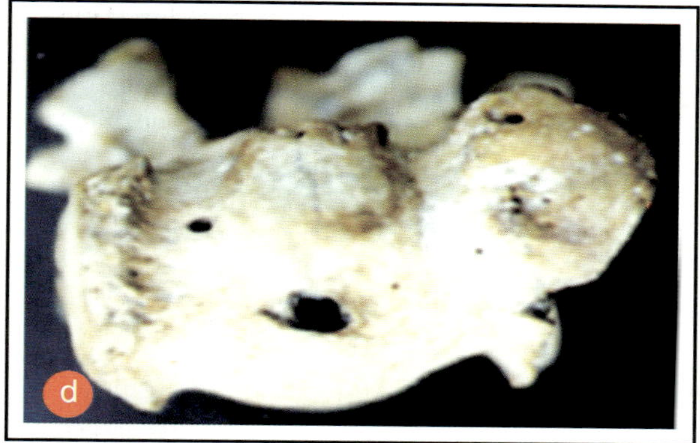

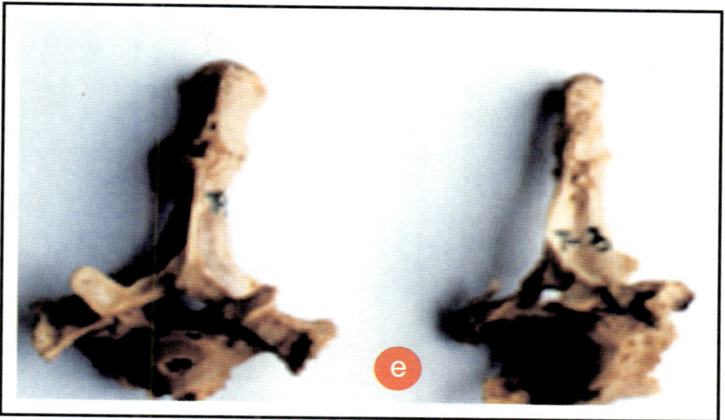

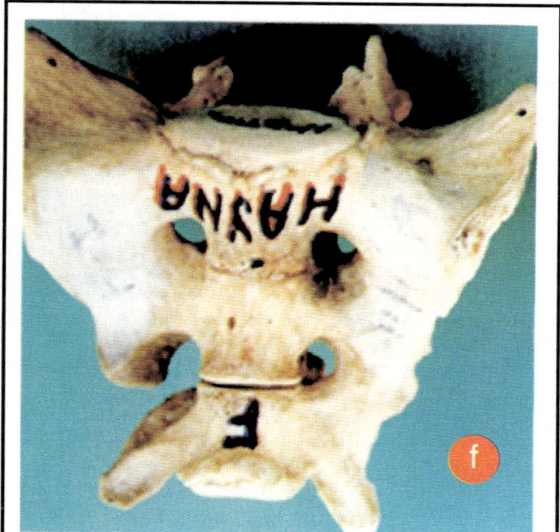

Figure 544: (d) Fusion between 11 and 12 th thoracic vertebrae and necrotic changes, (e) Fracture of spinal processes of thoracic vertebrae (healing in two shown). (f)Absence of union between second and third sacral vertebrae.

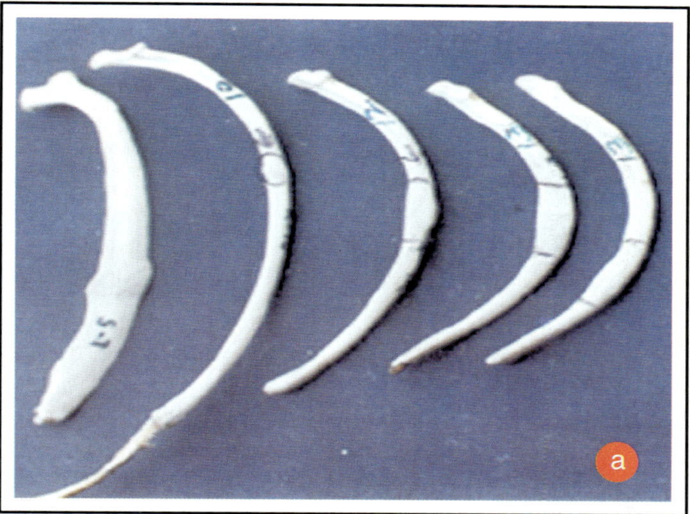

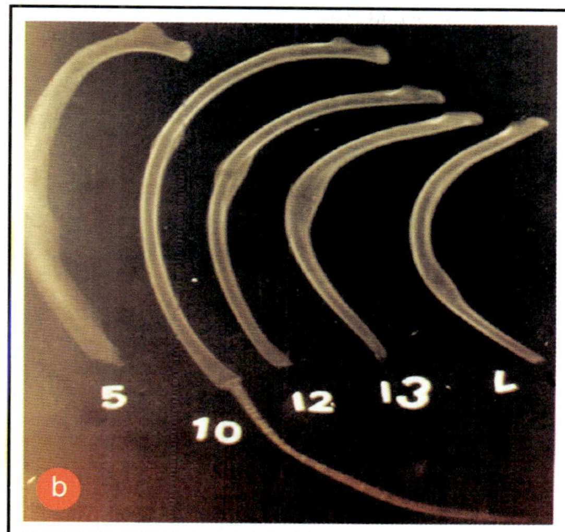

Figure 545: Ribs of a wolf (*C. lupus*) died in captivity showing: (a) Spontaneously healed fractures in 5th left,10th and 12th right ribs and in both 13 ribs. (b) Radiograph of (a) showing complete even healing of fractures.

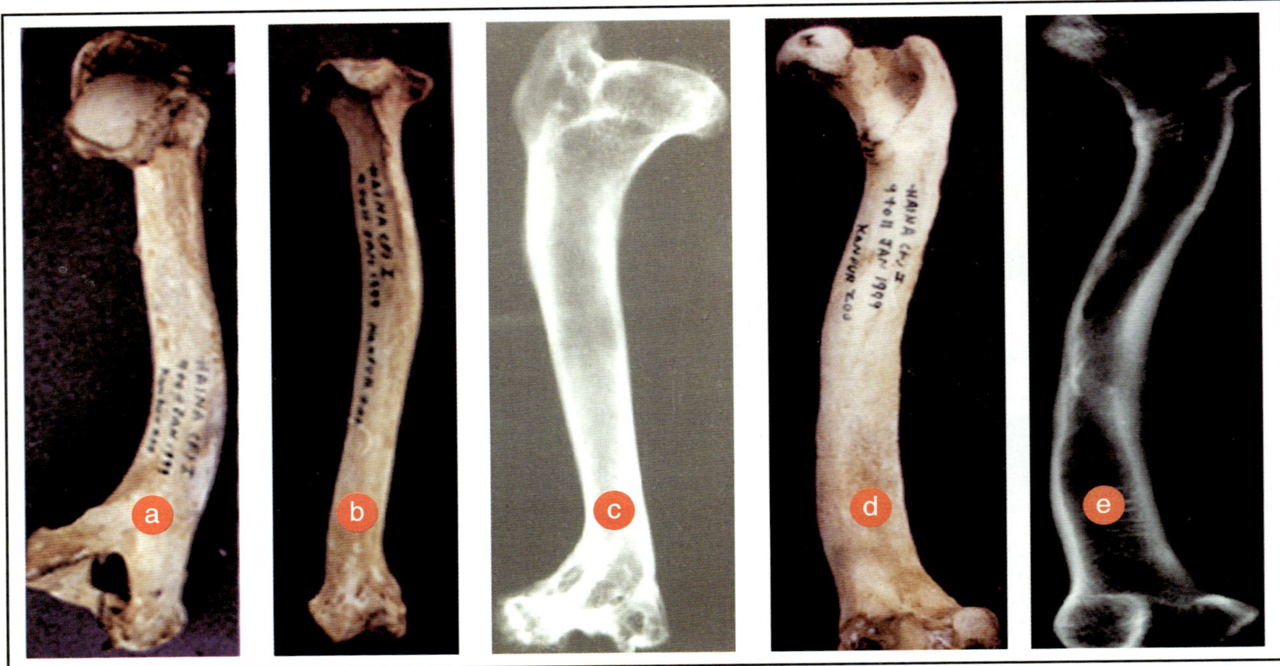

Figure 546: Photographs showing anomalies of long bones encountered in hyena (*H. hyaena*) died in captivity. (a) Formation of excrescences around the head of proximal extremity and condyles of distal extremity of humerus.Note shafts of humerous and radius(b) are slightly deviated in their normal course.(c) Radiograph of (a) showing density of variable thickness of the periosteum.(d) Femur shaft slightly deviated from its normal course. (e) Radiograph of (d) showing variable thickness of the periosteum.

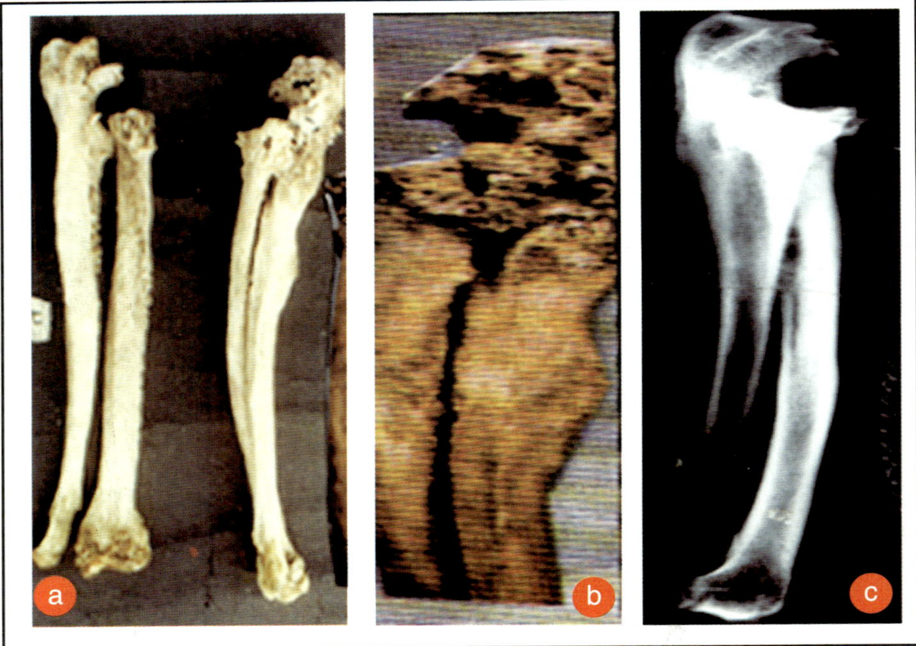

Figure 547: Photographs (a, b) showing osteophytic growths on proximal extremities of ulna and radius of hyena (*H. hyaena*), which suffered from spondyloarthopathy referred above. (c) Radiograph of (a) evidenced ankylosis of the joint.

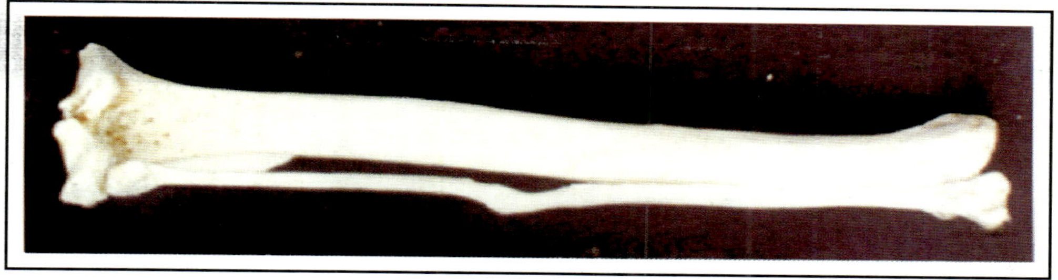

Figure 548: Photograph of tibia and fibula from wolf (*C. lupus*) died in captivity. Note shaft of fibula showing angular deformed as a result of uneven healed fracture in its middle.

Miscellaneous

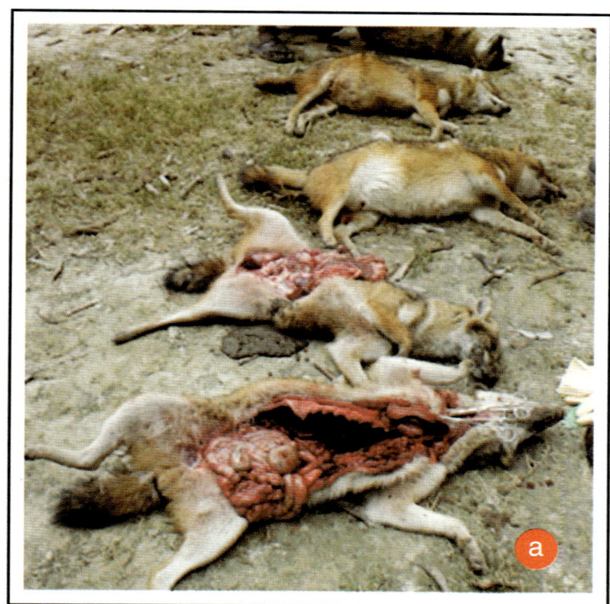

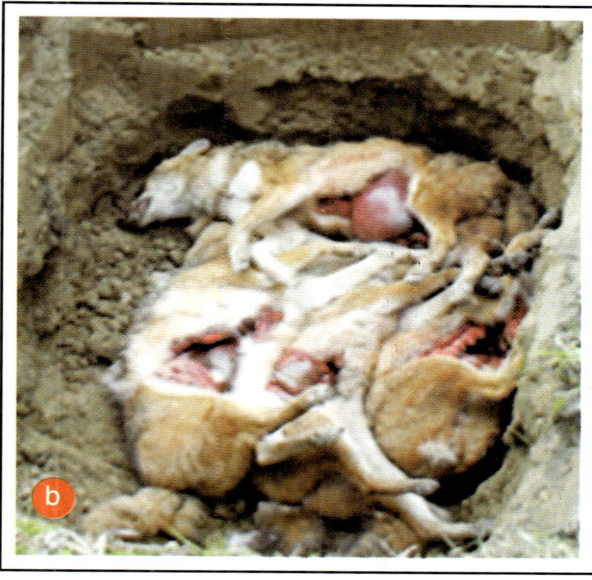

Figure 549: Photographs showing: (a) Four carcasses out of 16 wild jackals (*C. aureus*) that died due to DDT poisoning. (b) After necropsy examination carcasses being buried (Courtesy: Singh, K.K). Note:On 5th January 2008 in a particular location in Dhaurahra of north Kheri of Lakhimpur (U.P) fresh carcasses of 16 jackals have been found and DDT toxicity has been attributed for enmass death.

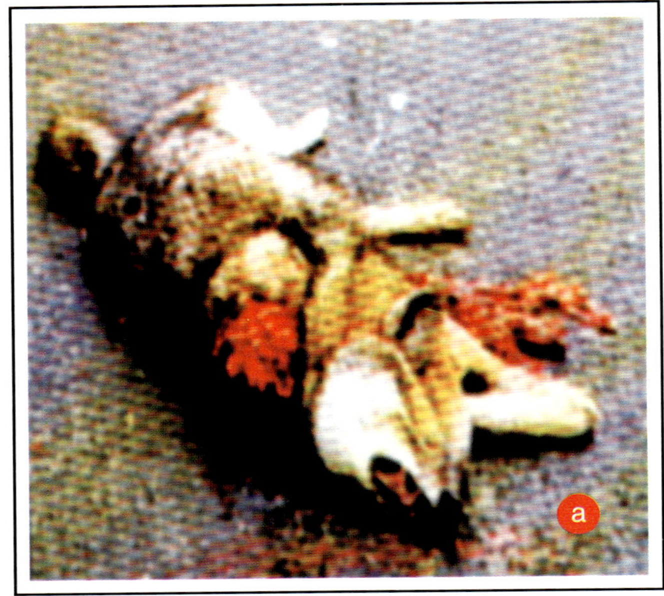

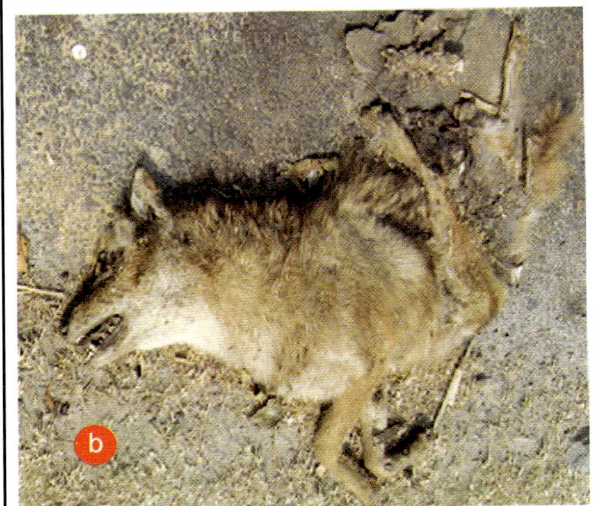

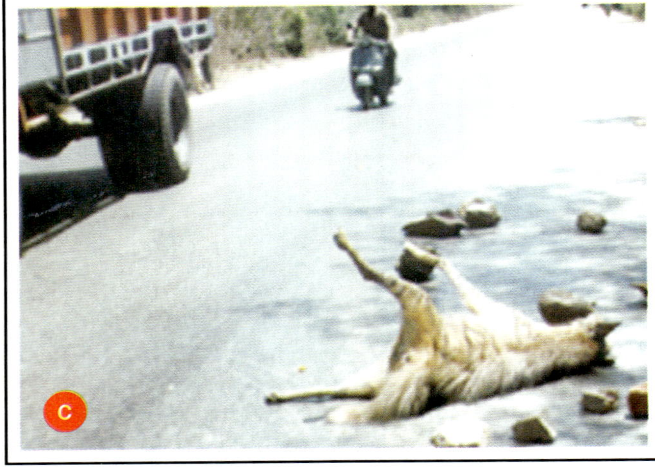

Figure 550: Accidental deaths : (a,b) Carcasses of crushed jackals (*C. aureus*) that had collided with speedy vehicles on high ways in Uttar Pradesh. (c) Carcass of hyena (*H. hyaena*) hit by a vehicle in Rajasthan.

Bears & Red Panda

Cardio-vascular System

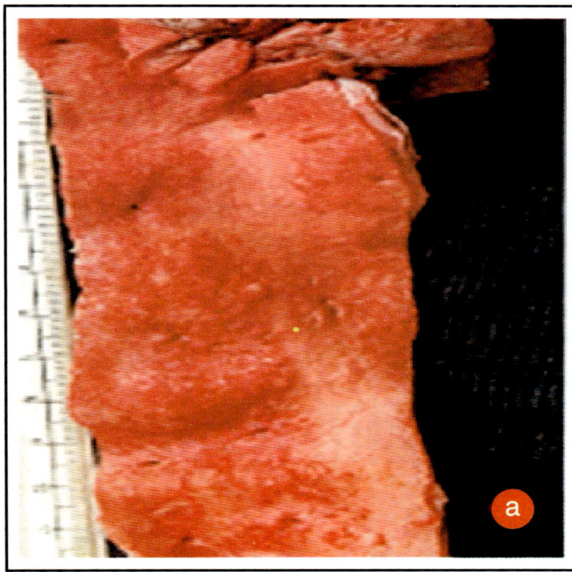

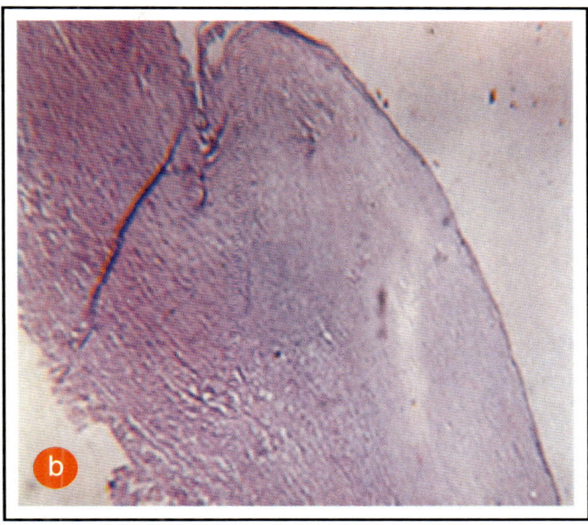

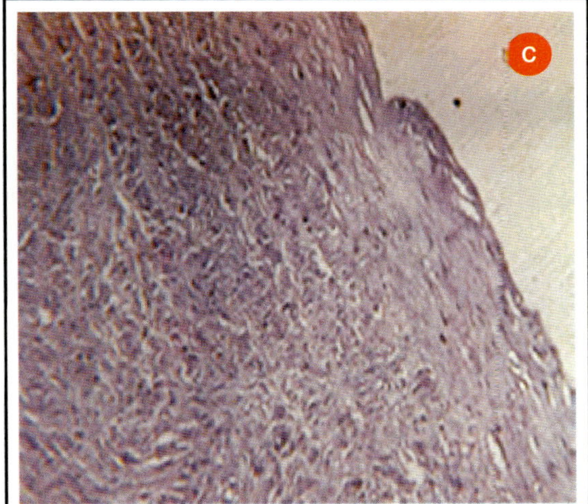

Figure 551: Atherosclerosis in sloth bear (*M.ursinus*) died in Zoological Garden,Guwahati, Assam. (a) Photograph showing sudanophilic intimal thickening in the aorta. Photomicrographs (b,c) showing Intimal thickening of aorta. H & E, x 100. (c) Same at higher magnification. (Nashiruddullah *et al.*, 2007).

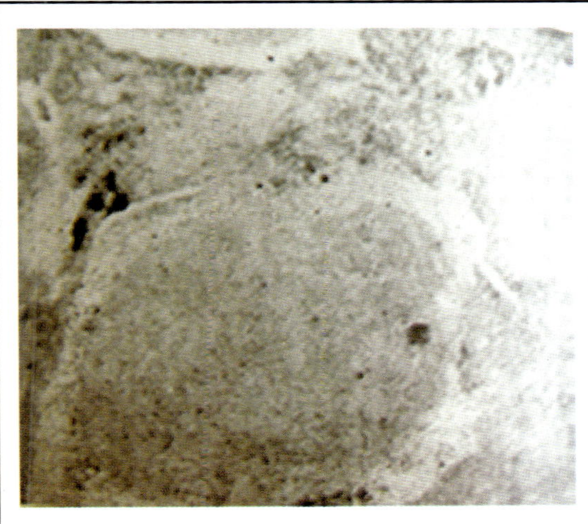

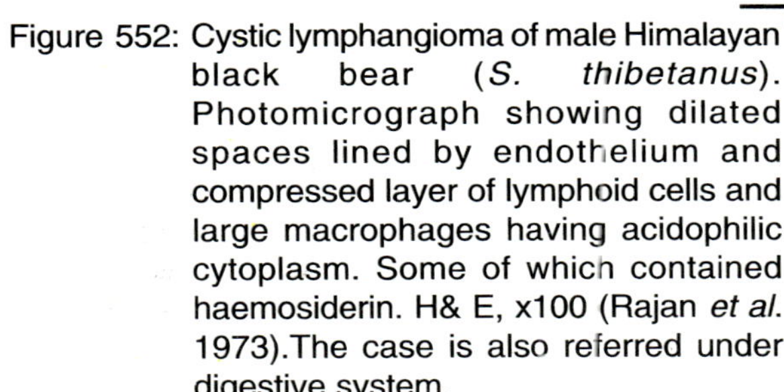

Figure 552: Cystic lymphangioma of male Himalayan black bear (*S. thibetanus*). Photomicrograph showing dilated spaces lined by endothelium and compressed layer of lymphoid cells and large macrophages having acidophilic cytoplasm. Some of which contained haemosiderin. H& E, x100 (Rajan *et al.* 1973).The case is also referred under digestive system.

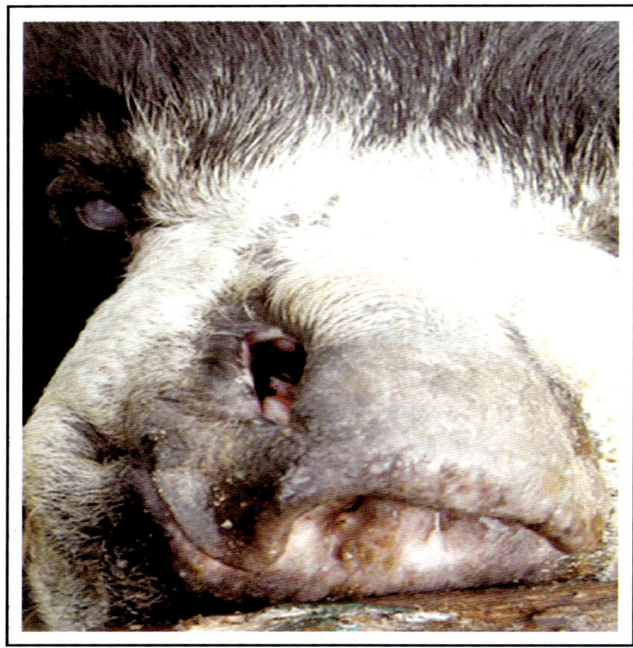

Figure 553: Photograph showing wound on the nostril of rescued sloth bear (*M. ursinus*) caused by nose ring. Note animal has also corneal opacity of right eye.

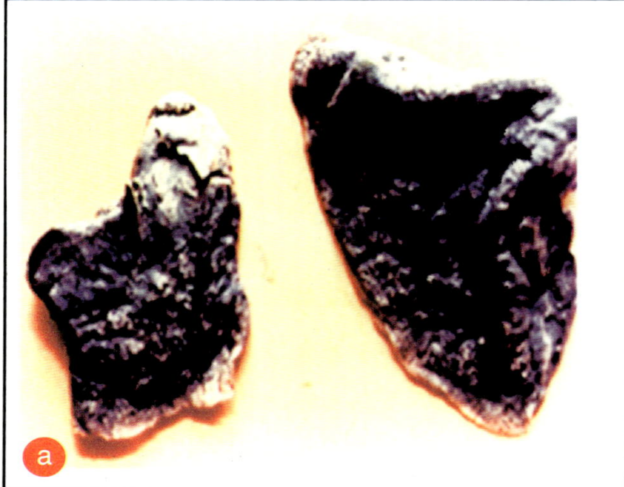

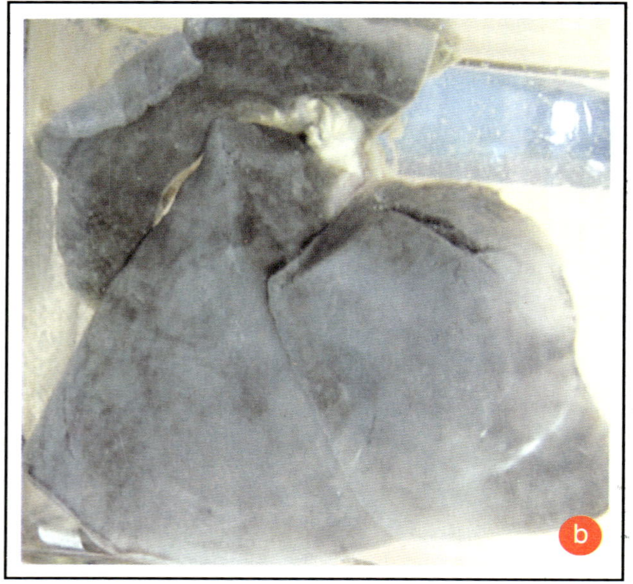

Figure 554: Photographs showing pneumoconosis of lungs encountered in: (a) Red panda (*A. fulgens*) died in captivity.(b) Sloth bear (*M. ursinus)* died in captivity.

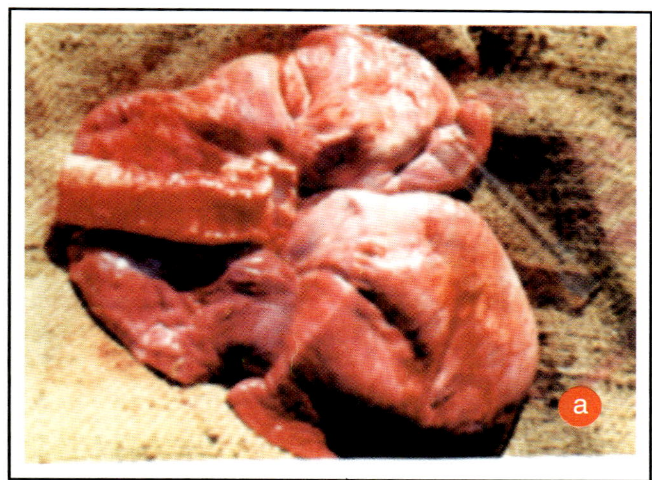

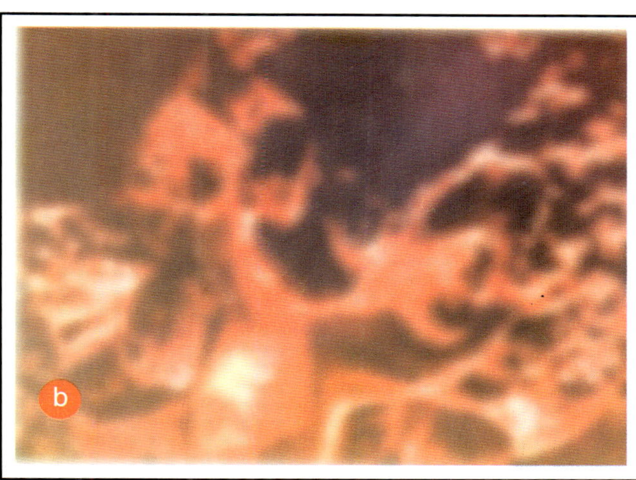

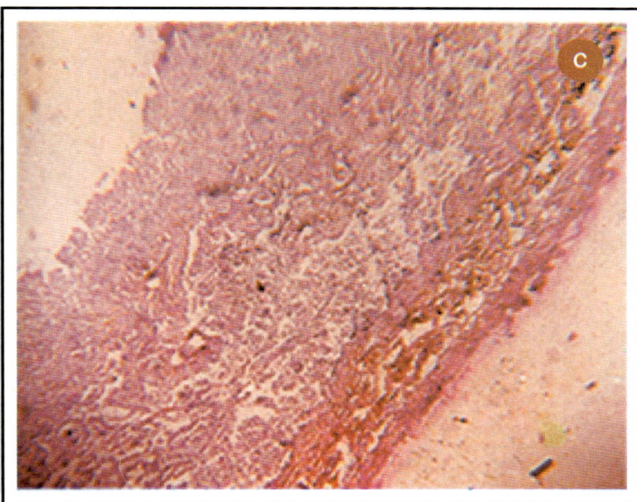

Figure 555: (a) Pneumonic lung of a sloth bear (*M. ursinus*) died of Aspiration pneumonia at Zoological Garden, Guwahati. Photographs showing: . (b) Cut section of (a) showing presence of foreign fluid content in lobes. (c) Photomicrograph of (a). (Nashiruddullah *et al.*, 2007). H & E x 70.

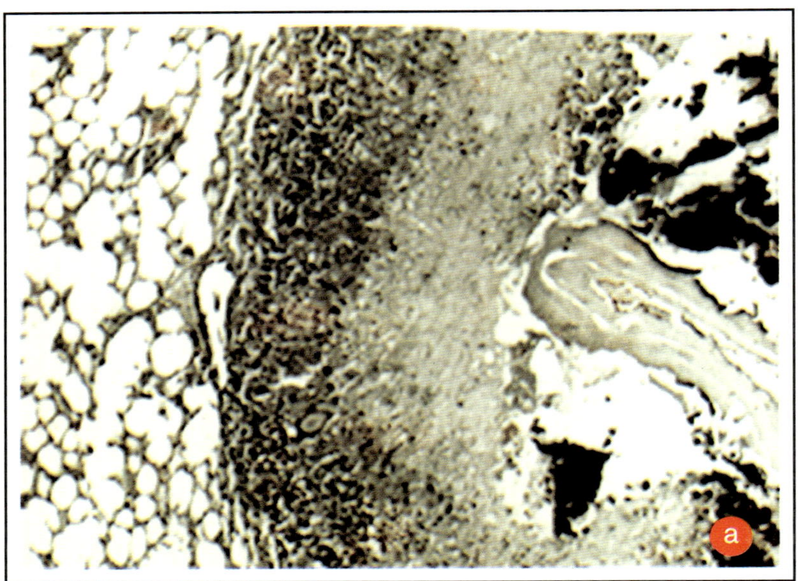

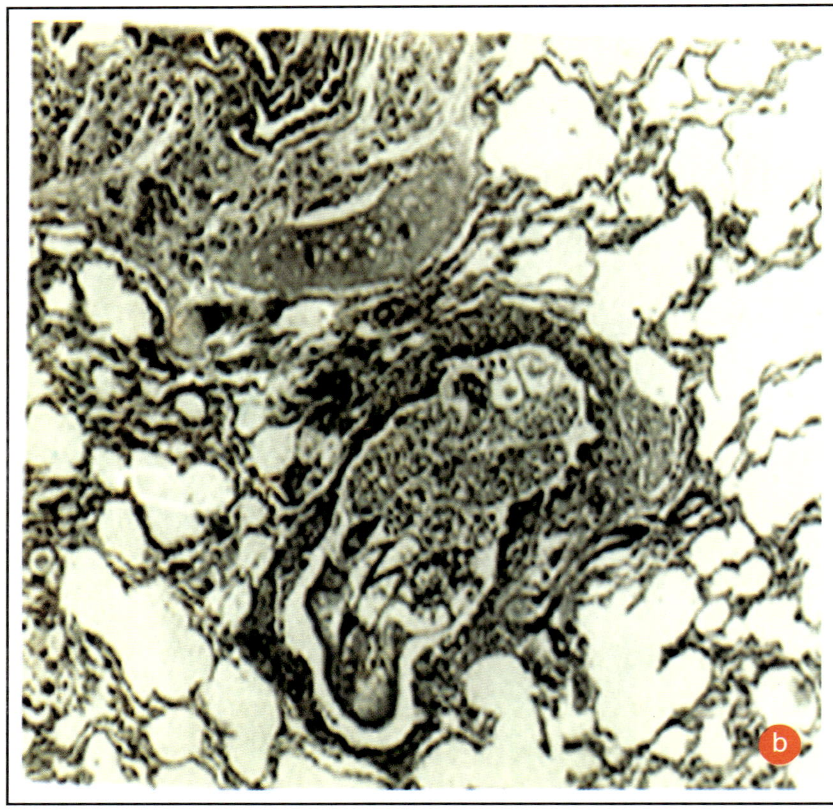

Figure 556: Parasitic pneumonia in red panda (*A. fulgens*) died in captivity. Photomicrographs showing: (a) Foreign body giant cell granulomatus reaction around the parasite in lung H & E, x 150. (b) Cross section of parasite in the bronchiole. x 150 (Courtesy: Parihar, N.S.).

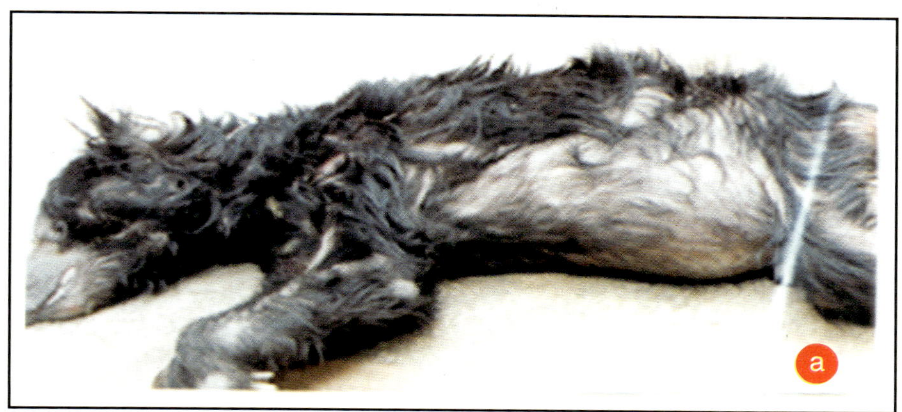

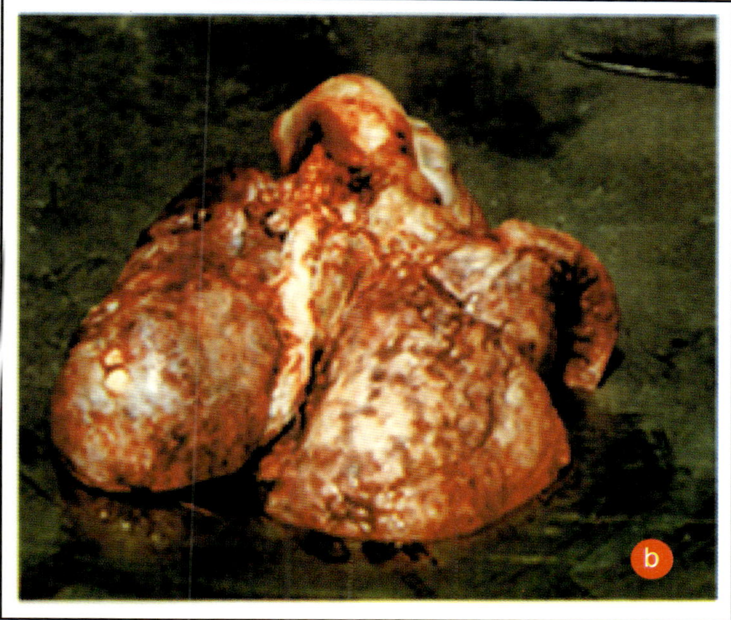

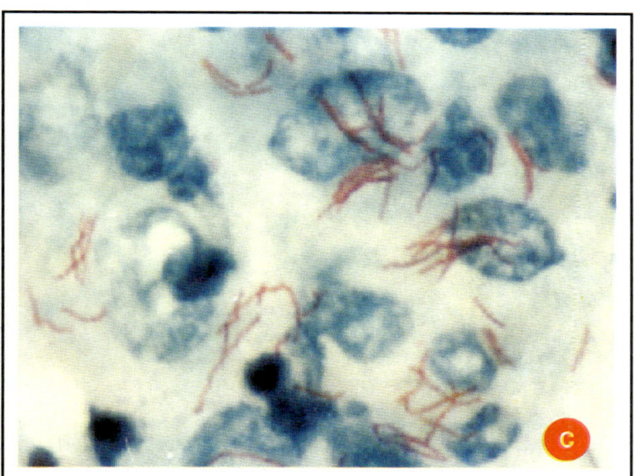

Figure 557: Photographs showing: (a) Carcass of emaciated sloth bear (*M. ursinus*) died due to tuberculosis at Bannerghatta National Park, Bangalore.(b) Caseated tuberculous nodules of various sizes in lungs of(a). (c) Masses of pink stained, beaded and slender rod like acid-fast bacilli. Z.N.Stain, x 1000 (Courtesy: Harish, B.R. & Ranukaprasad, C.).

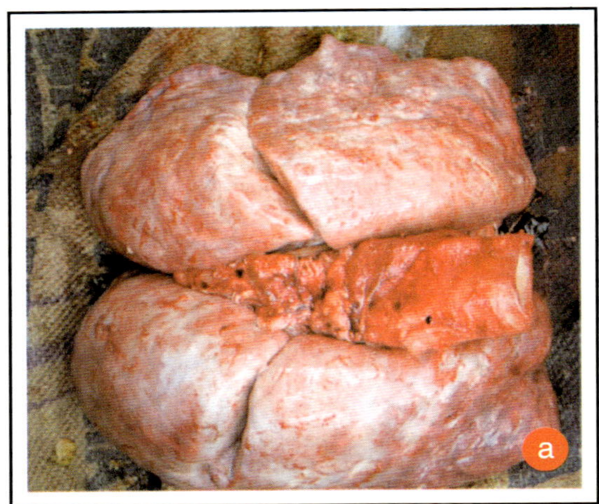

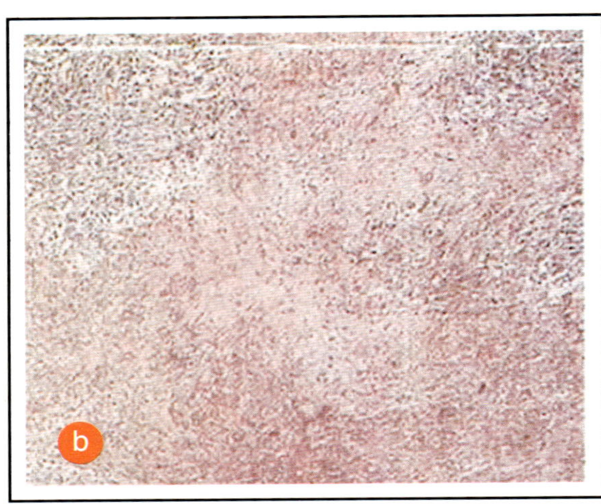

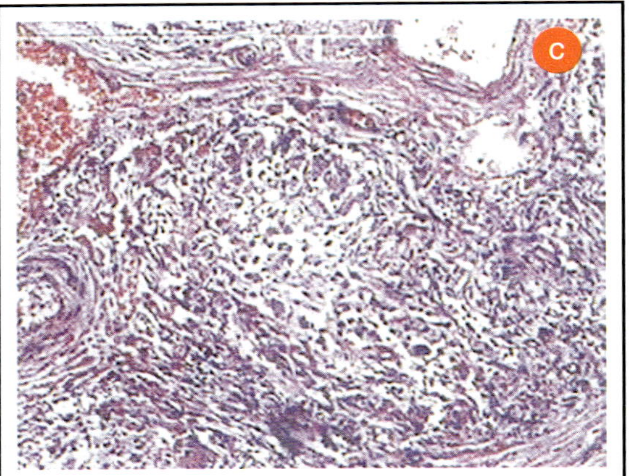

Figure 558: Photograph showing pulmonary tuberculosis in sloth bear (*M.uscinus*) died in Bear Rescue Center, Bannerghatta, Bangalore. Photomicrographs of lung showing tuberculous granulomas.(b) At lower magnification H & E x 100 (c) Higher magnification of (b) H & E, x 400 (Courtesy:Arun,A. Sah & Jai Anandh).

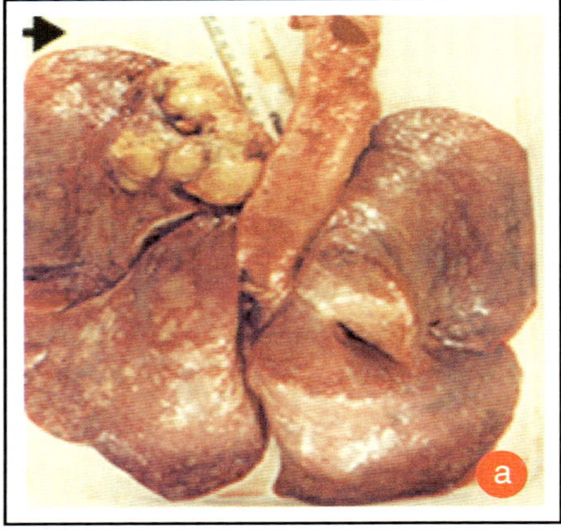

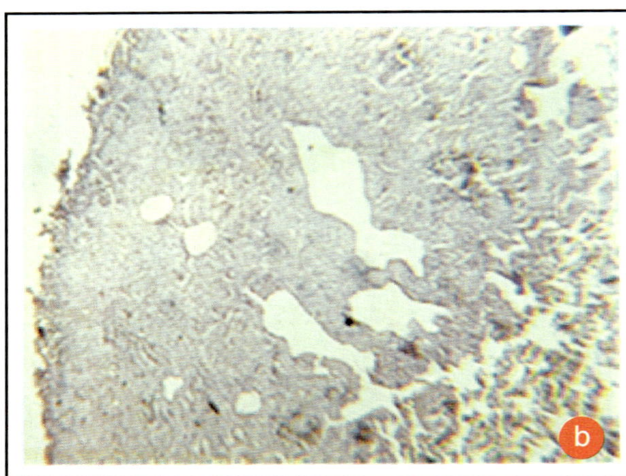

Figure 559: (a) Photograph showing growth in the lung of Himalayan black bear (*S. thibetanus*) died in captivity. (b) Photomicrograph of (a) showing histological changes characteristic of adenocarcinoma. H & E, x 100

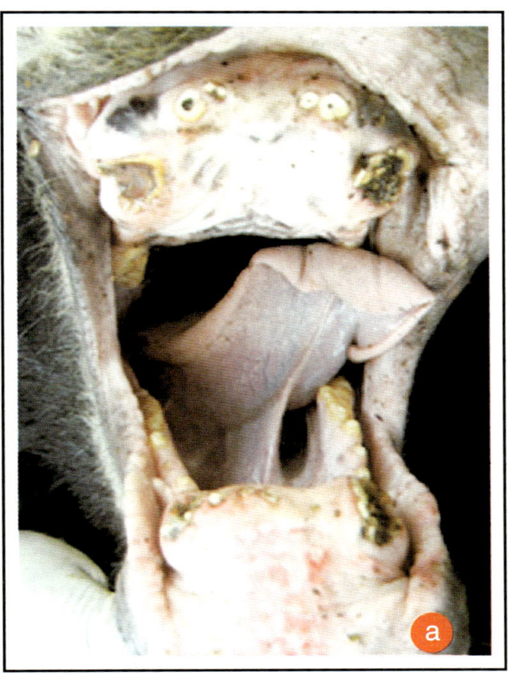

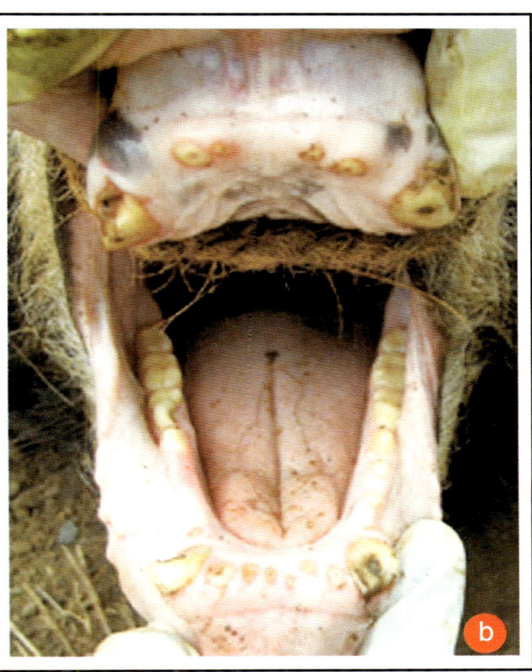

Figure 560: Photographs(a,b) showing heavy wear and loss of teeth in upper and lower jaws of sloth bear (*M. ursinus*)

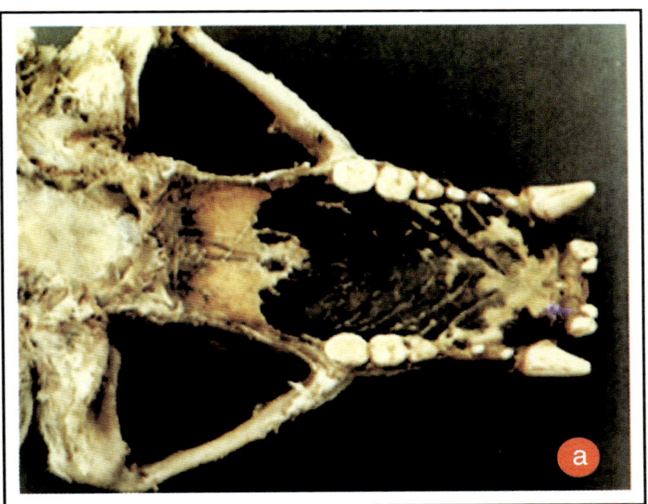

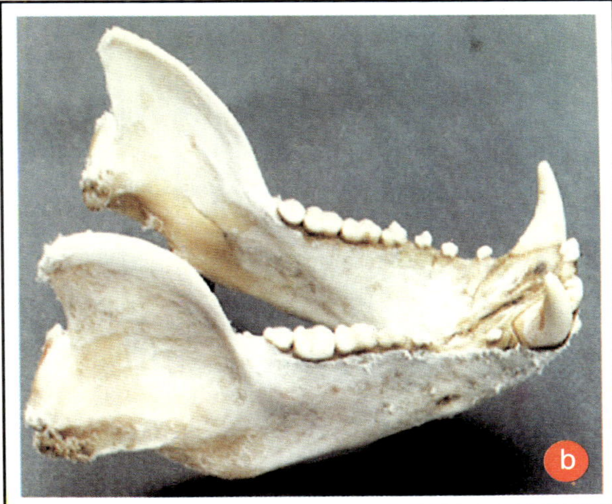

Figure 561: Photographs (a,b) of upper and lower jaws of sloth bear (*M. ursinus)* showing loss of central pair of incisors. Such loss is not uncommon in adult bear.

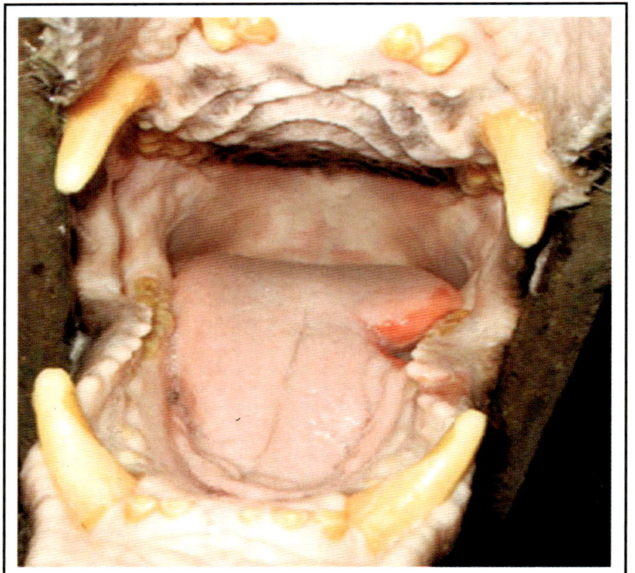

Figure 562: Photograph showing punctured wound on the left lateral border of the tongue and damaged the free border of the left lip caused due to low velocity bullet (of 9 mm dia.) in about 5- year-old sloth bear (*M.ursinus*). The case is also referred under integumentary system. (Arun. A. Sha, *et al.*, 2007a).

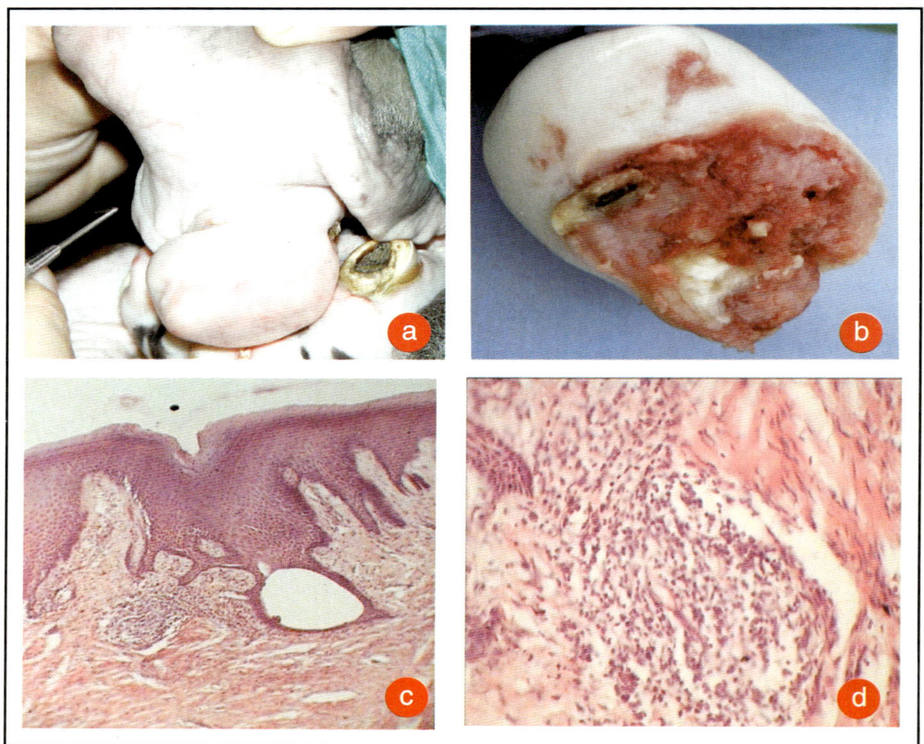

Figure 563: (a) Photograph showing round mass of growth in the oral cavity of rescued sloth bear (*M.ursinus*) cub.(b) Extirepated growth. Photomicrographs (c, d) of growth (a) showing gigantiform cementoma H & E, x 70 and x 200 (Arun. A. Sha *et al.*, 2007b).

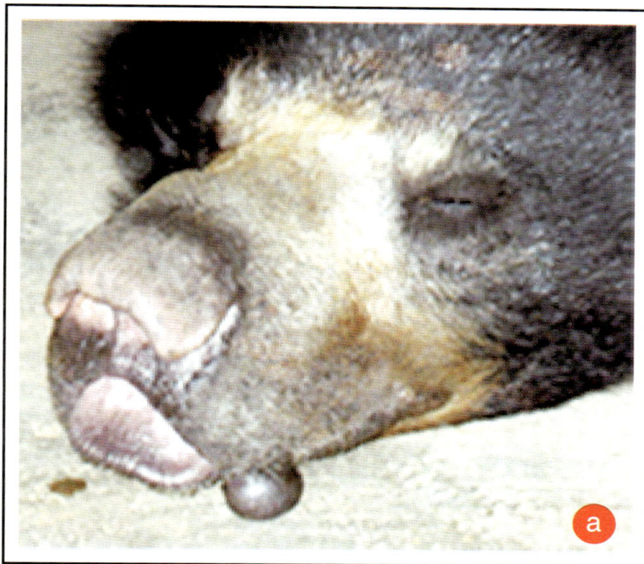

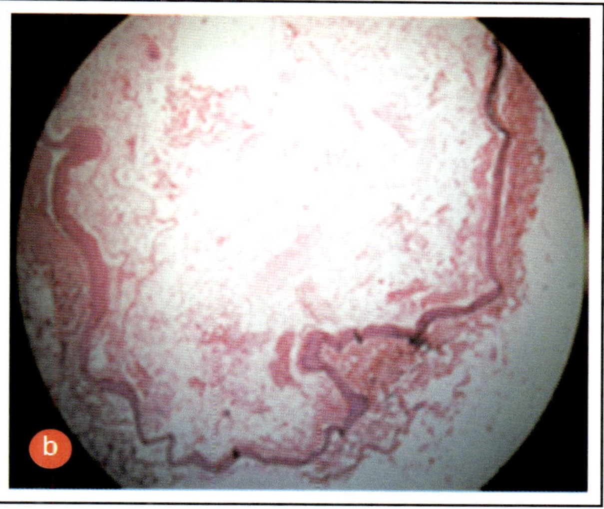

Figure 564: (a) Epidermoid cyst involving upper lip encountered in 13-Year-old male sloth bear (*M. ursinus*).(b) Photomicrograph showing cystic lining of keratinized squamous epithelium having prominent granular cell layer. Note presence of abundant orthokeratin which fills up the cystic lumen.The cyst was supported by loose connective tissue stroma. (Courtesy: Jadav,K.K).

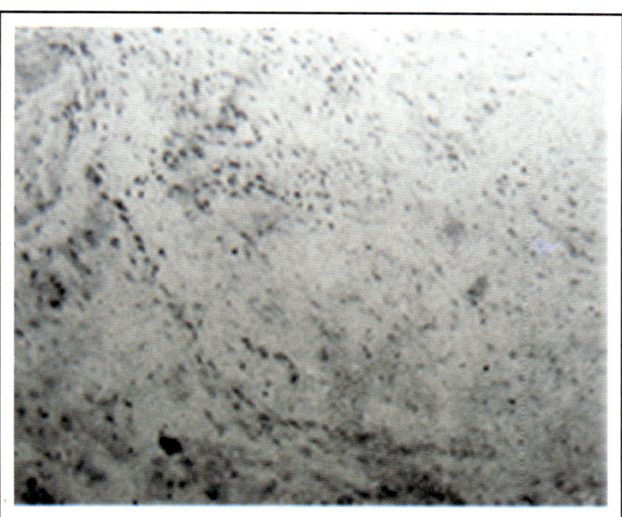

Figure 565: Squamous cell carcinoma of male black bear (*S. thibetanus*). Photomicrograph showing invasive proliferation of squamous epithelial cells and spicules of jaw bone embedded in the gingival growths. H& E, x100 (Rajan *et al.*, 1973).

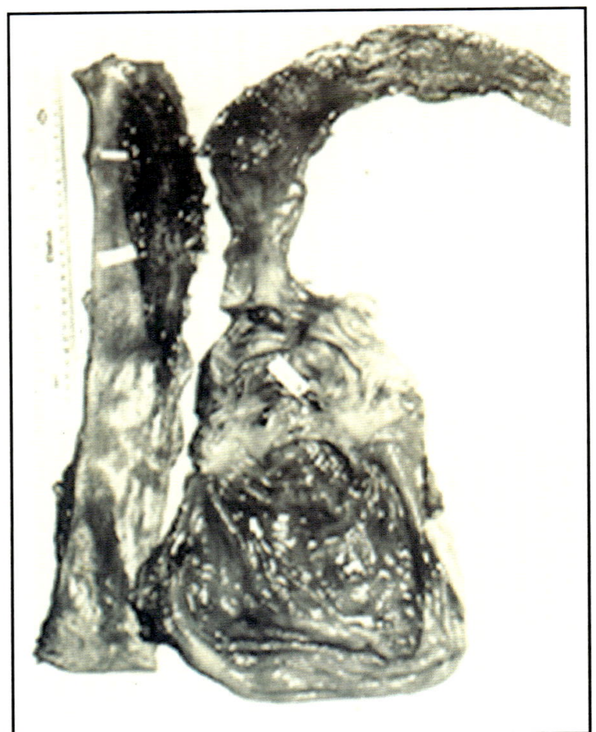

Figure 566: Photograph of oesophagus and stomach of Himalayan black bear (*S.thibetanus*) showing ulcers (also perforation) near cardiac end of stomach.

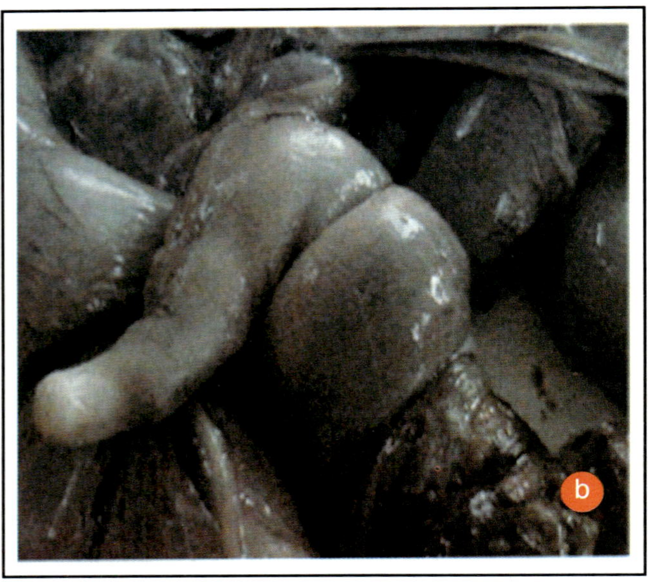

Figure 567 : Photographs showing intussusceptions in : (a) Ileum of sloth bear (*M. ursinus*) cub.(b) Large intestine of Himalayan black bear (*S. thibetanus*).

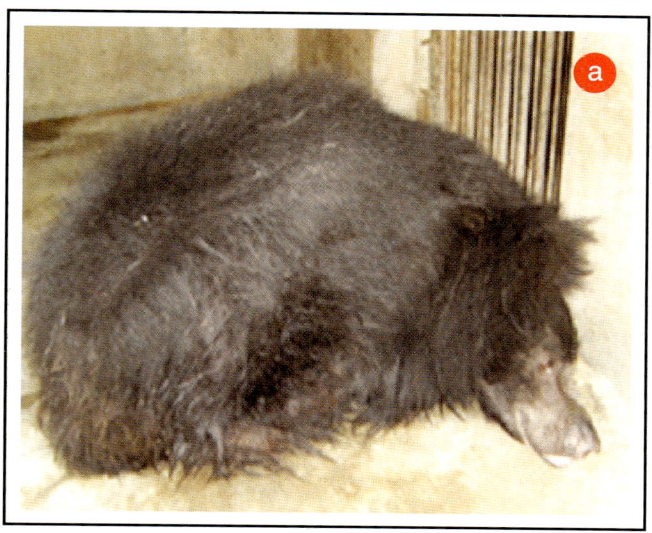

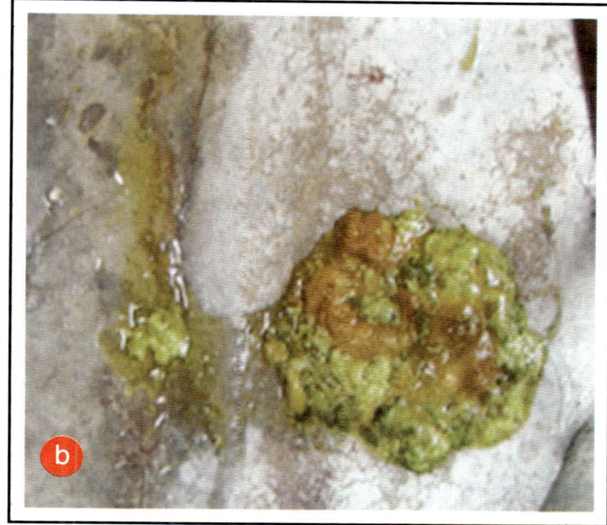

Figure 568: (a) Sloth bear (*M. ursinus*) suffering from enteritis in Zoological Garden, Lucknow (U.P.) (b) stool with blood and mucous.

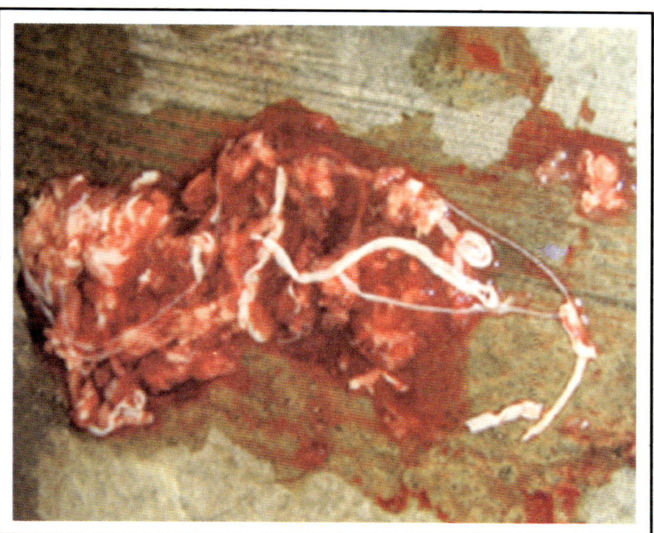

Figure 569 : Photograph showing bloody watery stools along with tape worms (21 July2007) passed by a sloth bear (*M. ursinus*) at Bear Rescue Centre, Bannerghatta, Bangalore.The animal had complaint of severe enteritis.

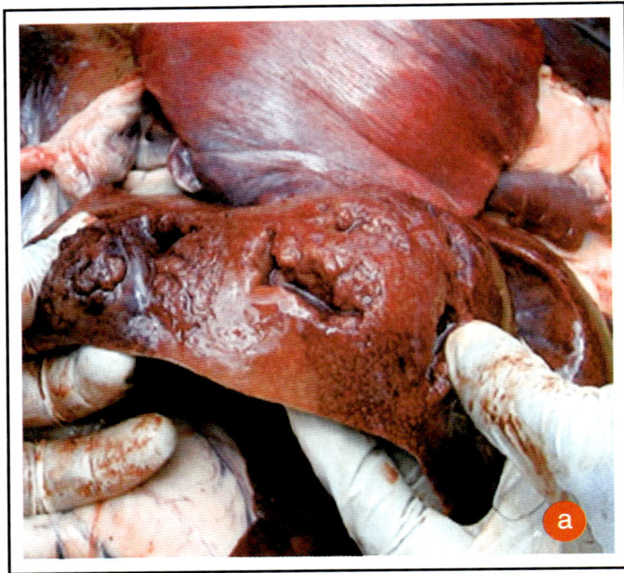

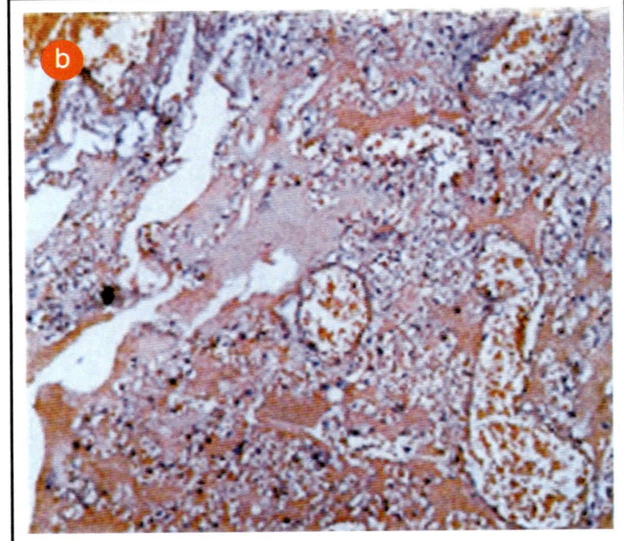

Figure 570: (a) Photograph showing soft and doughy texture liver in sloth bear (*M. ursinus*).(b) Photomicrograph of (a) showing lesions of hepatic degeneration (Courtesy:Arun A.Sha & Co-workers).

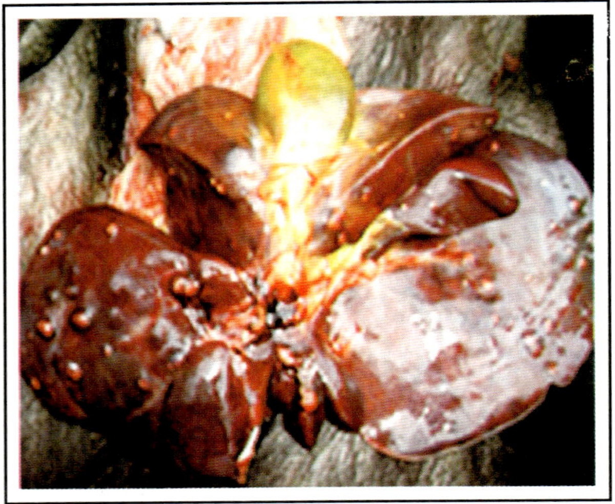

Figure 571: Photograph of liver of sloth bear (*M. ursinus*) died in captivity, showing small yellowish suppurative nodules (Courtesy: Arun, A. Sha),

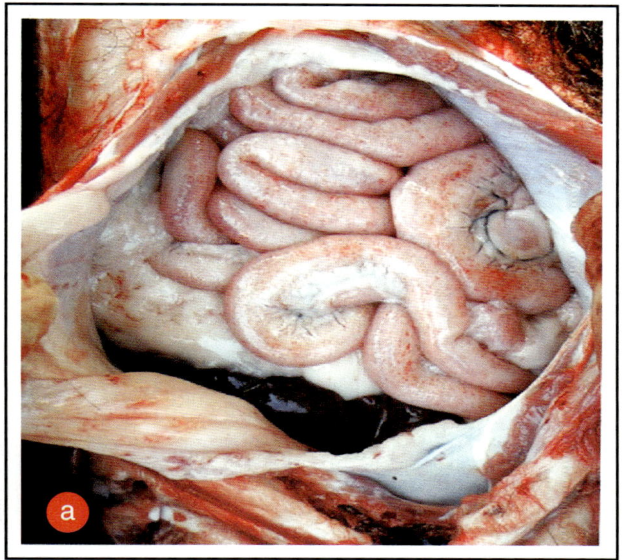

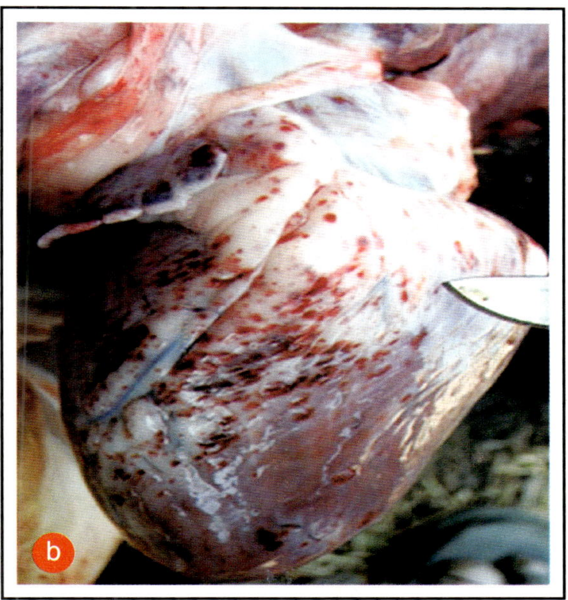

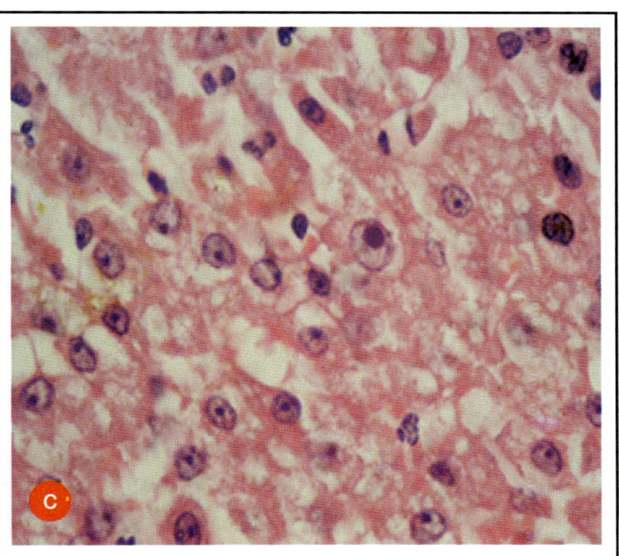

Figure 572: Infectious canine hepatitis (ICH) in sloth bear (*M.ursinus*) died at Bear Rescue Centre, Agra(U.P).Photographs (a,b) showing petechial haemorrhagic lesions in intestine and heart (Courtesy:Jadav,K.K & Illayaraja,S.).(c) Photomicrograph of liver showing ICH inclusion. H& E, x200 (Courtesy: Singh, R).

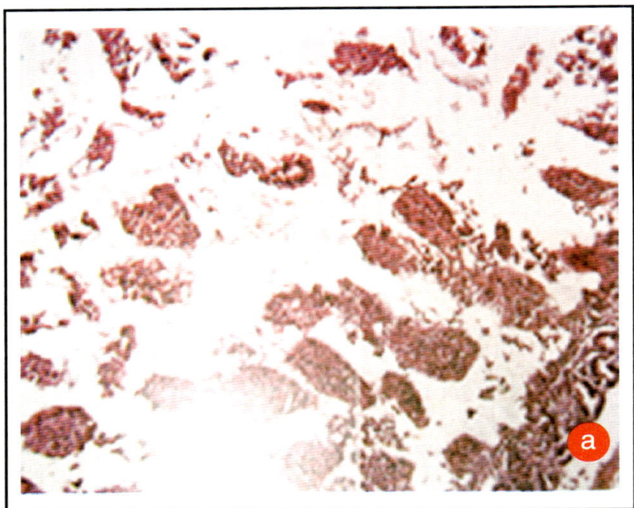

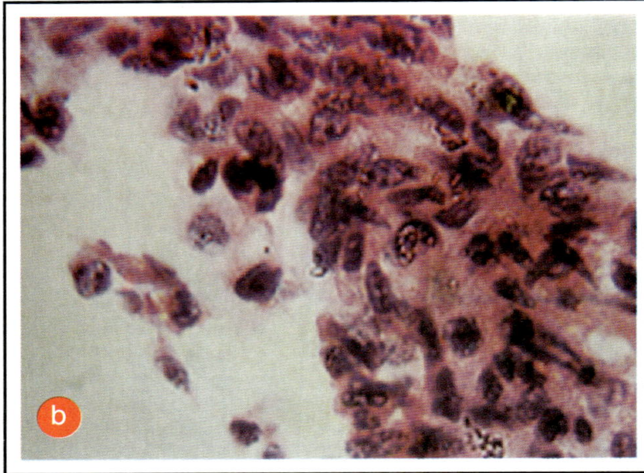

Figure 573: Panlecucopenia (FPL) in red panda (*Ailurus fulgens*). Photomicrographs showing: (a) Massive necrosis and sloughing of intestinal villus epithelium. H&E, x100 (b) Presence of eosinophilic intranuclear inclusion bodies in the epithelial cells of the intestine (inclusions were also seen in hepatic cells). H&E, x 500 (Chakraborty &Bhowmik, 1998).

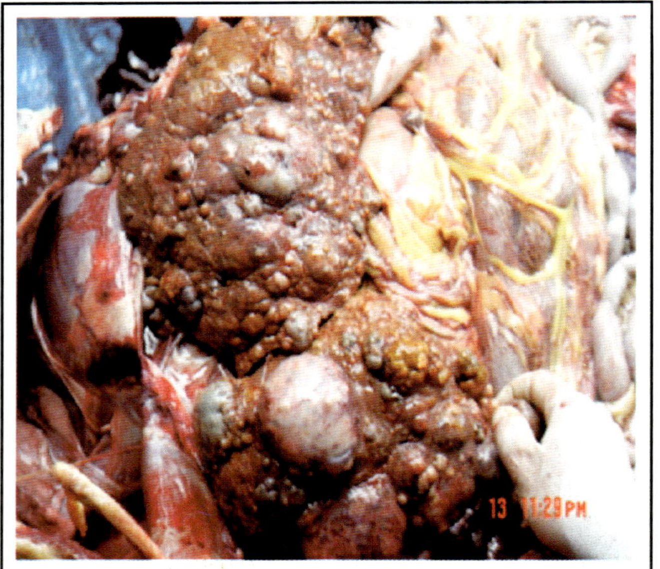

Figure 574: Photograph showing adenocarcinoma of liver of Himalayan black bear (*S. thibetanus*) died at Zoologcal Garden, Darjeeling (Courtesy: Deepak Sharma).

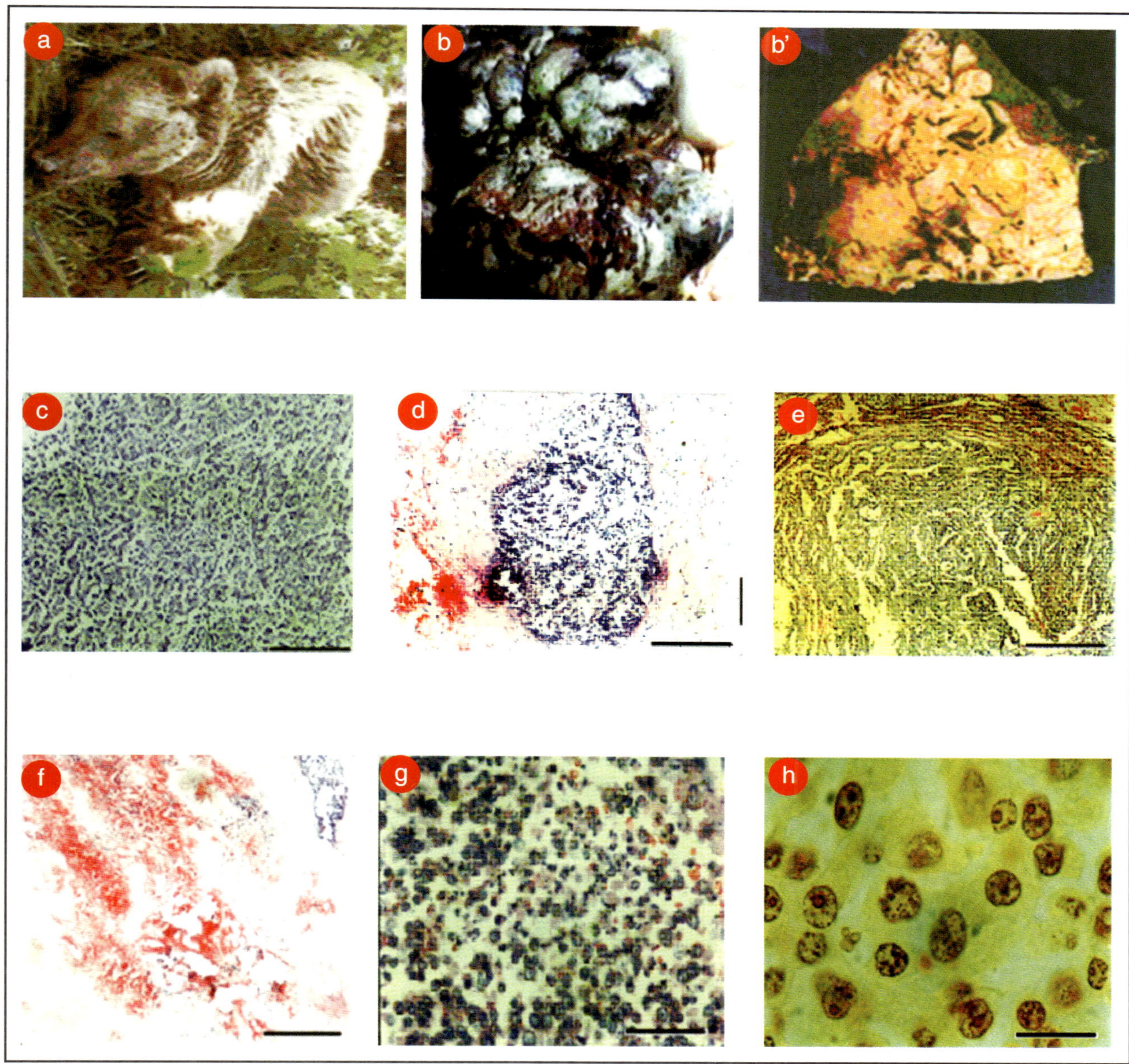

Figure 575: (a) Emaciated male Himalayan brown bear (*Ursus arctos isabellinus*) belonging to Dachigam National Park, Srinagar.(b.b') Photographs of liver of (a) showing yellowish-white to gray nodular growth measuring 24x25x23 cm and weighing about 14 kg. Photomicrographs(c-d) of (b) revealing: (c)Neoplastic cells arranged in cords. H& E, Bar =500µ. (d) Pseudoglandular pattern of hepatocytes. The hepatocytes at the periphery compressed. H&E, Bar = 500µ. (e) Papillary projection in the bile ductule with fibrosis around. H&E, Bar = 500µ. (f) Many cavernous spaces. H&E, Bar = 500µ.(g) Karyorrhexis and apoptotic bodies H&E, Bar = 200µ.(h) Sharp and evenly distributed AgNORs in the nuclei of the tumour cells.AgNOR staining, Bar = 20µ. AgNOR index 10.25±1.75 (Darzi *et al.*, 2007).

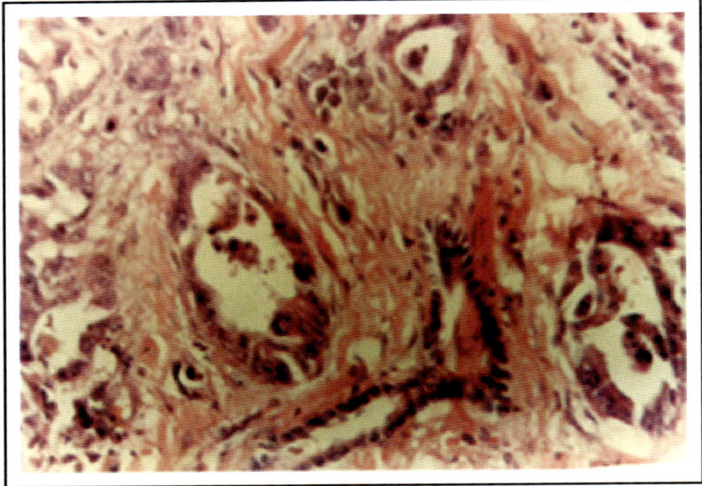

Figure 576: Photomicrograph showing cholangiocellular carcinoma in sloth bear (*M. ursinus*) died in captivity. H & E, x100. (Courtesy: Sharma, A.K.)

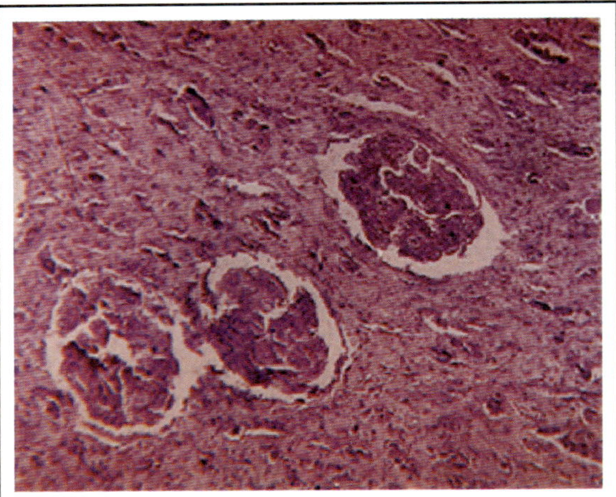

Figure 577: Chronic interstitial nephritis in Himalayan black bear (*S. thibetanus*) died in Zoological Garden, Guwahati (Assam). Photomicrograph showing massive fibrous tissue proliferation compressing the tubules. H&E, x100.

Reproductive System

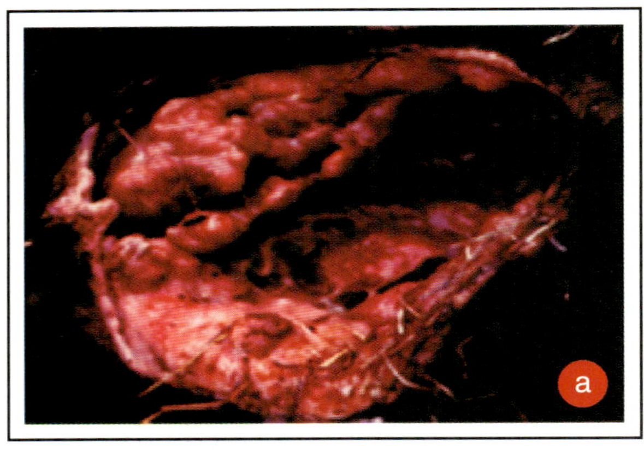

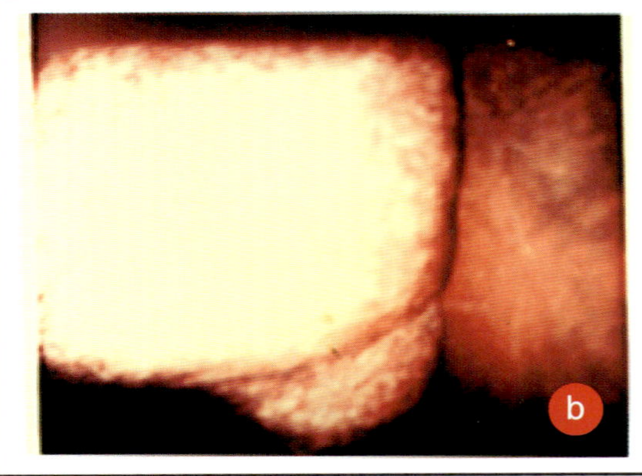

Figure 578: Photograph showing lacerated wound in testis of Himalayan bear (*S.thibetanus*).(b) Orchitis in another Himalayan black bear (*S.thibetanus*).

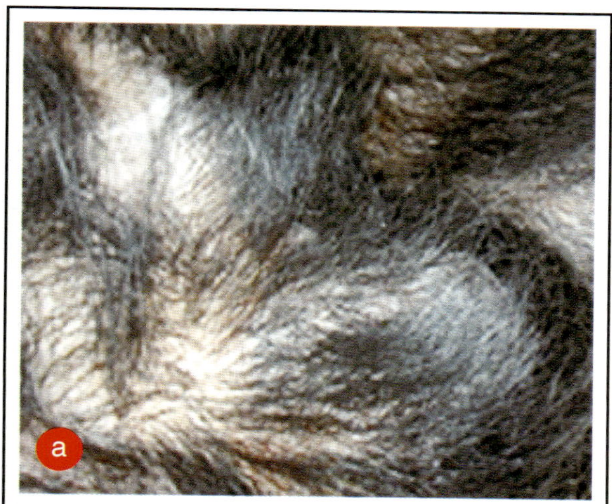

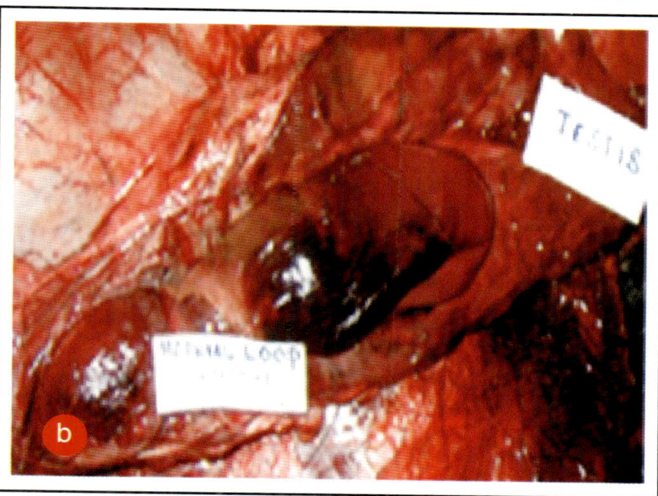

Figure 579: Unilateral scrotal hernia in a rescued sloth bear (*M. ursinus*).(a) Enlarged left testicle. (b) Operation of testicle and Surgical management of the condition .(Arun,A. Sha *et al.*. 2007c).

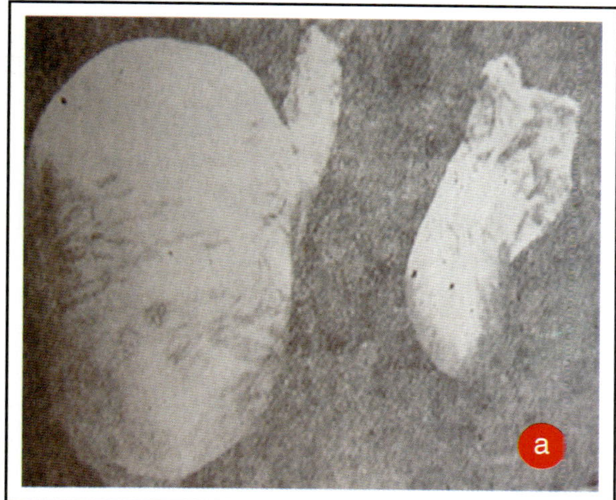

Figure 580: Haemangioma of testis of black bear (*S. thibetanus*). Photographs showing:(a) Tumorous left testis(20x30cm, and 300g) (b) Normal right testis 5x3.5 cm and 35g). (b) Photomicrograph of (a) showing numerous dilated capillaries containing erythrocytes. H&E, x 100 (Rajan *et al.*, 1973).

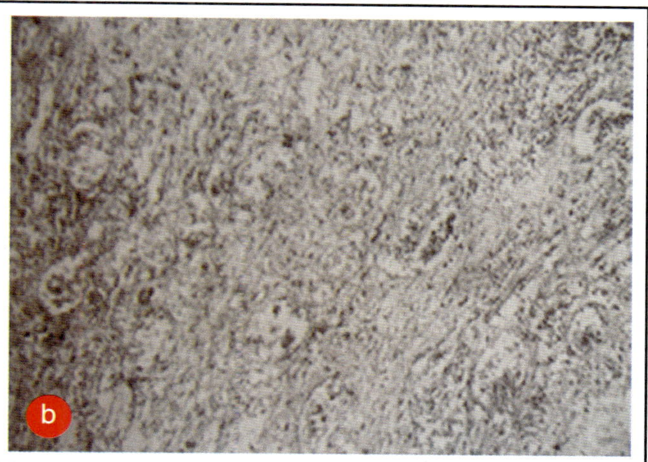

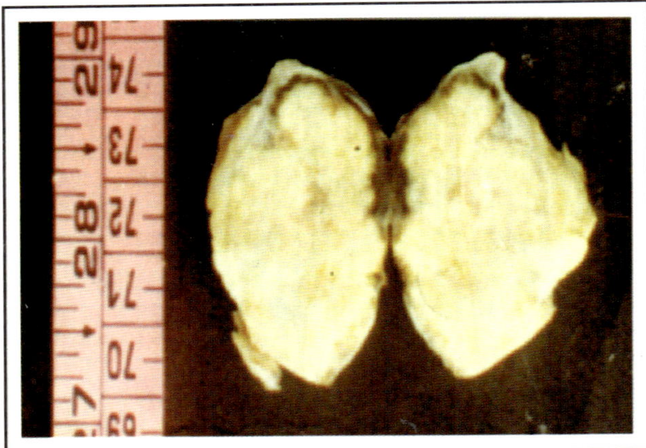

Figure 581 : Photograph of mammary gland tumour of from Malayan bear (*Helarctos malayanus*) died in captivity.

Nervous System

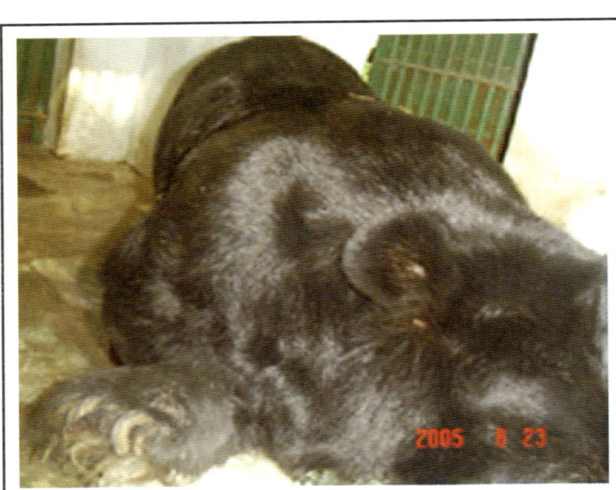

Figure 582: Himalayan black bear (*S. thibetanus*) suffering from paresis of fore limbs. Specific history remained untraced.

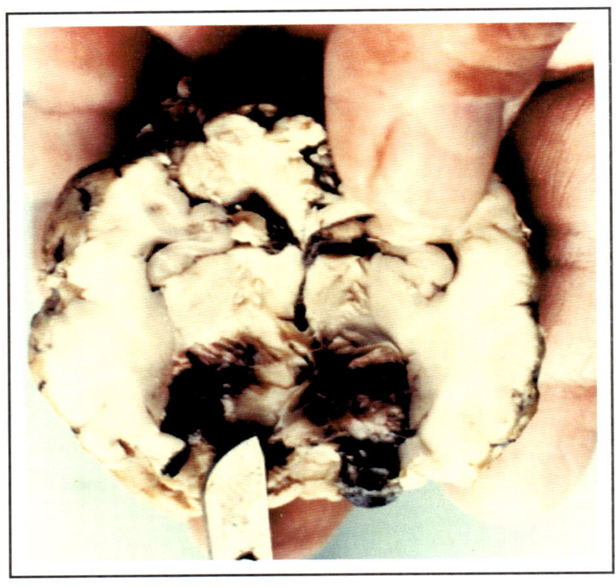

Figure 583 : Photograph showing blood clots in the brain of red panda (*A. fulgens*) died in captivity.

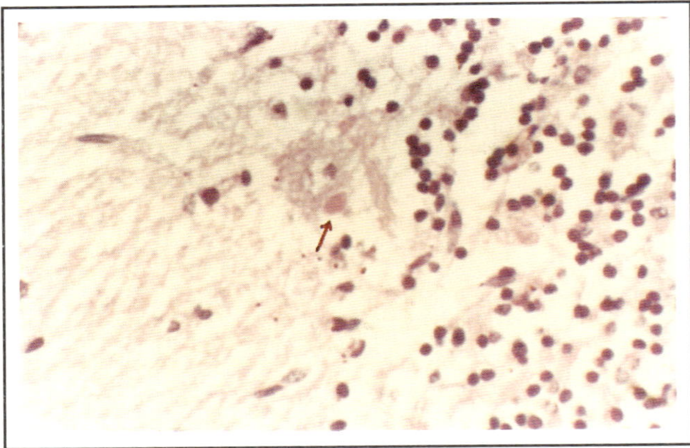

Figure 584 : Photomicrograph showing intra-cytoplasmic Negri body in a neuron (arrow) of the brain specimen of sloth bear (*M. ursinus*) died due to rabies at Bear Rescue Centre at Agra, Uttar Pradesh (Sharma *et al.*, 2004).

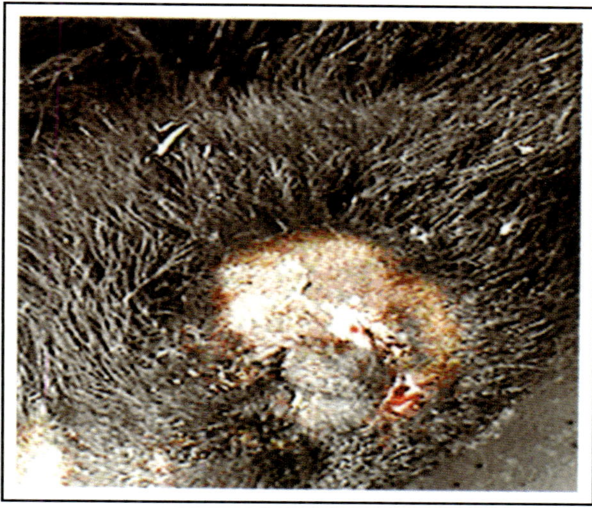

Figure 585 :Photograph showing damaged left eye of Himalayan black bear (*A. thibetanus*) (Courtesy: Kishtwaria, R.S.).

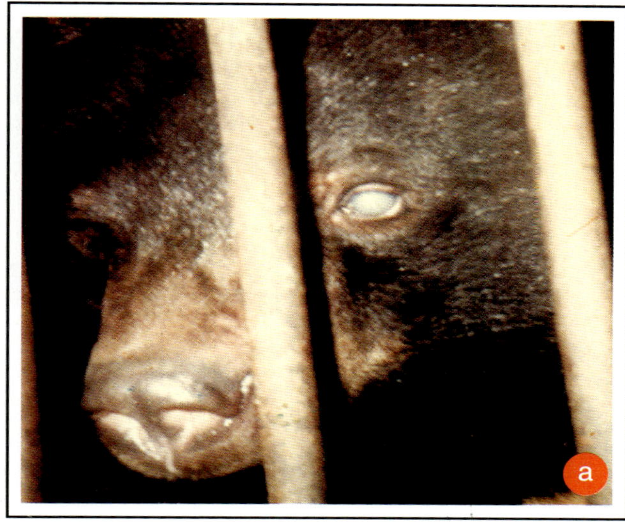

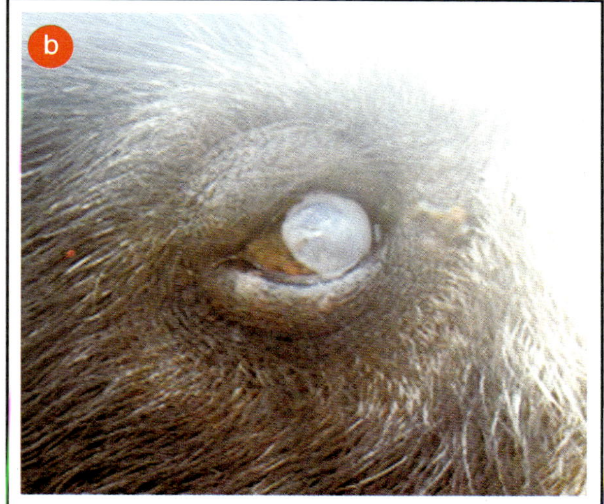

Figure 586: Photographs showing corneal opacity of left eye of: (a) Himalayan bear (*S. thibetanus*) belonging to National Zoological Park, New Delhi. (b) Rescued bear at a captive facility.

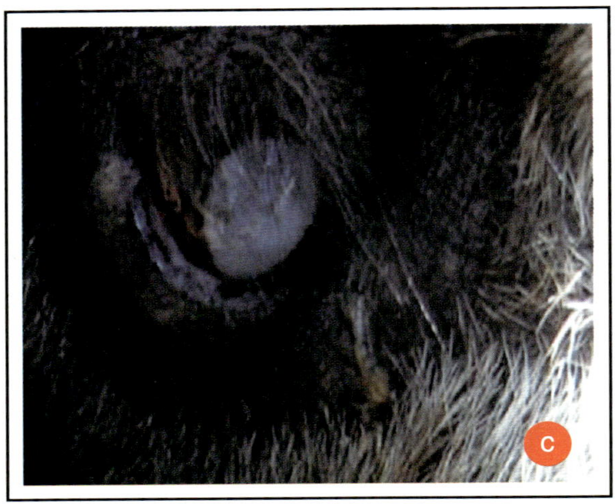

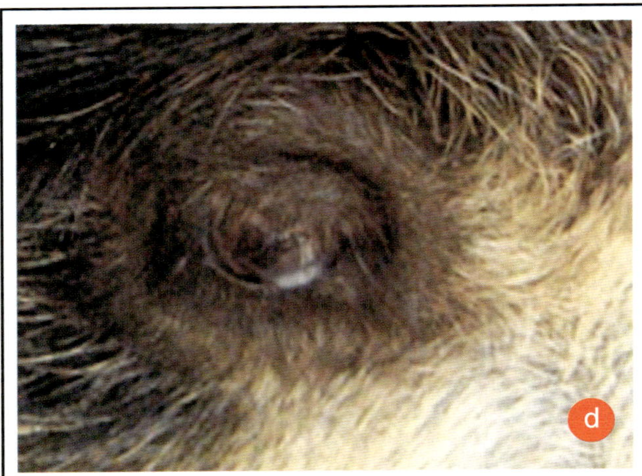

Figure 586: (c,d) Corneal opacity and keratitis in rescued sloth bears (*M. ursinus*) at Bear Rescue Centre, Bannerghatta, Bangalore (Courtesy: Arun, A. Sha).

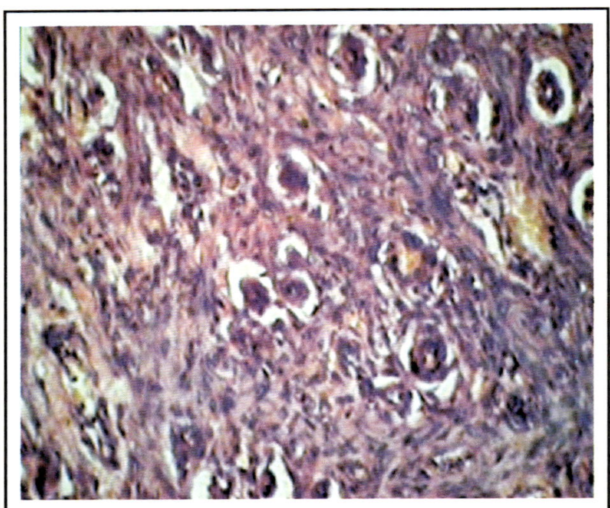

Figure 587: Photomicrograph showing capillary haemangioma in upper eyelid of 10- year- old male sloth bear (*M.ursinus*) at Bear Rescue Centre, Agra (U.P). H&Ex 40 (Courtesy: Illayaraja and Co-workers).

Integumentary System

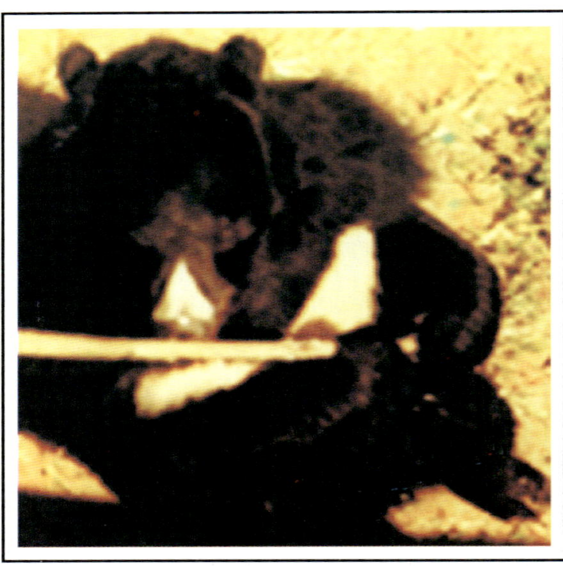

Figure 588: Himalayan black bear (*S.thibetanus*) having white skin on the nose in Zoological Garden, Guwahati, Assam.

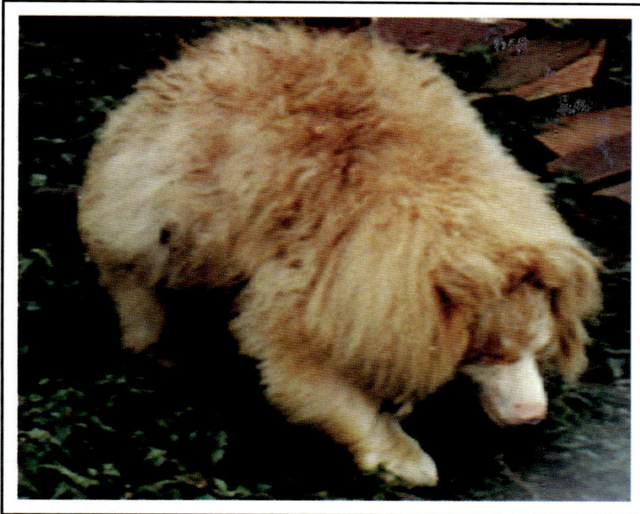

Figure 589: Albino white sloth bear (*M. ursinus*) in Bhopal Van Prani Uddyan (M.P).

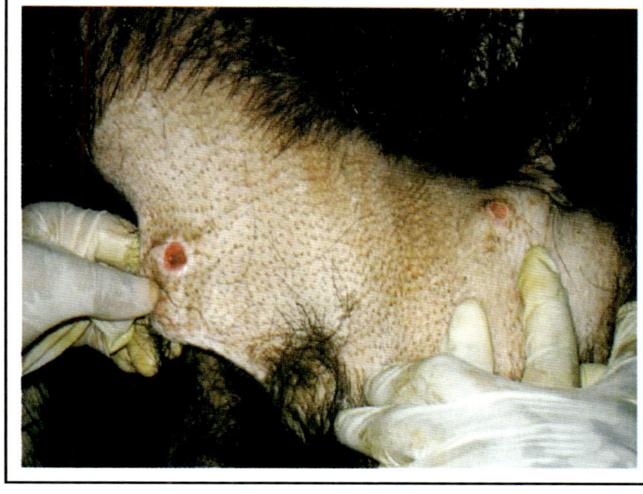

Figure 590: Photograph showing bullet punctured wounds in thigh region of sloth bear (*M. ursinus*). The wound at entry was 0.7 cm in dia.and at exit was 1.0 cm in dia.(Arun, A. Sha *et al.*, 2007a).

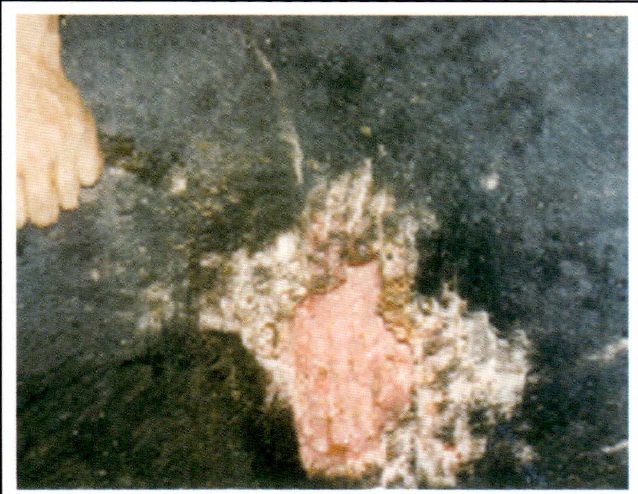

Figure 591 : Photograph showing laceration of skin and musc es at the elbow region in Himalayan blackbear (*S. thibetanus*) due to con specific infighting in captivity (Courtesy: Kishtwaria, R.S.)

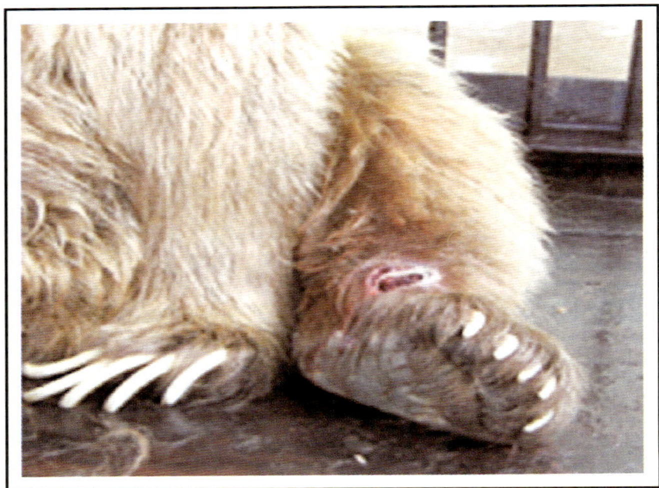

Figure 592: Photograph showing deep lacerated wound in left hind foot of brown bear (*Ursus arctos* sp.) at Zoological Garden, Mysore (Karnataka). Note bear has over grown nails.

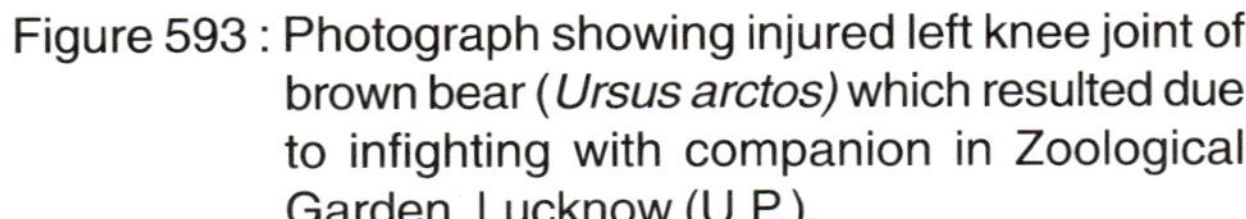

Figure 593 : Photograph showing injured left knee joint of brown bear (*Ursus arctos)* which resulted due to infighting with companion in Zoological Garden, Lucknow (U.P.).

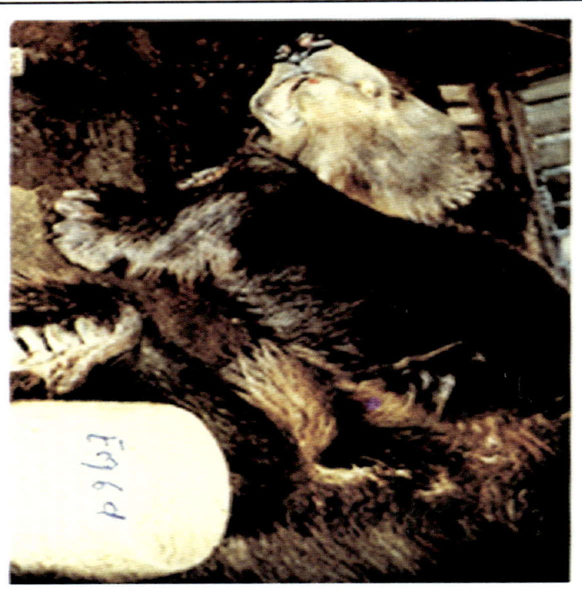

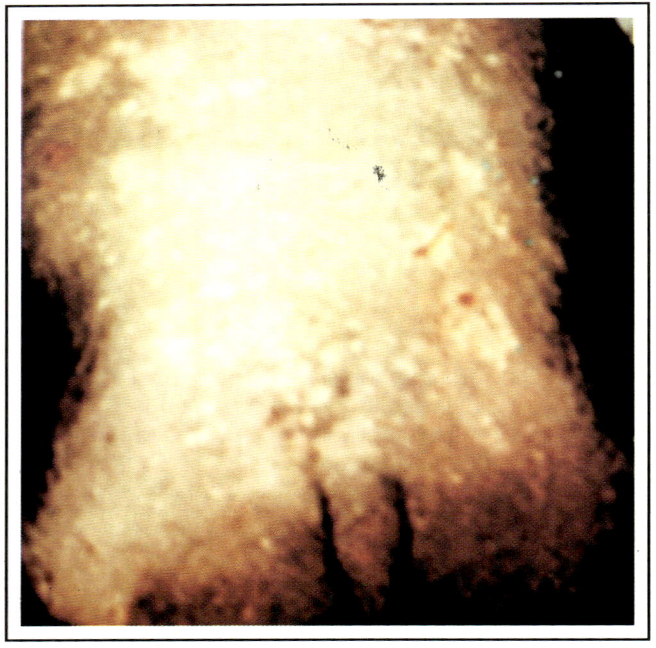

Figure 594: Alopecia affecting nearly half of the dorso-lateral aspect of body of the captive Himalayan black bear (*S.thibetanus*) caused by *Microsporum* sp.

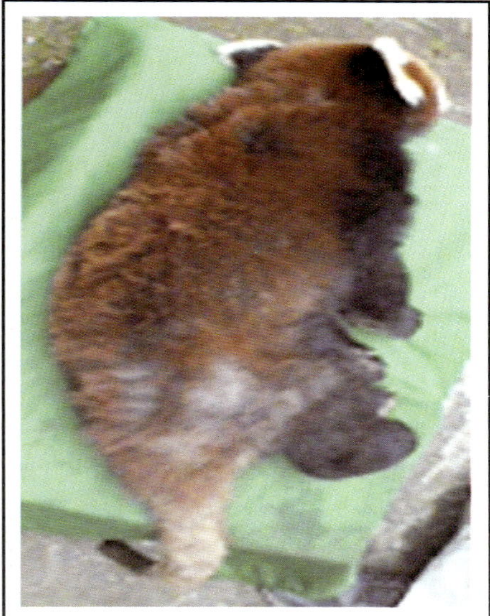

Figure 595: Sedated red panda (*A. fulgens*) showing alopecia at Zoological Garden, Gangtok, Sikkim.

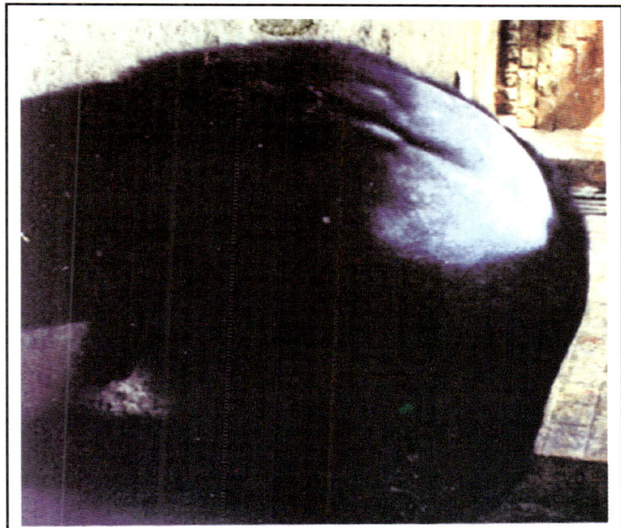

Figure 596: Chronic alopecia in its hind portion of a captive Himalayan black bear (*S.thibetanus*) related to hepato-toxicity.

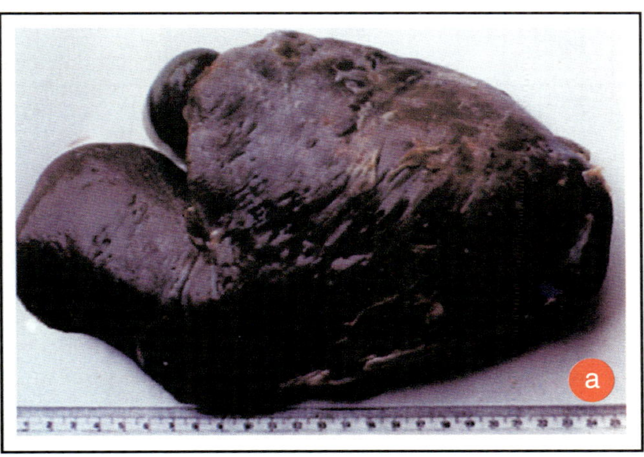

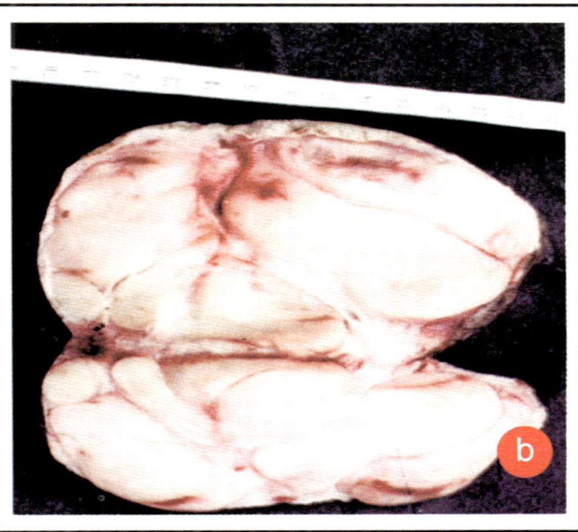

Figure 597: (a) Photograph showing a fibroma scaled 450 g and measured 12 cm in length,extirpated from lateral aspect of thorax of Himalayan bear (*S. thibetanus*). belonging to Zoological Garden, Almora (Uttarakhand).(b) Cut opened of (a).

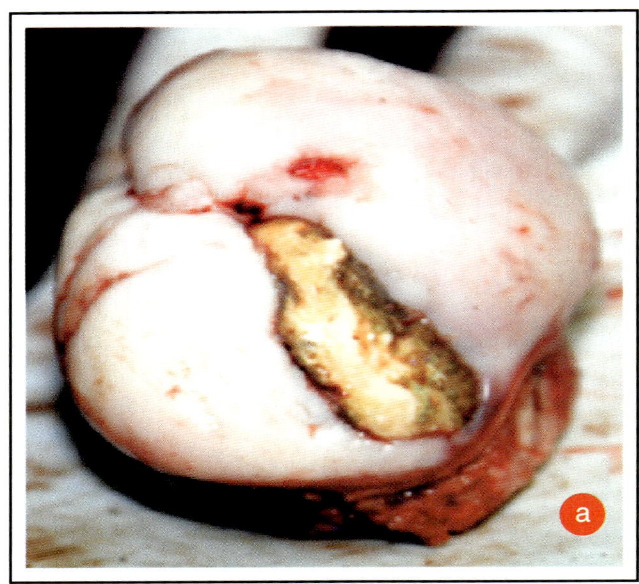

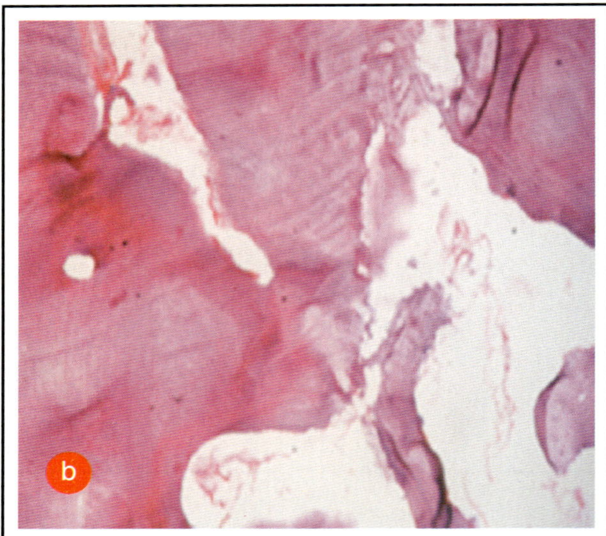

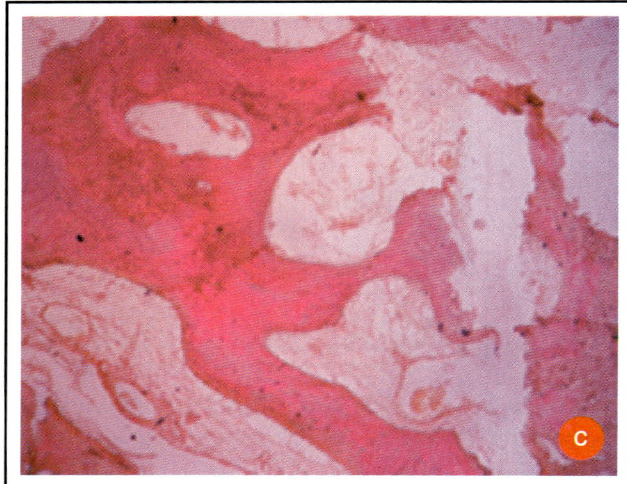

Figure 598: (a) Photograph showing a hard swelling in the canine region of maxilla and in the upper lip of 13-year-old sloth bear (*M. ursinus*) died in captivity. Photomicrographs (b,c) of (a) showing benign osteoblastoma (Arun, A. Sha *et al*., 2007d).

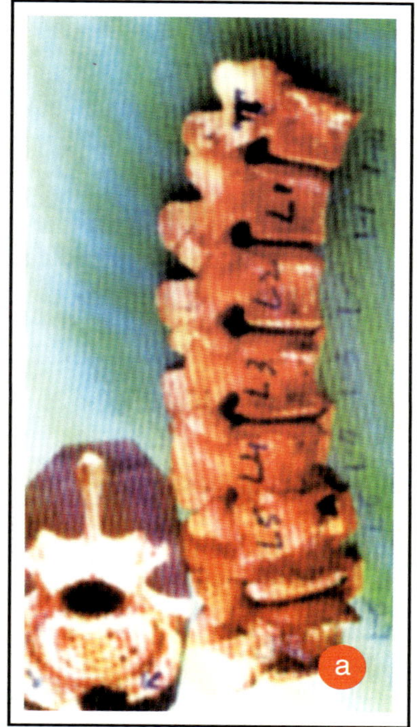

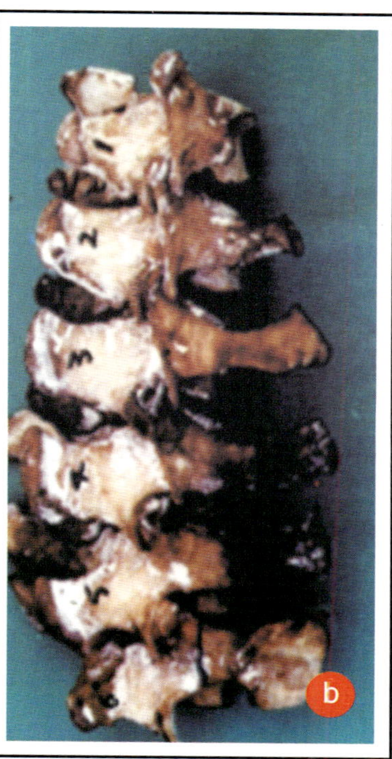

Figure 599: Lumbar vertebrae of Himalayan black bear (*S. thibetanus*) showing: (a) Ventro-lateral aspects of cranial margins of 3rd to 6th lumbar vertebrae having osteophytic growths. Also ventral aspect of the 6th lumbar had necrotic lesions.(b) Left transverse processes of 4th and 5th lumbar vertebrae atrophied. Right transverse process of sixth lumbar vertebra hypertrophied.

Figure 600: Photograph showing right transverse process hypertrophied and left transverse process hypotrohied encountered in last lumbar vertebra of sloth bear (*M. ursinus*) died in captivity.

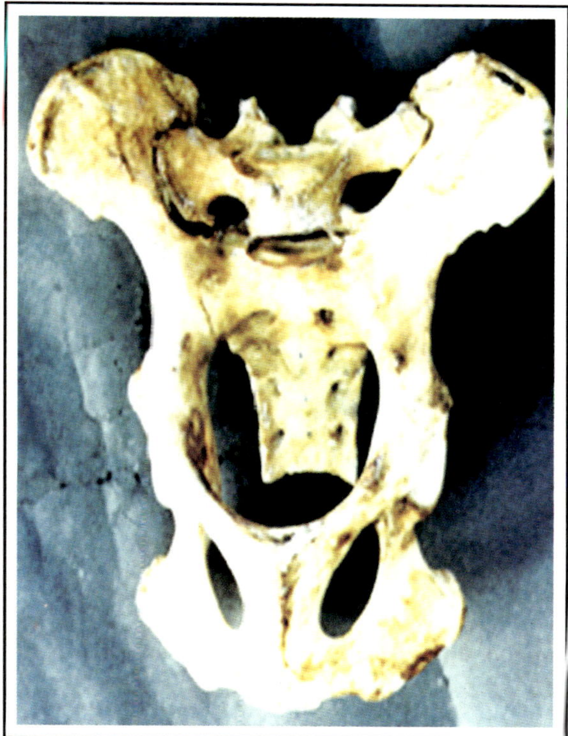

References

Large Cats

Arun A. Sha *et al.* (2007). Acute renal failure in Siberian tiger. Presentation in: *International Congress on Advances in Zoo & Wild Animals Health& Management, organized jointly by College of Vet Sc.& A.H.& AIZ&WV*, held from 26-27 April 2007 at SKUAS&T, Jammu (J&K).

Bhardwaj, R.M. and Chandra, C,J. (1991). Anterior luxation of eye lens in tiger. *Zoos Print. 6*:28.

Chanda, S.K. *et al.* (1995). Nodular lesions on the intestine of a tiger (*Panthera tigris*)- A case report. *Indian vet.J.* 72 :660-61.

Gajendragad, C. *et al.* (2004). A case of hydronephrosis in a tiger. *Indian J.Vet. Path.28*:145.

Gorhe, V.S. (1991). Root canal treatment in white tiger. A case report. *Zoos Print.*6 (11): 35.

Gupta, P.P. (1978) Infectious body hepatitis in a black panther (*Panthera pardus pardus*). Zbl. *Vet. Med.*B.25 :858.

Nashiruddullah, N. and Chakaraborty, A.(2003). Spontaneous neoplasms in captive wild carnivores of the Assam State Zoo. *Indian J. Vet. Path.* 27: 39-41.

Nashiruddullah, N. and Chakaraborty,A. (2006). Spontaneous aortic lesions in wild carnivores of Assam State Zoo. *Indian J. vet. Path.*30(2):46-48.

Nashiruddullah, N. *et al.* (2007). Pathological conditions and parasites affecting captive carnivores of Assam State Zoo. Presentation in: *International Congress on Advances in Zoo & Wild Animals Health& Management, organized jointly by College of Vet Sc.&A.H.& AIZ&WV*, held from 26-27 April 2007 at SKUAS&T, Jammu (J&K).

Parihar, N.S., Charan, K, and Chakravarty, I.B. (1976). Lipomatosis in a hunting cheetah (*Acinonyx jubatus*). *Indian J. Vet.Path.* 1:19-20.

Parihar, N.S and Srivastava, S.N. (1988). Bronchial hyperplasia in a tiger (*Panthera tigris*) *Indian J.Anim. Sc.* 58:230-33.

Paul, J.C. *et al.* (2002). Surgical management of squamous cell carcinoma of tail in a jaguar *Indian J.Anim.Hlth.41*:141-44.

Rajan A. *et al.* (1990). Renal carcinoma in a lion (*Panthera leo*). *Indian vet J.* 67:407.

Rajan A. *et al.* (1979). Pathological changes associated with senility in the endocrine glands of lions (*Panthera leo*) *Kerala J. Vet Sci.* 10:262-67.

Rao, A.T. and Acharjyo, L.N. (1971). A note on histopathology of lung of a leopard cat (*Felis bengalensis*) due to *Filaroides osleri.Indian J.Anim. Sci.* 41: 844-46.

Rao, A.T. and Acharjyo, L.N. (1993). Congenital malformations in wild animals at Nandan Kanan Zoo. *Indian J.Vet. Path.*17: 65-66.

Rao, A.T. and Acharjyo, L.N. (2002). Diseases of wild felids. Pub. Dept. Of Pathology, Orissa Veterinary College , Bhubneshwar-751003

Sen, N.K. and Chowdhuri, S. (1998).Trypanosoma in feline species. *Science & Culture.*14(8):363-64.

Sharma, A.K, Singh, N.D. and Arora, B.M. (2004) Certain pathological conditions diagnosed in wild mammals. *Indian Wildlife Year Book 3*:94-98.

Singh, B. *et al.* (1983). Infectious feline enteritis in panther cubs (*Panthera pardus*) *Indian J. Anim. Sci.* 53(8):921-24.

Somvanshi, R., Koul, G.L. and Biswas, J.C. (1987). Sarcocystis in a leopard (*Panthera pardus*) *Indian vet. Med.J.* 11:174-75.

Verma, R., Arora, B.M. and Iyer, P.R.K (1983). Cutaneous mycosis in a lion cub (*Panthera leo*) caused by *Candida tropicalis.* 7:63-65. .*Indian J. Vet. Path* 7:63-65.

Small Cats & Civets

Ashraf, N.V.K. (1992). Viverrine rarities in little known Indian Zoos *Print* 12 :26-27.

Nashiruddullah, N. and Chakaraborty,A.(2003). Spontaneous neoplasms in captive wild carnivores of the Assam State Zoo. *Indian J. Vet. Path.* 27: 39-41.

Nashiruddullah, N. and Chakaraborty, A. (2006). Spontaneous aortic lesions in wild carnivores of Assam State Zoo. *Indian J. Vet. Path.*30: 46-48.

Nashiruddullah, N. *et al.* (2007). Pathological conditions and parasites affecting captive carnivores of Assam State Zoo. Presentation in: *International Congress on Advances in Zoo & Wild Animals Health& Management, organized jointly by College of Vet Sc.&A.H.& AIZ&WV*, held from 26-27 April 2007 at SKUAS&T, Jammu (J&K).

Singh, R , Singh, K.P. and Arora, B .M. (2004). Spontaneous pancrearic islet amyloidodis in large civet (*Viverra zibetha*). *Indian Wildlife Year Book,* 3:100-103.

Valsala, K.V., Manmohan, S. and Rajan, A. (1995). Granulosa cell tunour in civetcat (*V. indica*). *Indian J. Vet. Path.*19:51-52.

Canids & Hyena

Nashiruddullah, N. *et al.* (2007). Pathological conditions and parasites affecting captive carnivores of Assam State Zoo. Presentation in *International Congress on Advances in Zoo & Wild Animals Health& Management, organized jointly by College of Vet Sc.&A.H.& AIZ&WV*, held from 26-27 April 2007 at SKUAS&T, Jammu (J&K).

Bears & Red Panda

Arun A.Sha et al. (2007a). Management of gunshot wound in a sloth bear (*Melursus ursinus*). Presentation in: *International Congress on Advances in Zoo & Wild Animals Health& Management,* organized jointly by College of Vet Sc.&A.H.& AIZ&WV, held from 26-27April 2007 at SKUAS&T, Jammu (J&K).

Arun. A.Sha (2007b). Gigantiform cementoma in a rescued sloth bear (*Melursus ursinus)*. Presentation in conference on "Bear information exchange for rehabilitators, Zoos & Sanctuaries (BIERZS),held from. 24-26 August 2007, at Pomona, CA.

Arun. A.Sha *et al.* (2007c). Unilateral scrotal hernia in a rescued sloth bear (*Melursus ursinus*). Presentation in conference on "Bear Information Exchange for Rehabilitators, Zoos & Sanctuaries (BIERZS), held from. 24-26 August 2007, at Pomona, CA.

Arun A.Sha *et al.* (2007d). Incidence and management of periepical abscess due to chronic infection in teeth in sloth bear (*Melursus ursinus*). Presentation in: *International Congress on Advances in Zoo & Wild Animals Health& Management, organized jointly by College of Vet Sc.&A.H.& AIZ&WV*, held from 26-27 April 2007 at SKUAS&T, Jammu (J&K).

Chakraborty, T. and Bhowmik, M.K. (1998) Panleucopenia in red panda (*Ailurus fulgens fulgens*) *Indian J. Anim. Hlth.37*: 63-64.

Darzi, M.M. *et al.* (2007). Histopathological identification of the molecular organizer regions and apoptiosis in a mixed hepatocellular and intrahepatic bile duct carcinoma of a Himalyan brown bear (*Ursus isabellinus*).

Nashiruddullah, N. *et al.* (2007). Pathological conditions and parasites affecting captive carnivores of Assam State Zoo. Presentation in: *International Congress on Advances in Zoo & Wild Animals Health& Management, organized jointly by College of Vet Sc.&A.H.& AIZ&WV*, held from 26-27 April 2007 at SKUAS&T, Jammu (J&K).

Rajan, C.G. Sivadas and Maryama, K.I. (1973). Neoplasms in the captive bears (*Melursus ursinus* and *Selenarctos thibetanus*). A report of three cases. *Ind. Vet. J.* 50:845-49.

Rao, A.T. and Acharjyo, L.N. (1993).Congenital malformations in wild animals at Nanadan Kanan Zoo, *Indian J. Vet. Path.*17:65-66.

Sharma, A.K *et al.* (2004). Certain pathological conditions diagnosed in wild mammals. *Indian Wildlife Year Book* 3:94-98.

NON-HUMAN PRIMATES

Introduction

The order consists of 12 families, which include 385 non- primate species. In India, 16 species are found, which belong to three families (Table 5). Two species are found in north India, five species in south India and 9 species in north east regions of the country. Most of them are endangered.

Table 5: Common and endangered non-human primate species and subspecies

Family,Sub-family	Genus	Species(Common and scientific names)
Lorisidae	*Loris*	Slender loris (*Loris lydekkerianus lydekkerianus; Loris l. malabaricus*)
	Nycticebus	Slow loris *(Nycticebus coucang)*
Cercopithecidae	*Macaca*	Lion-tailed macaque *(Macaca silenus*)
(i)Cercopithecinae		Pig -tailed macaque *(Macaca nemestrina leonina)*
		Arunachal macaque (*Macaca munzala*)
		Stump-tailed macaque (*Macaca speciosa*)
		Assamese macaque (*Macaca assamensis- M. a. assamensis; M. a. pelops*)
		Crab-eating macaque (*Macaca fascicularis*)
		Bonnet macaque (*Macaca radiata- M .r. radiata; M .rdiluta*)
		Rhesus monkey (*Macaca mulatta*)
(ii)*Colobinae*	*Semnopithecus* *Trachypithecus*	Common/Hanuman langur (*Semnopithecus entellus*- seven species)
		Nilgiri langur (*Trachypithecus johni*)
		Golden langur (*Trachypithecus geei*)
		Phayrei leaf langur (*Trachypithecus phayrei)*
		Capped langur (*Trachypithecus pileatus*)
Hylobatidae	*Hylobatus*	Hoolock gibbon *(Bunopithecus hoolock)*

Developmental anomalies: Birth of white colour rhesus monkeys (*M. mulatta*) in the wild is rare. Some of the specimens collected have been introduction into some of the captive facilities **(Figure 648)**. A black colour rhesus monkey (*M. mulatta*), frequenting in a troop seen nearby Nainital road forests could not be pictured. The congenital anomalies such as absence of gall bladder in a langur (*Semnopithecus entellus*), and ovary and fallopian tube **(Figure 638)** in Nilgiri langur (*Trachypithecus johnii*) died in captivity. One kidney atrophied, which also had tuberculous infection and another kidney hypertrophied was encountered **(Figure 632)** in Spider monkey (*Ateles geoffroy,* an exotic sp.). Similarly left contracted kidney and enlarged right kidney were encountered **(Figure 633)** in an adult chimpanzee (*Pan troglodytes,* an exotic species). They are postnatal acquired anomalies rather than congenital. Complete fusion of C-7and first thoracic vertebrae **(Figure 657)** and extremities of ulna and radius recorded **(Figure 662b)** in bonnet macaque (*Macaca radiata*) and regarded to be case of congenital anomaly. However, presence of notched anterior border observed in one of the scapulae **(Figure 662a)** of the very animal was not possible to co-rrelate as either congenital or post natal traumatic assault. The skeletal anomalies such as formation of osteophytic growths bridging vertebrae **(Figure 656)** in lion-tailed macaque (*M. silenus*) and fused mass of vertebrae in bonnet macaque (*M. radiata)* were difficult to interpret for definite etiology.

Eco-husbandry associated health hazards: Infanticide behaviour is reported in langurs. **Figure 649** presents a baby golden langur (*Trachypithecus geei*) assaulted by its male parent. Infighting in non-human primates is generally seen when unacquainted individuals meet and also to acquire dominance to possess estrus females. In captivity during feeding innocuous fighting is not uncommon. In apes, serious fighting has been observed **(Figure 650)**. Rhesus monkeys (*M. mulatta*) at large in metropolitan cities, stations, temples environment often suffer curs of electrocution **(Figure 660),** traffic accidents **(Figures 629,661)** and faulty enclosure **(Figure 618).**

Bone fractures in Zoo monkeys are usually husbandry management related problem **(Figures 663 to 666).** At times traumatic injuries are more severe and make animal permanently disable.

Heat stroke claimed more death cases in large exotic primate species such as chimpanzee (*Pan troglodytes*), organutan (*Ponogo pygmaeus*), and white-handed gibbon (*Hylobatus lar*) maintained in Zoos located in tropical environment. Pneumonoconiosis is not uncommon in monkeys **(Figures 605-606)** housed in captivity. Although rhesus monkeys (*M. mulatta*) are menace in metropolitan cities but poisoning or shooting **(Figure 645,660case-i)** in retaliation is rare because of religious sentiment of Hindu.

Nutritional and metabolic disorders: Pathological conditions relating to either nutritional or metabolic disorders are not uncommon in monkeys but we could not discern any such condition by picture. Miscellaneous conditions such as ossification in lung **(Figure 604)** of lion tailed macaque (*M. silenus*), protrusion of mandibular incisors **(Figure 616)** in hoolocks (*Bunopithecus* (*Hylobates) hoolock*). Wearing **(Figure 617)** and oligodentia are not uncommon in captive monkeys but their details remained unstudied. Similarly a lion -tailed macaque (*M. silenus*) died of tuberculosis had various types of skeletal lesions such as osteoporosis, bony hyperplasia, necrotic changes, fracture callus, etc **(Figure 667).** It was difficult to say any nutritional factor alone, be associated as the animal had generalized form of tuberculosis.

Diseases: (A) Infectious & Parasitic. Being native endangered primate species populations low in our zoos infectious and parasitic diseases information is less. Tuberculosis, salmonellosis, echinococcosis are of zoonotic importance. In captive monkeys, respiratory and alimentary disease complex claimed high number of deaths.

In primate species tuberculous lesions were both of caseated nodular form **(Figure 607,610)** as well as granulomatous form **(Figure 608,608).** Focal nodular lesions in organs are also not uncommon **(Figure 635, 636)**. In case of disseminated form of disease almost all the vital organs are involved **(Figures 626,641).** In a lion-tailed macaque (*M. silenus*) died of tuberculosis (pulmonary and kidney lesions) in captivity had various types of skeletal lesions such as osteoporosis, bony hyperplasia, necrotic changes, fracture callous, **(Figures 665, 667),** etc. It was difficult to relate those bones disorders either to tuberculous infection or nutritional factor.

Enteritis in Golden langur (*T. geei)* belonged to Manas Tiger Reserve, Assam marked for necrosis with infiltration of mononuclear cells in the intestine accompanied with focal hepatic lesion was diagnosed for *Samonella* infection **(Figure 623)**. Though haemorrhagic enteritis due to salmonella infection in common langur (*S. entellus*) was recorded but disease detection in a wild golden langur (*T. geei*) died in the Tiger Reserve itself is of great importance as the species being critically endangered. Suppurative nephritis caused due to *Streptococcus* sp. infection **(Figure 634)** in Golden langur (*T. geei*) has been recorded.

Pulmonary blastomycosis **(Figure 612)** in nilgiri langur *(T. johni)* and cryptoccosis **(Figure 613)** in rhesus monkey (*M. mulatta*) died in captivity are detailed. Pox in captive non-human primate species has rarely been recorded. Serological evidence of parainfluesnza-3 and measles infections are recorded in laboratory housed monkeys. Giant cell pneumonia is considered as the pathogonomic lesion of measles in primates and a case has been reported in an Assamese macaque. Kasanoor forest disease (KFD) has been recorded causing heavy morality in free ranging bonnet macaque (*M. radiata*) and common langurs but so far there appears to be no case report from the Zoo collections. *Blantidium coli* is of great concern in free living and captive primate species, however we had no specimen to demonstrate lesions (Arora, 2003).

Verminous pneumonia **(Figure 614)** has been documented in pig- tailed macaque (*M. nemestrina*). Pea sized nodular gross lesions encountered in the intestine of hoolock gibbon (*Bunopithecus hoolock*) were related to *Oesophagostomum acculeatum.* The detailed lesions included thickened mucosal lining, parasite protruding out of the nodule, which was surrounded by caseonecrotic lesions **(Figure 624).**

Echinococcus granulosus and *Faciola gigantica* **(Figure 627)** in liver are important findings encountered in common langur (*S. entellus*).

Certain systemic conditions registered based on gross clinico-pathological findings include, pericarditis, myocarditis, endocarditis, suppurative metritis (after abortion) etc.

Hyperkeratosis **(Figure 651)** and ecto-parasitic dermatitis **(Figure 653)** around the tail has been observed more common in rhesus monkeys (*M. mulatta*) particularly those frequent in human habitation. Complete alopecia was recorded in chimpanzee (*Pan troglodytes,* exotic species) being maintained in Zoological Garden, Mysore, however condition's raisen d'etre remained uninvestigated **(Figure 652).**

(B) Neoplasms: Occurrence of neoplasm is recorded in common and endangered non-human primate species but less frequently. Reported cases of neoplasms in certain species included are: bronchiogenic carcinoma **(Figure 615)** of lung of Common/Hanuman langur (*S. entellus*), Adenocarcinoma of stomach **(Figure 620)** of Capped langur (*T. pileatus*), adenoma of vagina **(Figure 642)** in bonnet macaque (*M. radiata*), endometrial adenocarcinoma of uterus **(Figure 643)** and seminoma **(Figure 644)** in lion tailed macaques (*M. silenus*).

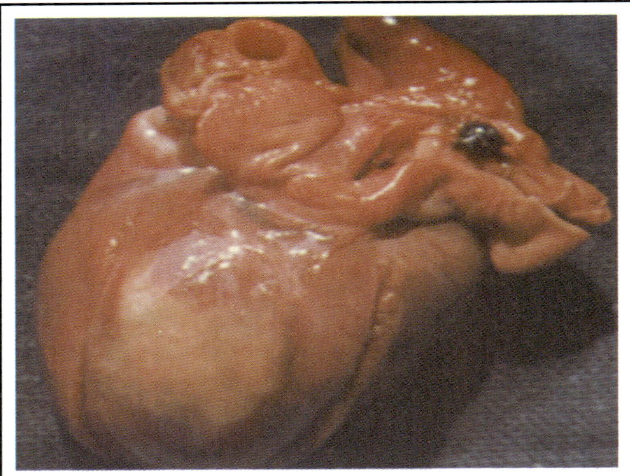

Figure 601: Photograph showing infarction in heart of slow loris (*N. coucang*).

Figure 602 :Photograph showing sudanophilic fatty streaks in aorta of monkey (*Macaque* sp.) died in captivity.

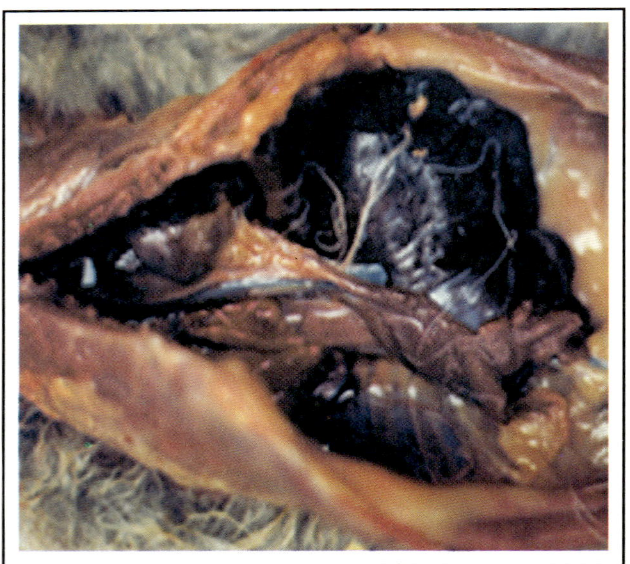

Figure 603: Photograph showing haemothorax in slow loris (*N. coucang*).Filarial worms seen in the thoracic cavity.

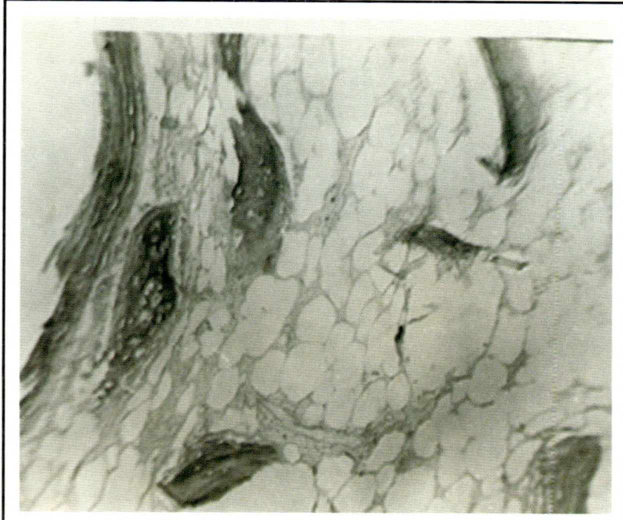

Figure 604: Photomicrograph showing ossification in lung of lion-tailed macaque (*M. silenus*) died in captivity. H&E,x70

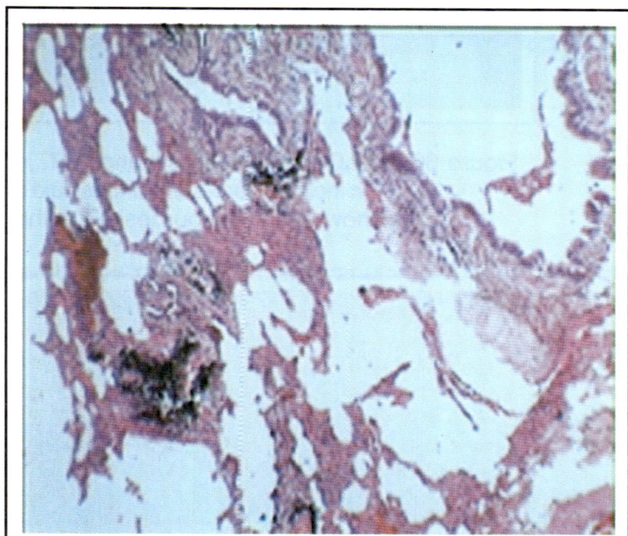

Figure 605: Photomicrograph showing pulmonary pneumonoconiosis encountered in common langur (*S. entellus*) died in captivity. H & E x 100

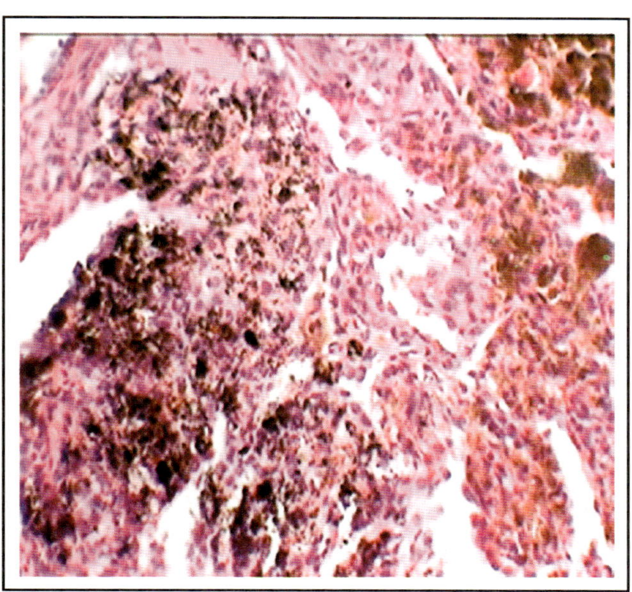

Figure 606: Photomicrograph showing pulmonary anthracosis and fibrosis in pig- tailed macaque (*M. nemestrina*) died in captivity. H & E, x 360.

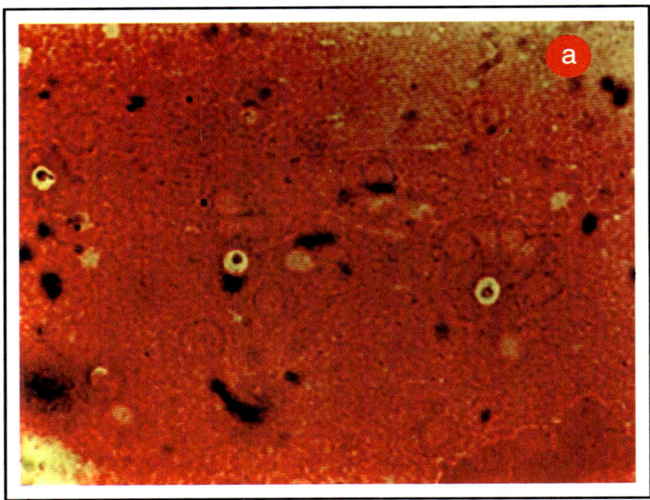

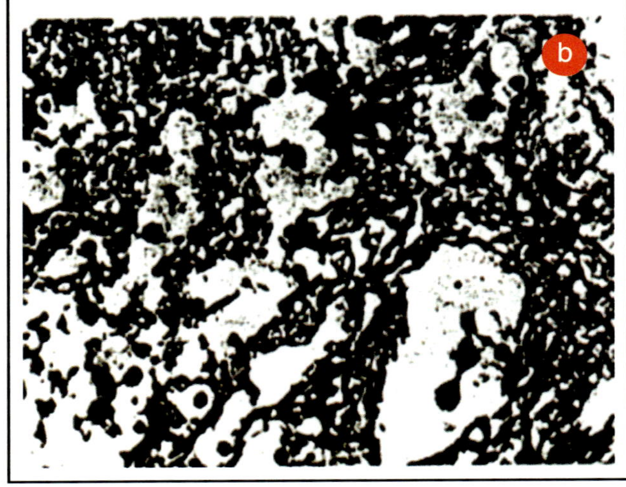

Figure 613: (a) Photomicrograph showing *C. neoformans* in impression smear from pneumonic lung of rhesus monkey (*M. mulatta*). (b) Photomicrograph of affected lung showing large mononuclear cell proliferation. Cryptoccocal cells are distributed throught the lung. PAS x 157.5 (Pal *et al.,* 1984)

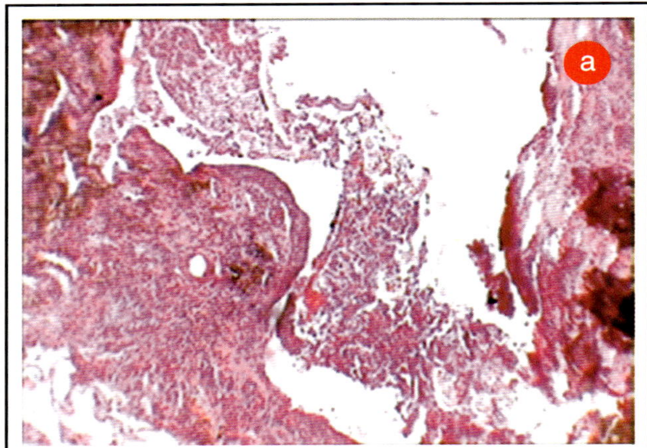

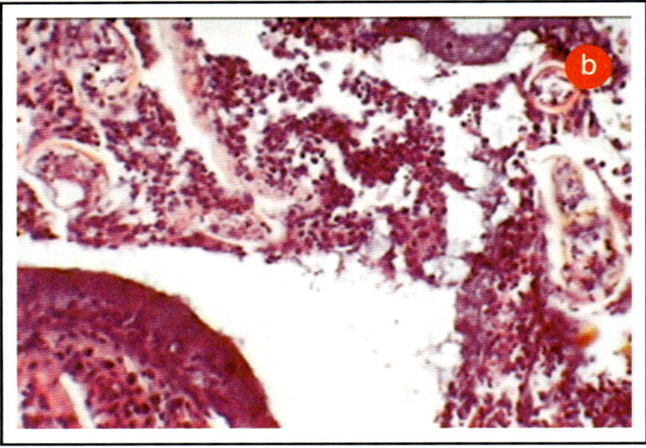

Figure 614: Photomicrograph of lung of pig- tailed macaque (*M. nemestrina*) showing verminous pneumonia. Exudate in the bronchi containing parasite eggs and sections of parasites. (a)H&E, x100 (b) H&E, x400

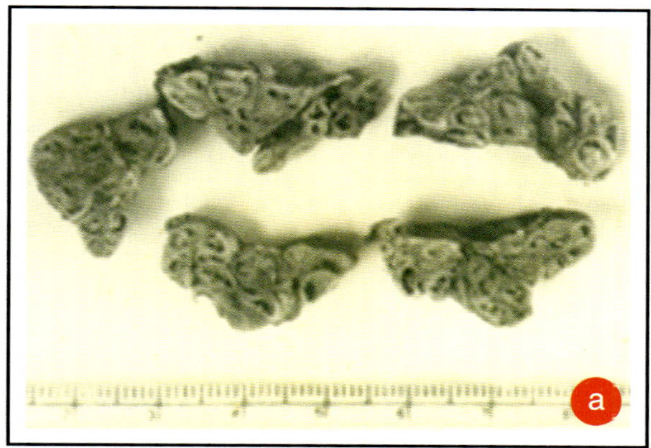

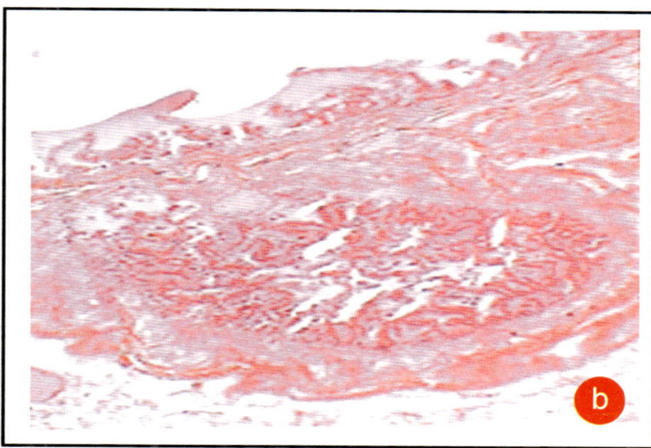

Figure 615: (a) Gross sections of lung of common langur (*S. entellus*) showing bronchiogenic carcinoma.(b) Photomicrograph of (a)showing papillary projections in the luminar bronchi. H&E,x100

Digestive System

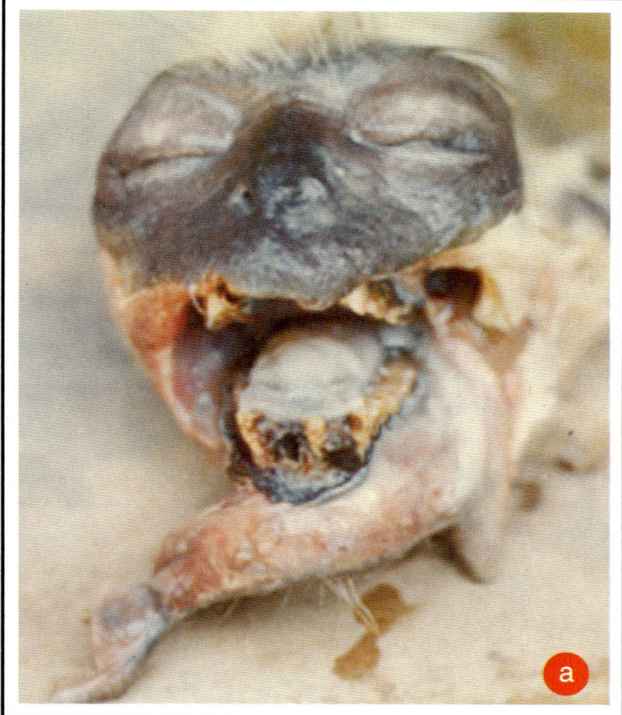

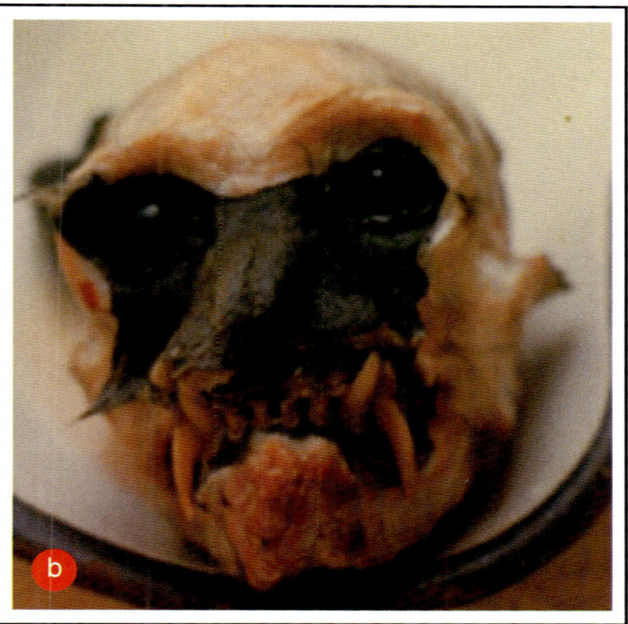

Figure 616: Photographs showing anomalies of oral cavity encountered in hoolock gibbons (*B. hylobates hoolock*) died in Zoological Garden, Guwahati (Assam): (a) Necrotic gingivitis resulting in loss of teeth. (b) Elongated canine teeth causing ulcerative lesions in the cheek.

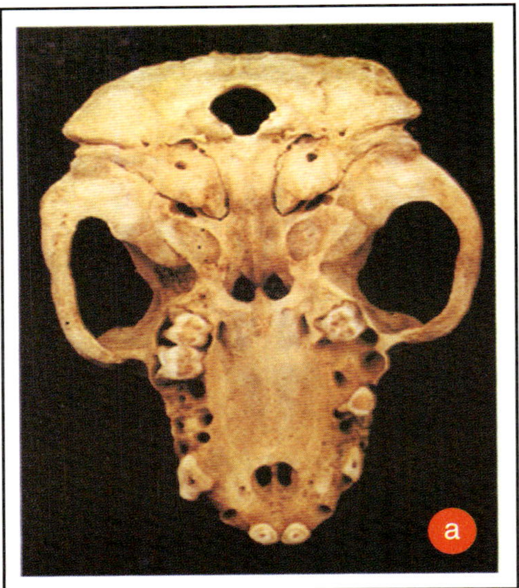

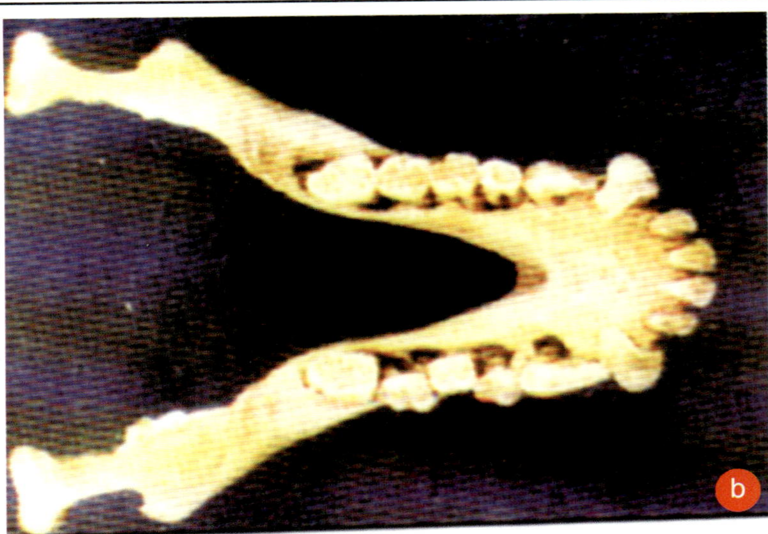

Figure 617: Photographs(a,b) showing wearing and loosing of teeth in upper and lower jaws of lion-tailed macaque (*M. silenus*) died in captivity.

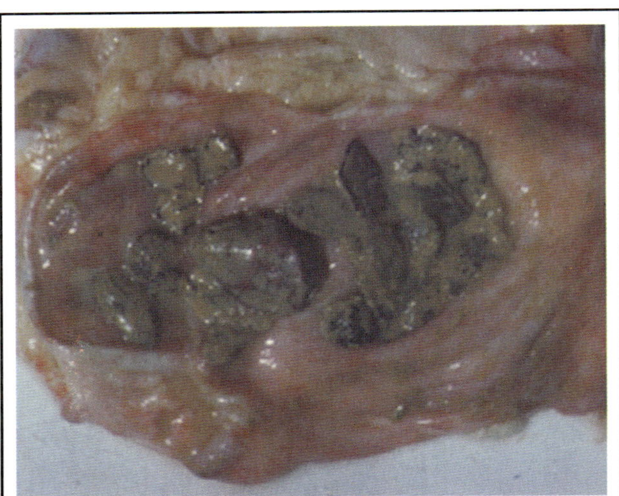

Figure 618: Photograph of stomach of chimpanzee (*Pan troglodytes*, an excotic sp.)showing dilatation at the pyloric end and a pouch. From pouch 21 numbers of rusted iron pieces, small stones and pieces of brick were recovered with ingesta.

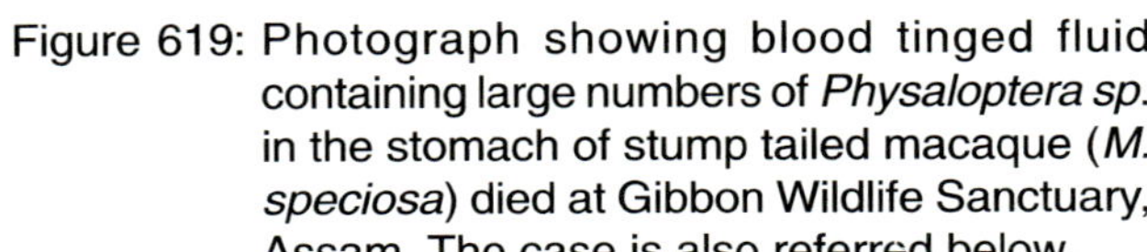

Figure 619: Photograph showing blood tinged fluid containing large numbers of *Physaloptera sp.* in the stomach of stump tailed macaque (*M. speciosa*) died at Gibbon Wildlife Sanctuary, Assam. The case is also referred below.

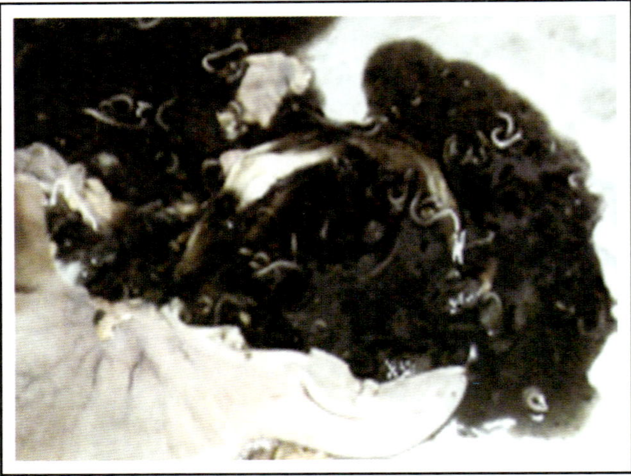

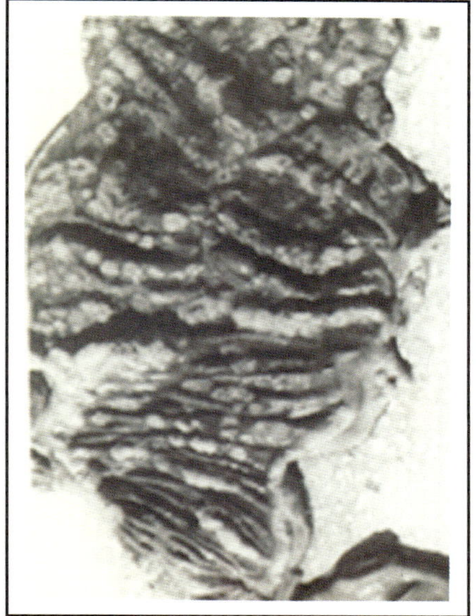

Figure 620: Photograph showing adenocarcinoma in the stomach of Capped langur (*T. pileatus*).Note the raised button like ulcerated nodules in linear pattern.

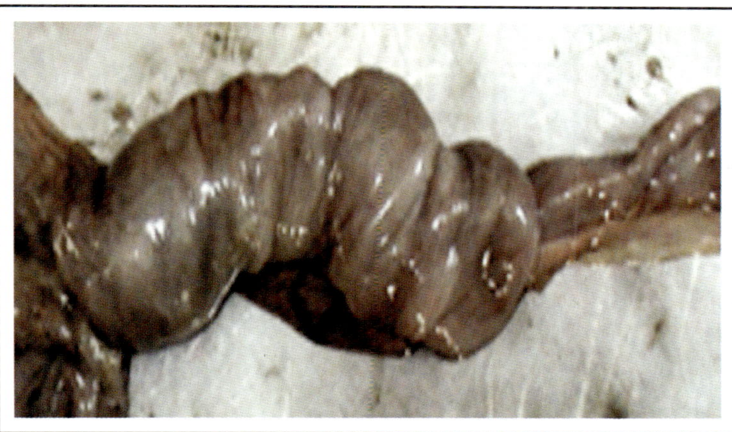

Figure 621: Photograph showing intussusception in the large intestine encountered in stump-tailed macaque (*M. speciosa*) died in Gibbon Wildlife Sanctuary, Assam.

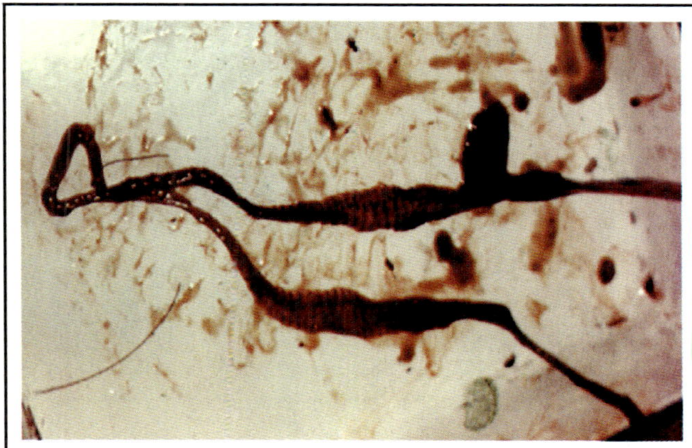

Figure 622: Photograph showing severe haemorrhagic lesion related to *Salmonella* infection in the intestine of common langur (*S. entellus*).

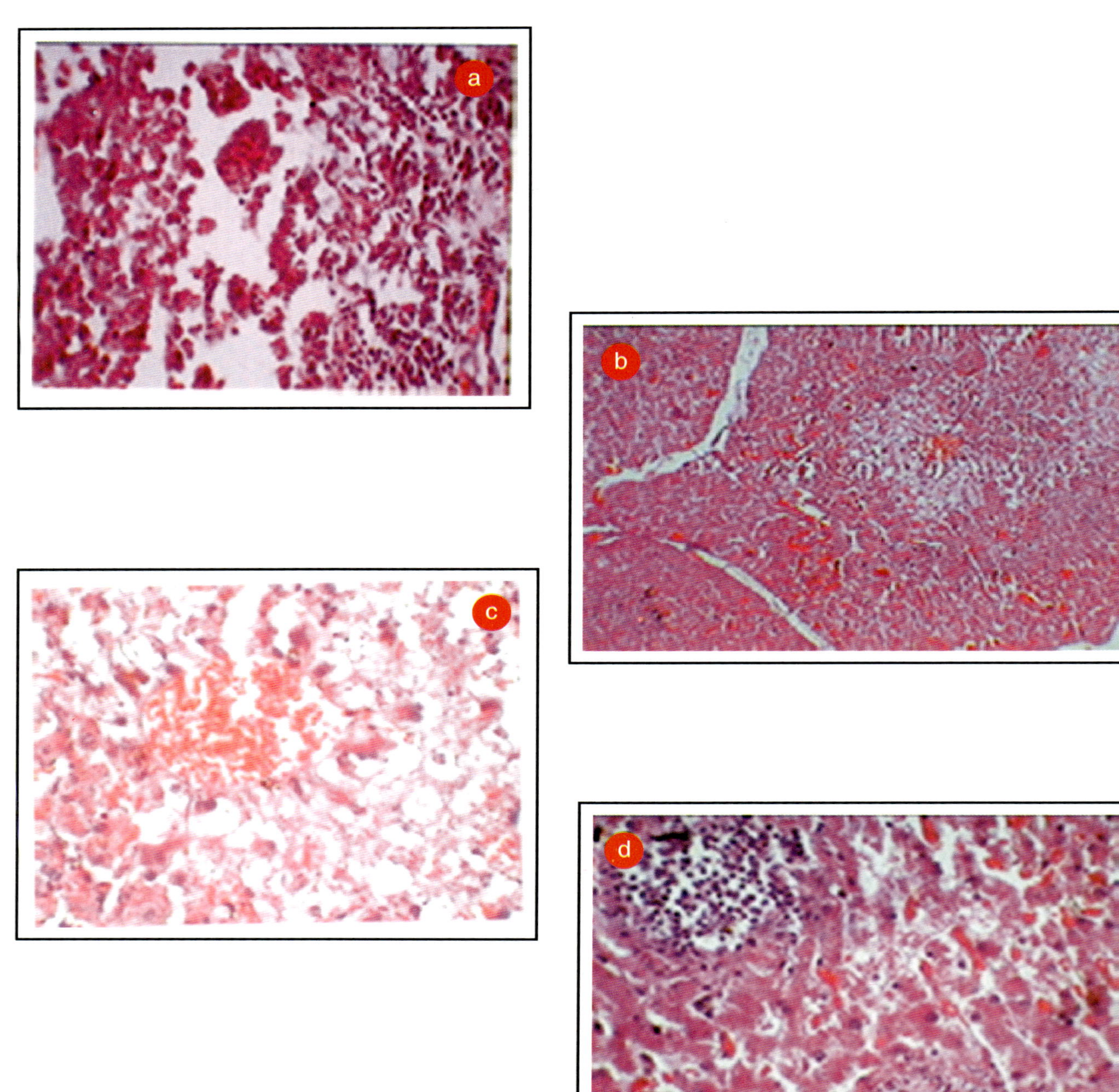

Figure 623: Salmonella enteritis in Golden langur (*T. geei*) Belonged to Manas Tiger Reserve, Assam. Photomicrograph showing: (a) Necrosis with infiltration of mononuclear cells in the intestine. H&E, x400. (b)Focal hepatic lesion accompanied by purulent infection. H&E, x100 (c) Centrilobular necrosis.H&E,x400. (d) Another view of (c).

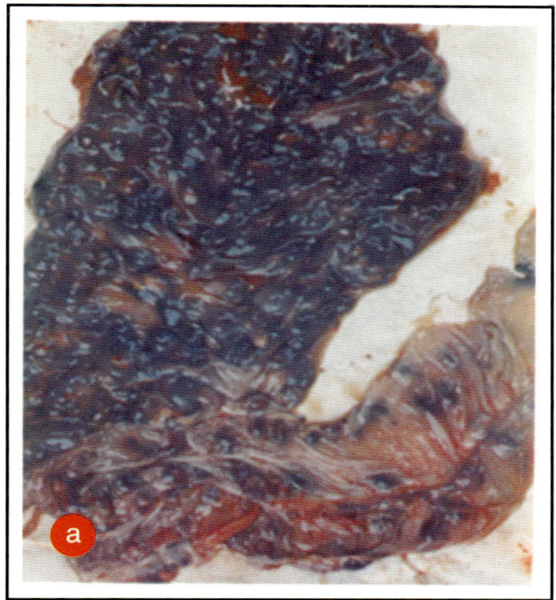

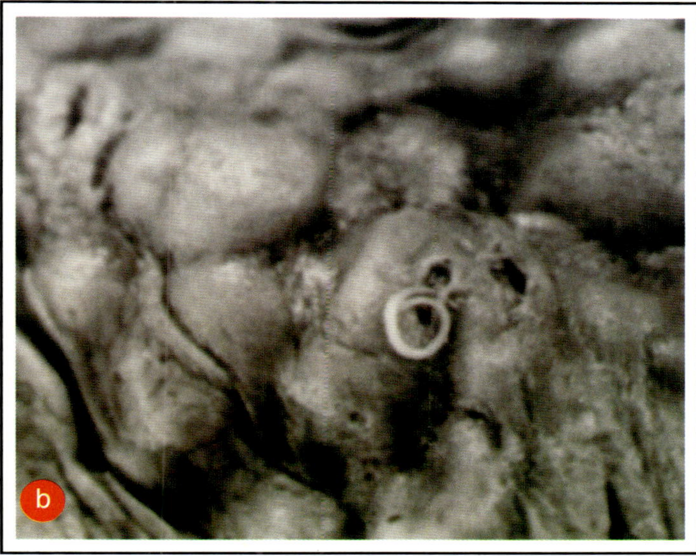

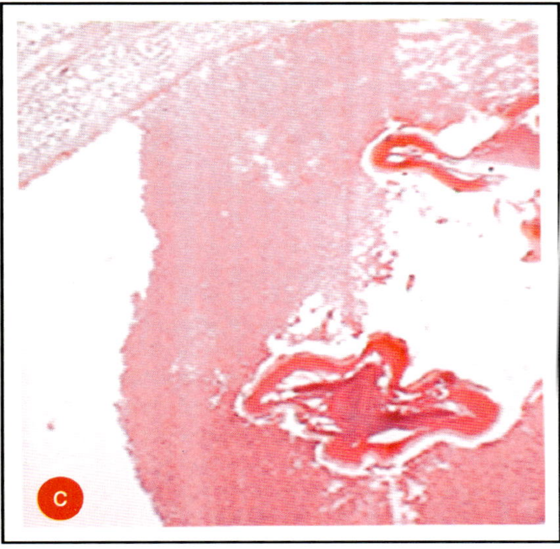

Figure 624: Photographs of large intestine from hoolock gibbon (*B. hoolock*) showing: (a) Pea sized nodules at the thickened mucosal lining. (b) *Oesophagostomum* sp. protruding out of the nodule. (c) Photomicrograph of cross section of *Oesophagostomum sp.* surrounded by caseonecrotic mass. H&E,x 100.

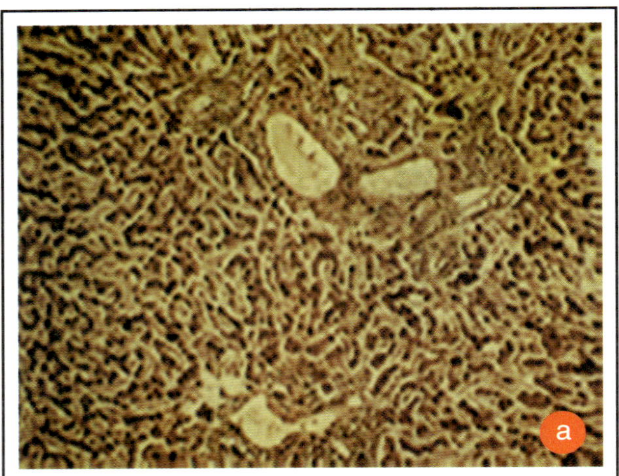

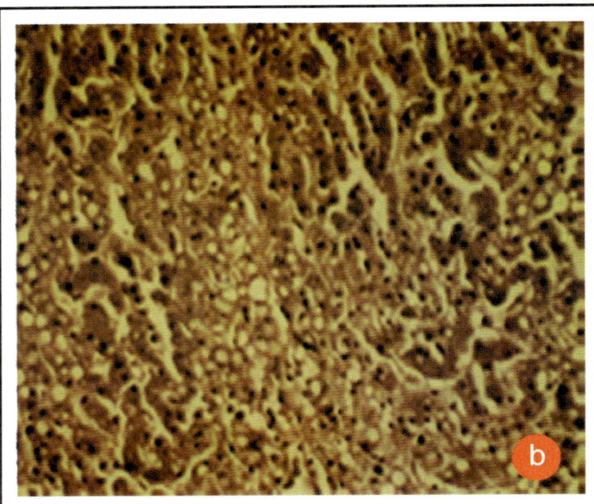

Figure 625: Photomicrographs of liver from Golden langur (*T. geei*) died in captivity showing: (a) Disrupted hepatic cords, dilated sinusoids and fibrocellular reaction in portal areas. H& E, x 100 (b) Heptocytes revealing presence of fat vacuoles in their cytoplasm. H&E, x160 (Patil, 2002).

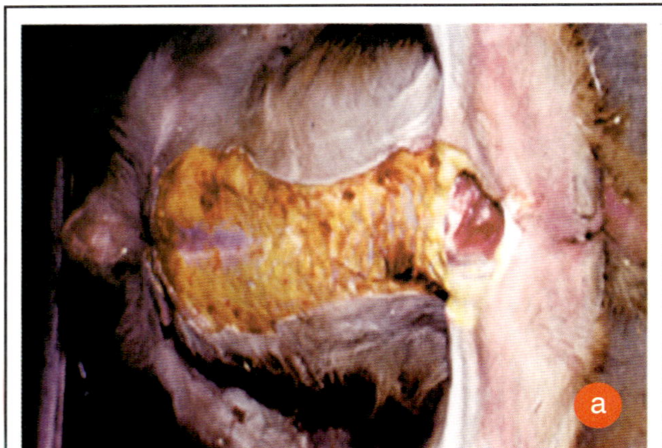

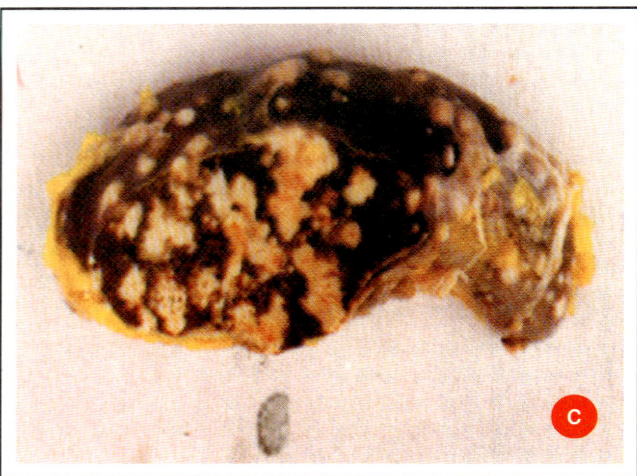

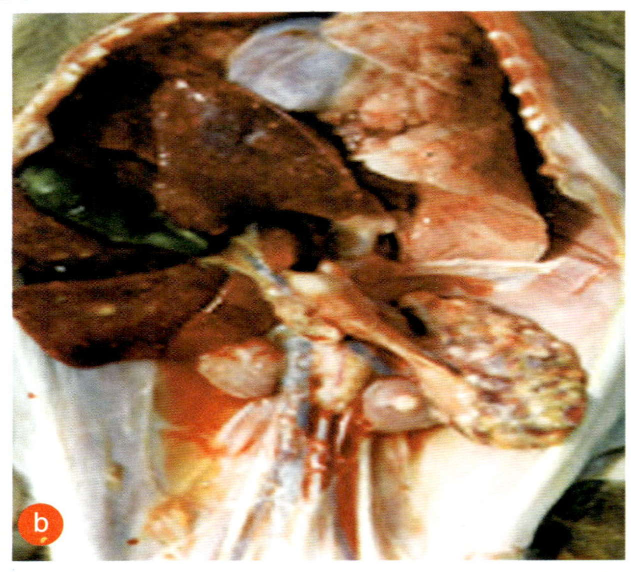

Figure 626: Dissection of debilitated female rhesus (*M. mulatta*) died in a free ranging troop showing presence of yellowish sheet of fat subcutaneously. (b) Tuberculous lesions in the liver, mesentery and lymph nodes.(c) Spleen studded with tuberculous nodules.The case is also referred under respiratory system and reproductive system.

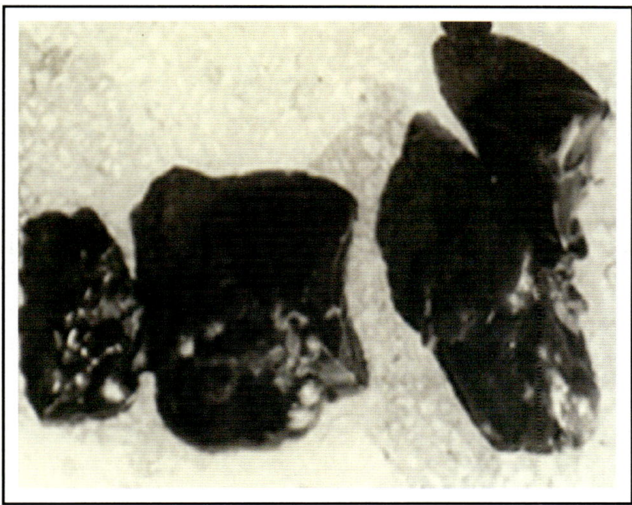

Figure 627: Nodular growths in the parietal surface of liver of common langur (*S. entellus*) caused by *Fascioloa gigantica.*

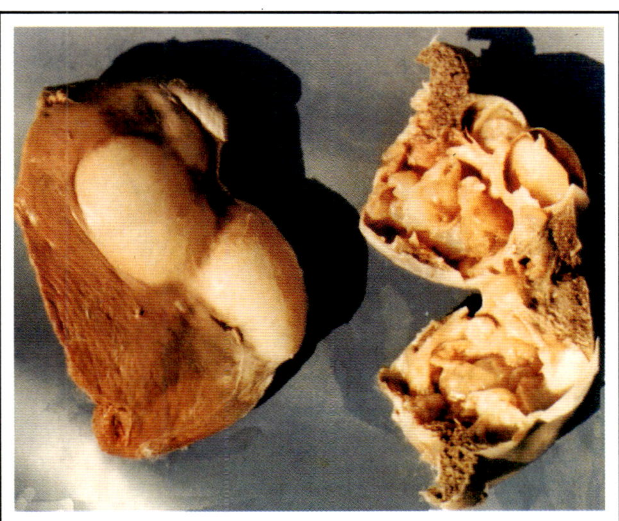

Figure 628: Cysts of *Echinicoccus granulosus* in the liver of langur (*S. entellus*) died at Zoological Garden, Lucknow (U.P).

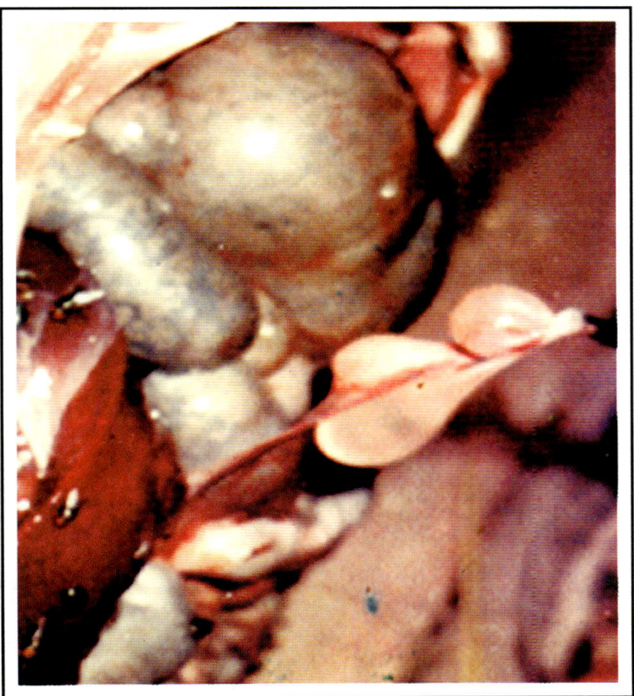

Figure 629: Cysts in the abdominal cavity of common langur (*P. entellus*) died after colliding with vehicle in Delhi city.

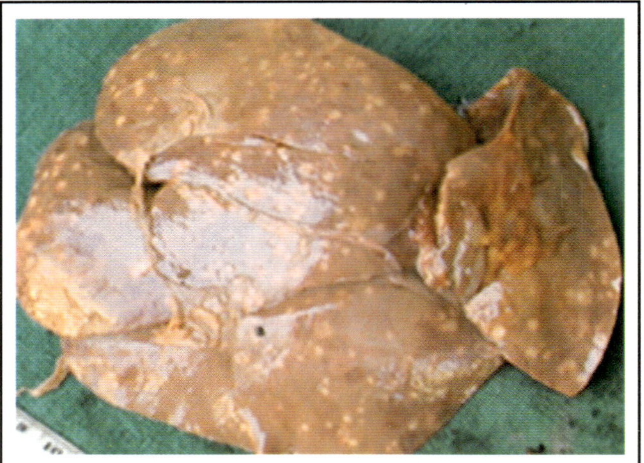

Figure 630: Liver of stump-tailed macaque (*M. speciosa*) died in Gibbon Wildlife Sanctuary, Assam. showing focal areas of necrosis and fibrosis resembling the lesion of “milk spot” as a result of parasitic migration .The case is also referred above for another condition.

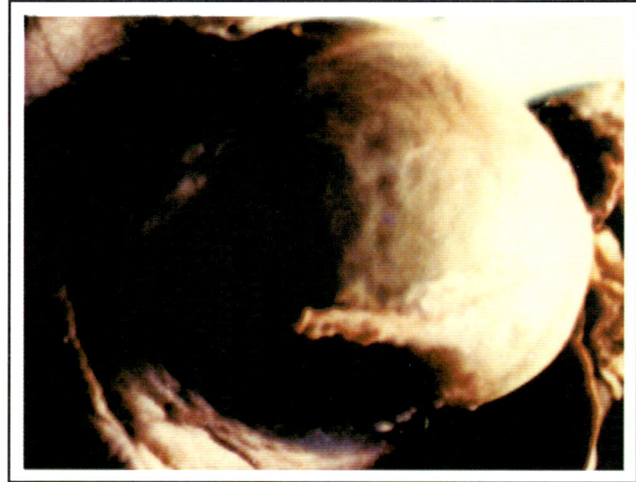

Figure 631: Photograph showing distended gall bladder due to obstruction in the bile duct encountered in young common langur (*S. entellus*) died in captivity.

Urinary System

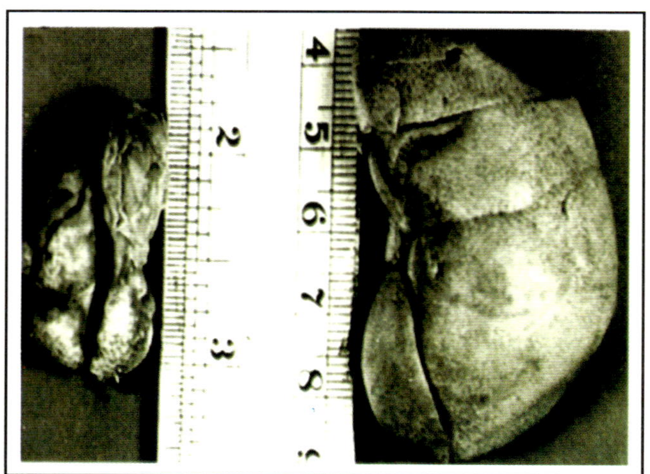

Figure 632: Left kidney arophied,also had tuberculous lesion and right kidney hypertrophied in Spider monkey (*Ateles geoffroy*, an exotic sp.) died in National Zoological Park,New Delhi.

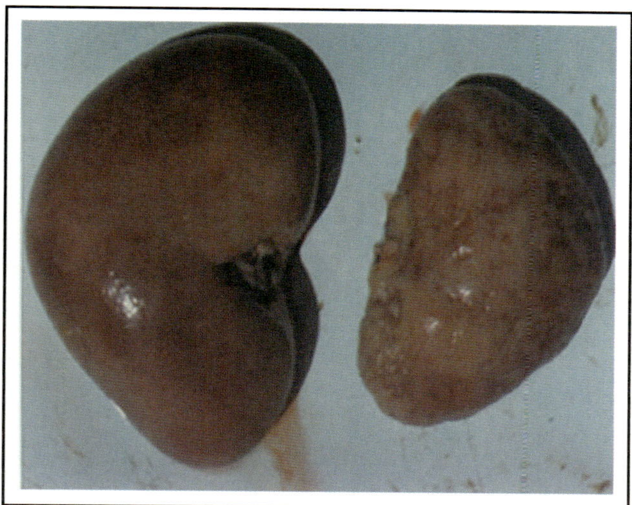

Figure 633: Photograph showing contracted small right kidney while the left kidney was hypertrophied found in chimpanzee (*Pan troglodytes*, an exotic sp.) died in captivity.

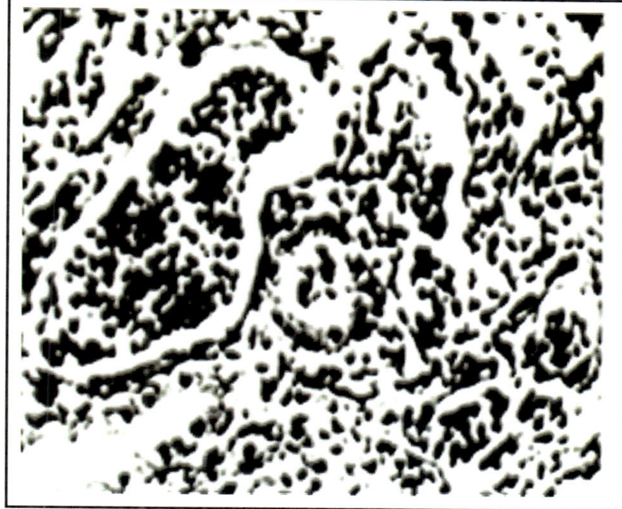

Figure 634: Photomicrograph showing suppurative nephritis related to *Streptococcus* sp. infection in Golden langur (*T. geei*). Note neutrophil aggregates in the tublar lumina and interstitial spaces. H & E,X 400 (Singh *et al.*, 1981).

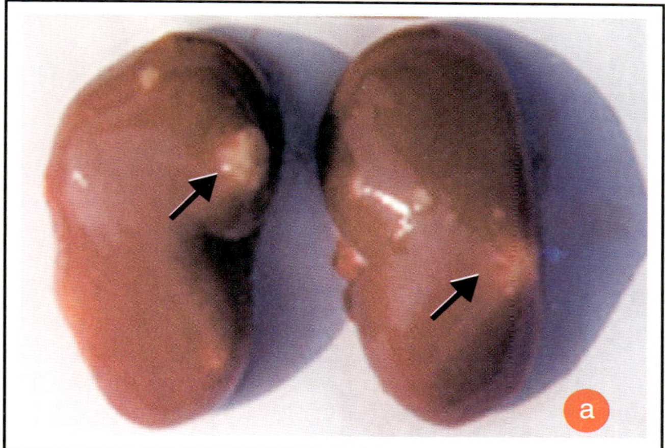

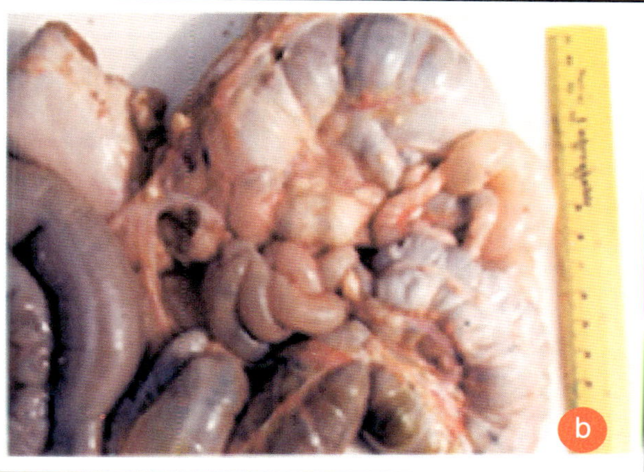

Figure 635: (a) Photographs showing tuberculous nodules in :(a) Kidneys. (b) Serosa of intestine of common langur (*S. entellus*) died in captivity.

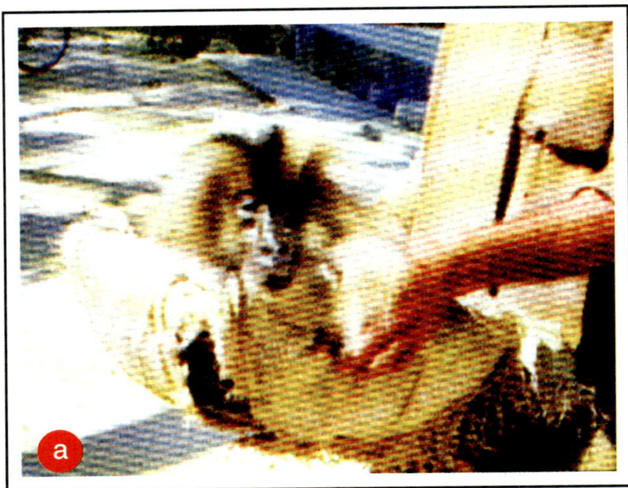

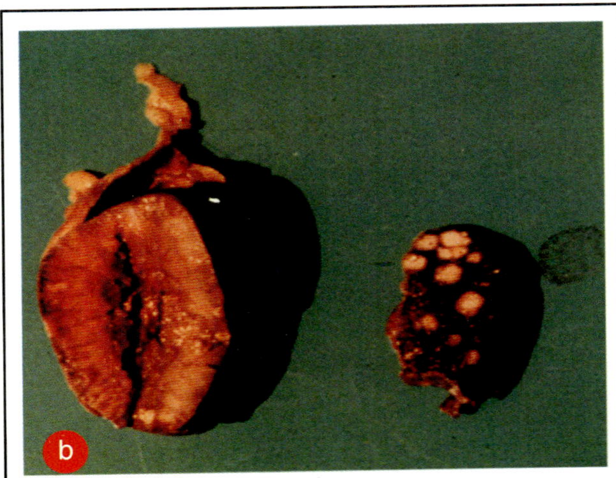

Figure 636: (a) Sick lion-tailed macaque (*M.silenus*) kept in basket at Kanpur Zoo Hospital suffering from tuberculosis. (b) Necropsy of (a) showed tuberculous nodules in kidney.

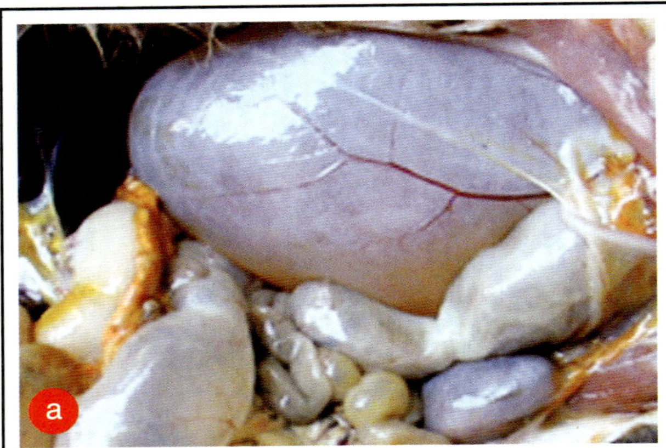

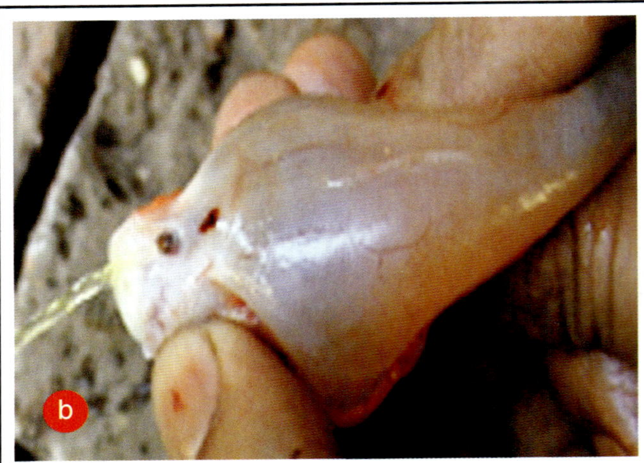

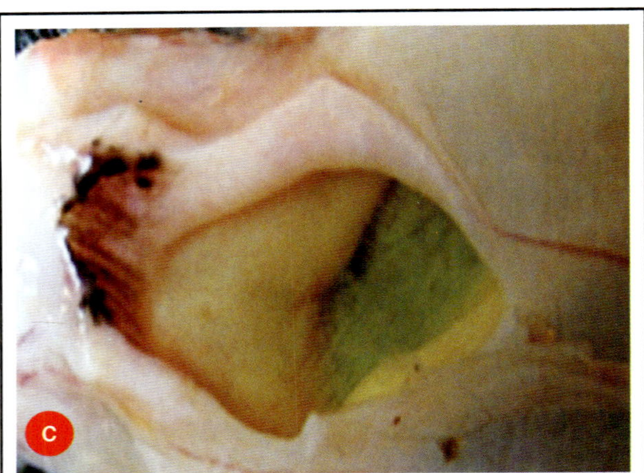

Figure 637: (a) Photograph showing distended urinary bladder displacing the visceral organs to left side of the abdomen in dissected slow loris (*N. caucang*) died in captivity.(b) On compression of bladder urine passing out with difficulty through the urinary meatus. (c) Opening of (b) showed haemorrhagic lesions in the urinary meatus.

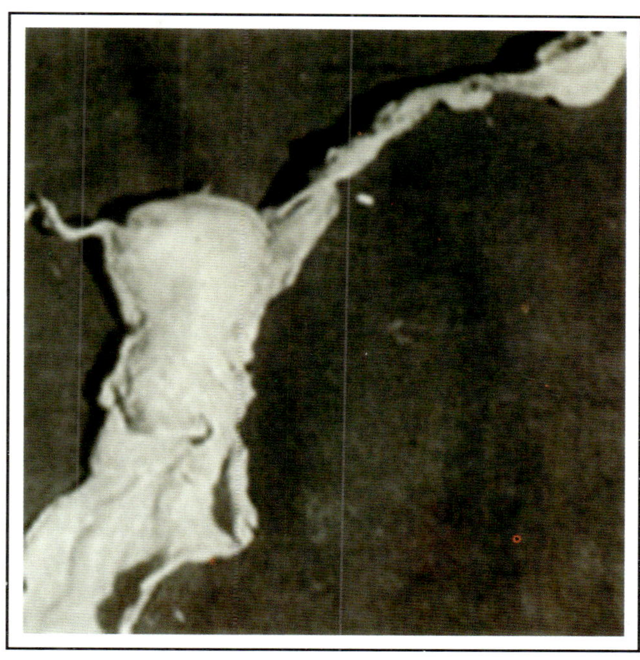

Figure 638: Photograph showing segmental aplasia in the genital tract of Nilgiri langurs (*T. johnii*). Left ovary missing and fallopian tube represented by a small blind tube.

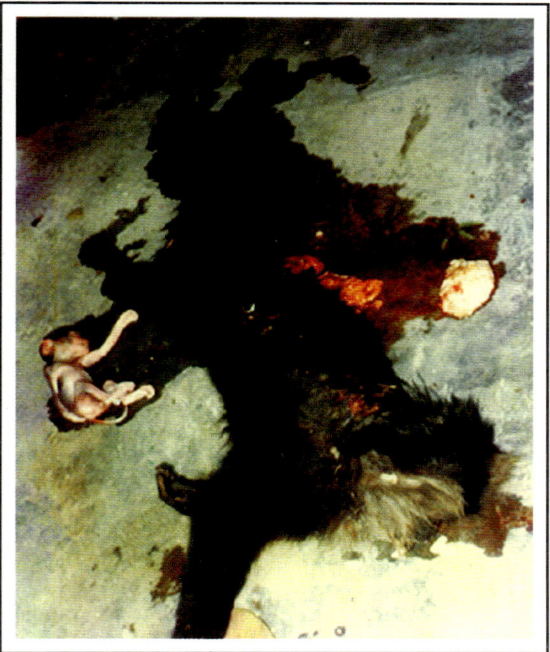

Figure 639: A female lion-tailed macaque (*M.silenus*) aborted immature fetus after she fell down accidently from the perching tree and succumbed instantaneously.

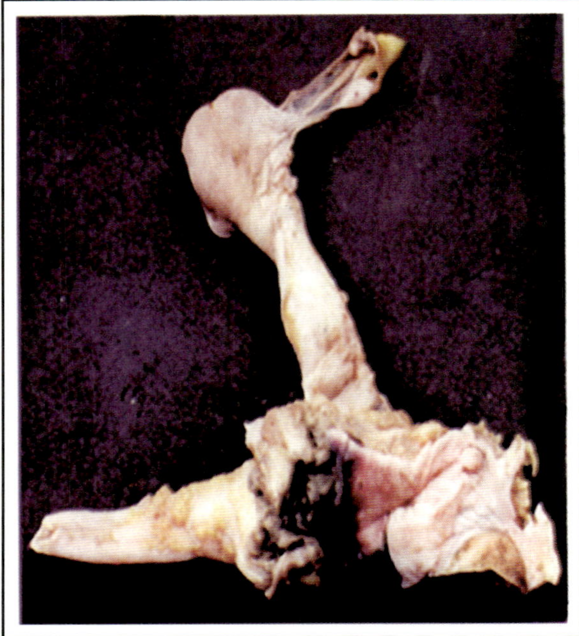

Figure 640: Tuberculous lesion in vagina of rhesus monkey (*M. mulatta*). The case is also referred under respiratory and digestive systems.

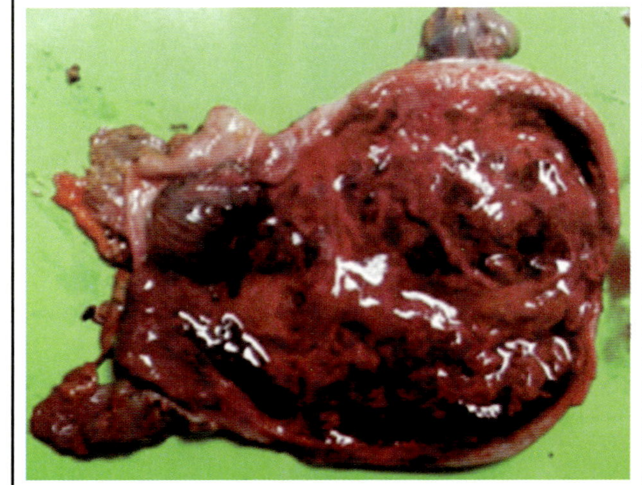

Figure 641: Photograph showing suppurative metritis after abortion in a common langur (*S. entellus*) died in captivity (Courtesy: Thirumurugan, R.)

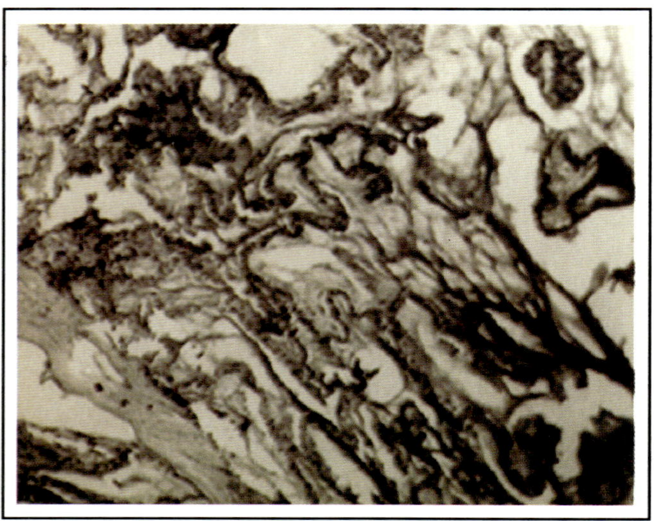

Figure 642: Photomicrograph showing adenoma of vagina encountered in bonnet macaque (*M. radiata*) died in captivity.

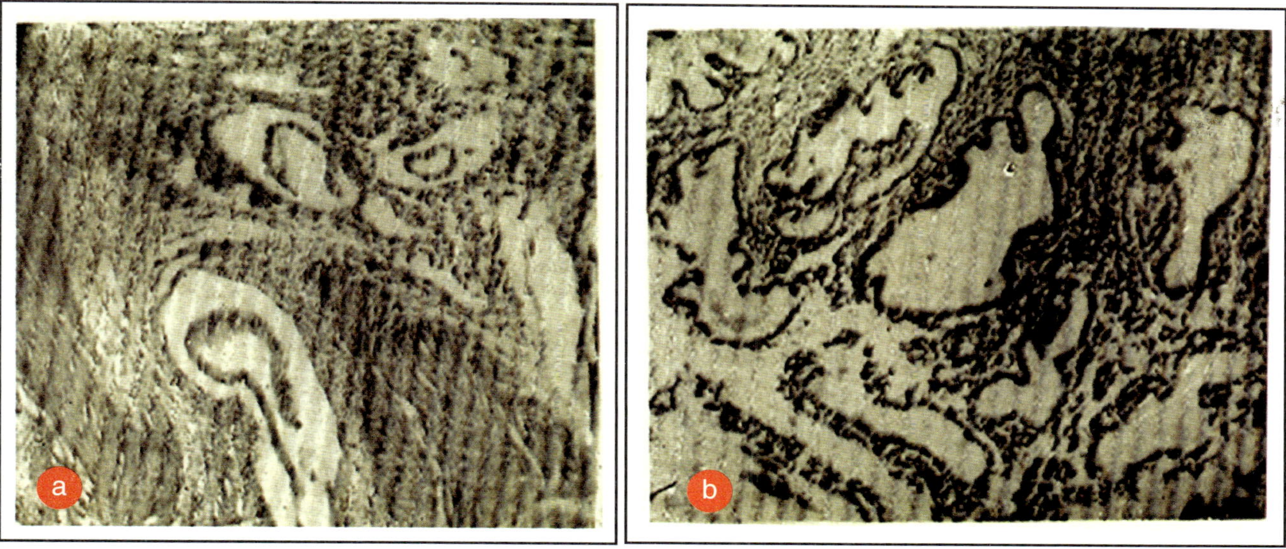

Figure 643: Endometrial adenocarcinoma in lion-tailed macaque (*M. silenus*). (a) Adenomatous tumorous tissue in the uterine musculature.(b).Papillary and thickened lining in some of the infiltrating structures in the uterine musculature. H & E x 100. (Parihar, 1976).

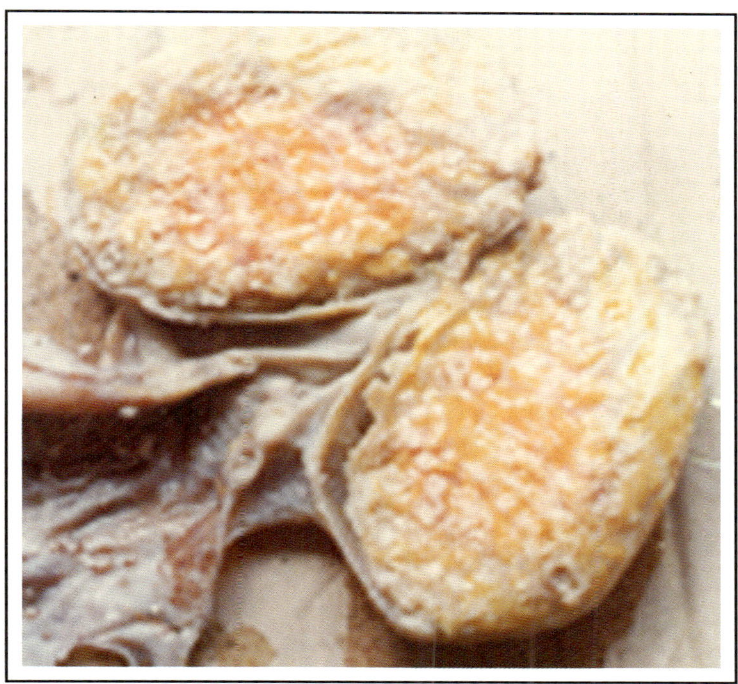

Figure 644: Photograph of unilateral seminoma encountered in lion-tailed macaque (*M. silenus*) died in captivity.

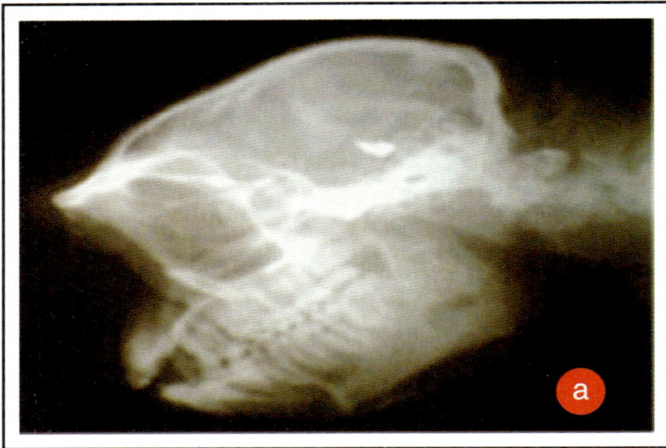

Figure 645: (a) Radiograph showing gun pellet lodged in the mid brain of a common langur (*S. entellus*).(b,c) C. T. scan of (a) revealed two pieces of bullet in the cranial cavity,one lying almost in the middle of raphe about 3.6 cm deep. (Kelewala *et al.*, 2007).

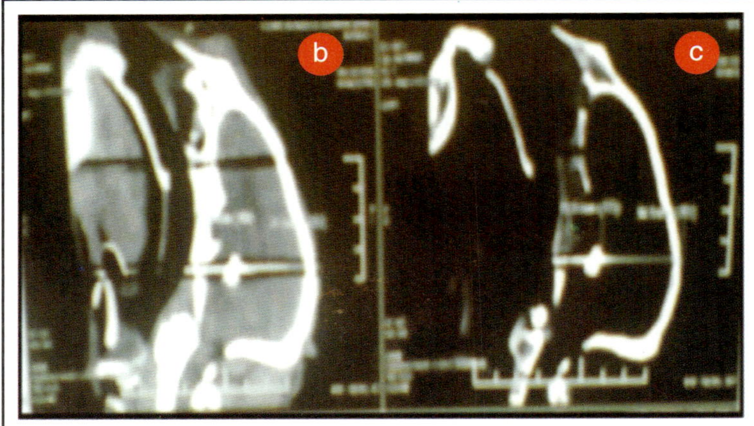

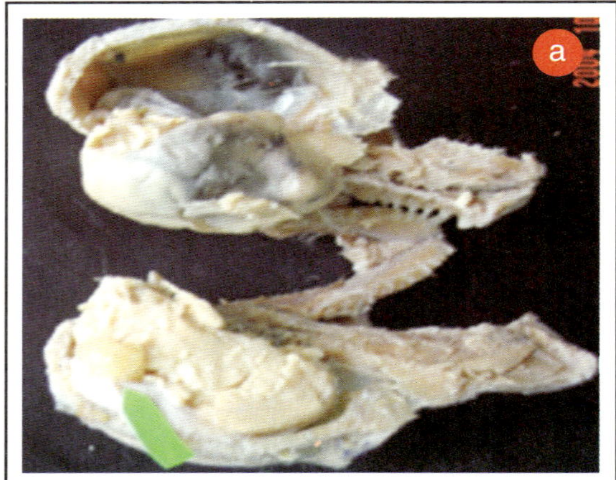

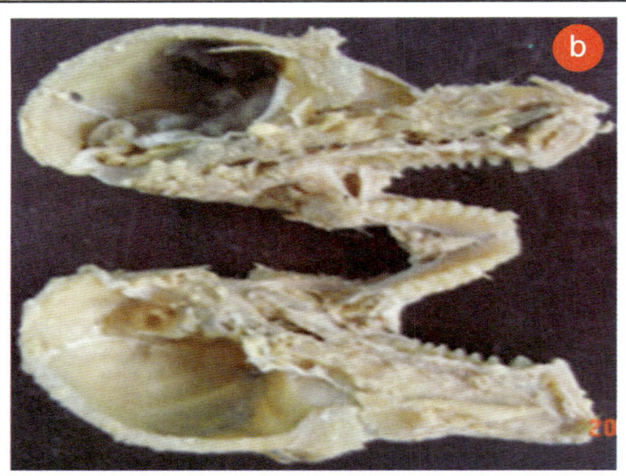

Figure 646: Photographs (a, b) of cranial cavity of slender loris (*L. lydekkerianus*) cut opened : (a) Left half having brain substance showing a round (sterile) cyst and the right half stained blackish due to haemorrhages. Cystic pressure on the brain might be the reason for fall of the animal from its perch and met with haemorrhagic lesions. (b) Emptied cranium with blackish discolouration.

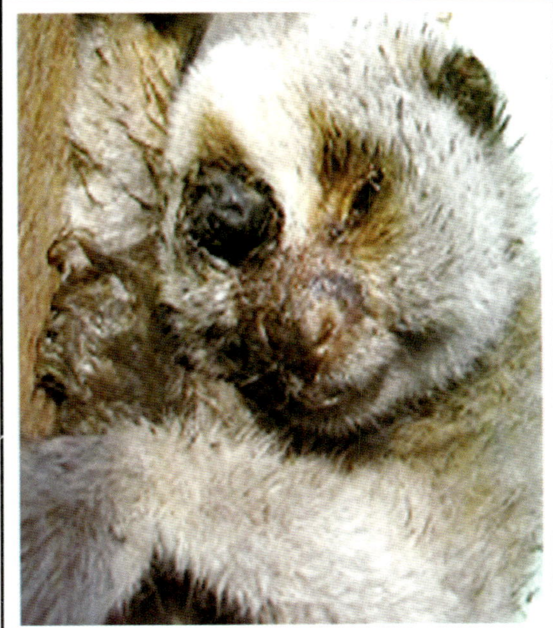

Sense Organ - Eye

Figure 647: Severely traumatized and damged right eye in a captive slow loris (*N. coucang*) caused by trauma (Courtesy: Talukdar, A. & Choudhury, B.)

Integumentary System

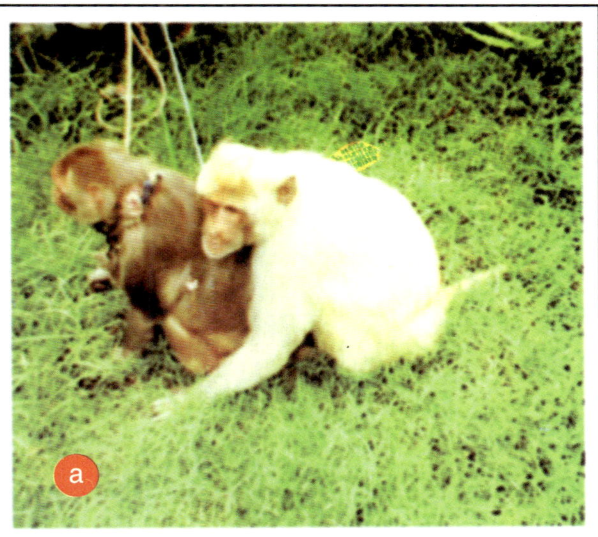

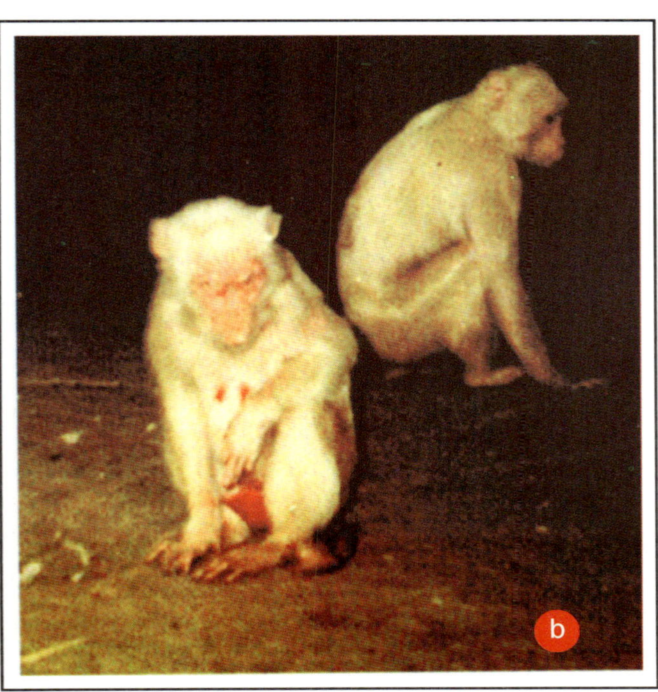

Figure 648: (a) A pair of rhesus monkey (*M. mulatta*) capture from the wild. Male white and female of normal colour.(b) A pair of albino (*M. mulatta*) male and female rhesus monkey at Z.G., Lucknow (U.P).

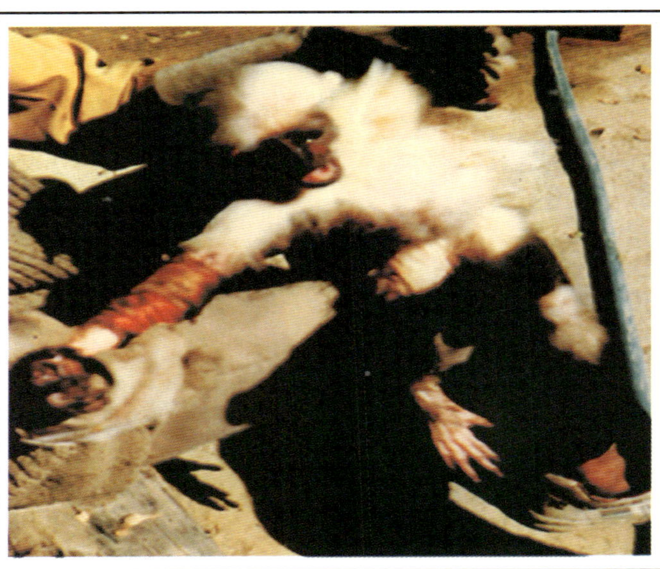

Figure 649: Photograph showing right hand of a golden baby langur (*T. geei*) bitten by its male parent in captivity.

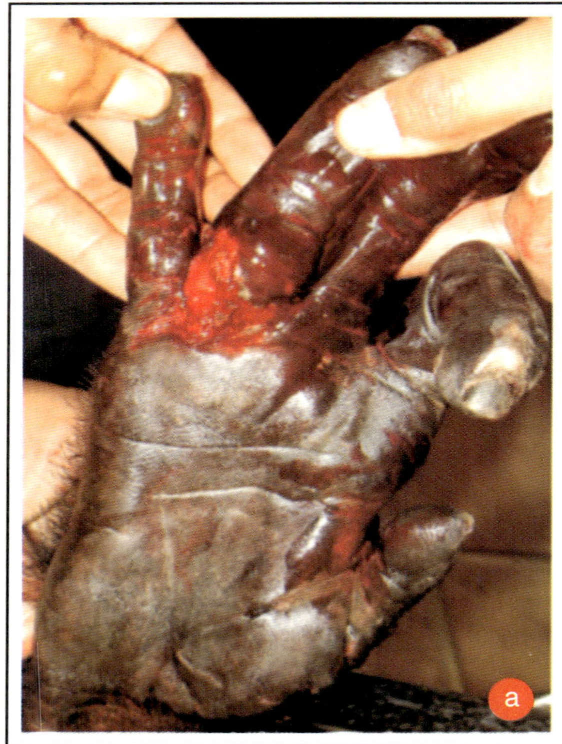

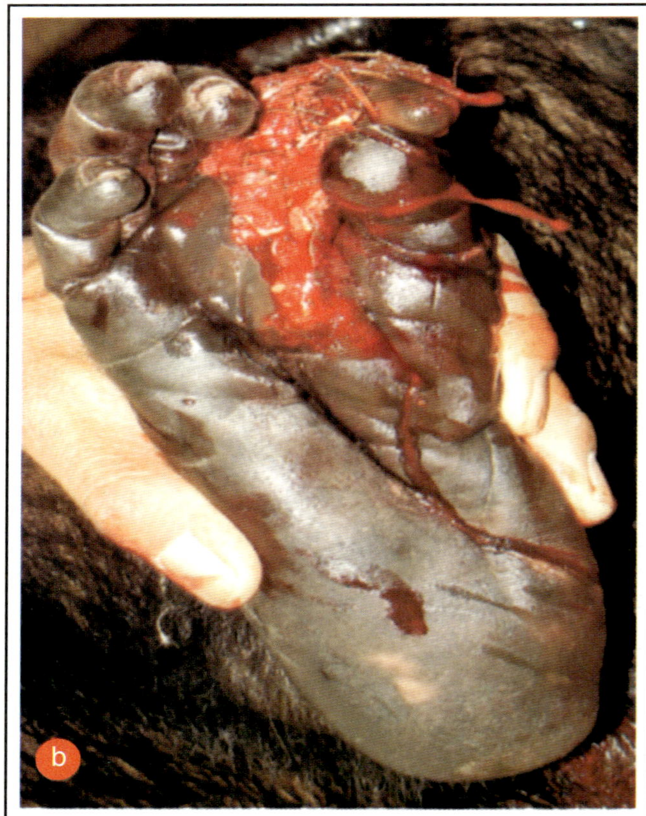

Figure 650: Photographs showing lacerations on the sole and fingers of right fore (a) and hind limbs (b) of chimpanzee (*Pan troglodytes*, an exotic sp.) following infighting at Zoological Garden, Mysore, Karnataka. (Courtesy: Nanjappa, K.A.).

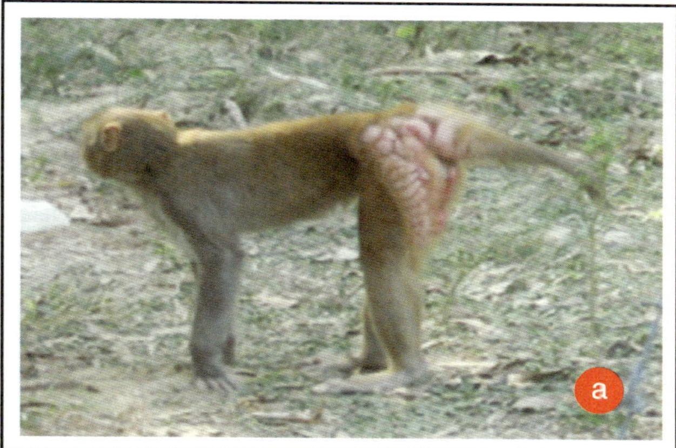

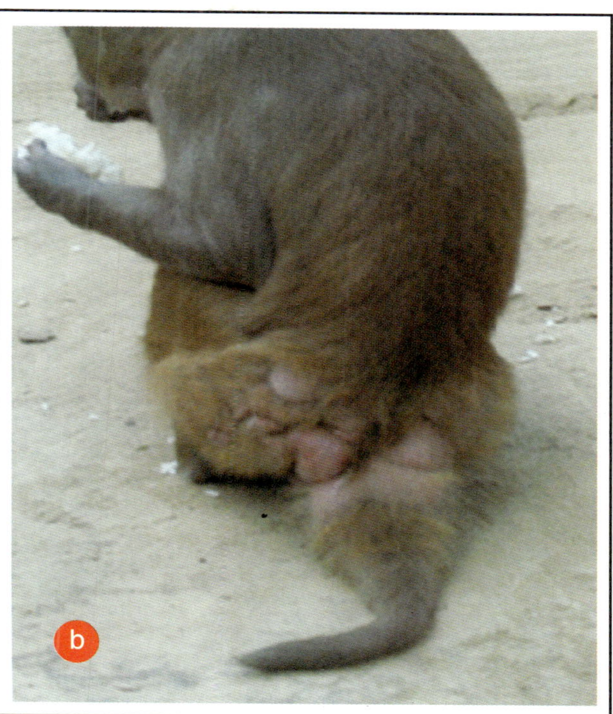

Figure 651: (a,b)Hyperkeratosis (thickened and corrugated skin folds) in free ranging rhesus monkeys (*M. mulatta*). In both the cases lesions were around base of the tail and extending to thigh and anal region.

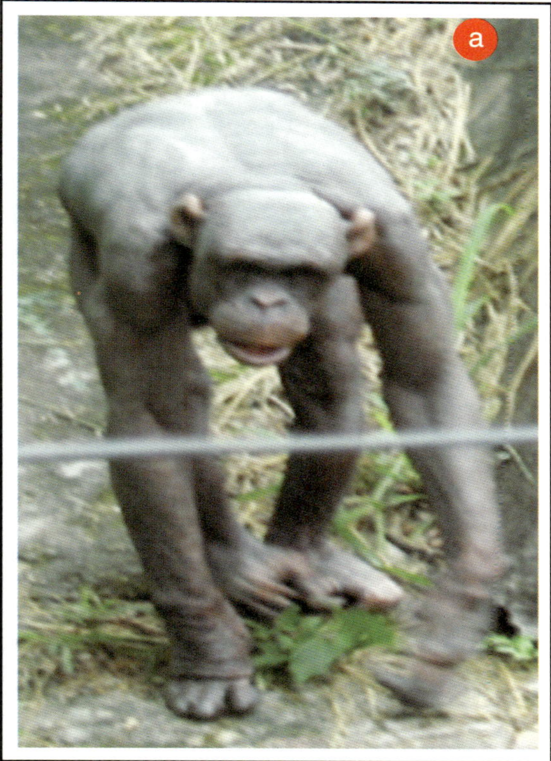

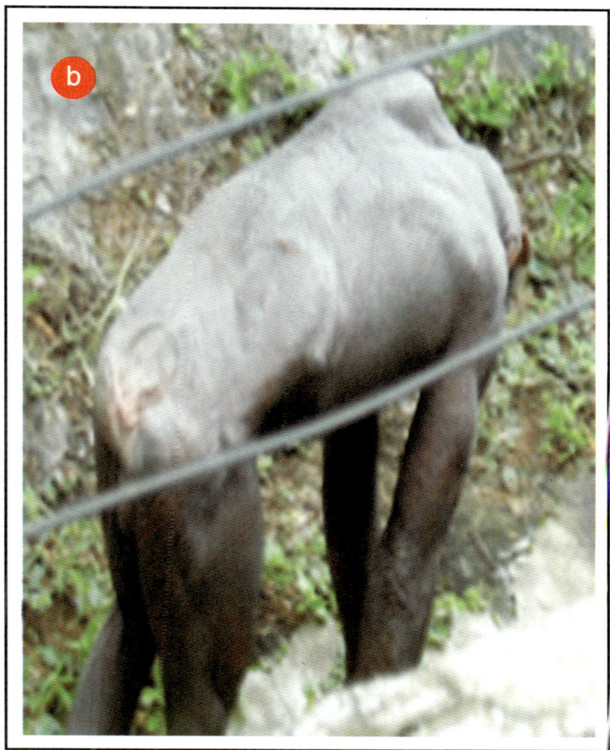

Figure 652: (a,b) Complete alopecia of chimpanzee (*Pan troglodytes*, an exotic sp.) at Zoological Garden, Mysore (Karnataka).

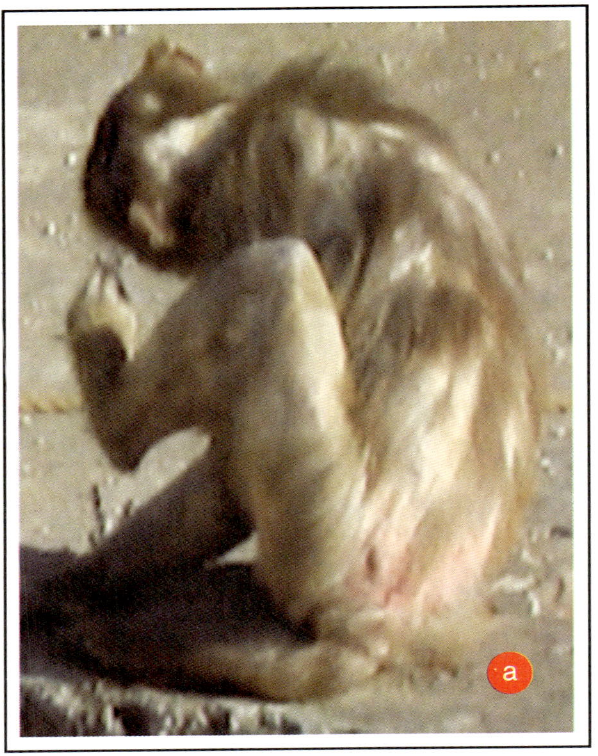

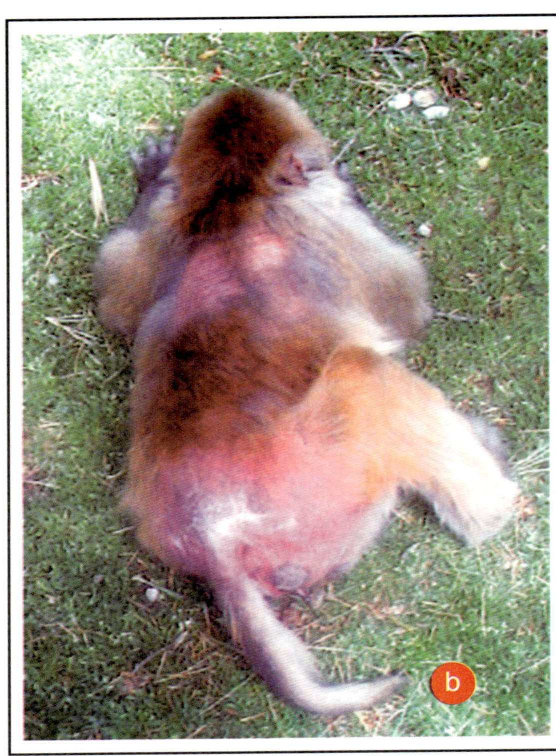

Figure 653: (a,b) Severe mite dermatitis in free ranging rhesus monkeys (*M. mulatta*).

Skeleton System

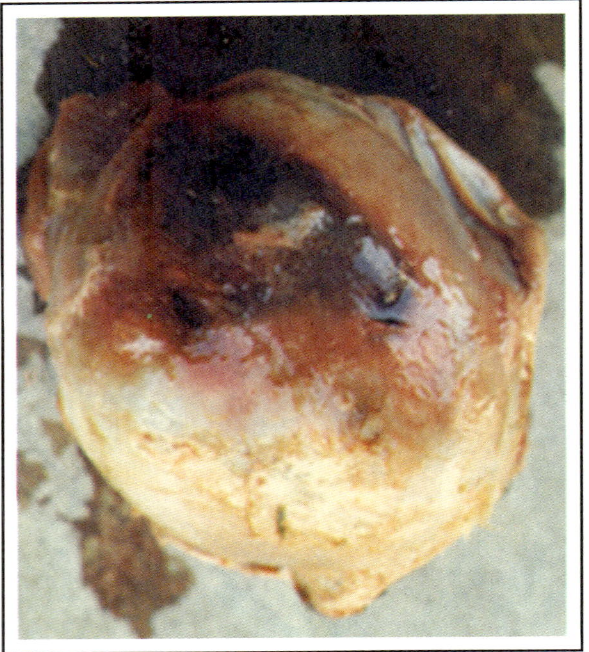

Figure 654: Photograph of skull of Capped langur (*T. pileatus*) showing fracture caused by infighting in captivity.

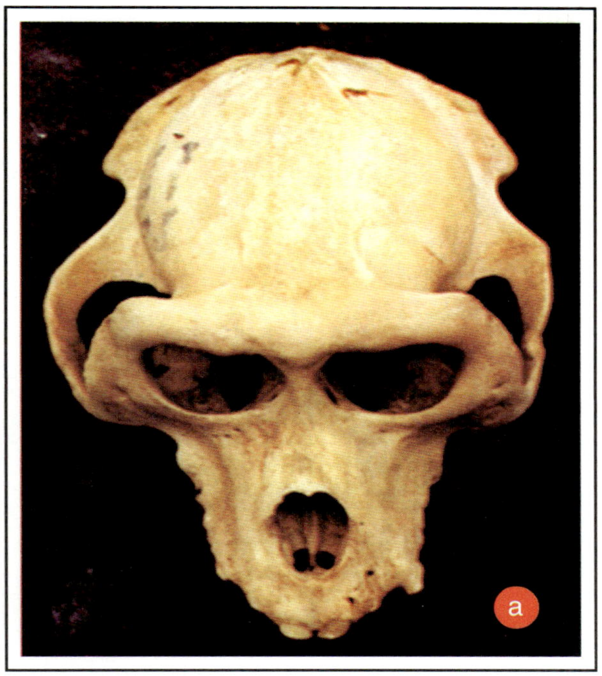

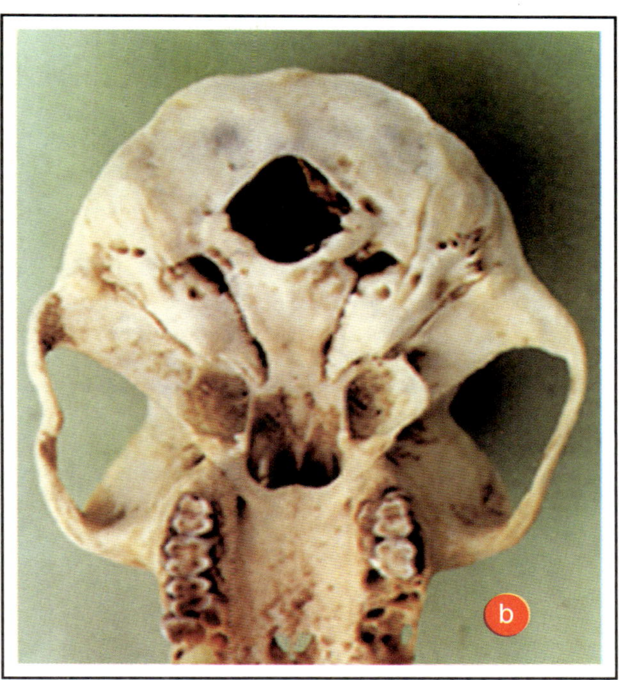

Figure 655: Photographs of skulls from macaque species died in captivity showing spontaneous perfect healing of fractures of left zygomatic archs in: (a) lion-tailed macaque (*M. silenus*) (b) Spectacle langur (*T. phayrei*).

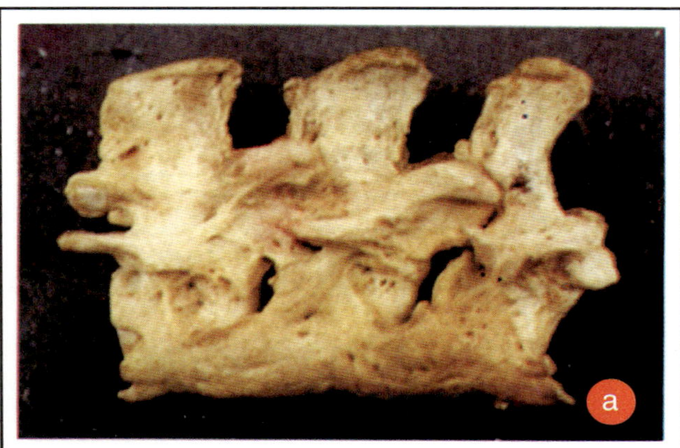

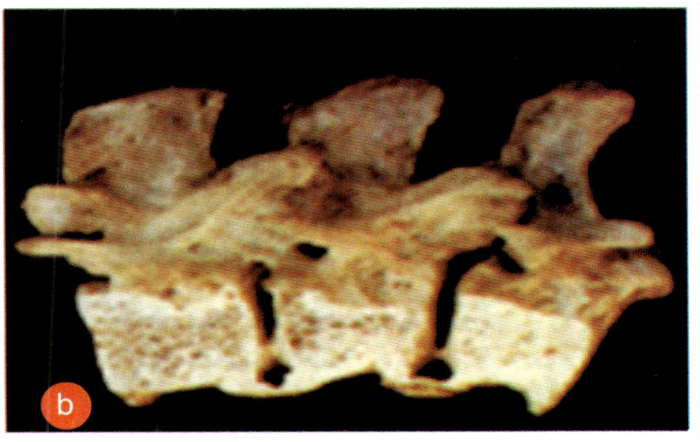

Figure 656: Photograph of a fused mass of 10 to 12 th thoracic vertebrae of lion tailed (*M. silenus*) died at National Zoological Park, showing osteophytic growths ventrally at cranial margin of each vertebra, which is bridging with caudal end of the proceeding vertebra. (b) Sagittal section of (a)showing osteophytic bridging between vertebrae.

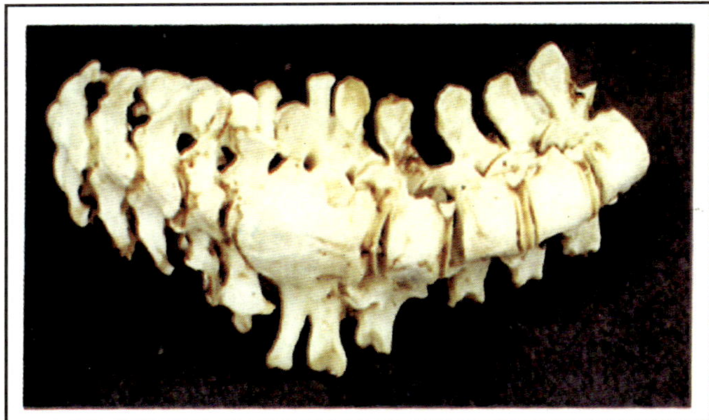

Figure 657: Photograph showing body of C-7 and body of the first thoracic vertebra fused as consolidated osseous mass in bonnet macaque (*M. radiata*) died in captivity. Note also bridging of their supra spinatous processes.

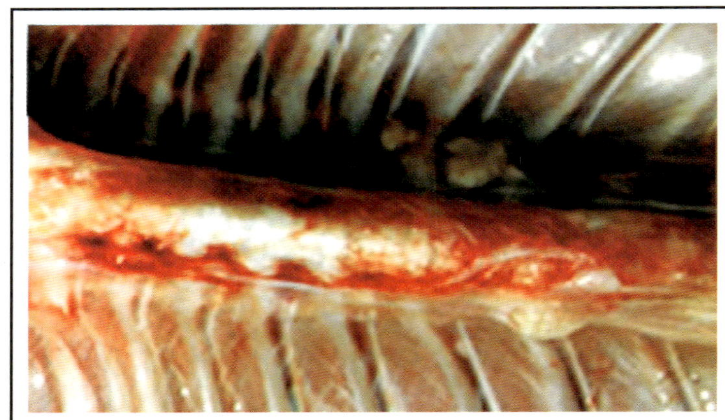

Figure 658: Tuberculous nodules over the vertebra and rib junction found in rhesus (*M. mulatta*) died in captivity.

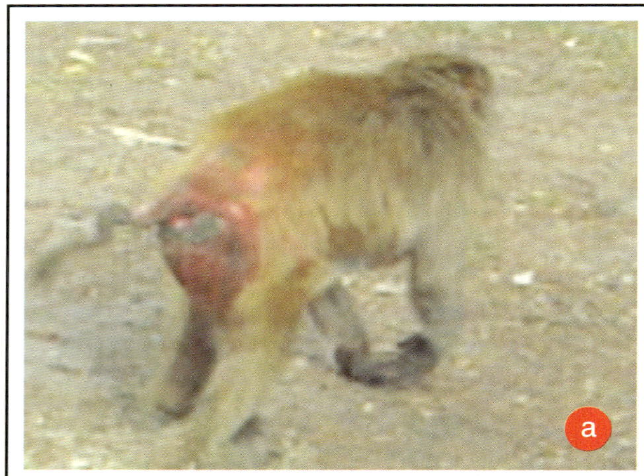

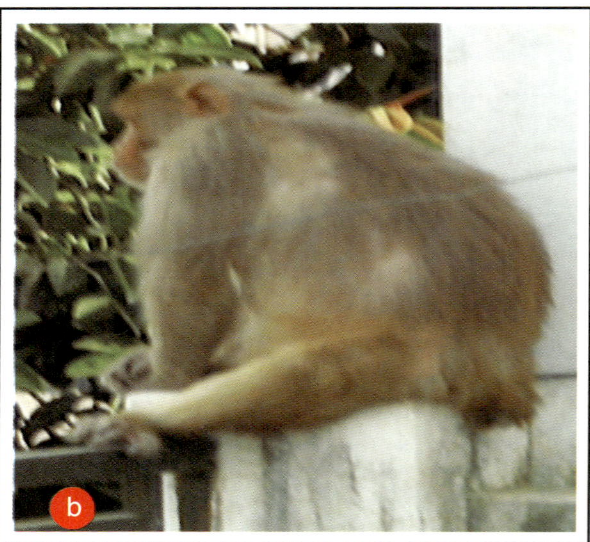

Figure 659: Tail anomalies in free ranging rhesus macaques (*M. mulatta*). (a) Twisted tail reported due its accidently trapping in electric cables.(b) Stump tail.

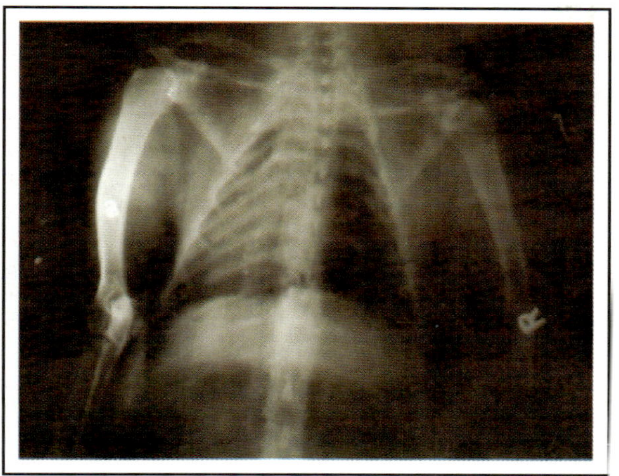

Case (i)

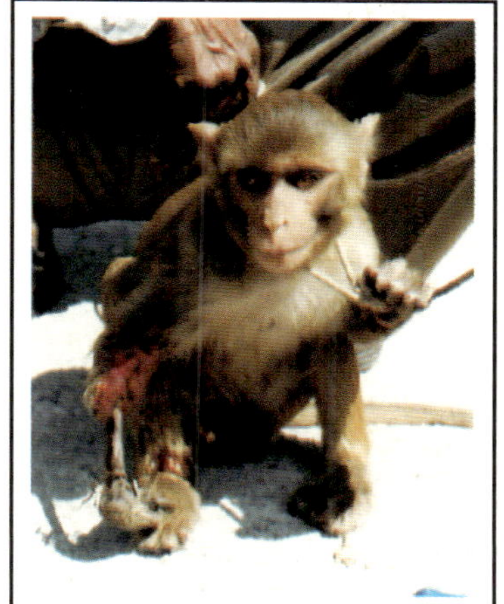

Case ii(a)

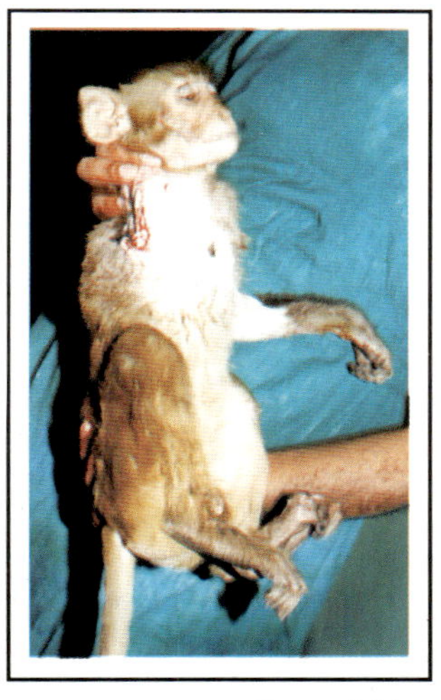
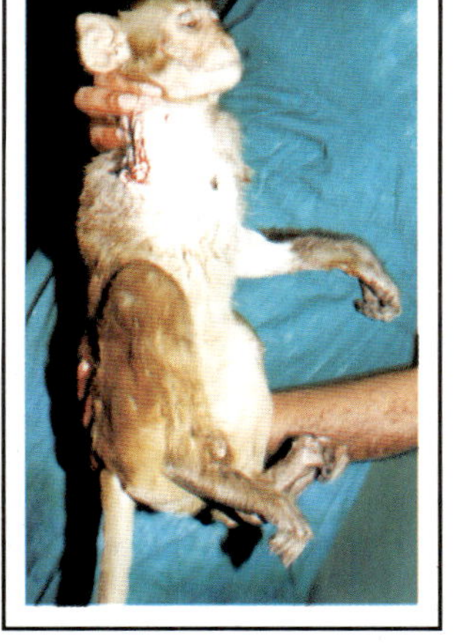

Case ii(b)

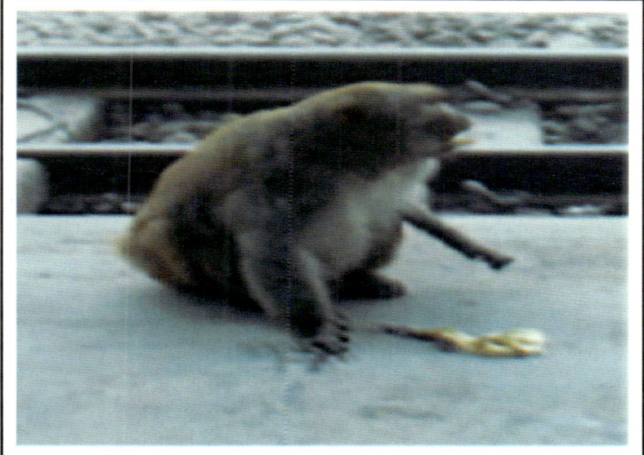

Case (iii)

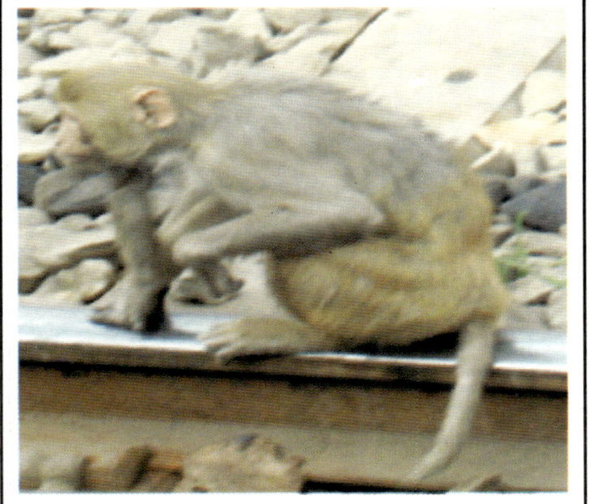

Case (iv)

Figure 660: Free ranging adult rhesus monkeys (*M. mulatta*) met with accidents.Case (i) Radiograph showing a pellet lodged in the forearm of rhesus monkey (*M. mulatta*). Case ii(a) Rhesus monkeys (*M. mulatta*) right fore arm electrocuted.(b) Arm of (a) amputed. Case (iii) Right fore arm hypotrophied and left arm slightly swollen. Case (iv) Left arm with wrist bones ankylosed. (Courtesy: Maiti, S.K. & Naveen Kumar, 2008)

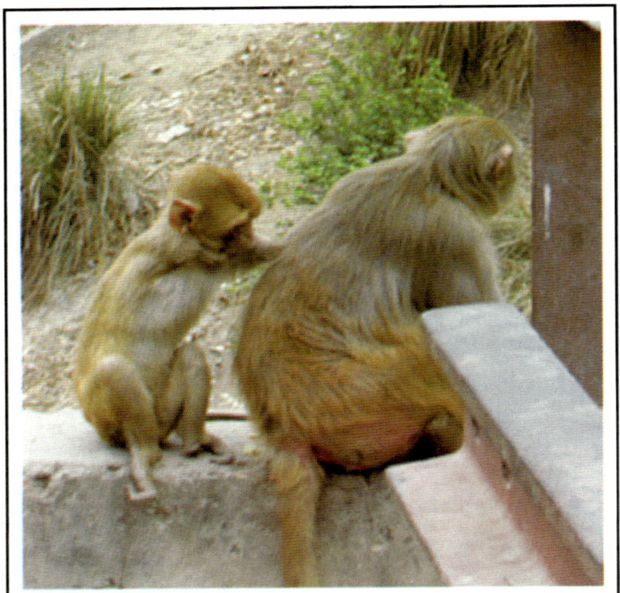

Figure 661: Rhesus macaque (*M.mulatta*) baby about 6-8 months old with mother at a railway station with its lower 2/3 right forearm lost and defective hind right foot. The monkey baby might have met with some accident.

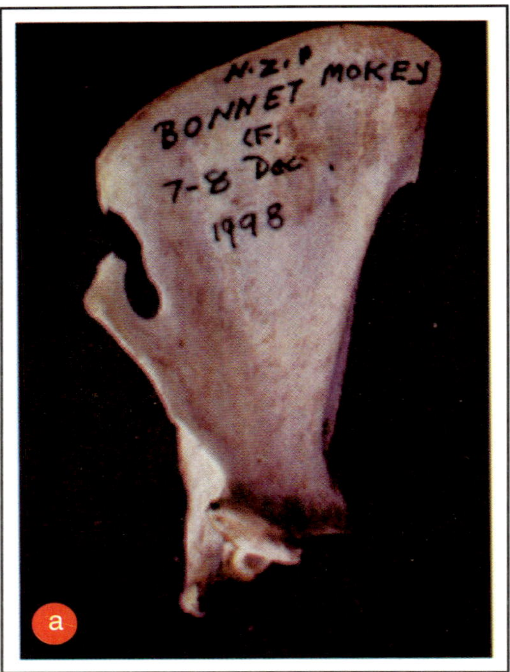

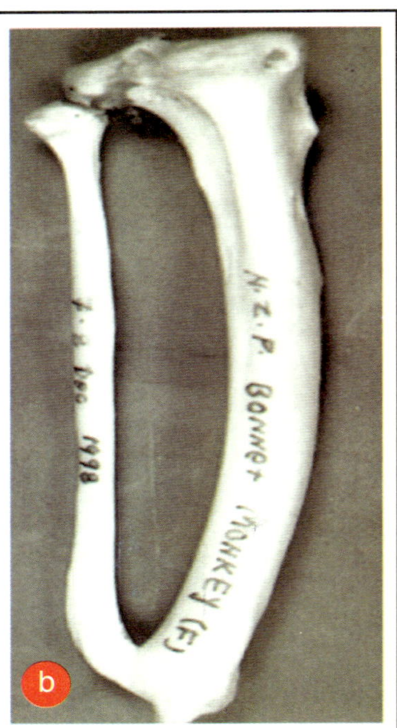

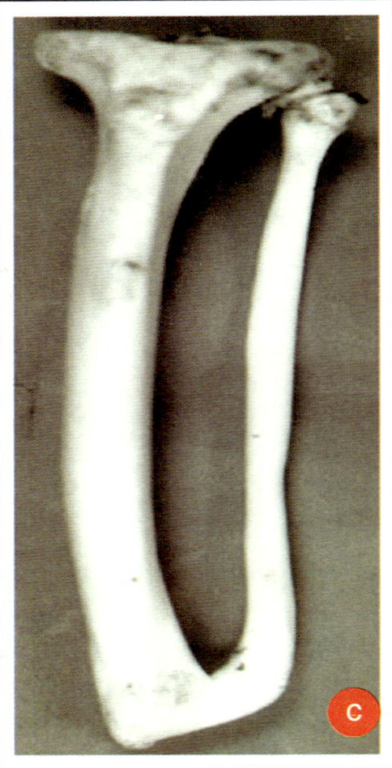

Figure 662: Long bone anomalies encountered in an adult female bonnet macaqus (*M. radiata*) died in captivity. Photograph showing (a) Notched anterior border of scapula.(b, b') Left tibia and fibula (lateral and medial views) fused at their lower extremities.

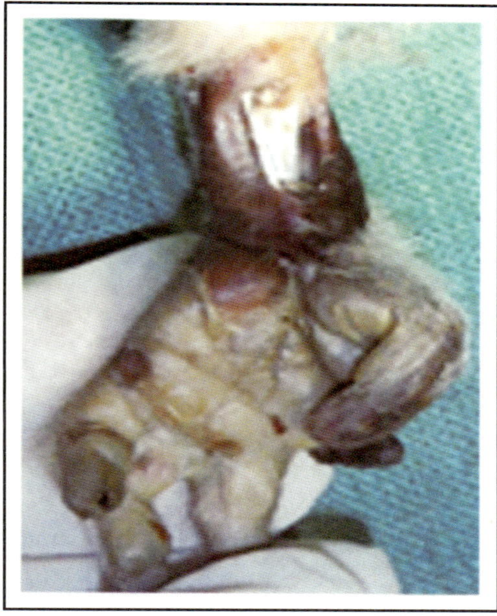

Figure 663: In a captive slow loris (*N.coucang*) gangrene developed in fractured right hand owing to tight bandage.

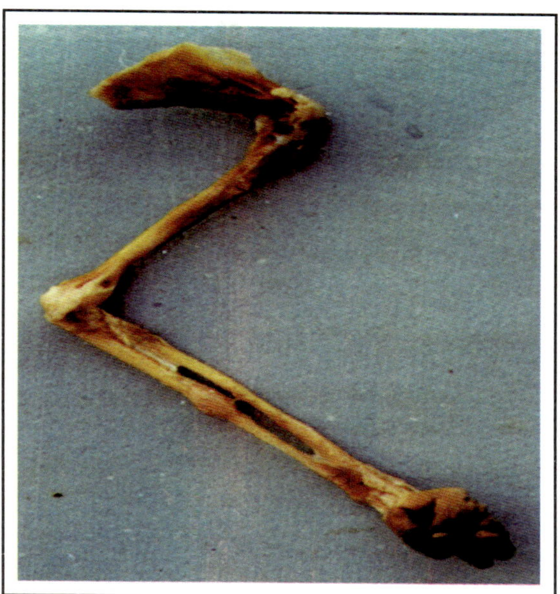

Figure 664: Photograph of fore limb of slow loris (*N.coucang*) died in captivity showing spontaneous healing of fracture in ulna.

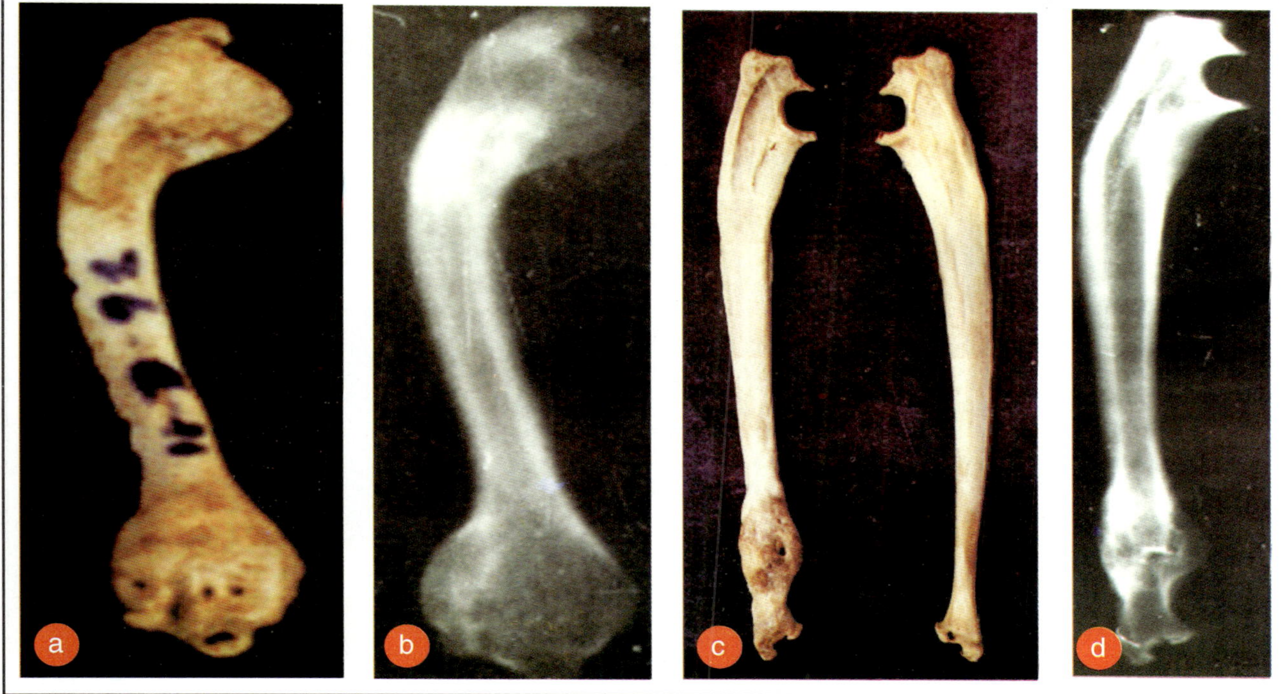

Figure 665: Photographs of fore leg of lion tailed macaque (*M. silenus*). (a) Humerus showing flared distal extremity (b) Radiograph of (a) showing obliteration of marrow cavity in the proximal third. (c) Photograph of right ulna showing persisting callus in its distal 3rd. (d) Radiograph of (c) showing unevenly healed fracture.

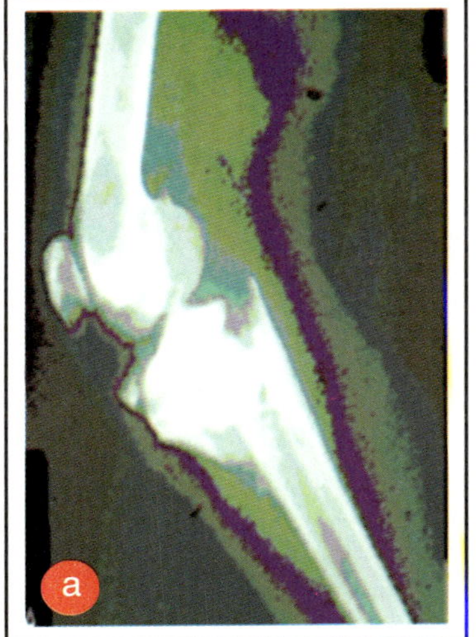

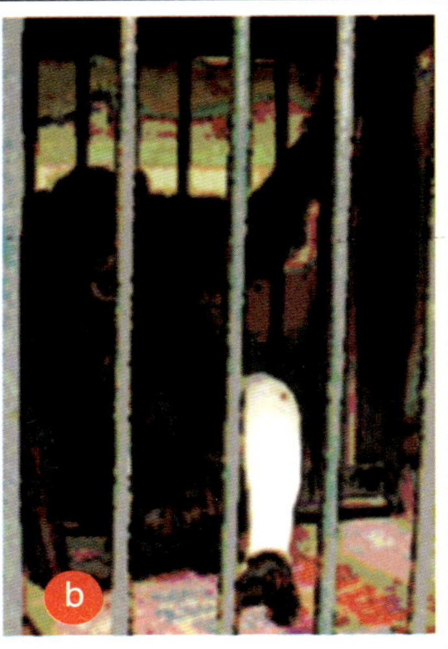

Figure 666: Surgical management of tibia fracture in a female chimpanzee (*Pan troglodytes*, an exotic sp.) at Zoological Garden, Mysore. (a) Radiograph showing multiple fractures in the proximal extremity of left tibia.(b) Fibre glass cast *in-situ* (Courtesy: Nanjappa, K.A).

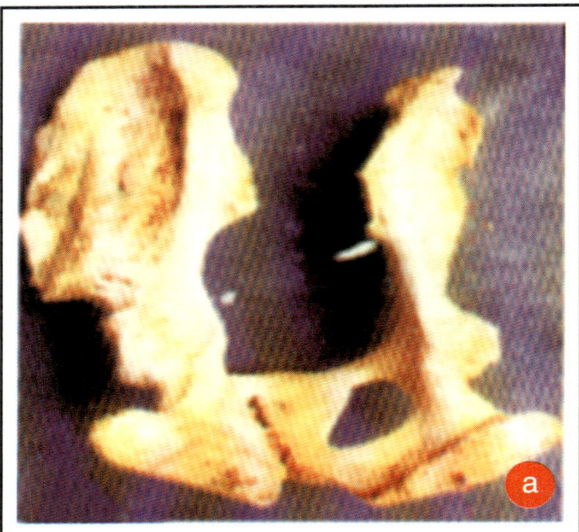

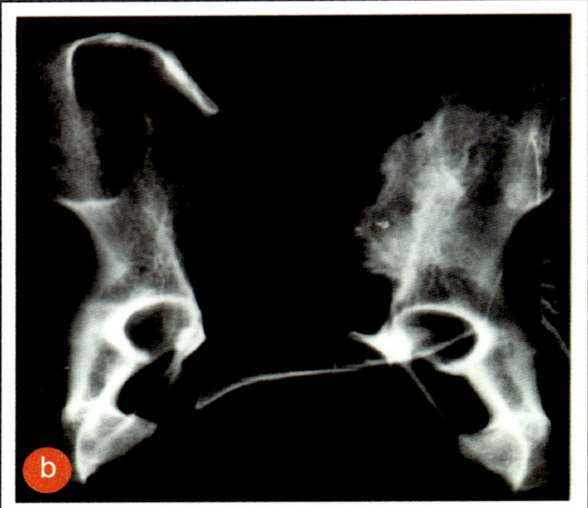

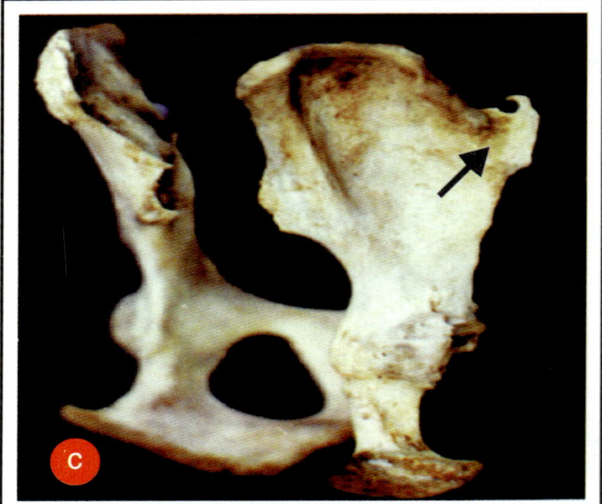

Figure 667: Photograph of pelvis of lion-tailed macaque (*M. silenus*).Wing of left ilium irregularly enlarged with obliterated gluteal concavity rough, pitted and with pores (b) Right tuber coxae had bony growths projecting forward.(c) Radiograph of pelvis showing osseous tissue of less density. Animal died of generalized form of tuberculosis.

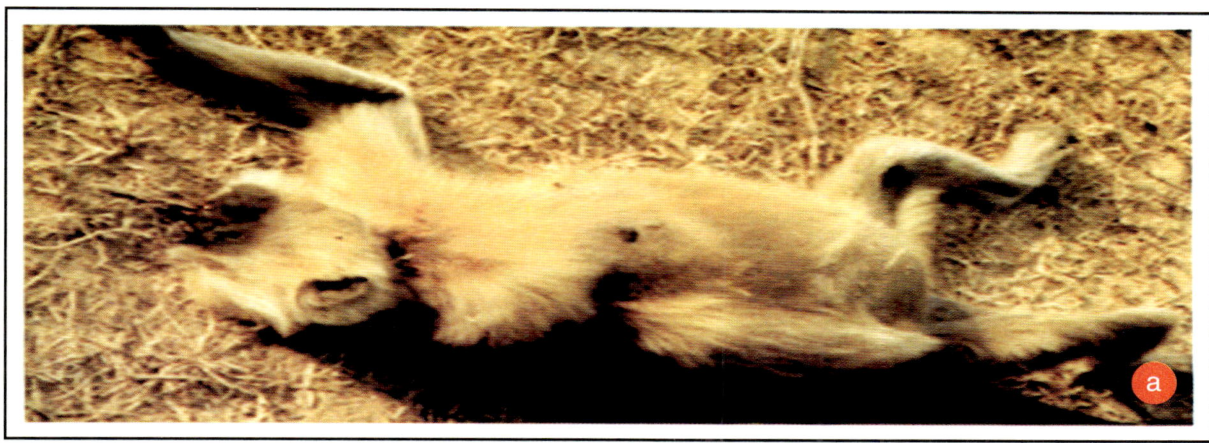

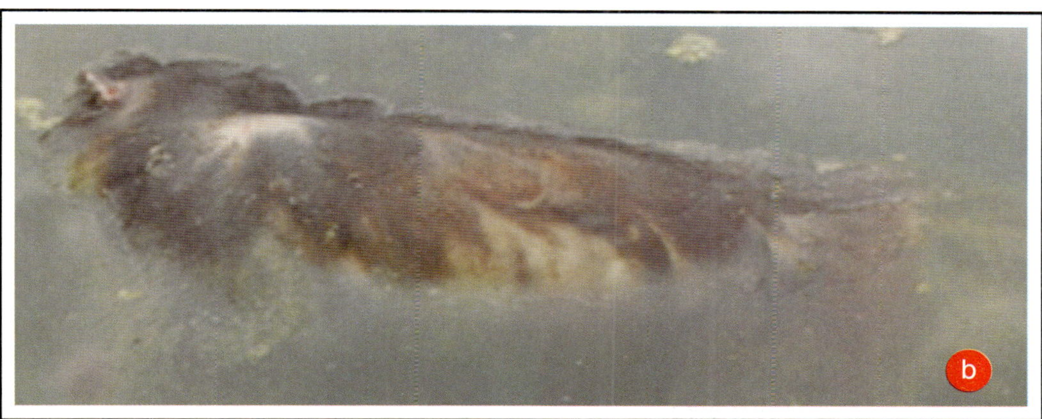

Figure 668: (a) A common langur (*S. entellus*) just fallen from a branch of the sal tree (about 40 feet high) in the forest and succumbed instantaneously. Incident occurred due to infighting between two males. (b) Carcass of rhesus macaque (*M. mulatta*) floating in a water harvesting pond.

References

Arora, B.M. (2003). Indian wildlife diseases and disorders. 1st Edition, Published by Association of Indian Zoo & Wildlife Veterinarians.

Kelewala, N.H. *et al.* (2007). A case report of bullet embedded in the mid brain of a Hanuman langur. Presentation in: *International Congress on Advances in Zoo & Wild Animals Health& Management, organized jointly by College of Vet Sc.&A.H.& AIZ&WV*, held from 26-27 April 2007 at SKUAS&T, Jammu (J&K).

Maiti, S.K. and Naveen kumar (2007-8). Anaesthesia in non-human primates. *Indian Wildlife Yearbook*, 5 &4:67-68.

Parihar, N.S. (1976). Endometrial adenocarcinoma in lion-tailed monkey (*Macaca silenus*). *Indian J. Vet. Path.* 1:19-20.

Patil, S. (2002) Studies on occurrence of diseases in certain wild mammalian and avian species in northern region of India, *M.V.Sc thesis, IVRI, Izatnagar (U.P).*

Pal, M. *et al.* (1984). Pulmonary cryptococcosis in a rhesus monkey (*Macaca mulatta*). Mykosen 27:309-12.

Singh, B. *et al.* (1981). Causes of mortality of some Zoo Animals. *Zbl. Vet. Med.* 28:596-602.

RODENTS AND PANGOLINS

Introduction

The Order Rodentia represents the largest order of mammals. It includes about 300 species under 44 genera under different families. Characteristics of the rodents are the four prominent incisor teeth, necessary for gnawing habit of the animals. Some of the species of family *Sciuridae* and *Hystrcidae* of Order Rodentia often embellish the zoo inventories. The Order Lagomorpha is distinct from Order Rodentia for having two pairs of incisors teeth. The only species in Zoological Garden being exhibit is wild hare (*Lupus nigricolis*). There are seven species of family *Manidae* in the Order Pholoidota; of which only three species namely Indian pangolin (*Manis crassicaudata*), Chinese pangolin (*M. pentadactyla*) and Malayan pangolin (*M. javanica*) are well known. Indian zoos often possess former two species but have poor inventories. Disease occurrence information in respect of rodent, lagomorph and pangolin species is almost negligible.

Developmental anomalies: No record of any congenital anomalies except birth of white and black colour variants in squirrels (*Funambulus penneti*). Both forms of porcupine (*Hystrix indica*) are well breeding in captivity. Due to space constraint photographs of white variant of porcupine (*Hystrix indica*) are included in this publication.

Eco-husbandry associated health hazards: In case of important species such as giant squirrels, hare, pangolins, though they are present in some of the zoos but are poorly studied, for their health problems. Predation of porcupines by the large cat in wild may sometimes prove to be fatal to the predator itself. One case each of porcupines predated by stray dog **(Figure 677a)** and crushed on the road by a motor vehicle is presented **(Figure 677b)**. Impact of some trauma was imputed for death of an adult wild black naped hare (*Lupus nigricolis*) as the necropsy findings showed presence of clotted blood over the heart and liver only **(Figure 671).**

Diseases: Except a case of pulmonary tuberculosis **(Figure 669)** and of intestinal serosal abscesses in giant squirrel (*Ratufa indica*) died in captivity **(Figure 670)** no other infectious conditions could be illustrated.The cases of helminthic infection included are: *Echinococcus granulosus* **(Figure 672)** in giant squirrel (*Ratufa indica*), *cysticercus fascilaris* and *Capillaria hepatica* **(Figures 673-674)** in wild rats (*Rattus narvagicus*). ecto parasitic dermatitis **(Figure 675)** in common porcupine (*Hystrix indica*) and soft tick infestation **(Figure 676)** without any apparent pathological effect in Chinese pangolin (*M. pentadactyla*) were detected.

RODENTS & PANGOLINS

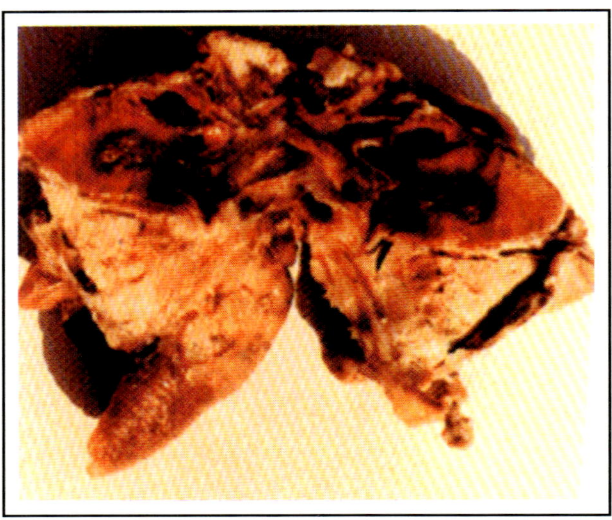

Figure 669: Photograph showing pulmonary tuberculous lesions in a giant squirrel (*Ratufa indica*) died in captivity.

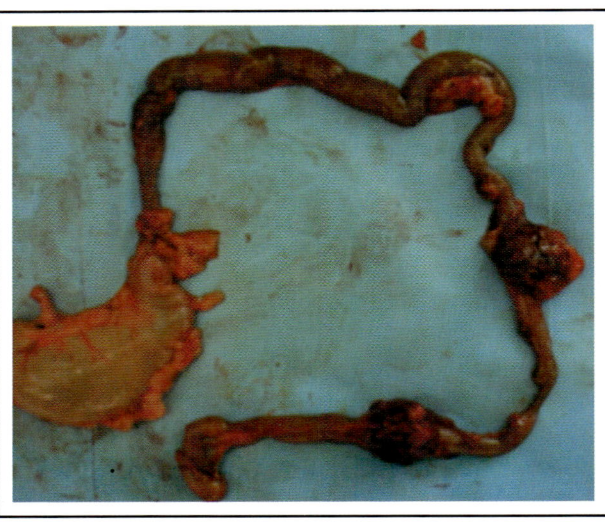

Figure 670: Photograph showing abscesses in the serosal surface of intestine of Indian giant squirrel (*Ratufa indica*) died in Zoological Park, Chennai (Courtesy: Thirumurugan, R).

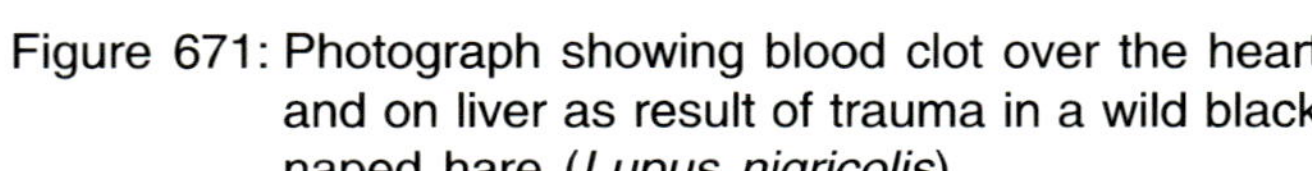

Figure 671: Photograph showing blood clot over the heart and on liver as result of trauma in a wild black naped hare (*Lupus nigricolis*).

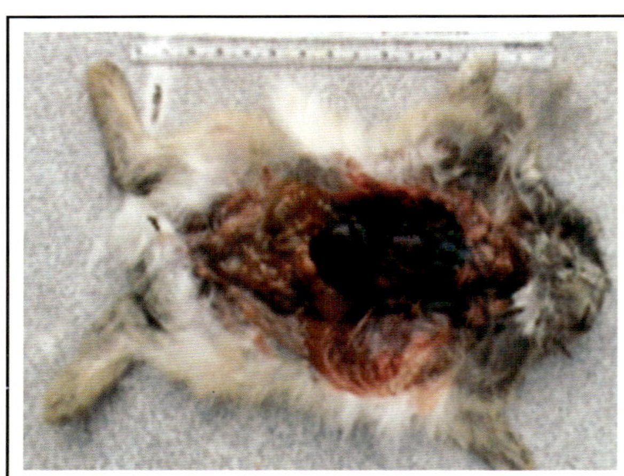

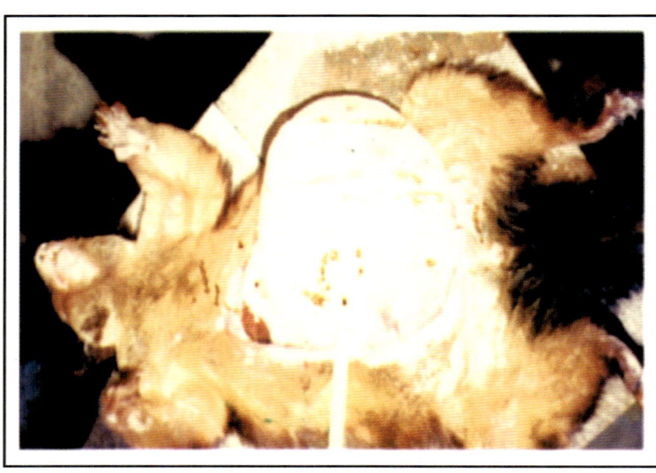

Figure 672: Photograph showing hydatid cyst of 122mm in diameter of *Echinococus granulosus* in the abdomen of Giant squirrel (*Ratufa indica*) died in captivity.

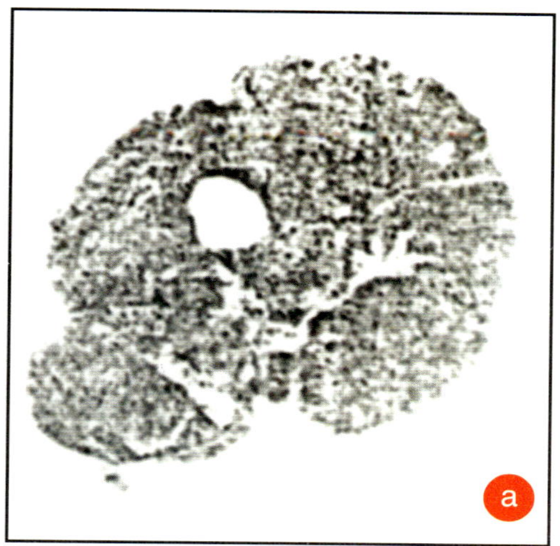

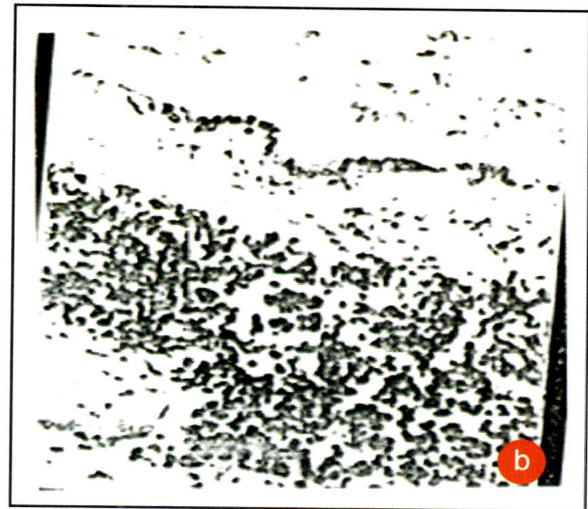

Figure 673: Photograph of liver from wild rat (*Rattus norvagicus*) showing about pea sized whitish cysts of *Cysticercus fasciolaris*. This infection is not uncommon in wild individuals.(b) Photomicrograph of (a) showing mononuclear cellular infiltration in the adjoining parenchyma to cysts. H&E, x250 (Somvanshi *et al.*, 1994).

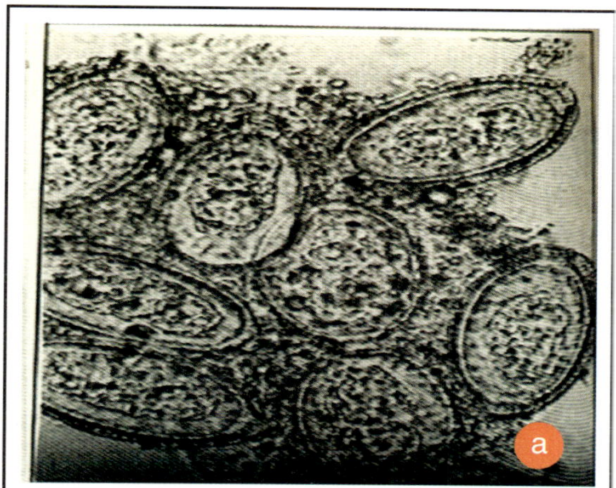

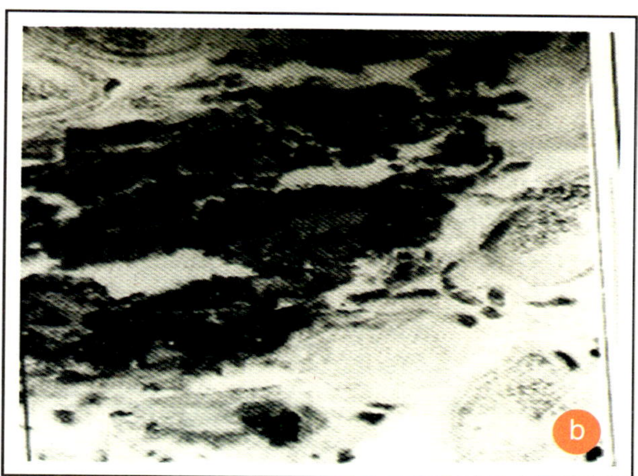

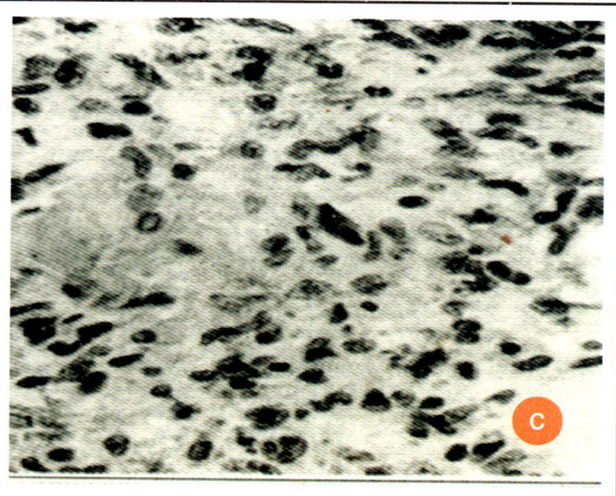

Figure 674: Spontaneous *Capillaria hepatica* infection in wild rats (*Rattus ratus*).Photographs showing:(a) Oval- thick- shelled bipolar plugged unsegmented eggs of *C. hepatica*. (b) Mesentric tissue reaction with mononulear cell infiltration H&E, x 200. (c) Calcification of degenerating eggs of *C. hepatica* and surrounding tissue. (Somvanshi *et al.*, 1995).

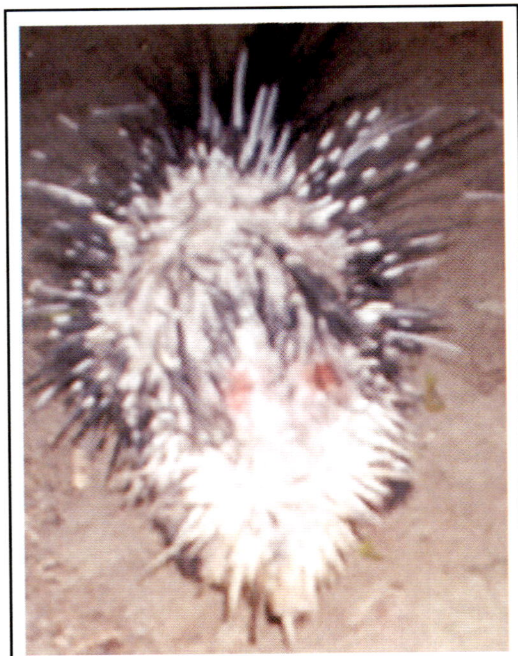

Figure 675: Photograph showing severe lesions of dermatitis in porcupine (*Hystrix indica*) belonged to Zoological Garden,Gwalior (M.P).

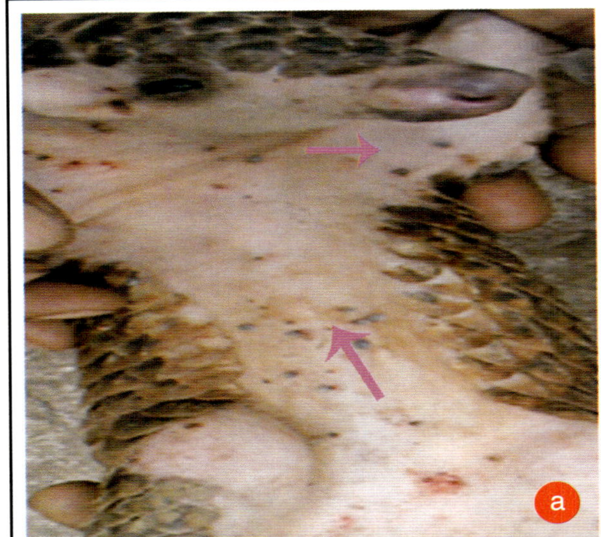

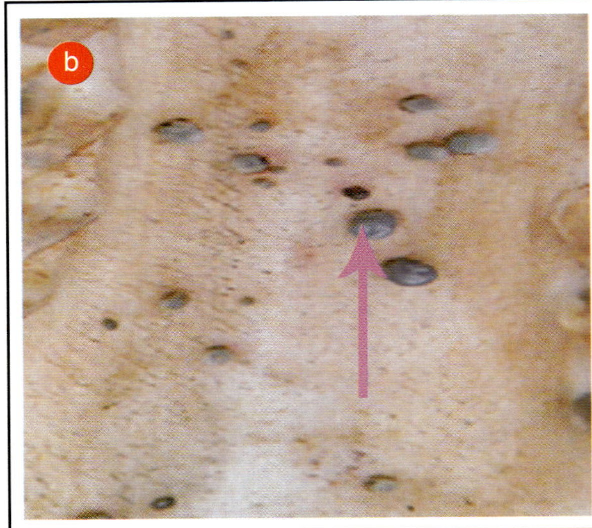

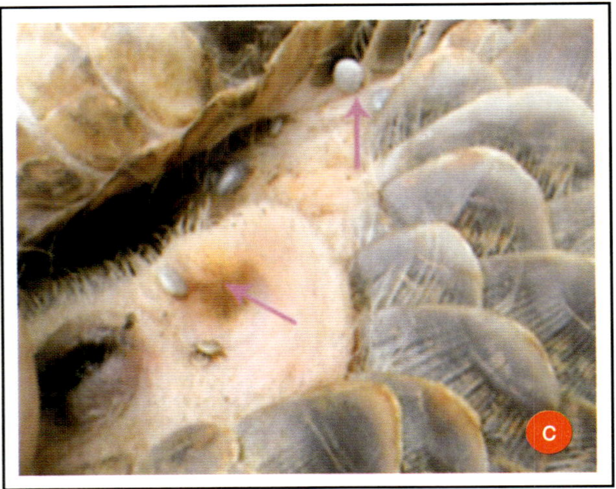

Figure 676: Photographs of a 2- month- old Chinese pangolin (*M. pentadactyla*) showing :(a,b) tick infestation in the ventral portion of the body. (c) Ticks in the ear and by the side of scales. (Courtesy: Shamistha Chakaraborty).

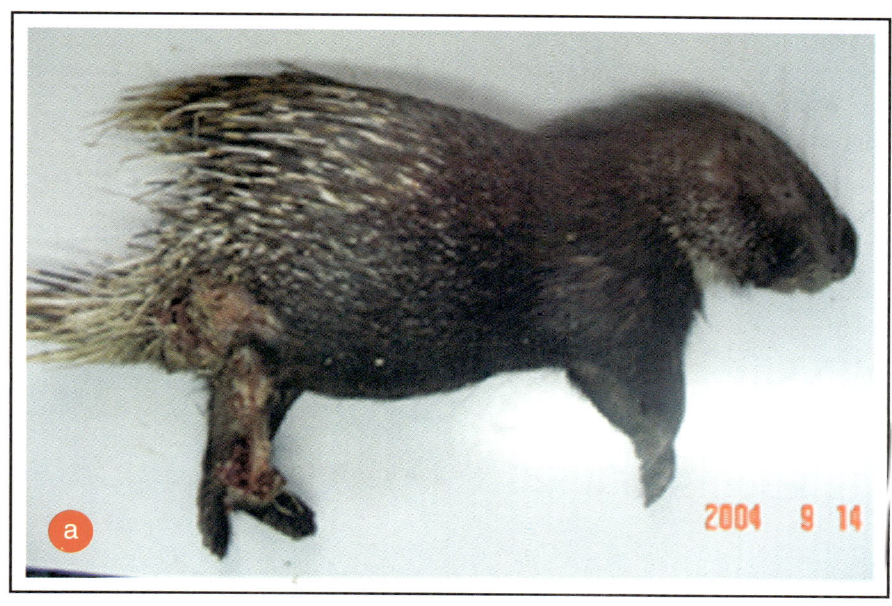

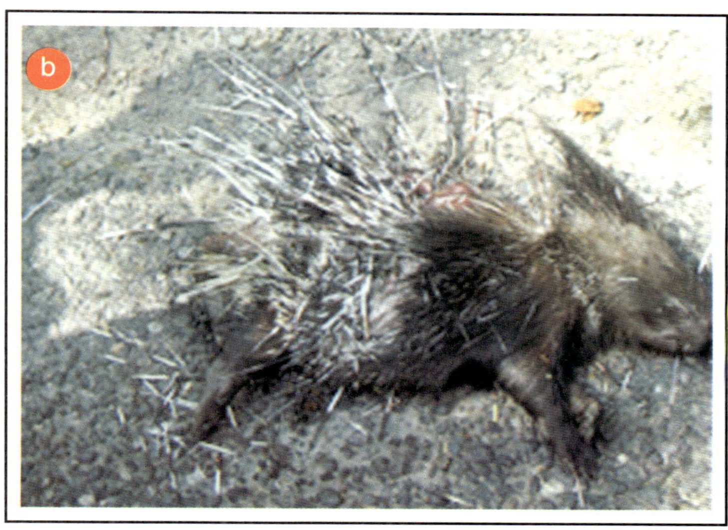

Figure 677: (a) Carcass of wild porcupine (*Hystrix indica*). It was killed by the stray dog. Note deep wounds on its right leg caused by dog bite. (b) Porcupine (*H. indica*) crushed under motor vehicle.

References

Somvanshi R. *et al.* (1994). Pathological changes associated with spontaneous cysticercus fasciolaris infected with wild rats. *Indian J. Comp. Microbiol Immunol. Infect. Dis.* 15(July& Oct.).

Somvanshi, R *et al.* (1995). Spontaneous *Capillaria hepatica* infection in wild rats, *Rattus ratus Indian J.Vet Path.* 19(1):44-45.

PERISSODACTYLIDS

Family: *Rhinocerotidae, Genus* -Rhinoceros

Species –Great Asian one –horned rhinoceros (*Rhinoceros unicornis*)

Family: *Equidae* Genus: *Equus.* Species/Sub species: (i) *Equus hemionus khur (ii) Equus hemionis kiang*

Introduction

India's current population of rhinoceros (*Rhinoceros unicornis*) is about 2200 in natural habitats and about 100 in captivity. Kaziranga National Park of Assam possesses about 85% of the wild population. Thus, the large number of rhinoceros existed in a single protected area, which is always exposed to flood catastrophy and poaching **(Figure 712).** The small populations of the species existing in Jaldapara Wildlife Sanctuary and Gorumara National Park of West Bengal, and in Dudwa N.P of Uttar Pradesh are enlarging but at the same time moving of animals out of the earmarked habitat areas is often confronted. Wild ass (*Equus hemionus khur)* maximum population in wild exists in Runn of Kuch of Gujarat and of *Equus hemionus kiang* in Tibet and Ladakh. Zebra (*Equus burchelii*) is exotic species and a good number exists in our Zoos but only there is limited pictorial documentation of its health problems. Studies on occurrence of diseases of rhinoceros (*R. unicornis*) and both subspecies of wild ass (*E. hemionus*) so far have not been taken off. Otherwise how death of several rhinoceroses between, 2001-2005 at Kaziranga National Park (Arora, 2007) have been ascribed to old age? Hence, pathological illustrations presented in the chapter remained inadequate in number.

Eco-husbandry associated health hazards: At times, fighting between tiger (*P. tigris*) and rhinoceros (*R. unicornis*) leave either one or both injured with severe multiple lacerated skin wounds. But it is the rhinoceros calf, which is mostly victim of tiger **(Figures 713,717).** Capture myopathy and superficial wounds on the maxillary and flank regions on account of improper and unsuitable transportation cage/crate are likely to be experienced **(Figures 714,720).**Con-specific conflicts during breeding season and at occasion of release of rhinoceroses into new population cannot be ruled out **(Figure 715)**. Infighting wounds in wild ass may prove fatal **(Figure 716)**. An adult female rhinoceros which was introduced in a natural habitat when tranquilized by an expert for radio collaring had fallen suddenly and suffered from fracture of knee joint and ribs, which were diagnosed after couple of days and despite huge medical aid she had died **(Figure 721)**. It was most painful experience for all of us.

Problem of enteroliths formation in the digestive tract **(Figures 685 to 686)** in zebra (*Equus brucheli*, an exotic sp.) in comparison to other equid species is more. The propensity of enteroliths formation in the species could be probably due to excess amount of magnesium and phosphorus consumed in diet consist of wheat bran and sluggish movement of the intestine as animal being in confinement without any predator threat nearby. Rarely problem of stomach impaction in rhinoceros due to inferior quality of food may be faced **(Figure 687).** Rhinoceros may eat any object lying in its enclosure. Impaction of colon due to sand has caused death of two rhinoceroses in a zoo (Arora, 2003). Among the reproductive problems encountered ,pictorial presentation of dystocia due to mal presentation of the foetus has been made, one case each of wild ass (*E. hemionus khur*) and rhinoceros (*R. unicornis*) maintained at two different zoos **(Figures 700 to 701)**.

Diseases. (A) Infectious & Parasitic: Not many infectious diseases affecting rhinoceros (*R. unicornis*) populations are recognized. Tuberculosis, pasteurellosis, anthrax, salmonellosis **(Figure 689)**, rabies (**Figure 708**) are the important infectious diseases recorded in rhinoceroses.

Haemorrhagic gastro-enteritis in rhinoceros (*R. unicornis*) died in captivity was related to *Salmonella* sp. infection **(Figure 689)**. Nodular and ulcerative lesions on the large intestinal mucosal surface with severe oedema were related to mixed infection of *E.coli* and *Candida* sp. in rhinoceros (*R. unicornis*) calves **(Figure 691)**. A case of *Staphylococcus pyogens* mastitis **(Figure 702)** in a recently calved rhinoceros (*R. unicornis*) was recorded, which appears to be the first report. After the outbreaks of African horse sickness in wild ass (*E. hemionus khur*) in 1961and 1962 no other infectious diseases has been encountered in the wild population of species. However, certain infectious diseases recorded in native and exotic equine species in zoological facilities are cited here and illustrated pictorially. For example, pulmonary nocardiosis (**Figure 680**) and orchitis due to botryomycosis **(Figure 703)** in Zebra (*Equus burchelii*, an exotic sp.), Strangle **(Figure 681),** and rabies **(Figure706)** in wild asses (*E. hemionus khur*). There have been rabies cases in rhinoceros (*R. unicornis*). A case of *Balantidium coli* was recorded in rhinoceros calf died in captivity **(Figure 692).**

Of helminthic infections massive load of *Anoplacephala sp.* **(Figure 696)** was found in rhinoceroses (*R. unicornis*) died in captivity and in wild, which may not alone be the primary cause of severe enteritis. A case of liver fluke (*F. gigantica*) in rhinoceros (*R. unicornis*) died in wild **(Figure 695)** appears to be the first report. A case of verminous pneumonia due to *Dictyocalus arnfieldi* **(Figure 682)** in Zebra (*E. burchelii,* an exotic sp.) is presented.

(B) Neoplasms: Only few reports of neoplasms such as intrahepatic bile duct carcinoma **(Figure 698)**, adenoma of intestine **(Figure 699)**, uterine adenocarcinoma **(Figure 705)** in rhinoceros (*R. unicornis*) are illustrated. For more information on the neoplasms of perissodactylids, readers may consult Indian Wildlife Diseases & Disorders by Arora (2003).

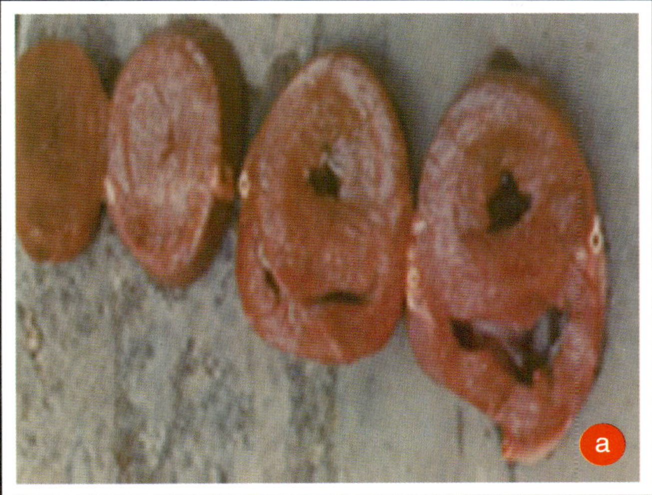

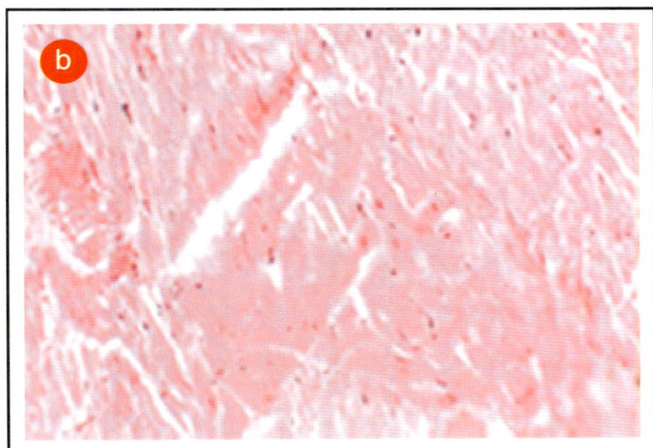

Figure 678: (a)Photograph of sections of heart of wild rhinoceros (*R. unicornis*) calf showing haemorrhages in capture myopathy. (b) Photomicrograph of (a) showing hyalin degeneration and haemorrhages in cardiac muscle. H&E, x400.

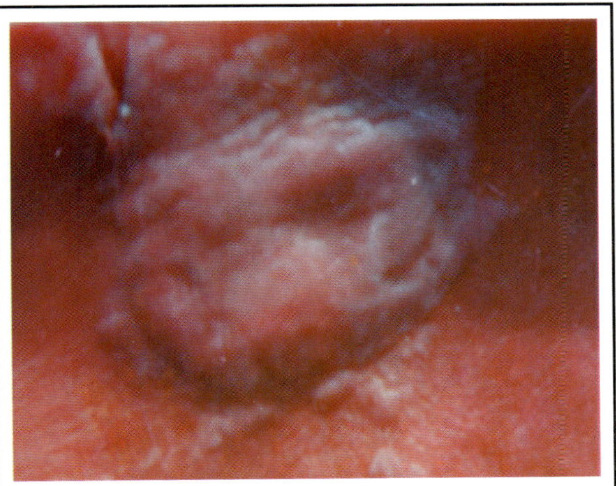

Figure 679: Photograph showing sudanophilic artheromatous plaque in the arch of abdominal aorta of zebra (*Equus burchelii*,an exotic species) in Zoological Garden, Guwahati, Assam.

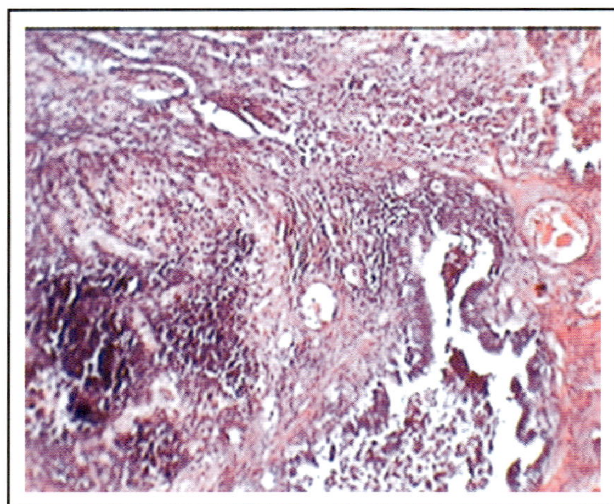

Figure 680: Photomicrograph of lung of Zebra (*Equus burchelii*, an exotic sp.) showing Nocardial pulmonary abscess. Note basophilic granules with irregular border. H&E, x100.

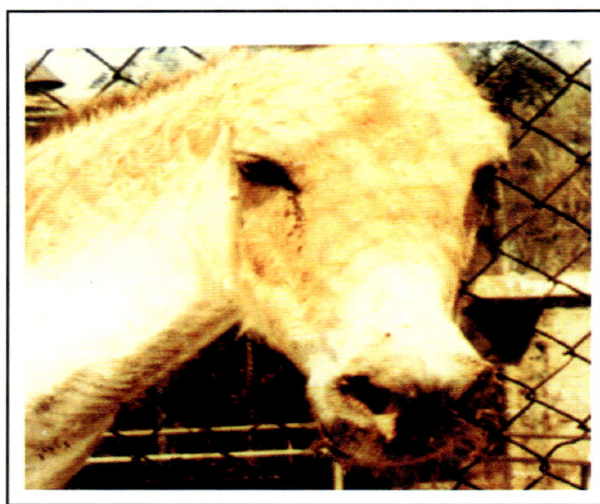

Figure 681: Wild ass (*E. hemionus khur*) suffering from strangles (*Streptococcus equi*). Note thick slightly yellowish purulent discharge from the nostrils.

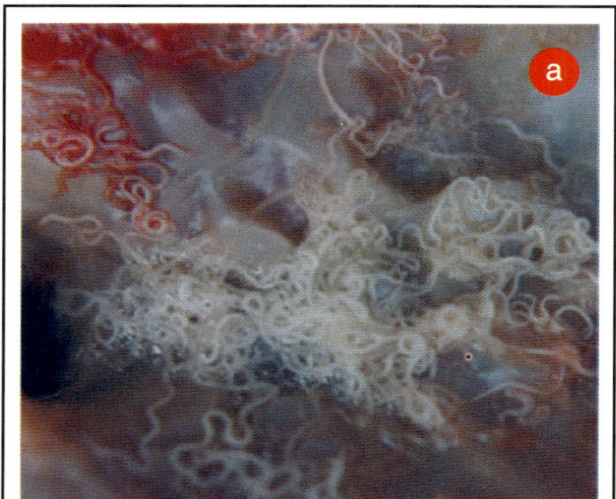

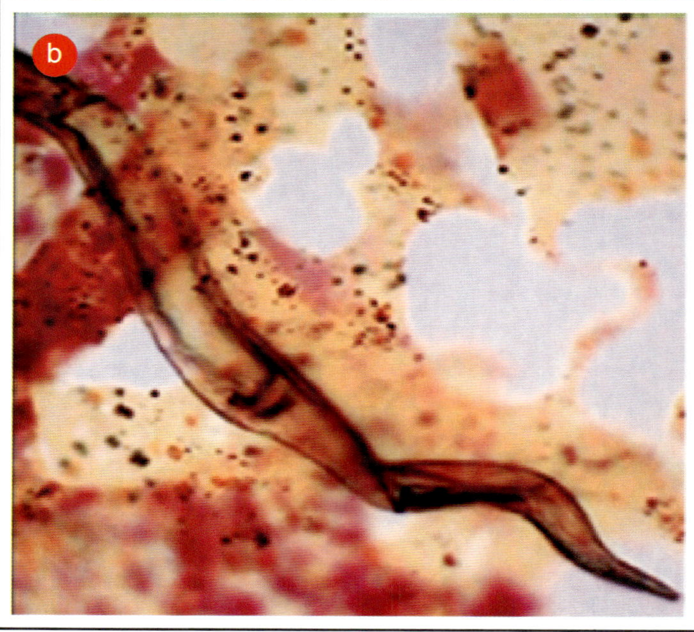

Figure 682: Photograph showing clumps of *Dictyocaulus arnfieldi* mixed with blood tinged froth in bronchi of zebra (*Equus burchelii*, an exotic sp.) died in captivity. Photomicrographs showing;(b) *Dictyocaulus arnfieldi* larva in the lung H.& E, x400.

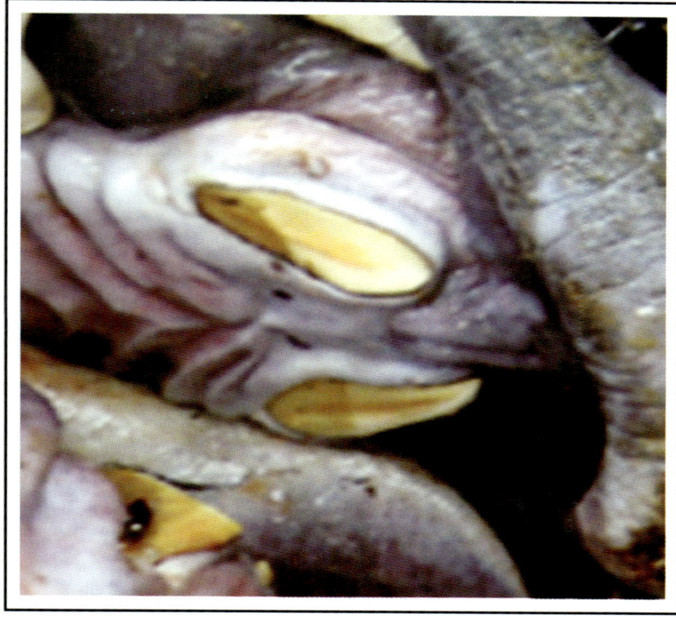

Figure 683: Photograph showing complete wearing of upper incisors in captive rhinoceros (*R. unicornis*).

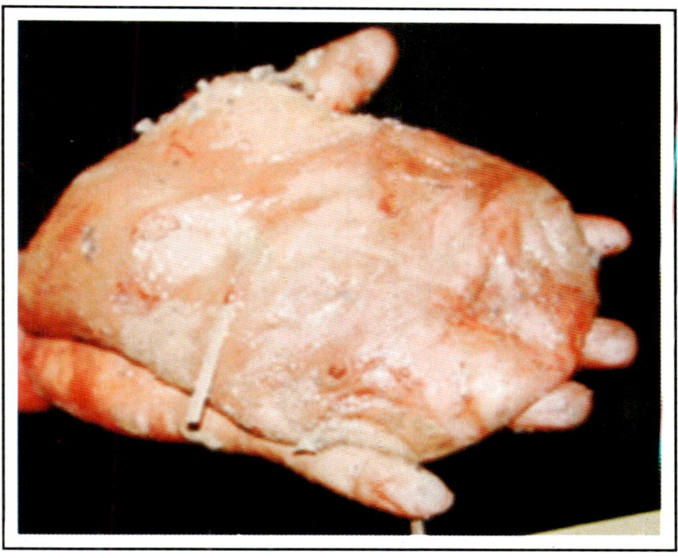

Figure 684: Photograph showing pustular vesicles on the dorsal surface of tongue of rhinoceros (*R. unicornis*) died at Zoological Park, Kanpur (U.P).

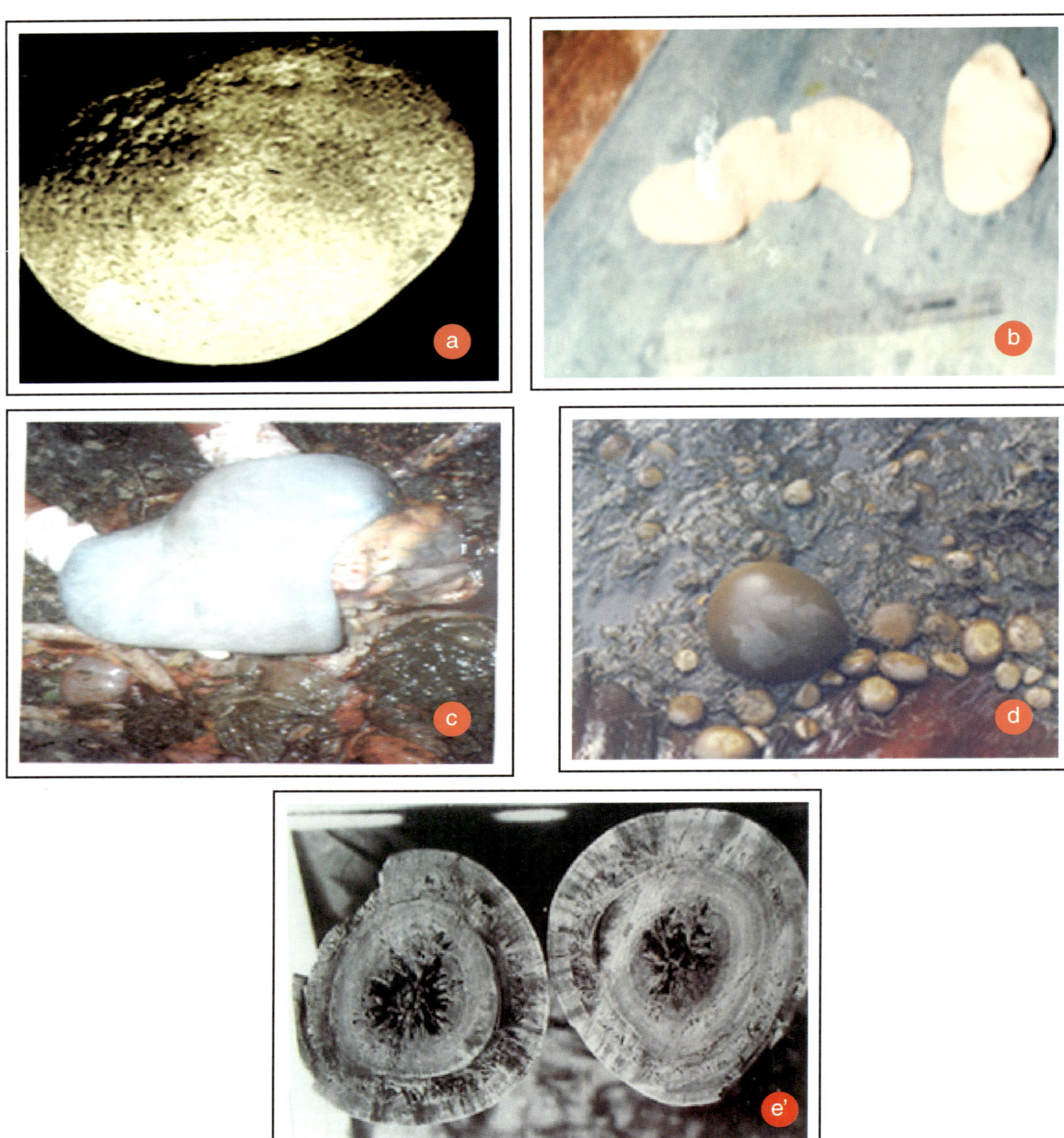

Figure 685: Enteroliths of different shapes and sizes from the large intestines of zebras (*Equus bruchelii*, an exotic sp.) died in Indian captive facilities:(a) Round like stone weighing 6.5 kg, (b) Cylindrical, (c) Saddle shaped, 1.2 kg. (d) Sandy and stone type. (d') Cut section of a large enterolith of (d).

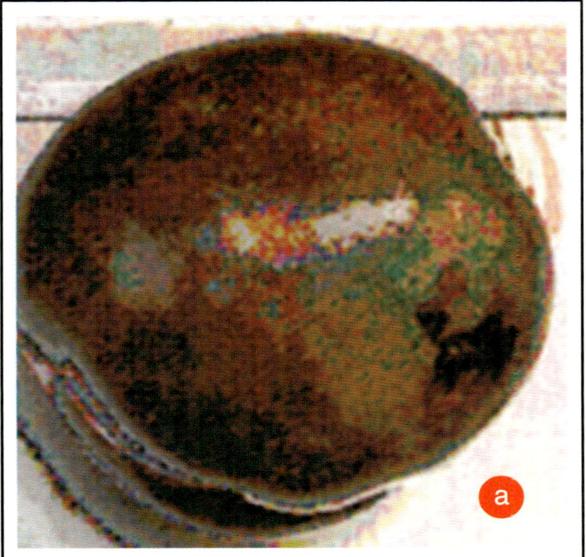

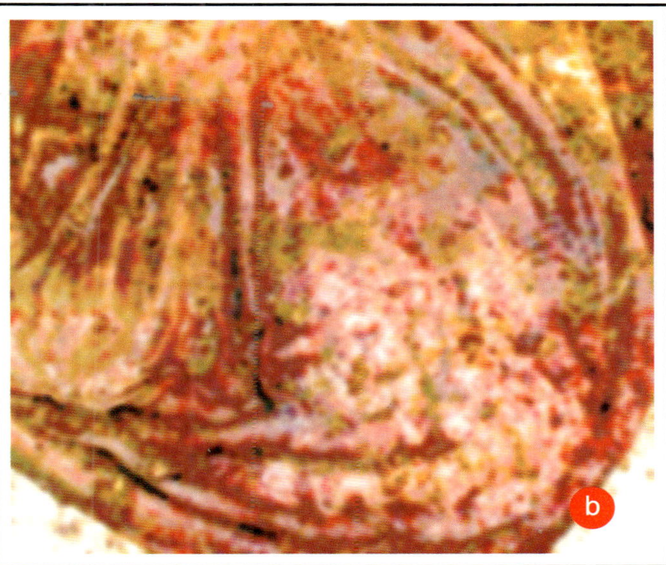

Figure 686 : Photograph showing (a) An enterolith causing intestinal obstruction and severe enteritis (b) in zebra (*Equus bruchelii*, an exotic sp.) died in Zoological facility Bangalore (Courtesy: Harish, B.R.).

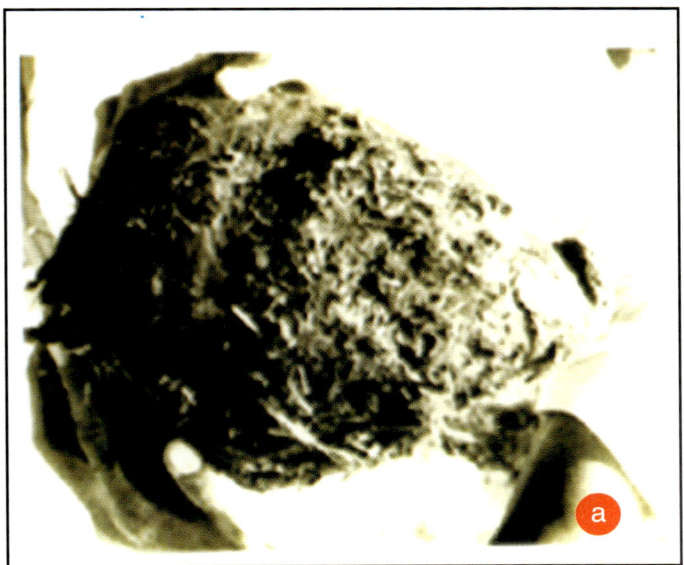

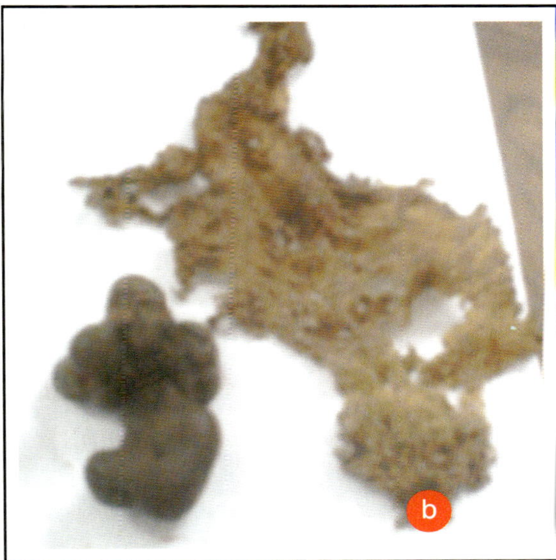

Figure 687 : Photographs of fecolith which caused impaction of: (a) Stomach in rhinoceros (*R. unicornis*) died at National Zoological Park, New Delhi. (b) Intestine of Zebra (*Equus burchelii*, an exotic sp.) died at Zoological Park, Patna, Bihar (Courtsey: Ajay, S.K.).

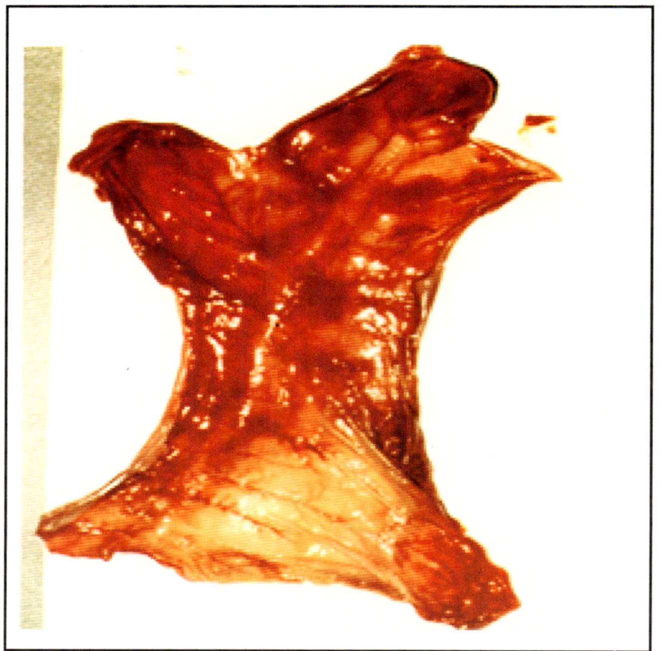

Figure 688: Intestinal mucosa showing severe haemorrhages and congestion in wild ass (*E.h.khur*) died of rabies. The case is also referred under nervous system.

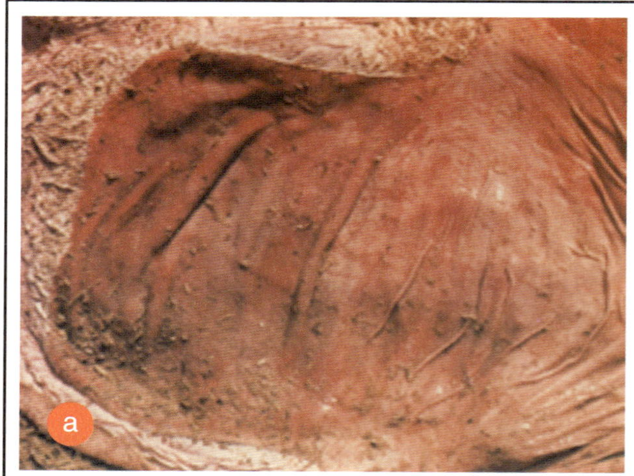

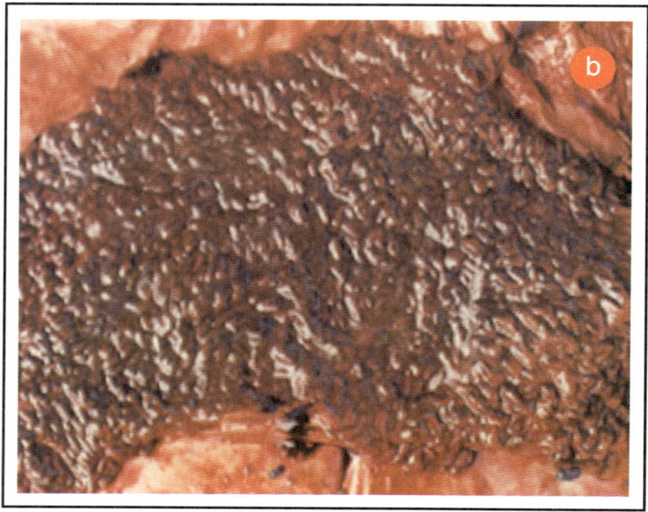

Figure 689: Haemorrhagic gastro-enteritis in rhinoceros (*R. unicornis*) died in captivity. Photographs showing haemorrhages in the (a) glandular part of the stomach and (b) intestine. Lesions are attributed to *Salmonella* infection.

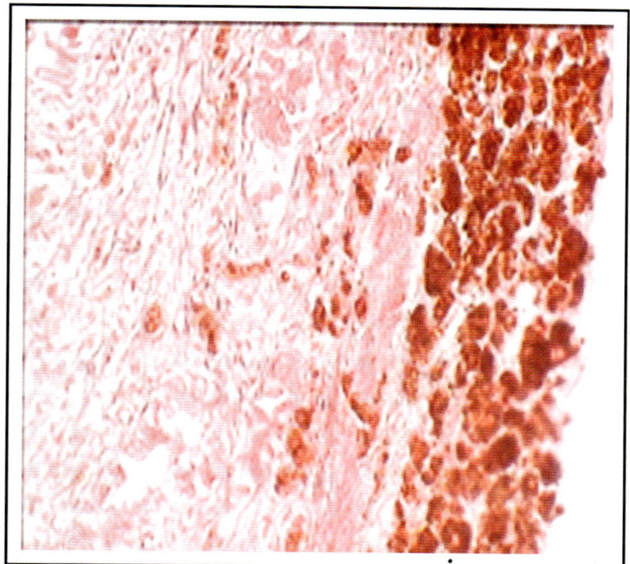

Figure 690: Photomicrograph of ileum of rhinoceros (*R. unicornis*) showing haemosiderin pigmention in the mucosa. H&E, x 400.

Figure 691: Photograph of large intestine of rhinoceros (*R. unicornis*) calf showing nodular and ulcerative lesions on the mucosal surface with severe oedema in mixed infection of *E.coli* and *Candida* sp.

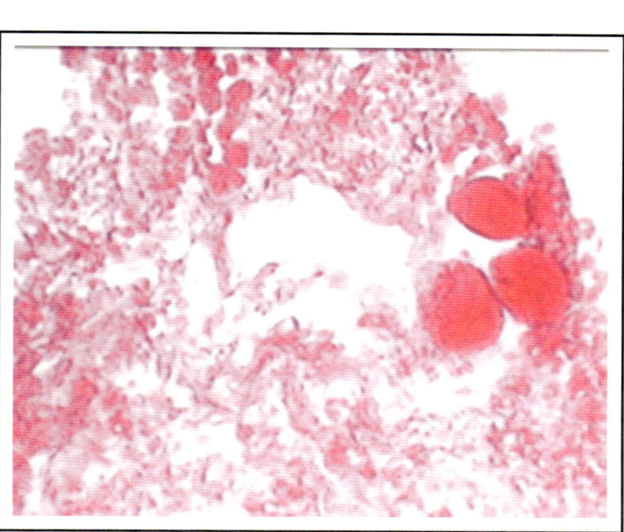

Figure 692: Photomicrograph of large intestine from rhinoceros (*R. unicornis*) showing *Balantidium coli* infection. H&E, x 400.

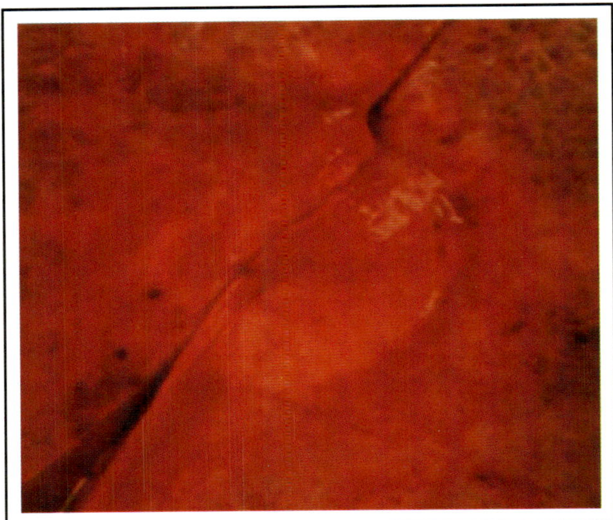

Figure 693: Photograph showing tuberculous nodule in the liver of rhinoceros (*R. unicornis*) .

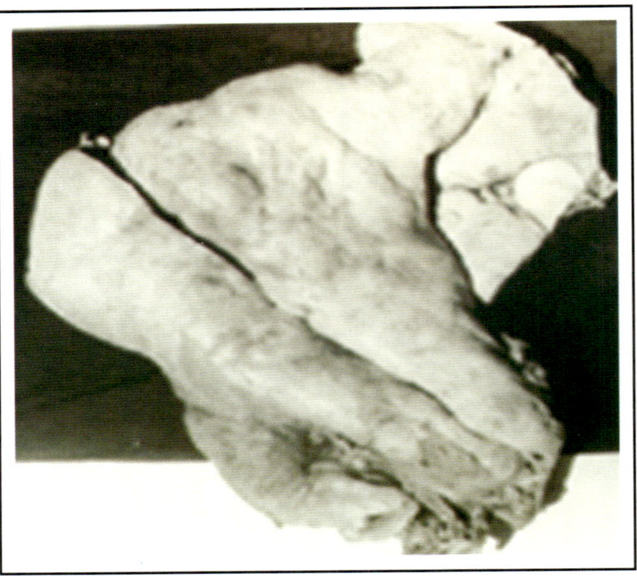

Figure 694: Photograph showing enlarged mesenteric lymph node filled with pus due to botryomycosis in Zebra (*Equus brucheli*,an exotic sp.) formation fixed specimen.

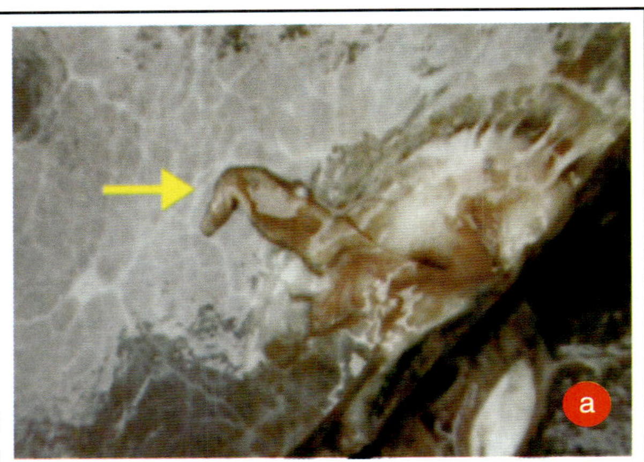

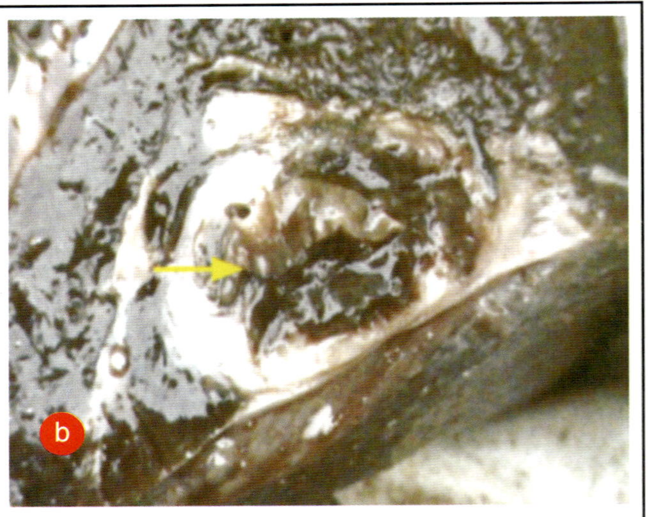

Figure 695: Photographs showing :(a) *Fasciola gigantica* in the liver of rhinoceros (*R. unicornis*) died in the Pobitora Wildlife Sanctuary, Assam (b) Necrotic mass cut open in the liver with *F. gigantica.*

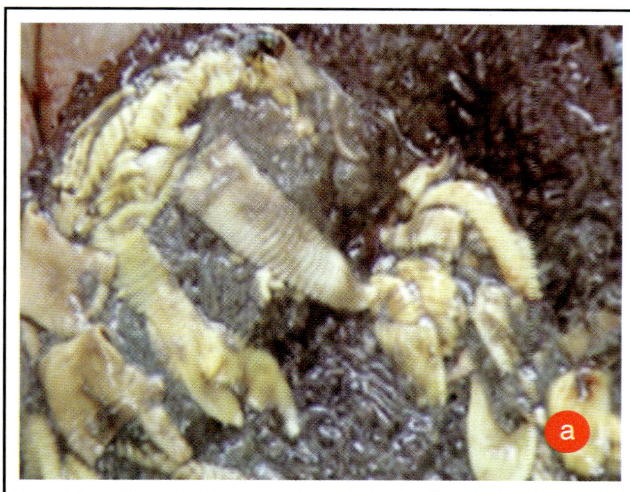

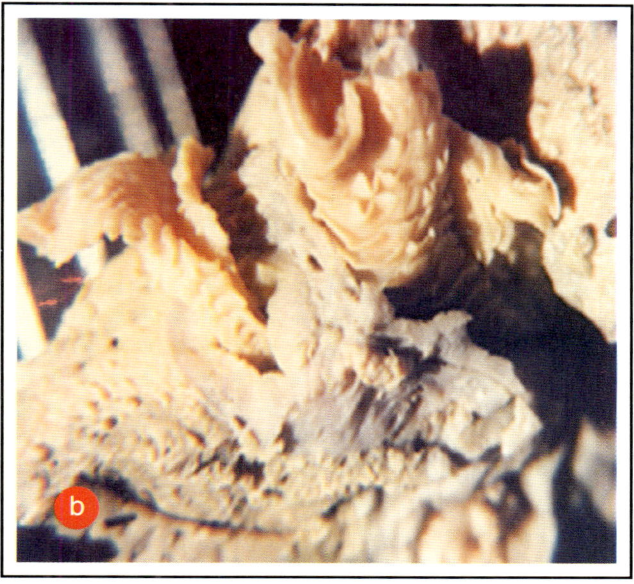

Figure 696: Photograph showing: (a) Massive *Anoplocephala sp.* tape worms in ntestine of rhinoceros (*R. unicornis*) died in Kaziranga NationalPark, Assam. (b) Also *Anoplocephala sp.* in the bile duct of (a).

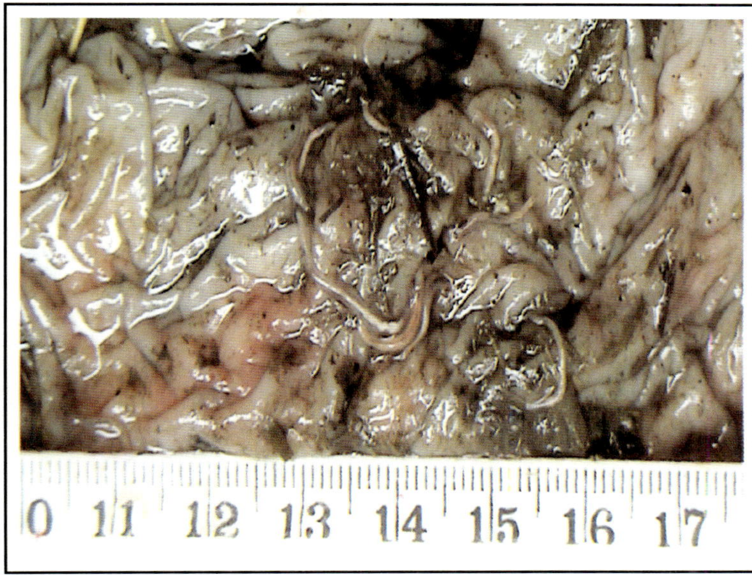

Figure 697. *Chabertia* sp in the small intestine of rhinoceros (*R. unicornis*) died in the Pobitora Wildlife Sanctuary, Assam.

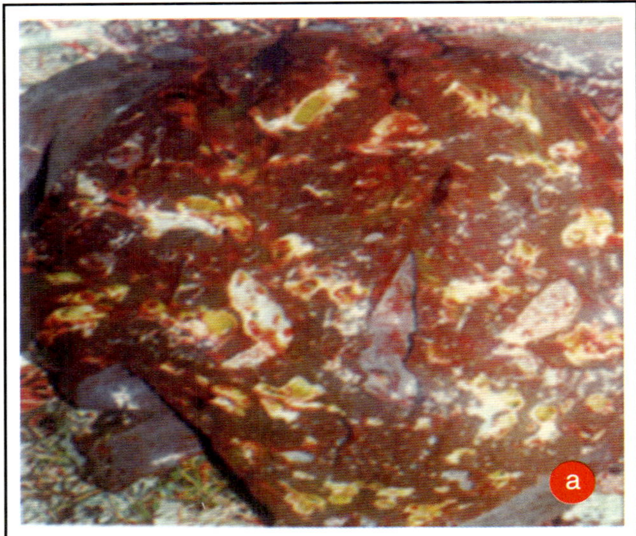

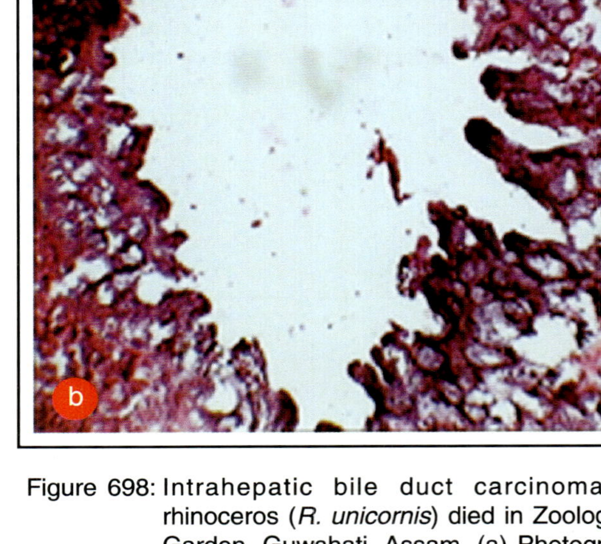

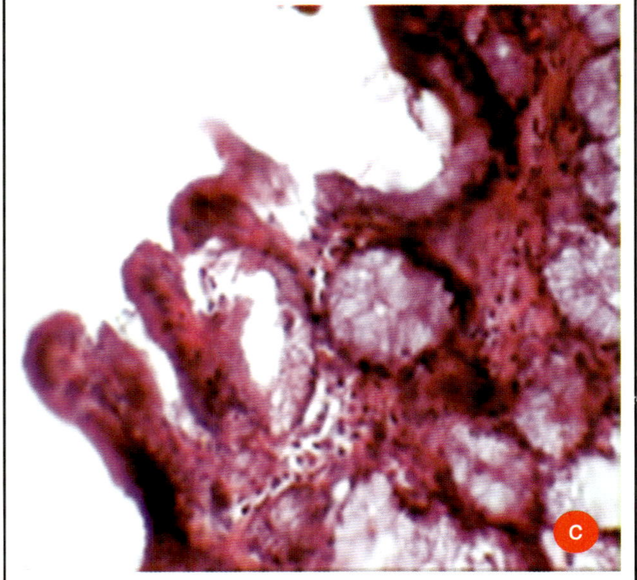

Figure 698: Intrahepatic bile duct carcinoma in rhinoceros (*R. unicornis*) died in Zoological Garden, Guwahati, Assam. (a) Photograph of segital section of liver showing extensive proliferation of new bile ducts filled with bile. (b) Photomicrograph showing characteristic histological changes of biliary epithelium with typical papillary projections and acini formation. H&E, x 100 (c) Higher magnification of (b) showing basophilic mucin in the lumen of neoplastic tubules/ acini.The nuclei are round or oval and vascular.H&E, x 400.

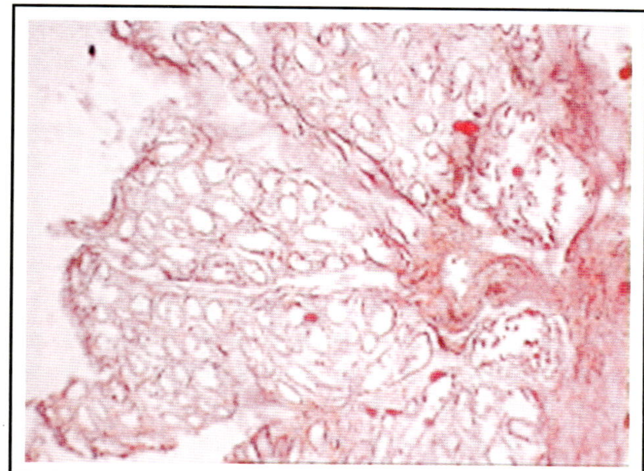

Figure 699: Photomicrograph of intestine of rhinoceros (*R. unicornis*) showing adenoma. H&E, x100.

Reproductive System

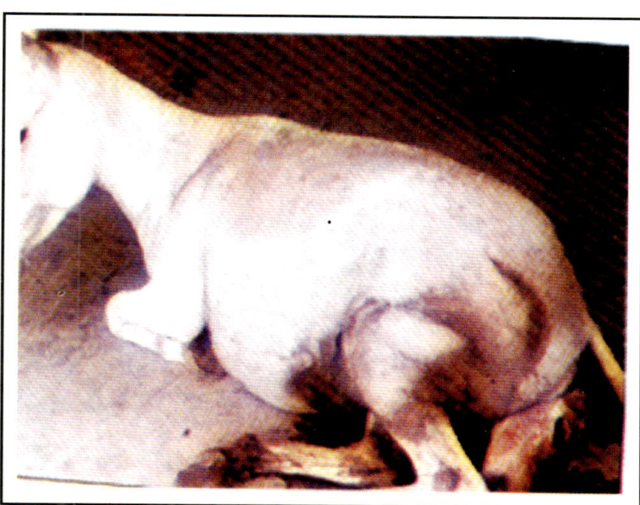

Figure 700: Dystocia in wild ass (*E. h. khur*) due to mal presentation of foetus in captivity (Courtesy: Jani, R.G.).

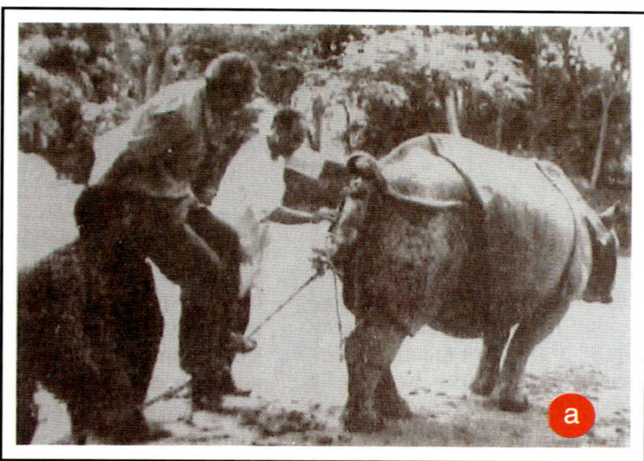

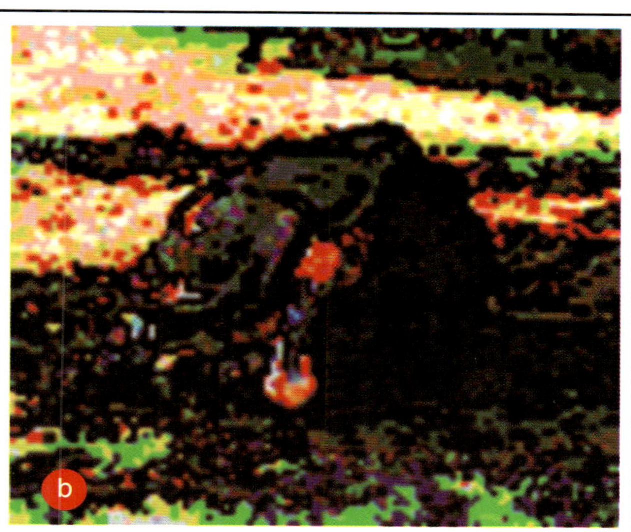

Figure 701: (a) Dystocia in rhinoceros (*R. unicornis*) belonged to Z.G.Guwahati, Assam. Photograph showing extraction of dead foetus manually. (Tamuli *et al.,* 2000) (b) A female rhinoceros (*R. unicornis*) in labour pain just prior to calving in Biological Park, Patna (Bihar).(Courtesy: Ajay, S.K.).

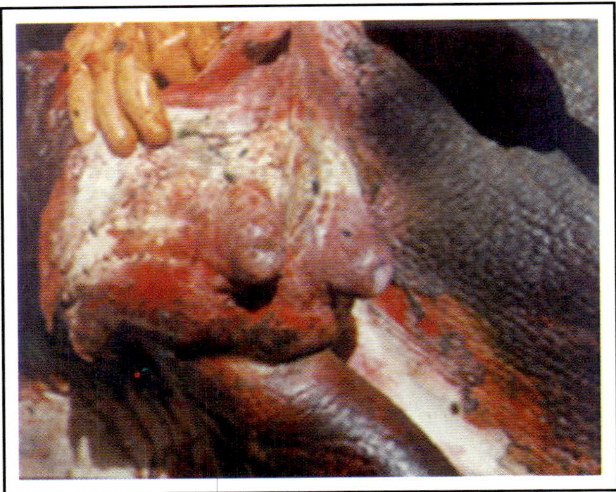

Figure 702: Photograph showing swollen udder due to *Staphylococcus pyogenes* mastitis. in rhinoceros (*R. unicornis*) died in Zoological garden, Guwahati (Assam).

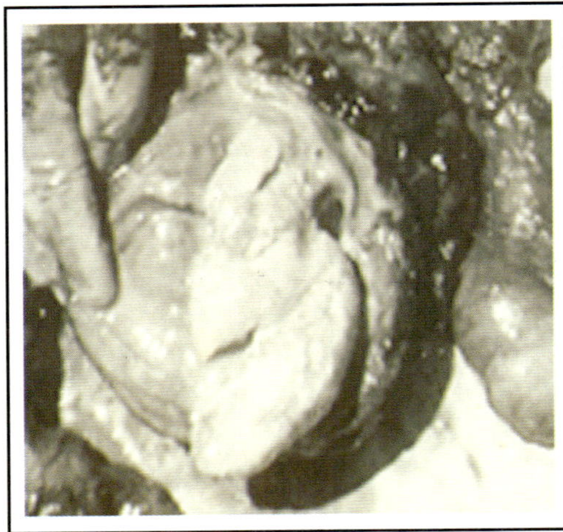

Figure 703: Enlarged testis, due to botryomycosis abscessation in Zebra (*Equus brucheli*,an exotic sp.) died in Zoological Garden, Guwahati, Assam.

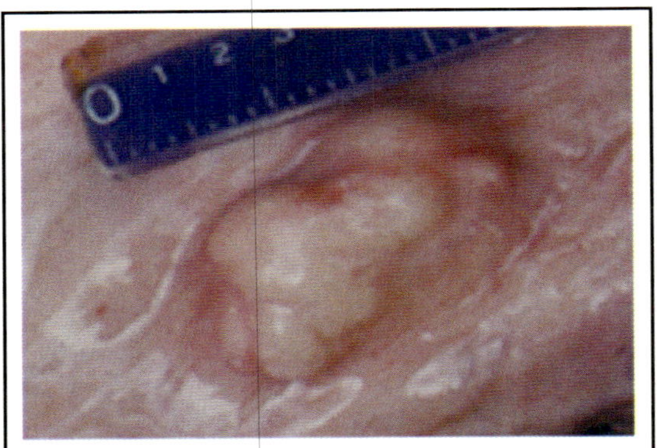

Figure 704. Photograph showing fibroma on the serosal surface of uterus.

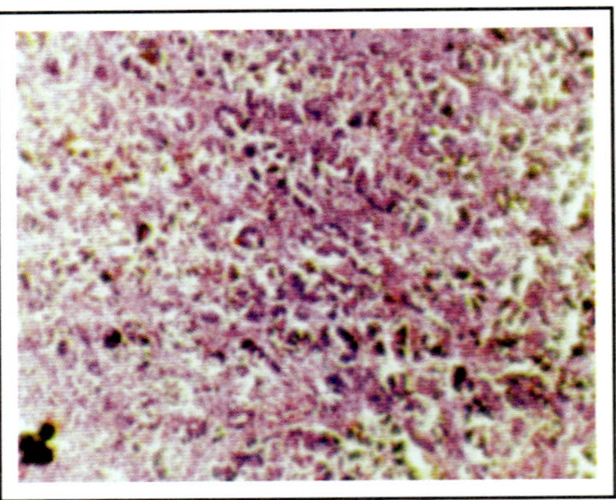

Figure 705. Photomicrograph of uterine adenocarcinoma in rhino (*R. unicornis*). Note the glandular pattern (Courtesy: Panda, S.K. & Nath, I.).

Nervous System

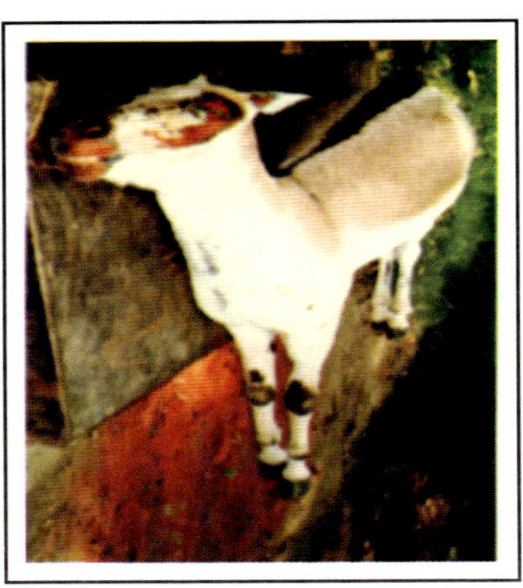

Figure 706: Wild ass (*E. h.khur*) died of rabies at National Zoological Park,New Delhi after clinical course of 8 days.

Figure 707: Severe congestion of brain encountered in rhinoceros (*R.unicornis*) without attributed to any factor involved.

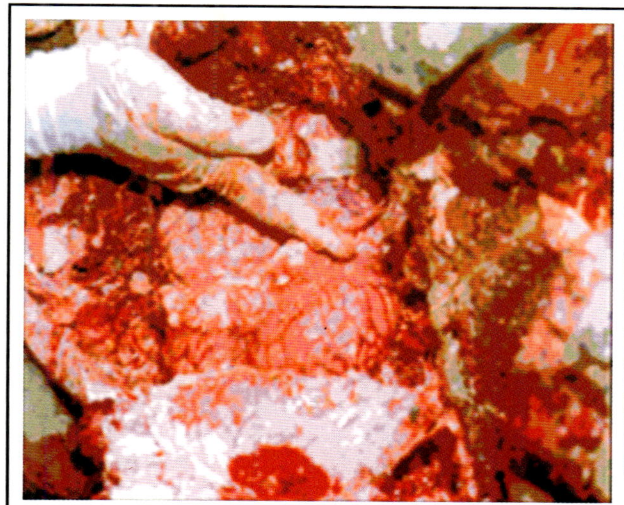

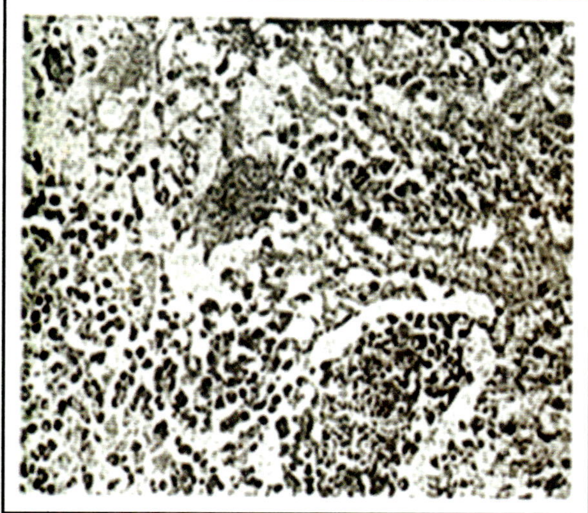

Case (i)a

Case (i)b

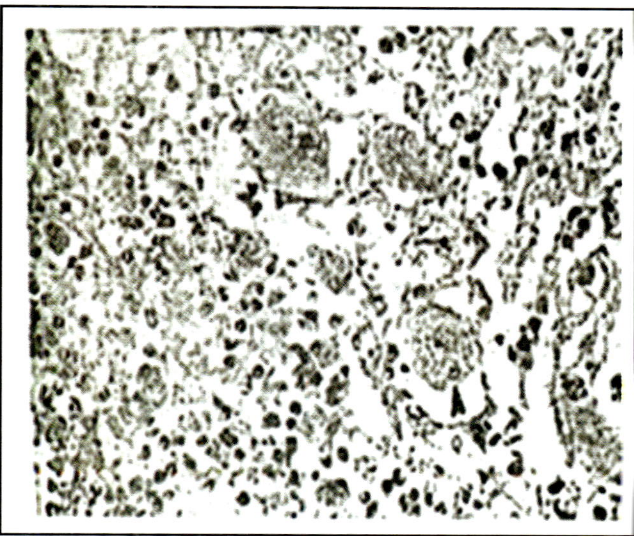

Case (ii)

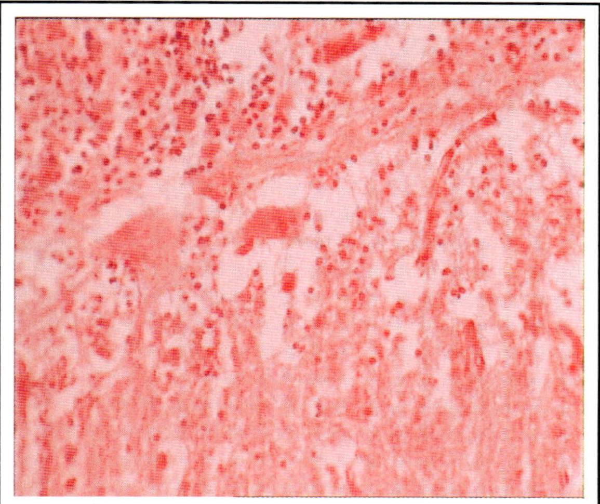

Figure 708: Case (i)a Photomicrograph of brain from rhinoceros (*R. unicornis*) died in Zoological Garden, Lucknow (U.P.) showing: (a) Perivascular cuffing and Negri bodies in neuron. H&E, x 950 (b) Negri body (spear) in a Purkinje cell of cerebellum and a degenerated neuron (arrow) Schleifstein's stain. x 950 (Mukherjee *et al.*, 1984). Case (ii): Negri body in a Purkinje cell of cerebellum of a rhinoceros died at Z.G. Guwahati, Assam. H&E x 400 (Rahman *et al.*, 2004).

Sense Organs

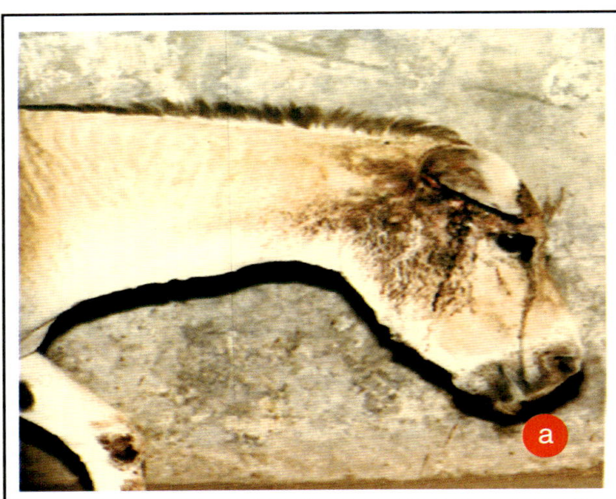

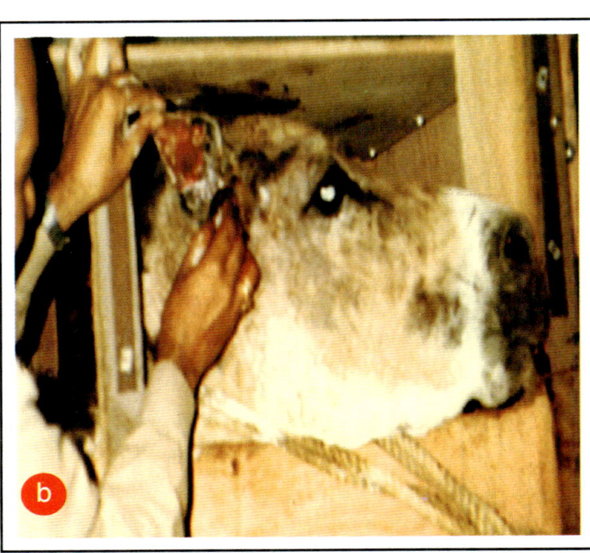

Figure 709: Photographs (a,b) showing ear lesions suspected of Stephanofilarial infection in a wild ass (*E. hemionus khur*) in a captive facility.

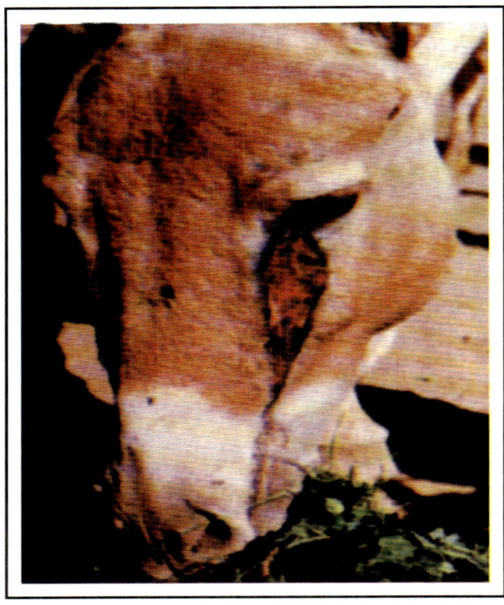

Figure 710: Wild ass (*E. hemionus khur*) showing ulcerative lesions extending downwards from inner canthus of eye. *Alternaria sp*. and *Penicillinum* sp. were isolated on cultural examination, but the specific etiology could not be related. This condition was said to recur in rainy season in all stock of wild ass being maintained at Zoological Garden, Junagarh (Gujarat).

Integumentary System

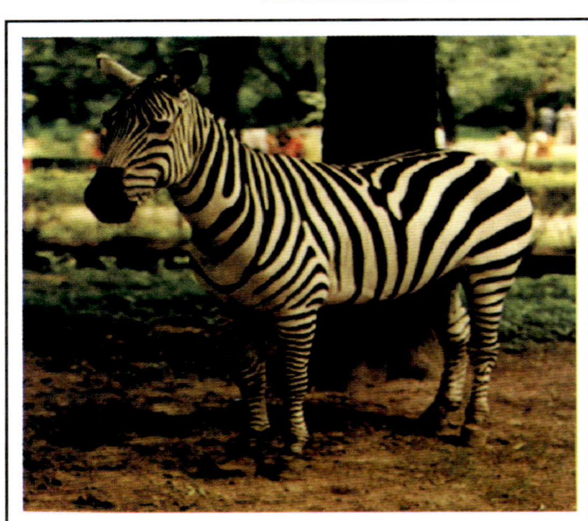

Figure 711: Zebra (*Equus brucheli*,an exotic sp.) in Zoological Garden, Kanpur (U.P.) has tendency of hooves over growing.

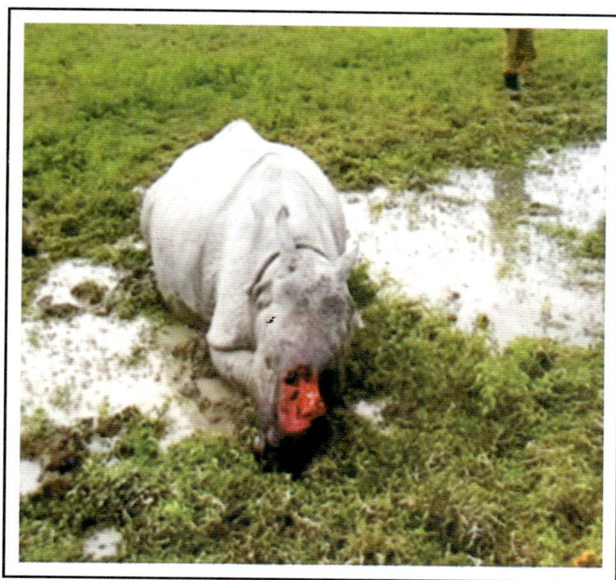

Figure 712: Poacher cut the horn of rhinoceros (*R. unicornis*) in Kaziranga National Park of Assam.

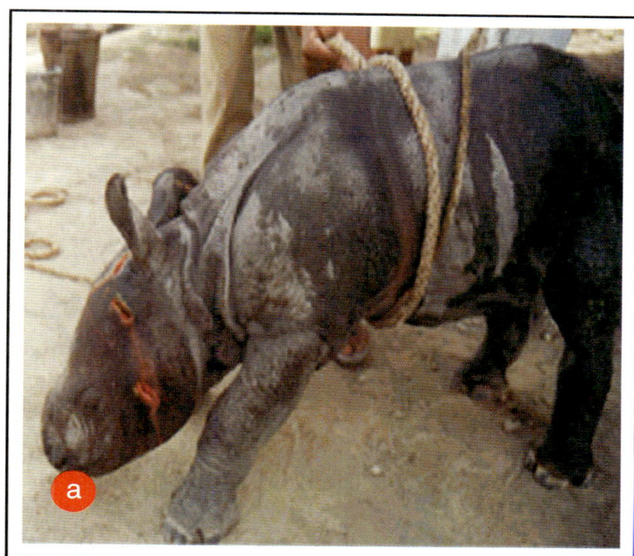

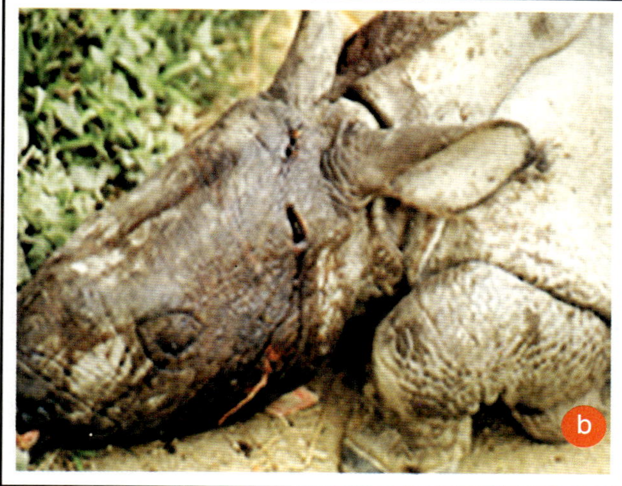

Figure 713: The predator injured rhinoceros (*R. unicornis*) calves (a,b) rescued from Kaziranga National Park. Note lacerated wounds on the left side of face(a) and mandible. (Courtesy : Talukdar, A.)

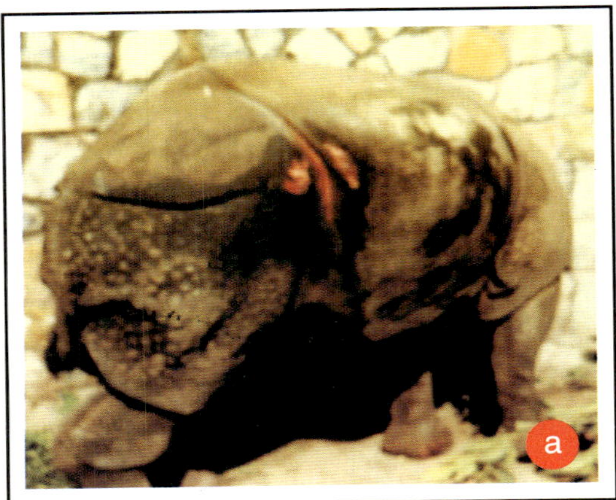

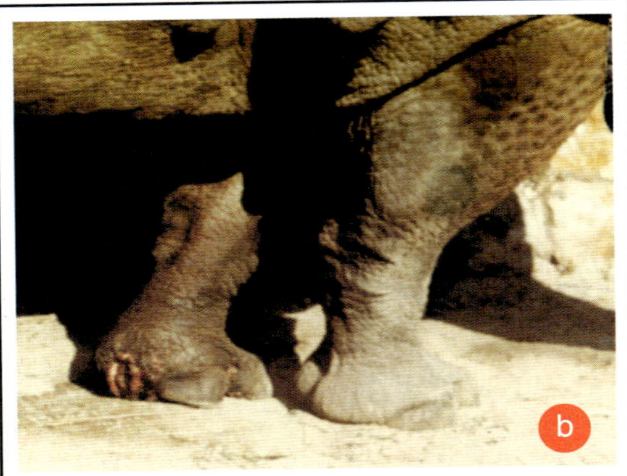

Figure 714: Photographs(a, b) showing lacerations of skin of rhinoceros (*R. unicornis*) over the external angle of the ilium, flank and back of the left hind foot. The lesions had developed as a result of striking and rubbing against the transportation crate during long journey by road.

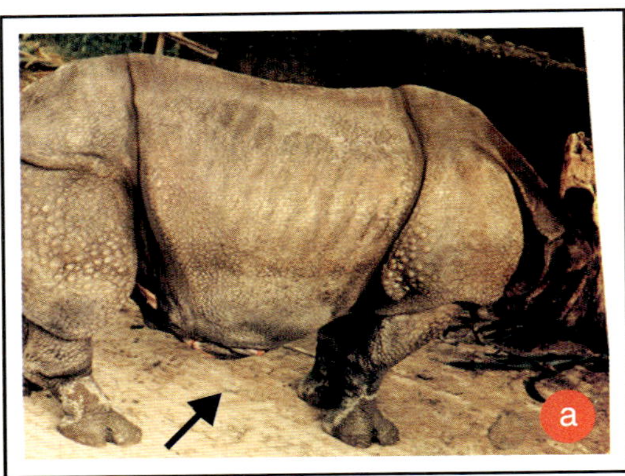

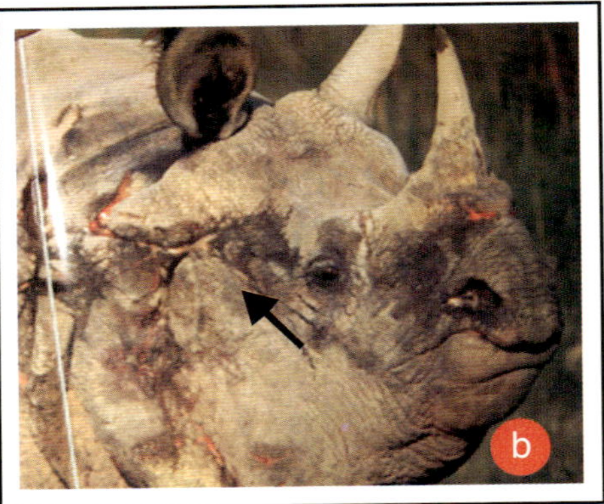

Figure 715: Photographs showing (a) healed up lacerated wounds in rhinoceros (*R. unicornis*) on the ventral surface of abdomen of captive rhinoceros inflicted by resident wild male upon its release in Dudhwa National Park, Uttar Pradesh. (b) Another case showing infighting wounds on the face and base of horn (Bedi & Bedi, 1984)

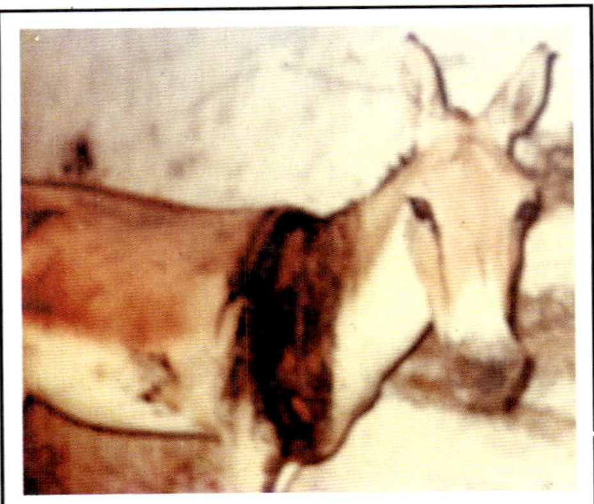

Figure 716: Photograph showing wounds on the withers of an adult female wild ass (*E. hemionis khur*) due to biting by her male partner at National Zoological Park, New Delhi. Later on the animal died of tetanus.

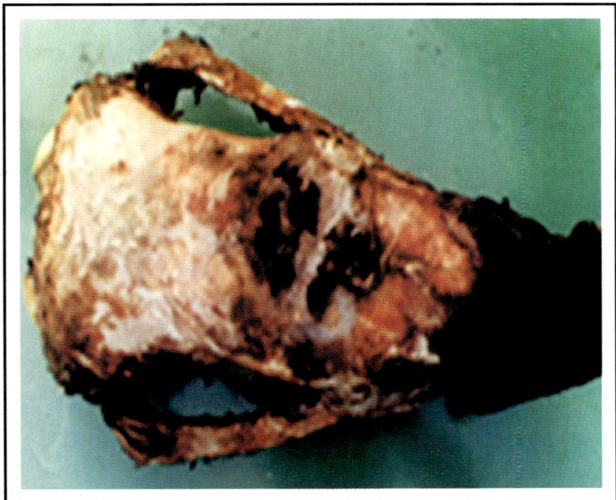

Figure 717: Photograph of skull of rhinoceros (*R. unicornis*) calf showing tearing of frontal bone due to attack by tiger (*P. tigris*) in National Park, Dudwa (U.P.).

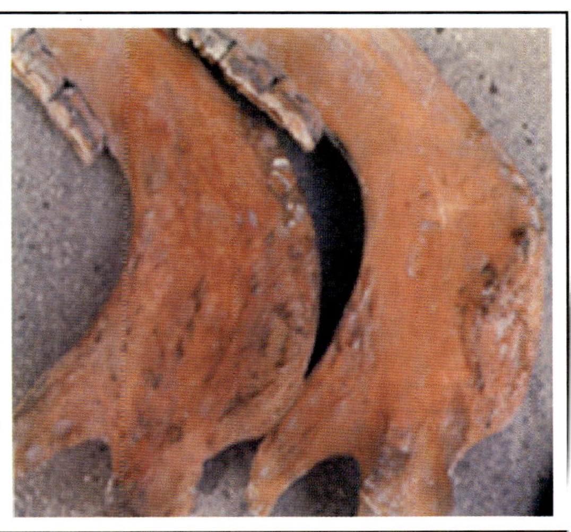

Figure 718: Photograph of rhinoceros (*R. unicornis*) mandible from Kaziranga N.P., showing degenerative lesions extending upwards from lower borders.

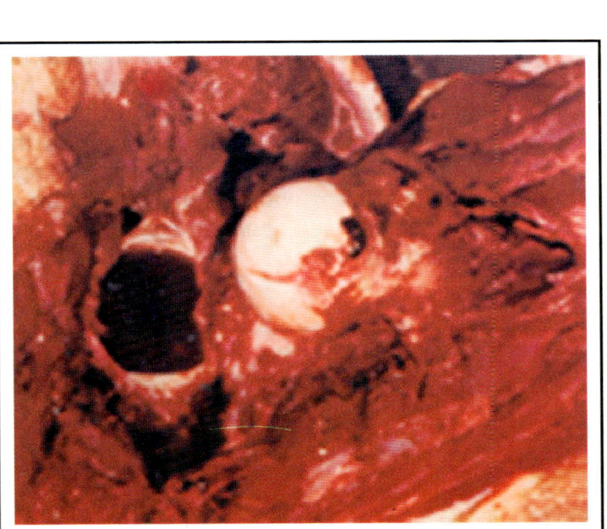

Figure 719: Photograph showing detached head of femur out of acetabular fossa filled with blood encountered in rhinoceros (*R. unicornis*) calf belonged to Kaziranga National Park, Assam which had caused due to trauma.

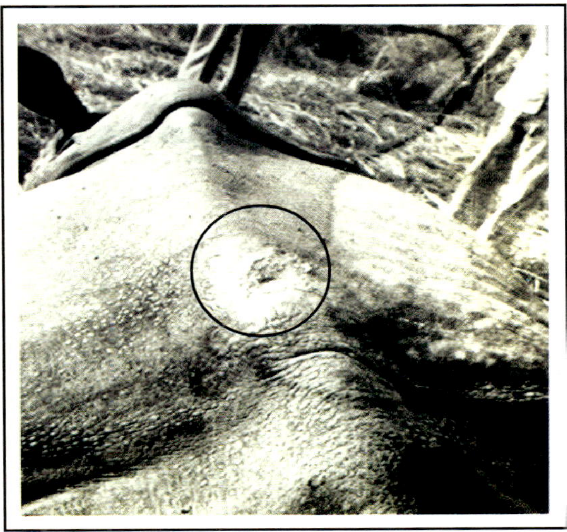

Figure 720: An adult female rhinoceros (*R. unicornis*) introduced in National Park, Dudwa (U.P.) had a chronic large wound in its croup region suffered during transportation.

PROBOSCIDS

Family: *Elephantidae*

Genus: *Elephas*

Species: Indian elephant (*Elephas maximus*)

Genus: *Laxodont* Species: African elephant (*Laxodont africana*)

Introduction

India has only one species of elephant (*Elephas maximus)* under order *Proboscidea*, which has been domesticated since ancient times. The Zoological Parks/Gardens and Rescue centers have no breeding obligation. Presently the country has 11 wild elephant reserves inhabiting nearly 28000 heads of Indian elephant (*Elephas maximus*). Recently, domesticated elephant (*E. maximus*) has also been included under the WPA and its registration has become a legal requirement. In captivity elephants are maintained by four agencies namely, State forest departments, Zoological Parks/ Gardens, temples and circuses. In forest camps elephant numbers is around 482, maximum number being with Kaziranga National Park (Assam). With private individuals number may be 2500-3000, being maximum 1800 numbers in Assam. This chapter includes clinical and pathological illustrations of certain diseases and disorders of Indian elephants (*Elephas maximus*).

Eco-husbandry associated health hazards: In wild these include accidental collision with trains passing through reserves, inter and intra species conflict injuries and electrocution and poisoning in retaliation besides poaching.

(a) Accidents: Accidental collisions of wild elephants with trains **(Figure 784)** passing through species reserves of Uttarakhand and Assam alleged for high mortality. This is because of species possessing a quite different sensory (vision, hearing, touch, feeling, etc) and ethological traits. For example, elephants despite of acute vision are handicapped in making use of this sense to a degree equal to most other animals due to shortness of its neck, which does not permit the head being turned sideways sufficiently to see the objects. Further, the limited field of vision is due to small size of eyes supplied with small size of optic nerves and less number of muscles to move the eye. Possessing of acute smelling and partial keen hearing power animal is able to perceive the danger existing quite nearby only. Electrocution mortality either accidental or caused due to malicious intension is considered to be the other most important factor for loss in wild elephants. Accidental electrocution deaths occurred when an adult elephant touches the live electric transmission wires and if others come to rescue the companion also met the same fate. Deaths of 16 wild elephants in Karnataka were attributed to accidental electrocution when they went out of forests to satiate their huge dietary need **(Figures 798-799)**. This matter needs to be looked judiciously. If reserve has no short of fodder and number of elephants has not increased over the carrying capacity then why elephants leave the reserve and move to agriculture field and human dwelling areas?.

Certain accidents in elephant calves (*E. maximus*) are illustrated. Tiger attacks wild elephant calf (*E. maximus*) stealthily, which may or may not be gainful **(Figure 768).** Elephant calf while playing may suffer from certain problems, such as getting its head trapped between forked tree stems **(Figure 795),** fall into trench or well **(Figure 796)** or get injured its trunk tip which later on becomes a severe problem **(Figure 724).** Intestinal intussusceptions **(Figure 735)** and radial paralysis following fracture of radial bones have also been encountered **(Figure 789).** Capture myopathy and fracture in course of restraint and translocation operations at times are fatal **(Figure 797)**. In case of capture myopathy severe internal haemorrhages may occur **(Figure 738)**. At the face of lack of circumstantial evidence leg bone dislocations or fractures in case of wild cow elephant could be perceived due to slipping and falling **(Figures 788, 790- 791)** while transecting difficult terrain, mounting by forbidden tusker and in tuskers during infighting mostly. An elephant while marching on the traffic road in dark hours of the day.may get hit by an automobile **(Figure 785).**

(b) Poaching: This is a major threat to conservation of wild elephant populations as tuskers are killed for the tusks **(Figure 786)**.

(c) Poisoning: More cases of poisoning of wild elephants were recorded in Assam. During August 2001 to January 2002 in Nameri National Park 9 wild elephants died of Organo-phosphorous (Demecron) poisoning and again in October-November, 2002 three elephants at Sonitpur district died of carbamate insecticide poisoning. Probably these poisoning cases might be the result of "man-elephant conflict." In captivity due to workers attrition with management poisoning of elephants with Zinc phosphide has been committed **(Figures 733,752)**.

(d) In captive elephants over growth of cuticle-hyperkeratosis **(Figure 762)** at the site of fattering, cuticular splitting **(Figure 763)**,overgrown and cracking of nails **(Figures 764),** over worn and cracked sole and heel **(Figure 765)** due to their housing in chronically wet and dirty conditions and inadequate exercise are related to husbandry management shortcomings. If pressure necrosis lesions are not cared seriously may prove fatal **(Figure 769).** Out of the three cases of allergic dermatitis encountered in elephants belonged to Kaziranga National Park and Pobitora Wildlife Sanctuary, type of skin lesions of one case are illustrated (**Figure 778**). The cases were successfully treated with parentral administration of antihistaminic drug. Allergic dermatitis may occur due to contact of animal body with some toxic plant, or when such plants are consumed along with fodder, insects bite, and also in captivity when drugs such as phenothiazine preparation are administered.

(e) Miscellaneous: Dystocia in cows stationed at forest camps has occasionally being recorded. Some reports indicate atherosclerosis, diabetes in captive elephants. Stomach impaction (**Figure734**) and nepharolithiasis **(Figure 750 to 751)** are registered in captive elephants but rarely.

Diseases. (A) Infectious & parasitic: There appears to be no project on morbidity and mortality investigations related to bacterial, viral and mycotic disease conditions in wild elephant populations. Some clinico-pathological illustrations of some diseases of wild and captive elephants are presented.

(a) Cardiovascular system: Anthrax (*Bacillus anthracis*) and Haemorrhagic septicaemia (*Pasteurella multocida*) are the only two bacterial diseases **(Figures 723,726)** recorded to cause septicaemic lesions in young as well as adult elephants. Per acute cases of deaths are often mistaken for snakebite. Diagnosis is made by microscopic examination of blood smear and culture from discharges. Colibacillosis occur in newborn orphan elephant calves, which do not get colostrums. Young elephants when exposed to heavy dose of *E.coli* under poor hygienic condition may fell sick, and die of septicaemia.

The only blood protozoan infection, first known in elephants appear to be *Trypnosoma evansi.* The blood fluke *Bivitellobilharzia nairi* is reported causing chronic wasting disease in elephant. *Onchocerca* sp. has also been demonstrated histologically in the aorta. None of these could be pictorially depicted in the Atlas.

(b) Respiratory system: A case of acute pasteurellosis (*P. multocida*) in elephant is presented **(Figure 726).** Indian literature in the Hindu mythology (2000BC) furnishes the evidence that tuberculosis was encountered in elephants. Pulmonary form of disease is more commonly encountered **(Figure 727)**. The disseminated form includes lesions in large intestine and mesenteric lymph nodes. The lesions usually described are caseated nodules/ abscesses (rather than granulomas) encircled by fibrous tissue capsule, lymphocytes and macrophages without giant cells. Lesions lack calcification and there be poor cellular response. In addition to bovine and human strains; a worker from abroad has identified another strain, *Mycobacterium elephantis.*

Pulmonary blastomycosis in elephant (*E. maximus*) died at Forest Camp of Kaziranga National Park, Assam appears to be the first report **(Figure 728).**

(c) Digestive system: A rescued elephant calf died of salmonella enteritis. Spleenomegaly was also concurrent finding **(Figure 741).** Colibacillosis and salmonellosis (*Solmonella javiana, S.butantam, S.weltervreden, S.typhimurium*) have been attributed as the major causes of elephant calf mortality. Signs associated with salmonellosis include diarrhea, sometime containing blood and mucus, loss of appetite, weakness and fever. Post mortem, gross lesions include haemorrhagic gastritis and enteritis **(Figure 740)**. Intestinal haemorrhagic lesions were diagnosed for enterotoxaema in an elephant **(Figure 742)** died in captivity. However, details of the cultural and histological findings were unavailable.

Except foot and mouth disease (FMD), no other viral disease affecting oral cavity is recorded. The disease causes ulcerative lesions **(Figure 731)** on the tongue, upper palate, rima orifis (besides trunk and at the junction of skin and nails and sole of the feet).

Pox in elephants has been described. Pustules formation on buccal mucosa, tongue, and ventral portion of the trunk besides the external body lesions were mentioned (Chandrasekharan, 1989). A case of: extensive lesions of non-tuberculous granulomatous hepatitis in wild elephant (*E. maximus*) died in Cauvery Wildlife Sanctuary, Karnataka has been documented **(Figure 743).**

Among the helminthic diseases, hepatic fasciolosis due to *Fasciola jacksoni* **(Figures 746 to 748)** causes damage of liver and bile duct severely in elephants and disease morbidity is reflected as chronic wasting condition. To understand pathogenesis of *Fasciola jacksoni*, its electron microscopic study was conducted **(Figure 749).**

(e) Urinary system: Leptospiral infection is only serologically evidenced. Cases of nepharitis of undetermined specific etiologies are often described (Arora, 2003).

(f) Reproductive system: Following dystocia and abortion cases have been reported in elephants stationed at forest camps. Infectious metritis/ endometritis cases are related to *Corynebacterium* sp. infection. Postmortem of a cow elephant died in captivity showed metritis with ulcerative lesions **(Figure 753)** and had *Pseudomonas aeurogenosa* infection in feet lesions.

(f) Nervous system: Sporadic cases of tetanus (*Clostridium tetani)* are recorded. First case of rabies in Indian elephant attributed to bites of rabid dogs was documented by Evans (1910). Disease in captive and wild elephants histopathologically diagnosed in a young elephant died in the forest of Karnataka and one case each died in elephants Forest Camp of Kaziranga National Park, Assam and Forest Camp of Corbett National Park, Uttarakhand **(Figures 757i&ii,758).**

(g) Sense organs: *Thelazia sp.* occurs in the elephant's eyes. From the available literature (Arora, 2003) it appears that the eye lesions such as corneal opacity, conjunctivitis, keratitis **(Figures, 759-761)** have not been investigated for specific etiology.

(h) Integumentary system: Pododermatitis causes much trouble to the captive elephants **(Figures 772 to 774).** *Pseudomonas* and *Proteus* organisms have been cultured from the suppurative lesions of foot. Cases of cutaneous abscess formation in forest camp elephants are encountered **(Figures 769-770).** From the suppurative skin lesions acid-fast organisms indistinguishable from Tb bacilli were demonstrated in smear examination

Mycotic dermatitis in elephant (*E. maximus*) related to *Trichophyton* sp. infection **(Figure 776)**. Similar lesions such as scaling and dryness of skin **(Figure777)** noted in 7-8 weeks old elephant calf rescued from wild housed at Zoological Garden, Mysore (Karnataka).

Occurrence of cutaneous filarial worm infection in elephants **(Figure 779b)** is more common in Assam.

Several tick species infestation in elephants is not uncommon. Both nymph and the adult stages are infective and cause biting injury; sucking of blood. In forest camp elephants cutaneous infestation with elephant louse, *Haematomyzus elephantis* is marked for pruritis, dryness of skin and scale formation **(Figure 780).** Besides the skin infestation caused in an elephant by the hard ticks, their penetration into rectal folds caused lesion on the mucosa **(Figure 781).**

Myiasis: The biting flies *Stomoxys, Tabanus, Haematopota* and *Chrysops* are common to cause severe irritation, loss of blood and to transmit mechanically *Trypanosoma* infection to elephant. The larvae of non-biting fly *Cobboldia elephantis* occur in the stomach of elephants but are also found in the lungs of an elephant. Another larva of fly similar to *Cobboldia elephantis* but have smaller size is seen in some elephants of North-eastern part of the country. The lesions produced by this are the eruption of small nodular growths over the skin and on pressure the larva comes out. Probably these are dipterous larva.

(B) Neoplasms: They are poorly studied in elephants. The cases illustrated include papillomatous growths **(Figure 783)** on the trunk of an elephant calf and hard growths diagnosed as fibroma **(Figure 782)** over the legs in an adult captive elephant (*E. maximus*).

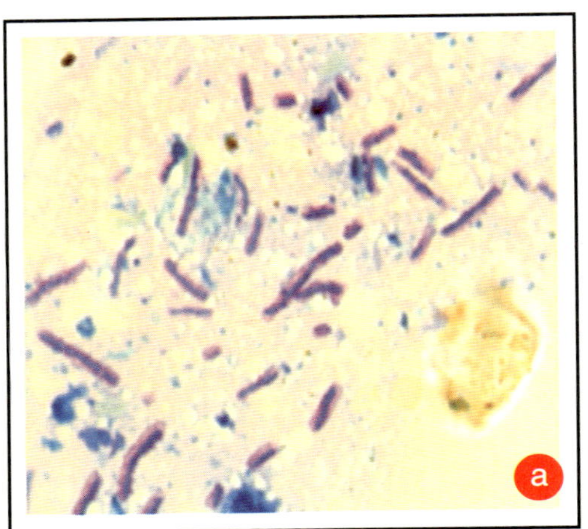

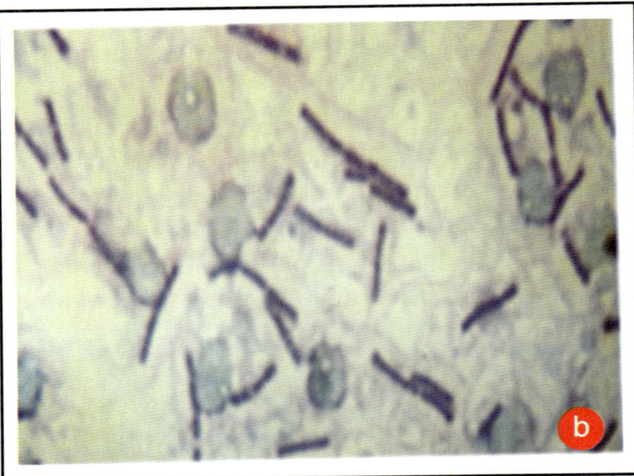

Figure 723: Photographs (a,b) of blood smears from elephants (*E. maximus*) died in wild showing *Anthrax bacilli*. (Courtesy: IVRI Regional Centre, Kolkata).

Respiratory System

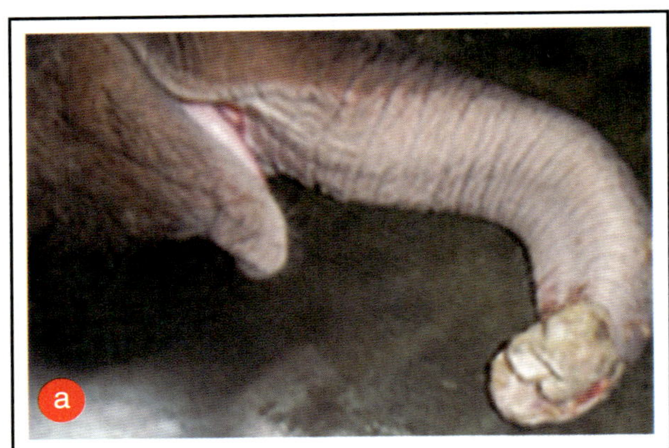

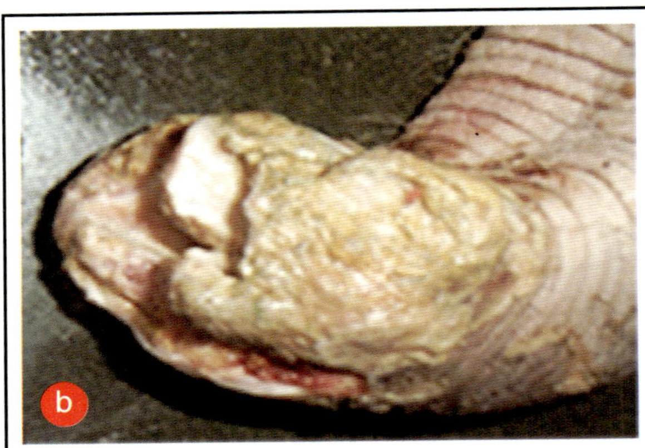

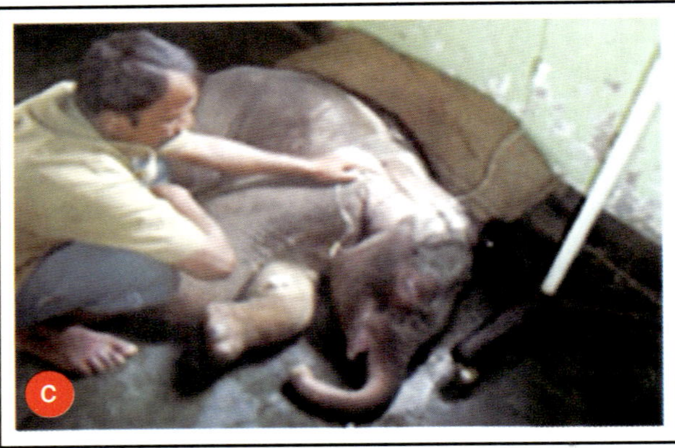

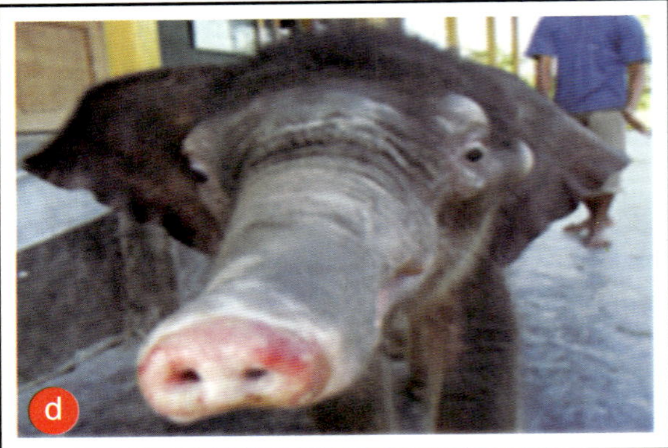

Figure 724: Photographs (a, b) showing extensively injured anterior portion of trunk in one month old rescued wild elephant (*E. maximus*) calf. (c) Calf under sedation for treatment. (d) Improved condition trunk after 15 days of treatment (Talukdar & Choudhury, 2007).

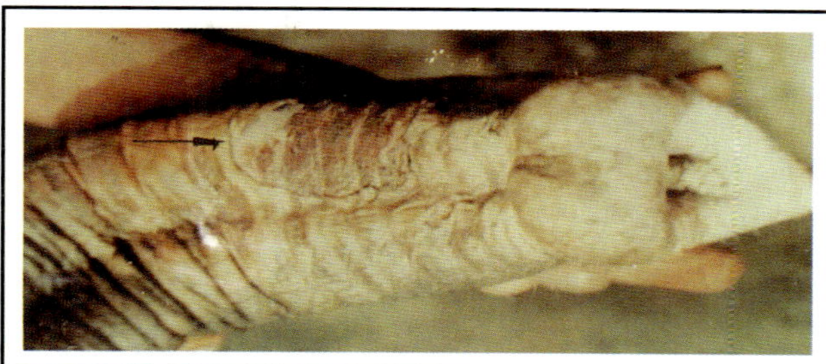

Case (i)

Figure 725: Photographs showing Foot & Mouth Disease lesions on the trunk of the elephant (*E. maximus*). Case (i) Courtesy : Sharma, *et al.* 1994. Case (ii) Anon. Source could not be traced

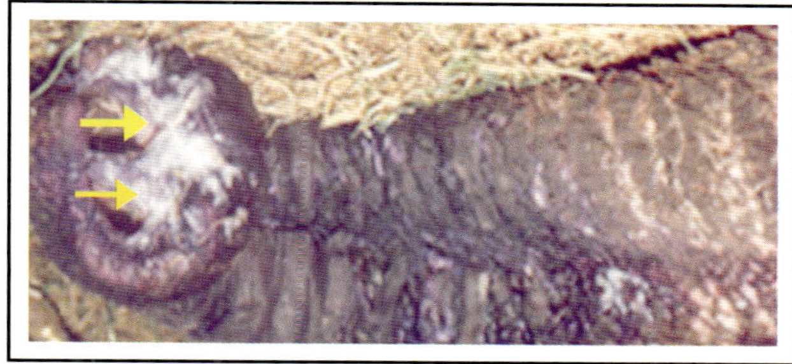

Case (ii)

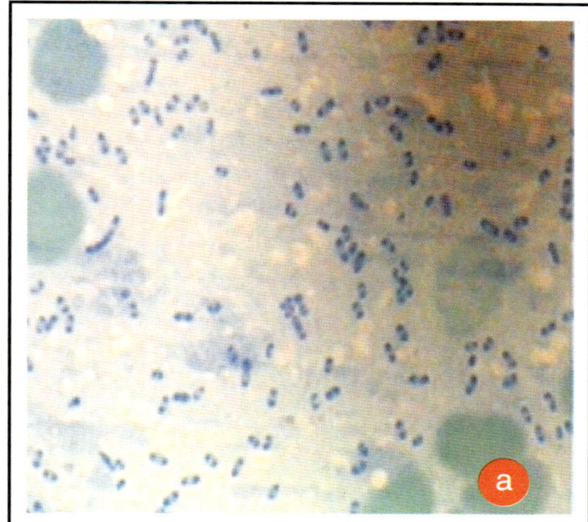

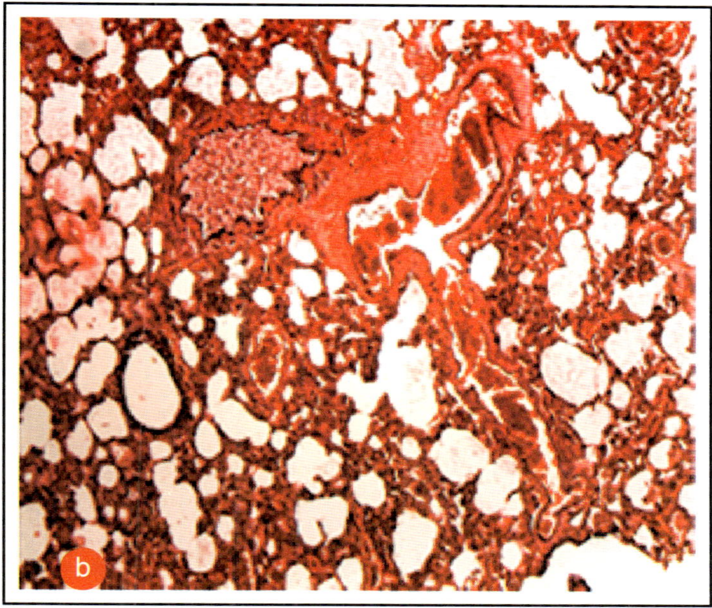

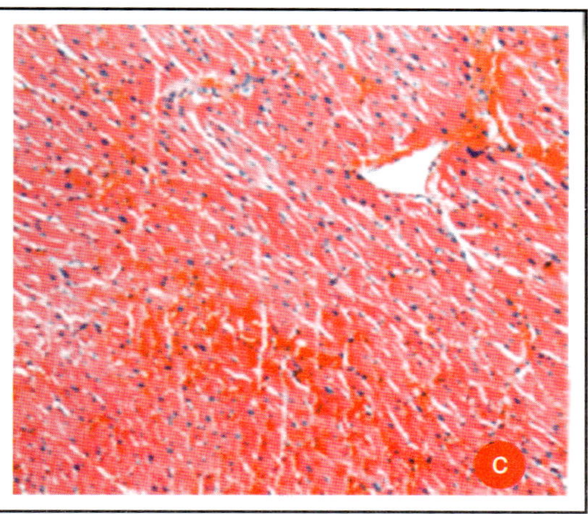

Figure 726: (a) Impression smear from lung of elephant (*E. maximus*) showing bipolar organisms morphologically akin to *Pasteurella* sp. Photomicrographs (b,c) of lung from (a) showing acute endothelial damage and infiltration of RBCs in the interstitial spaces of muscle fibers and alveolar spaces in lung and heart. (Courtesy: Harish, B.R.).

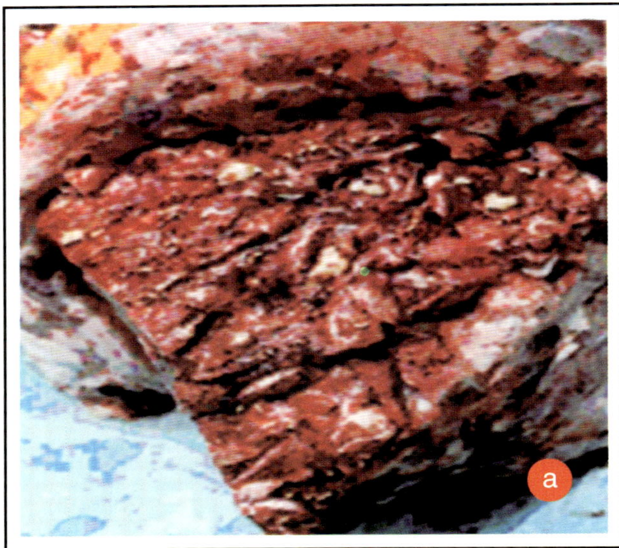

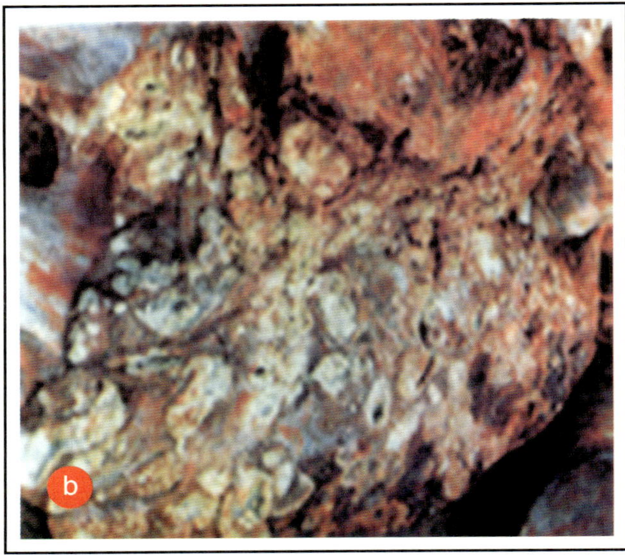

Figure 727: Photographs showing pulmonary tuberculous nodules in lung of elephant (*E. maximus*) died in captivity. (a) Courtesy: Harish, B. R. (b) Chandrasekharan (1989).

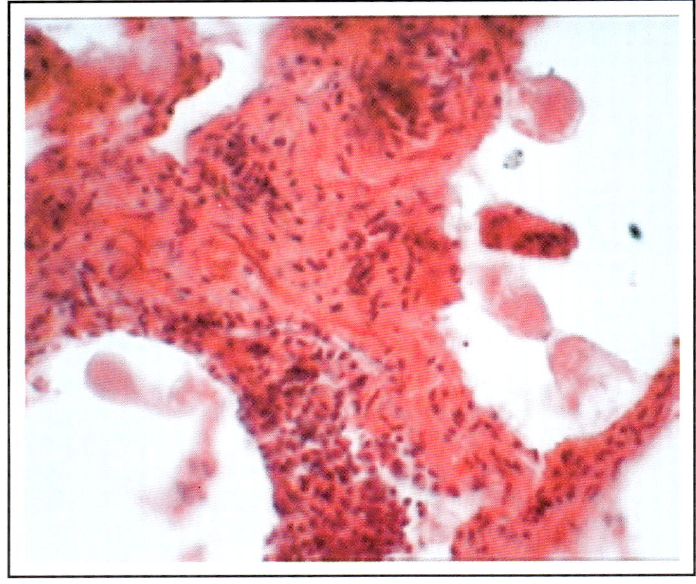

Figure 728: Pulmonary blastomycosis in elephant (*E. maximus*) died at Forest camp of Kaziranga National Park, Assam. Photomicrograph showing budding yeast cells in the alveoli. The buds have a broad basal attachment to the parent cell. H&E, x 400.

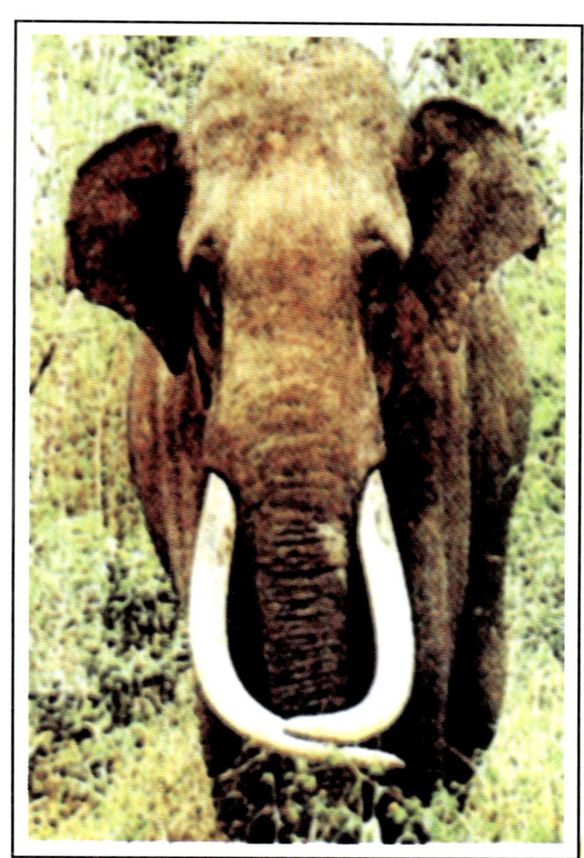

Figure 729 : Elephant (*E. maximus*) tusks curved and joining each other in their lower third length (Desai, A. 1989).

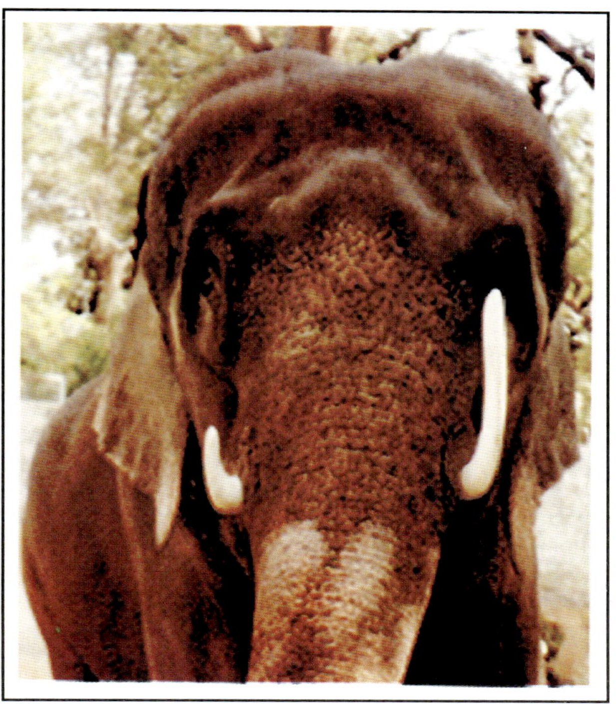

Figure 730: Elephant (*E. maximus*) with upward bent tusks. Note right tusk is smaller and thinner than the left.

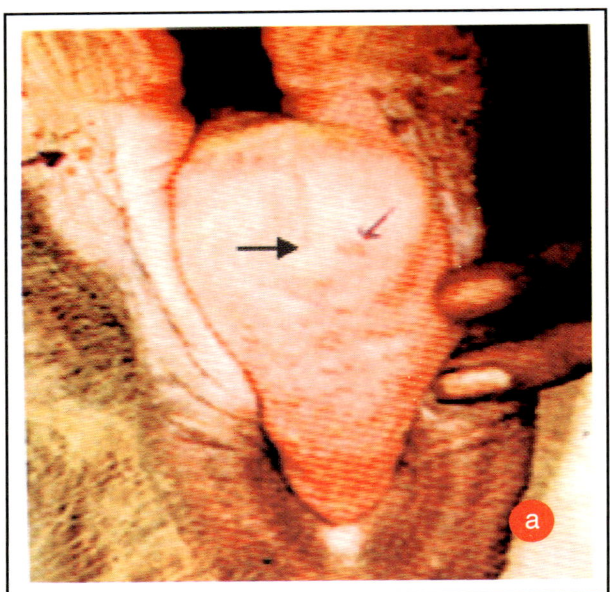

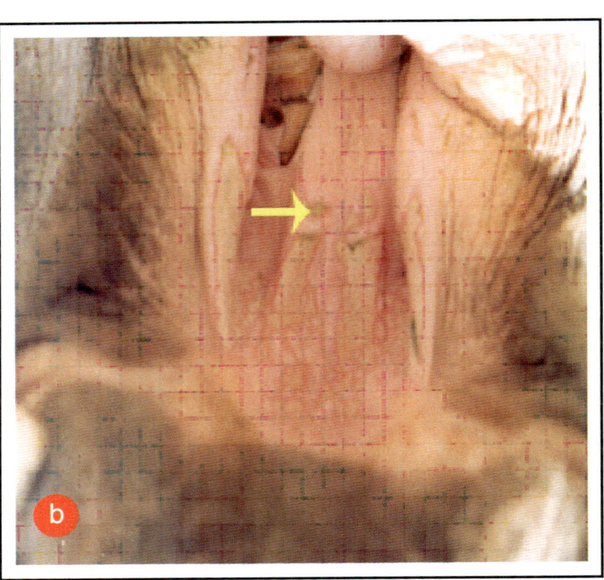

Figure 731: Photographs (a, b) of tongue of elephant (*E. maximus*) calf showing vesicular lesions and erupted vesicles (arrow) on the tongue and rima oris due to FMD virus type 'O' infection (Sharma, D.K. *et al.,* 1994).

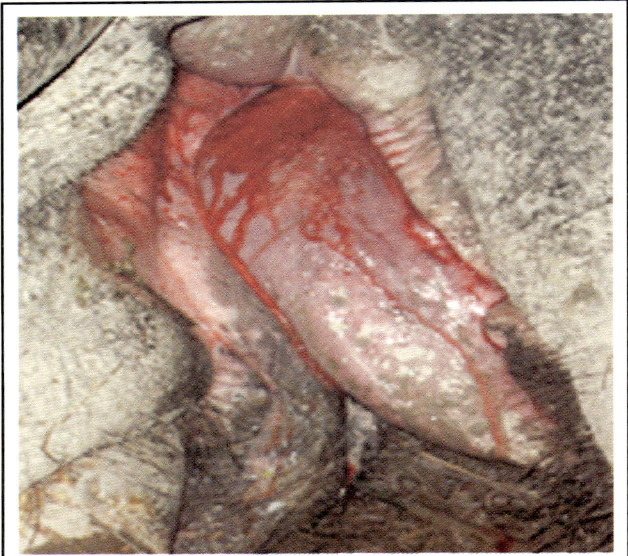

Figure 732: Photograph showing protrusion of tongue and oozing of blood from the mouth suspected organophosphorus poisoning in wild elephant (Courtesy: Boro,P.K.).

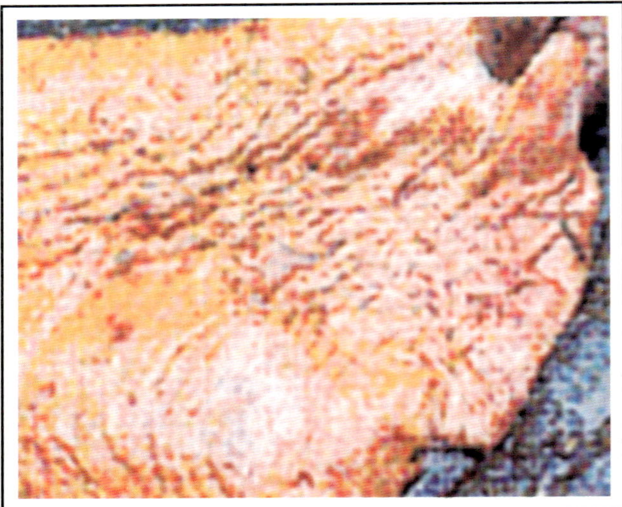

Figure 733 : Photograph showing ulcers in the stomach of elephant (*E. maximus*) died in Zoological Garden Mysore (Karanataka) related to Zinc phosphide poisoning. The case is also referred under urinary system (Courtesy: Harish, B,R.).

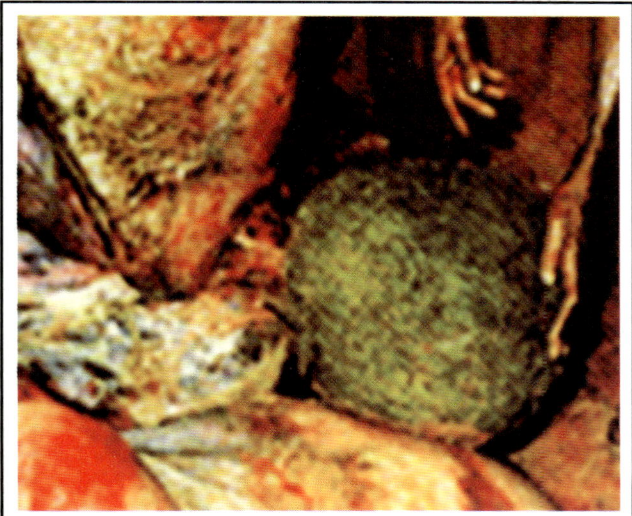

Figure 734 : Rupture of colon in elephant (*E.maximus*) caused due to impacted plant fibrous contents (Chandrasekharan, 1989).

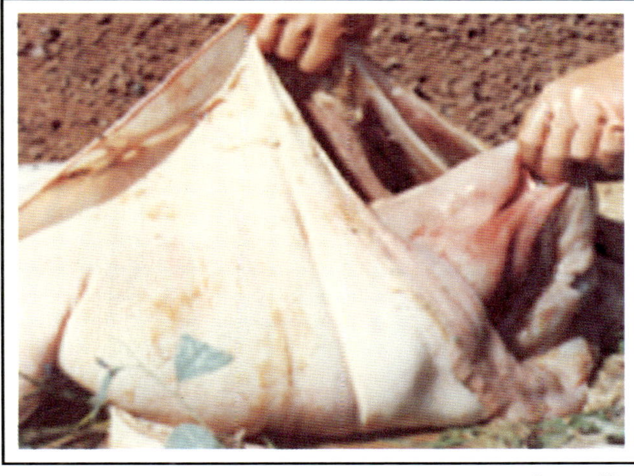

Case (i)

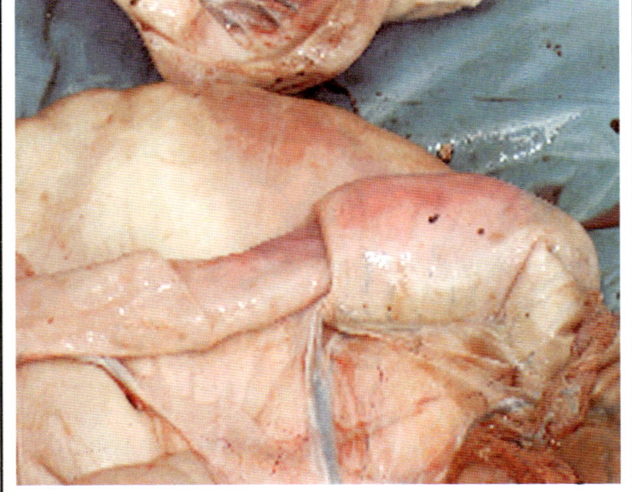

Case (ii)

Figure 735: Intussusceptions in elephants (*E. maximus*). Case(i) Necropsy of an adult elephant in Zoological Garden, Guwahati (Assam) showed about 80-90 cm anterior part of the small intestine invaginated into the posterior part of the intestine along with mesentery. The serosal surface of the invaginated part showed necrosis and deposition of fibrinous flakes over it. Case (ii) About 3 months old elephant calf rescued from Manas National Park (Assam) and maintained in captivity had developed severe diarrhoea after a week, which could not be cured and calf had died. Necropsy showed telescopic invagination of intestine (ileo-ileal). (Courtesy: Sarma, K.K.).

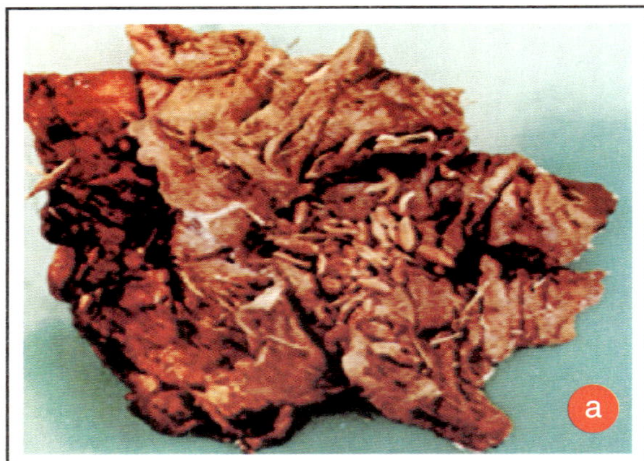

Figure 736: Photograph showing a large number of bots in the stomach of elephants (*E.maximus*) died in : (a) Wild.(b) Captivity. (Courtesy: Jacob Alexander and Easwaran, E.K.).

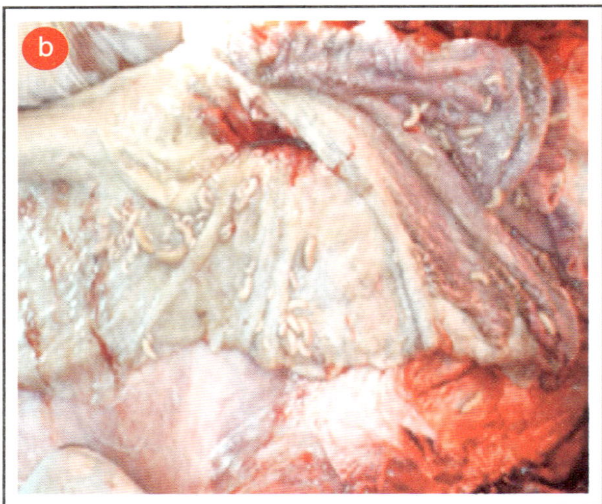

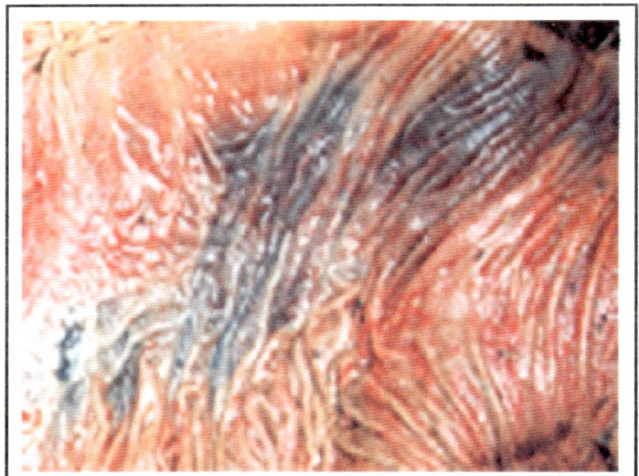

Figure 737: Photograph showing haemorrhagic gastritis in an adult elephant (*E. maximus*) died in Zoological Garden, Guwahati.

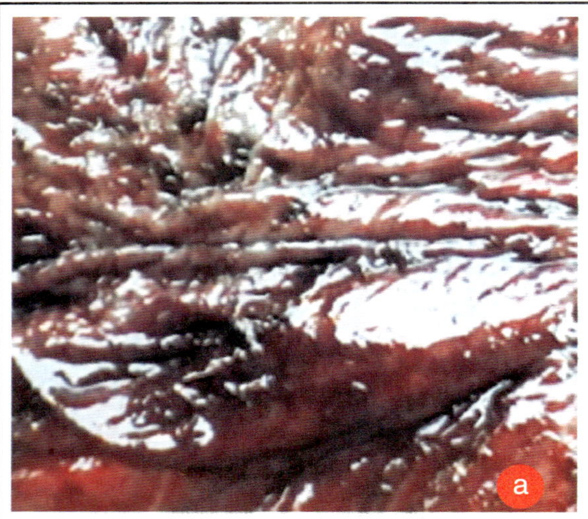

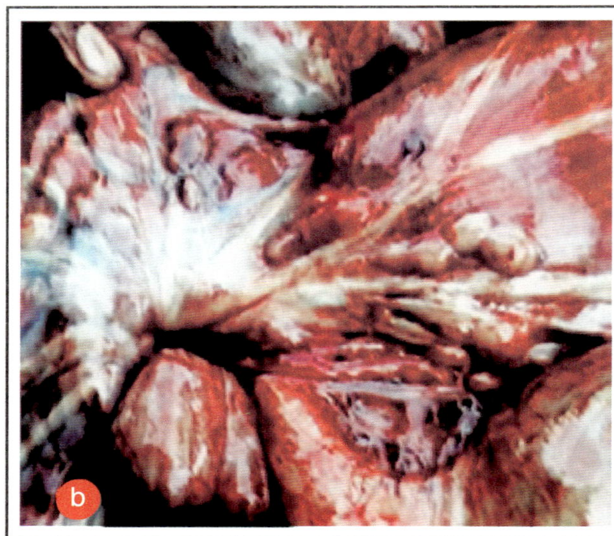

Figure 738: Photographs (a,b) showing haemorrhagic enteritis and haemorrhages in mesentery in elephant calf died during rescue from the flood in Kaziranga N.P., Assam (Courtesy: Abhijit, Bhowal)

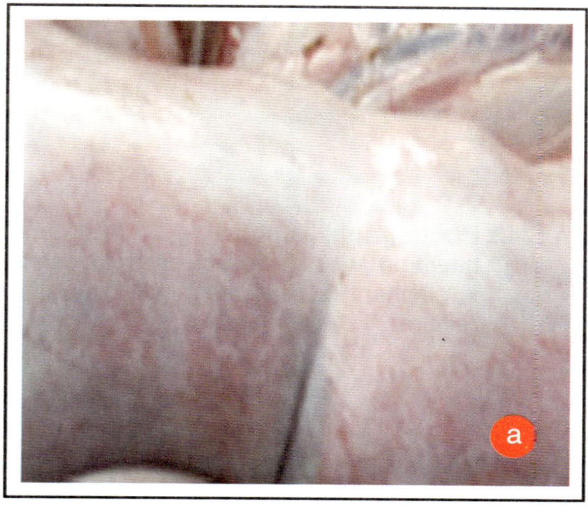

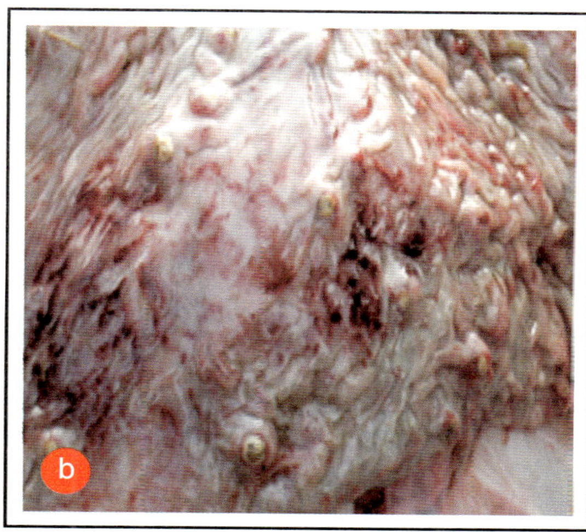

Figure 739: Enteritis in elephant (*E. maximus*) calf. Photographs (a,b) showing congestion of serosal surface of intestine and small necrotic nodular lesions on intestinal mucosa (Courtesy: Abhijit, Bhowal).

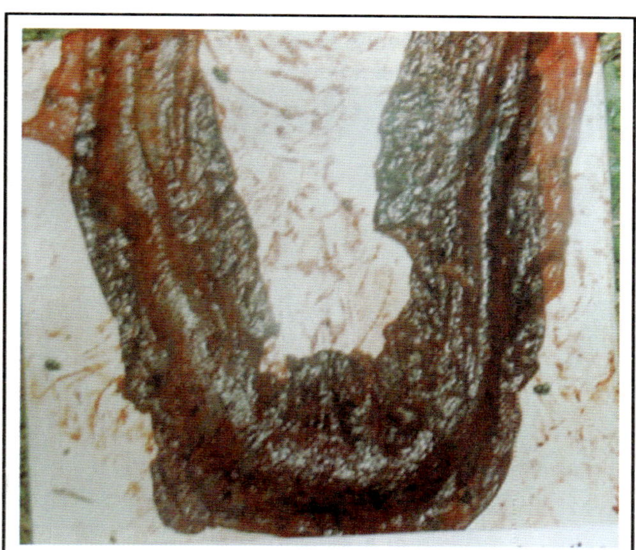

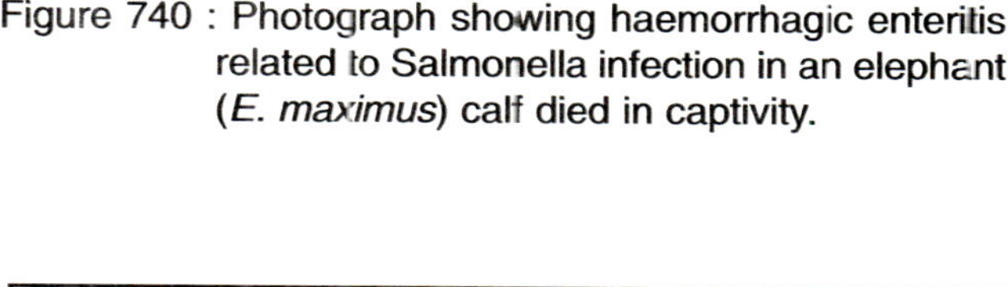

Figure 740 : Photograph showing haemorrhagic enteritis related to Salmonella infection in an elephant (*E. maximus*) calf died in captivity.

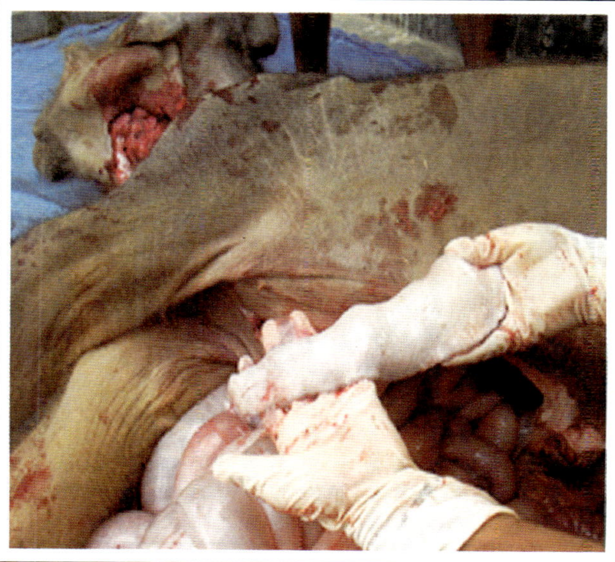

Figure 741: Spleenomegaly in rescued elephant (*E. maximus*) calf died of *Salmonella* infection at CWR & C, Kaziranga, Assam. (Courtesy: Choudhury, B.& Talukdar, A.).

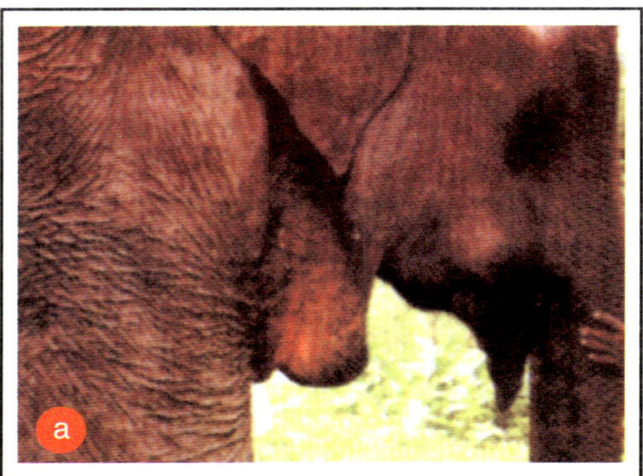

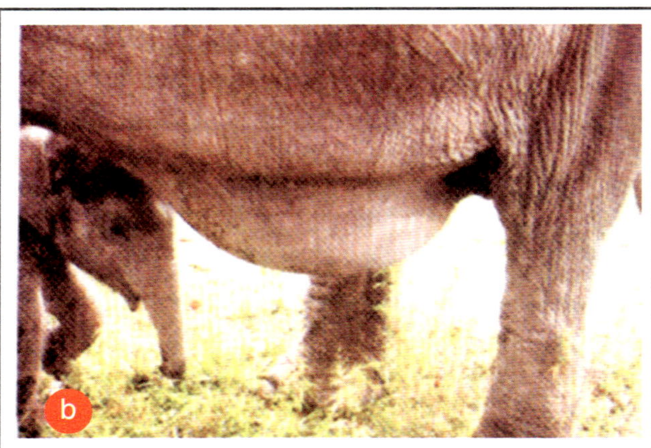

Figure 747: Photographs showing:(a) Submandibular oedma in a cow elephant affected with *Fasciola jacksoni* (b) Ventral oedema in abdominal region in freshly calved cow affected with *Fasciola jacksoni* (Sarma *et al.*, 2005).

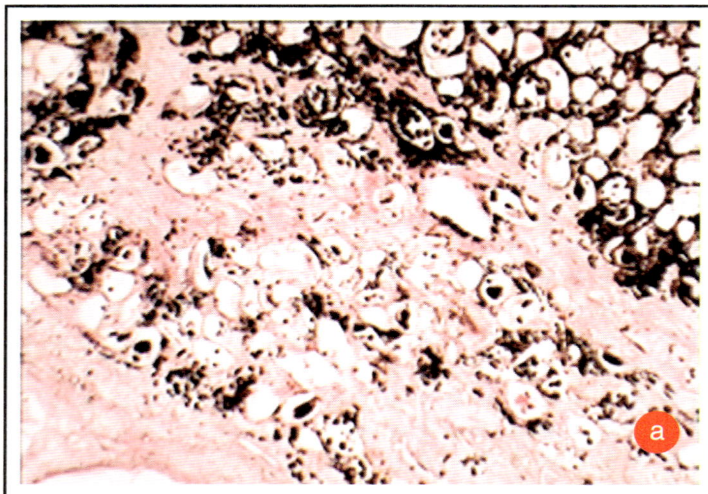

Figure 748: Elephant (*E. maximus*): Photomicrographs showing:(a) Fibrosed bile duct containing large number of *Fasciola jacksoni* eggs trapped within the necrotic debris. H&Ex100. (b)Higher magnification of (a) x400.

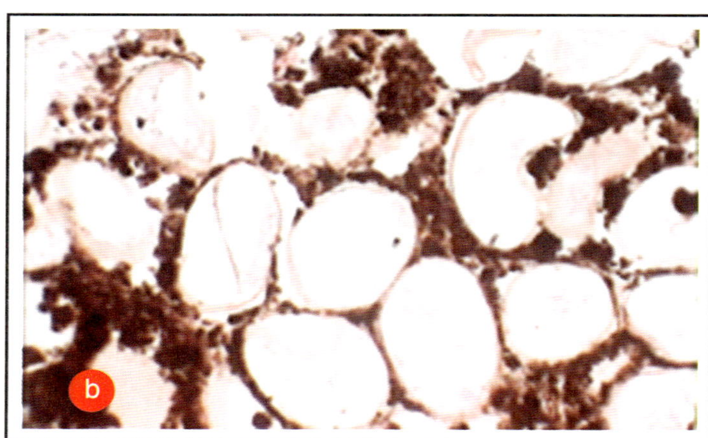

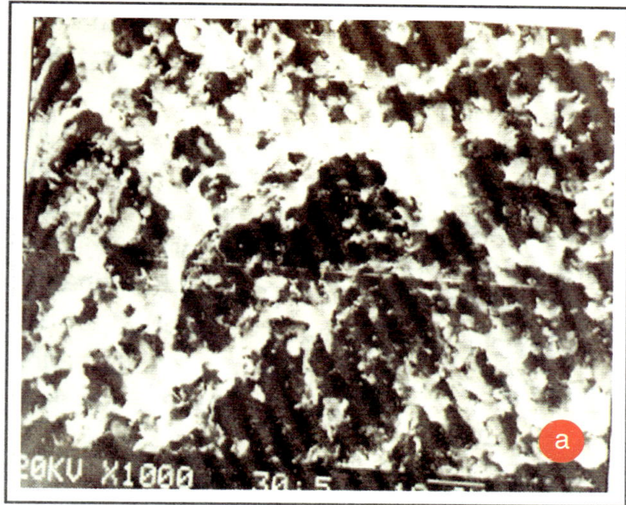

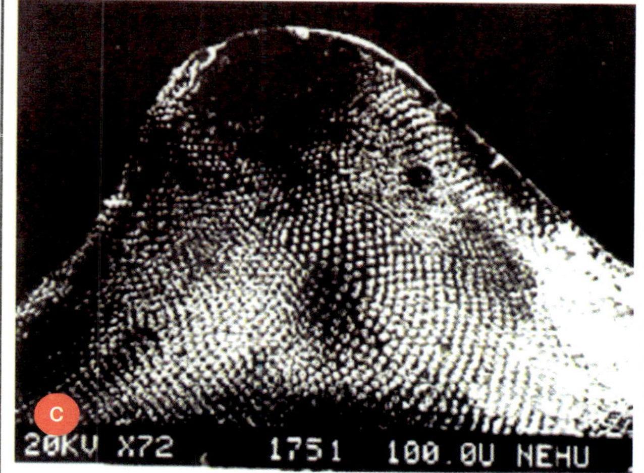

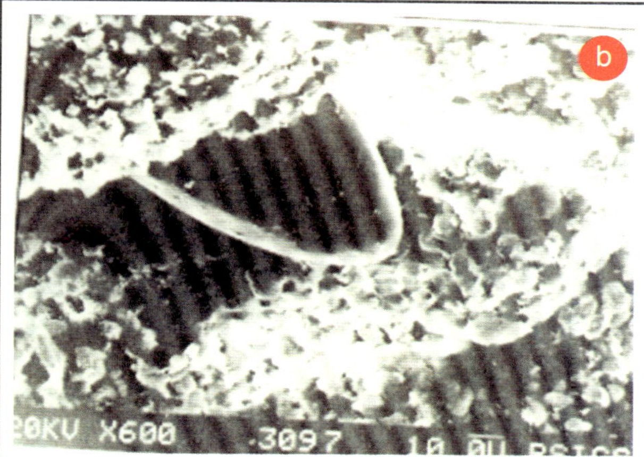

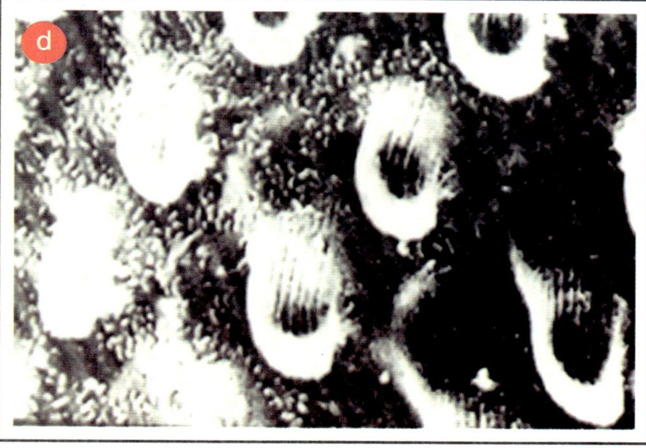

Figure 749: (a) SEM view of *Fasciola jacksoni* infected distorted biliary epithelium which turned into homogenous mass. x 1000. (b) SEM showing an egg of *F. jacksoni* trapped in the necrotic mass of bile duct x 600. (c) SEM of dorsal surface of *F. jacksoni*. Note presence of spines all over the body of the parasite x72. (d) SEM view of higher magnification of spines x 1200.

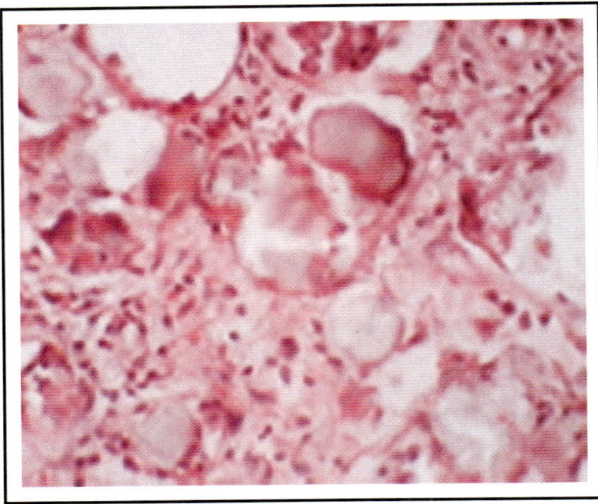

Figure 750: Photomicrograph of kidney of elephant (*E. maximus*) showing calcium oxalate crystals within the tubules. H&E, x400.

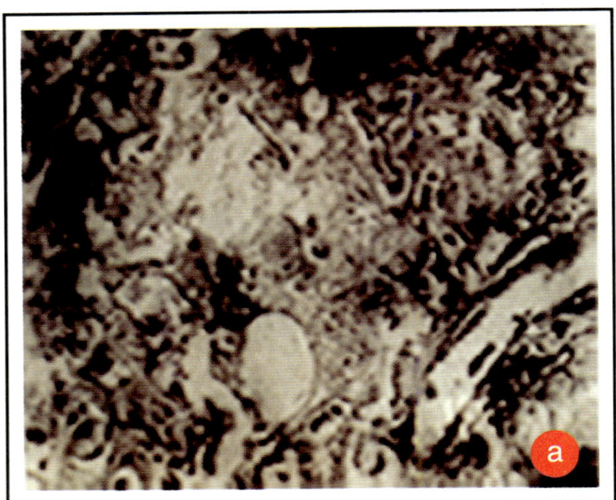

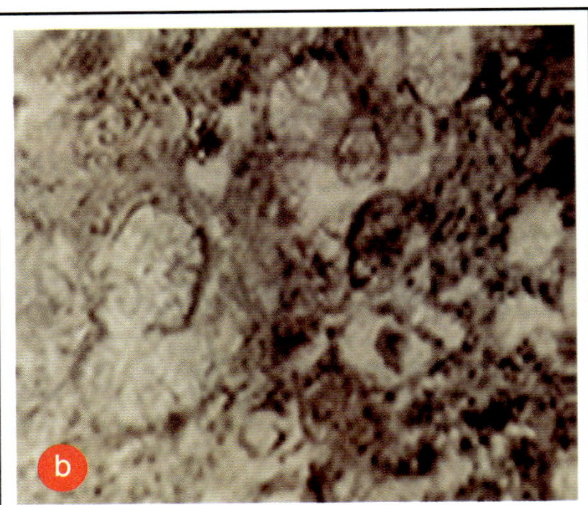

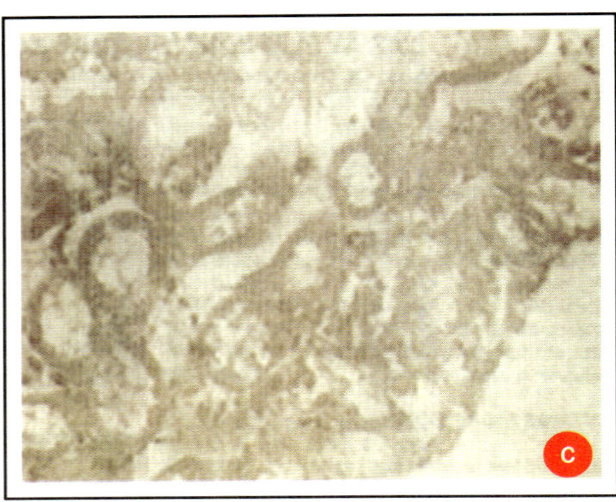

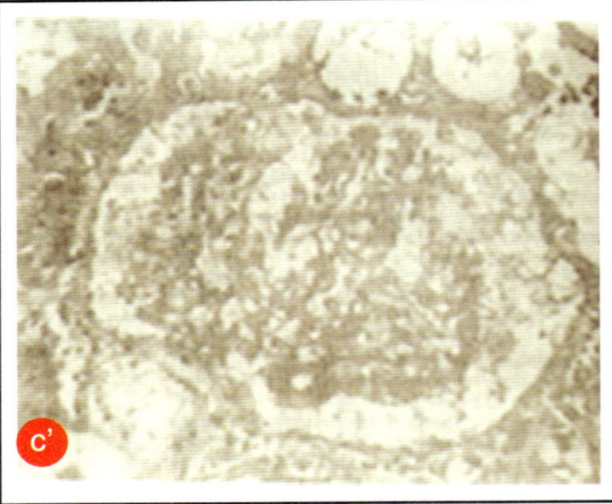

Figure 751: Photomicrographs (a, b) showing rosette shaped crystals in the tubules, free crystals in the interstitial spaces and cystic dilatation with fibrosis.(a) H&E,x 100 (b) H & E, x 200. (c, c') Nephrotic changes in the renal tubules.H&E x 200. Coagulative necrosis of the lining epithelium of renal tubules. Note presence of fibrinous deposits in the Bowman's spaces. H& E, x 200 (Islam Saidul *et. al.*,1996).

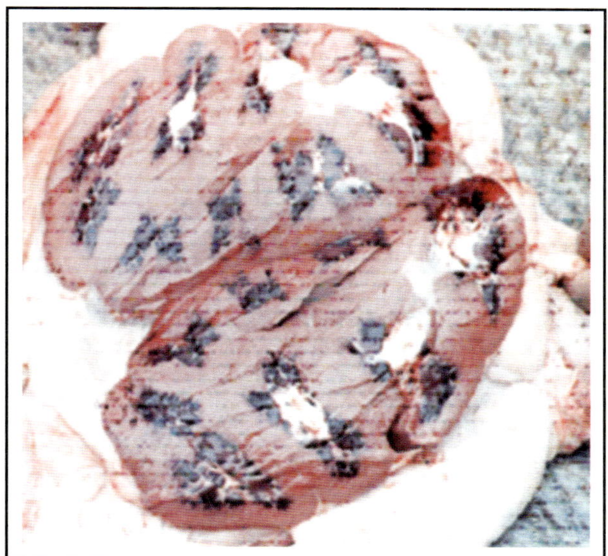

Figure 752: Massive haemorrhages and congestion in the medullo-corticular region of the kidney encountered in elephant (*E.maximus*) died of Zinc phosphide poisoning at Zoological Garden Mysore ,Karnataka. (Courtesy: Harish, B.R.& Ranukaprasad, C.).

Reproductive System

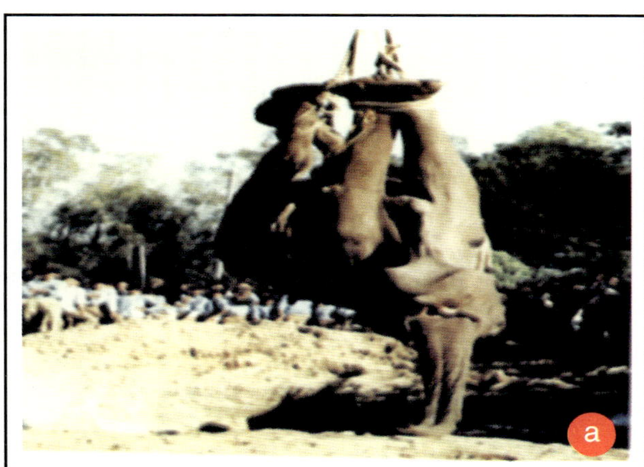

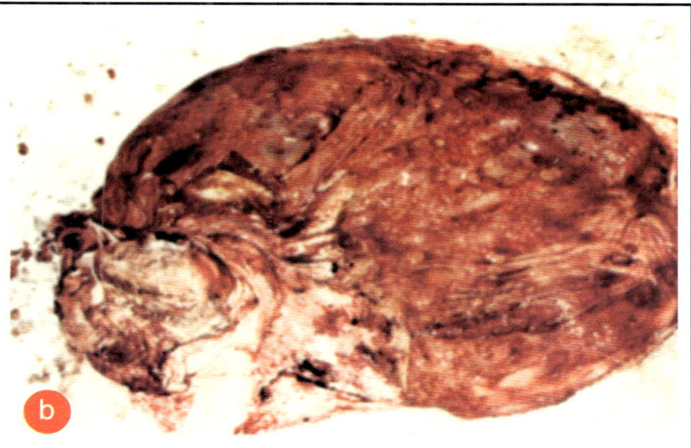

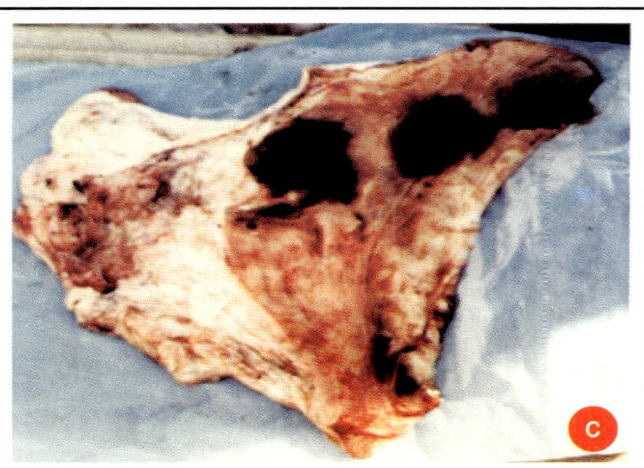

Figure 753: (a)Carcass of an adult elephant (*E. maximus*) cow being shifted to conduct postmortem examination and burying. Necropsy showed:(b) Haemorrhagic lesions of uterus. (c) Ulcerative lesions of uterine mucosa.

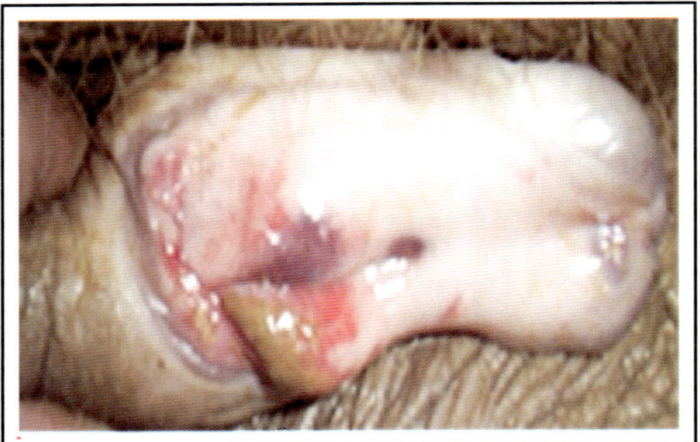

Figure 754: Photograph of vagina of elephant (*E. maximus*) showing haemorrhagic lesions.

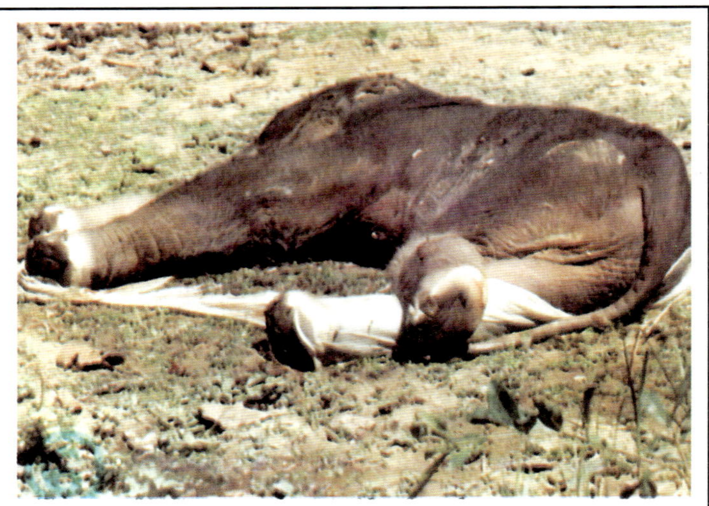

Figure 755: Carcass of elephant calf, which died of dystocia in elephant cow maintained at Forest Camp, National Park, Dudwa (U.P).

Nervous System

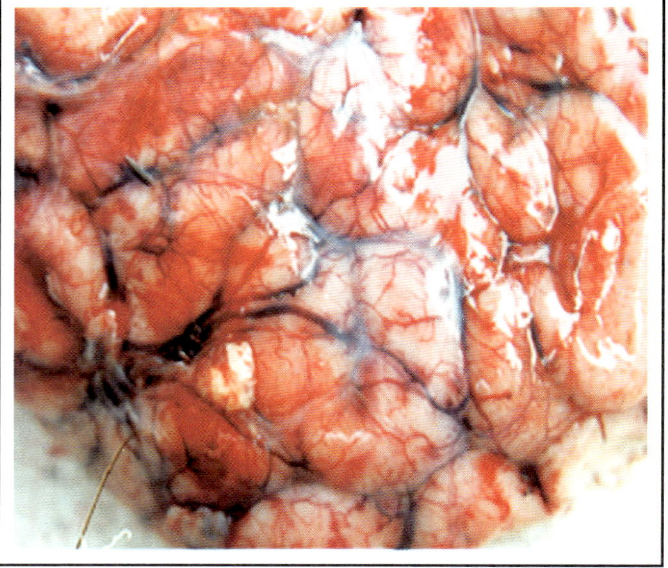

Figure 756 : Photograph of brain of elephant (*E. maximus*) showing congestion. The specific cause remained undermined.

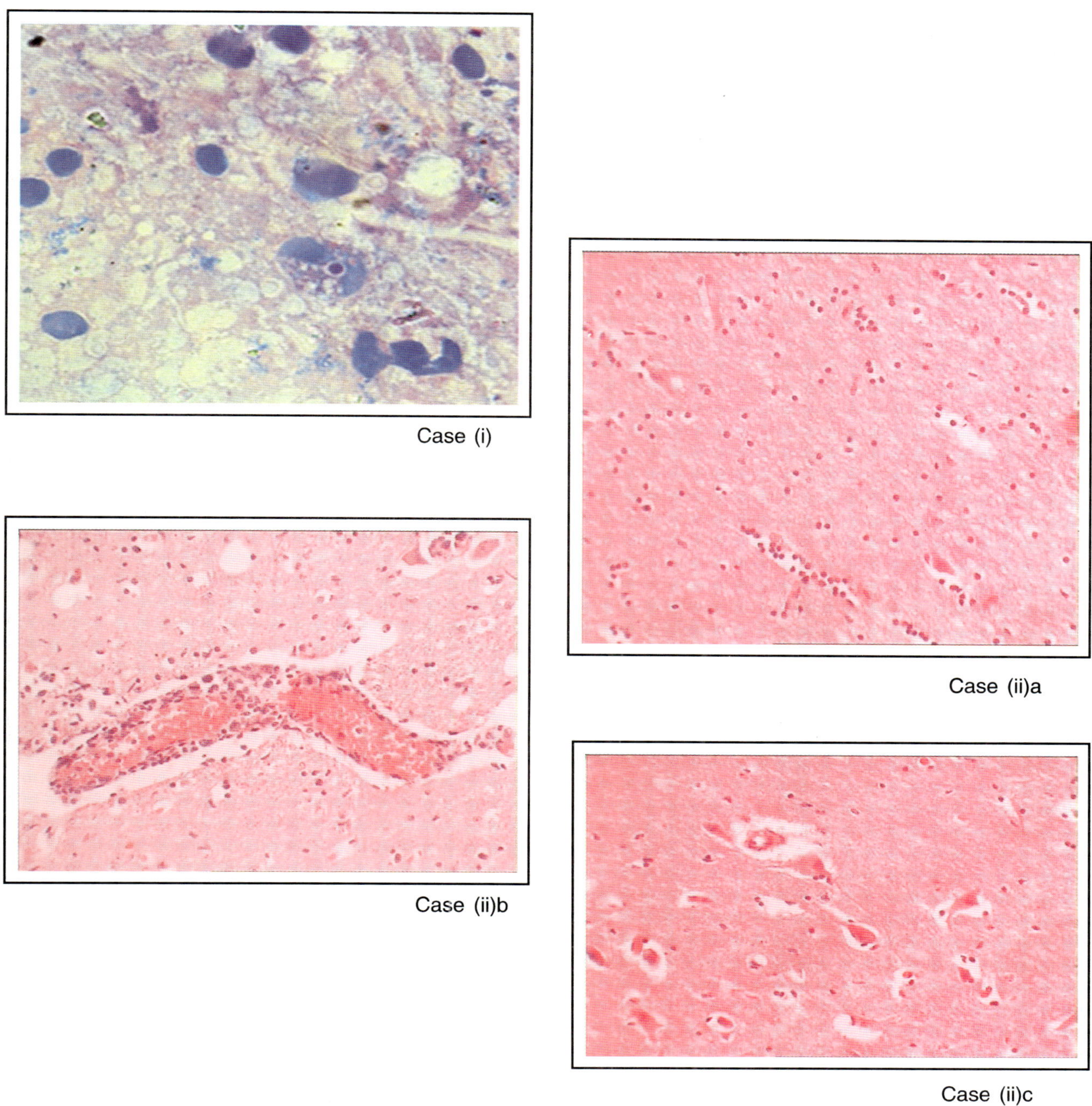

Figure 757: Case (i): Photomicrograph of brain of wild elephant (*E.maximus*) died of rabies showing Negri bodies (Courtesy: Institute of Animal Health & Biologicals Bangalore, Kanataka). Case (ii): Photomicrographs of cerebellum of an elephant died in forest camp of Manas National Park, Assam showing: (a) Accumulation of glia cells. H&E,x400 (b) Perivascular cuffing. H&E,x400 (c) Negri bodies in the cerebellum. H&E,x400.

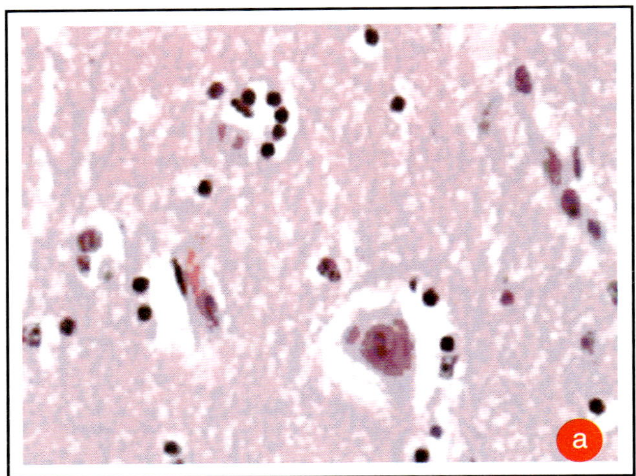

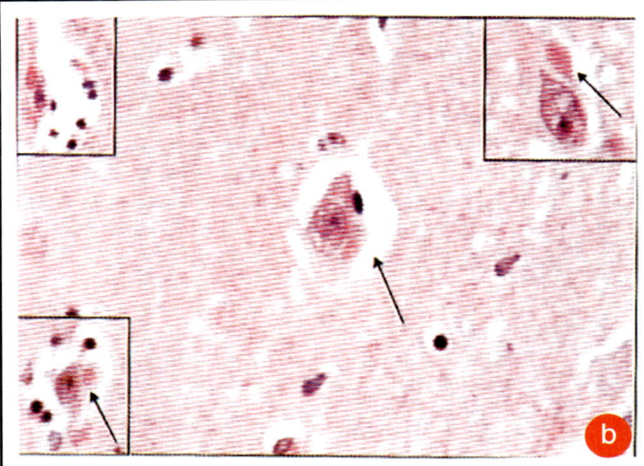

Figure 758: Photomicrographs of brain showing: (a) Neuronal degeneration with increased perineuronal space. Negri body (arrow head) and satellitosis. H&E,x400 (b) Increased perineuronal space and presence of various shapes of Negri bodies in the neurons (arrow). H& E, x400 (Courtesy: Sharma, A.K.).

Sense Organs - Eye

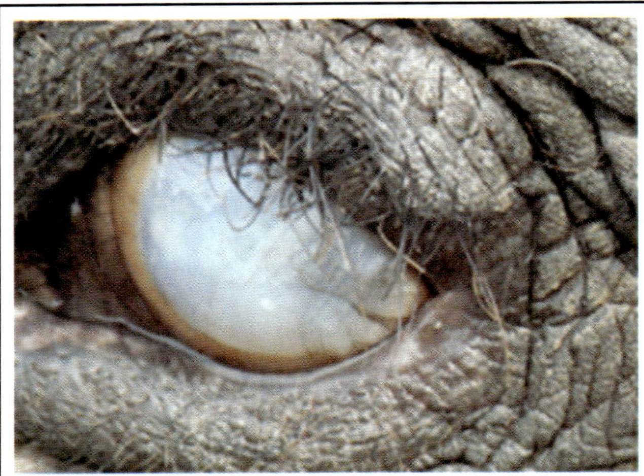

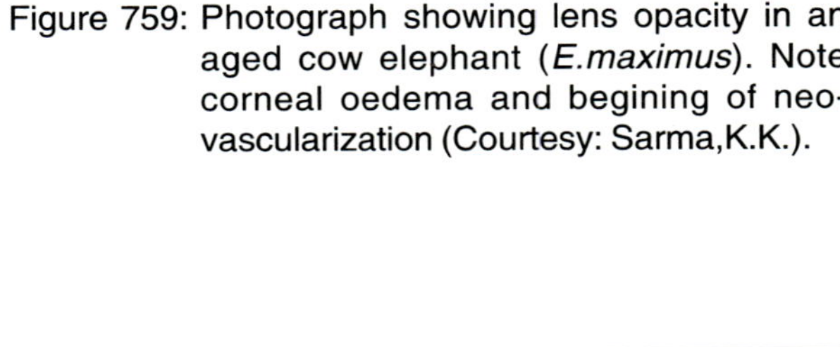

Figure 759: Photograph showing lens opacity in an aged cow elephant (*E.maximus*). Note corneal oedema and begining of neo-vascularization (Courtesy: Sarma,K.K.).

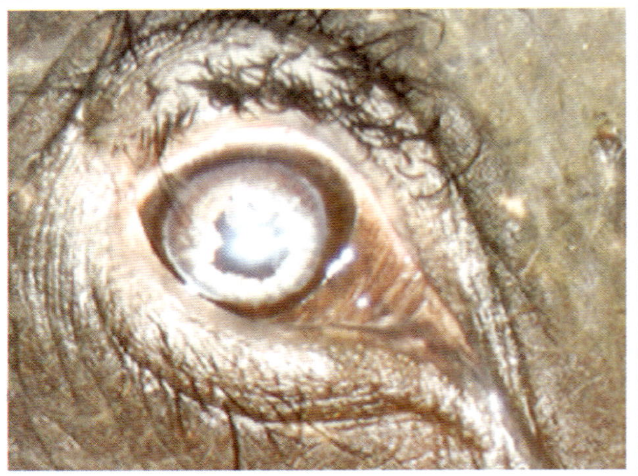

Figure 760: Photograph showing complete corneal opacity in an adult elephant (*E.maximus*).

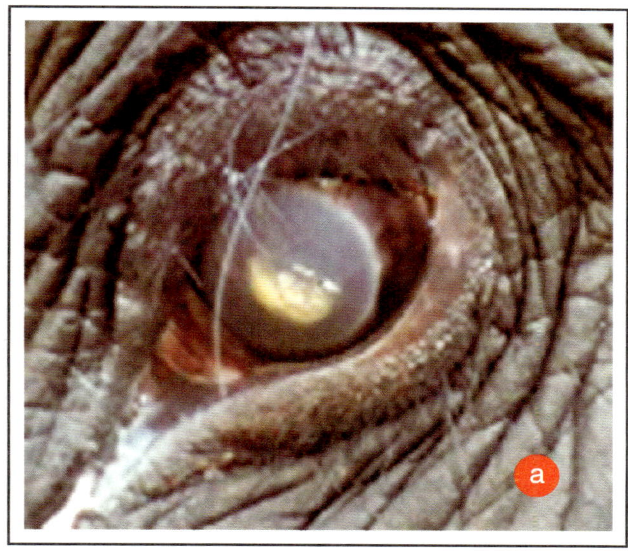

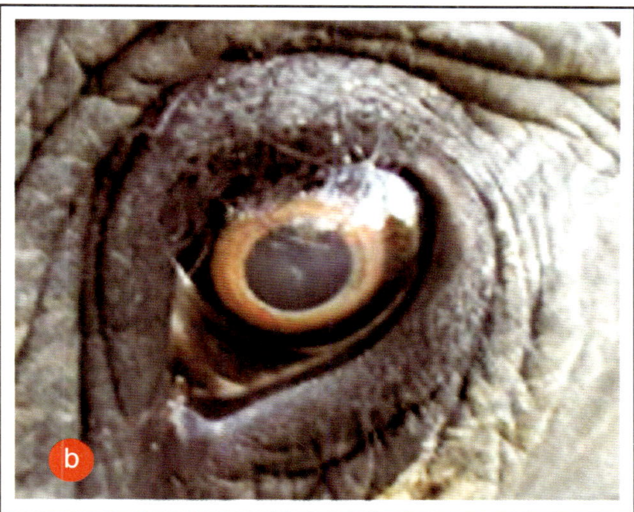

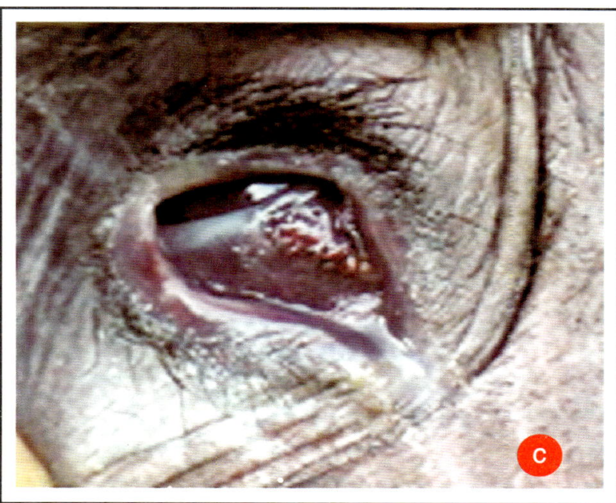

Figure 761: Eye problems in captive elephants (*E.maximus*). Photographs showing:(a) Corneal opacity and damaged lens, (b)Cataract (c) Conjunctivitis related to bacterial infection. (Courtesy:Talukdar, A.)

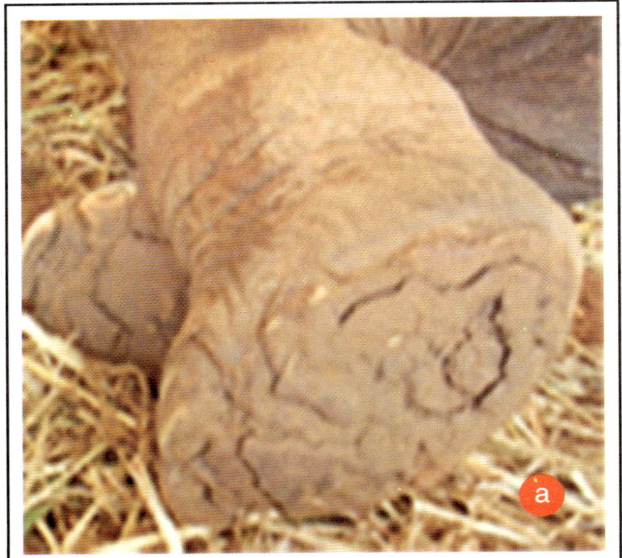

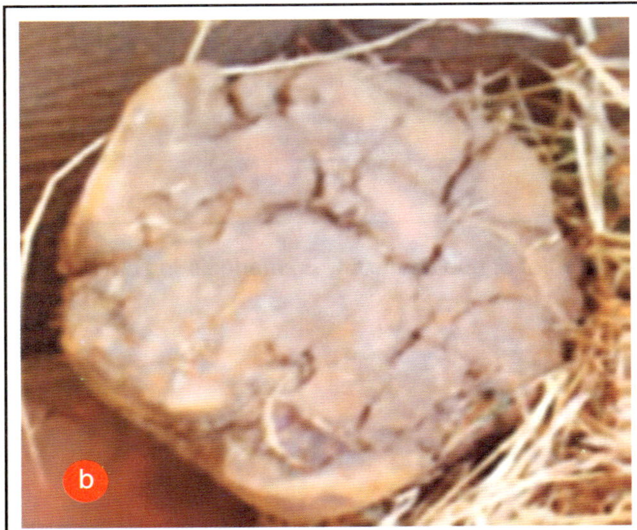

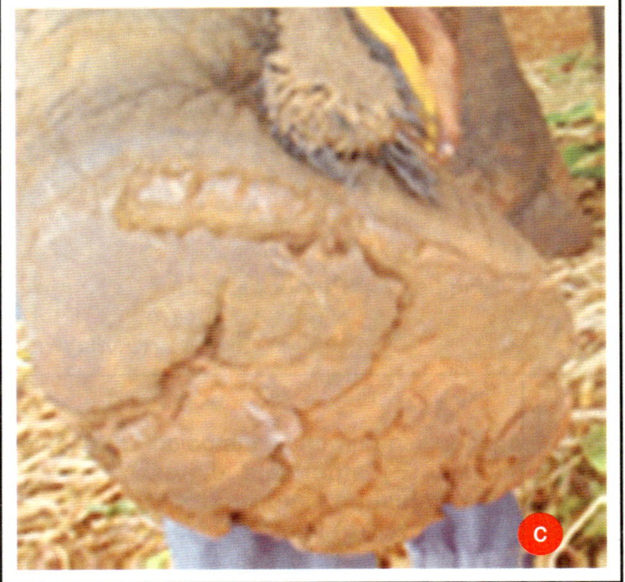

Figure 765: Photographs (a-c) showing cracks and sloughing in foot soles due to un-natural flooring provision to elephants (*E. maximus*).

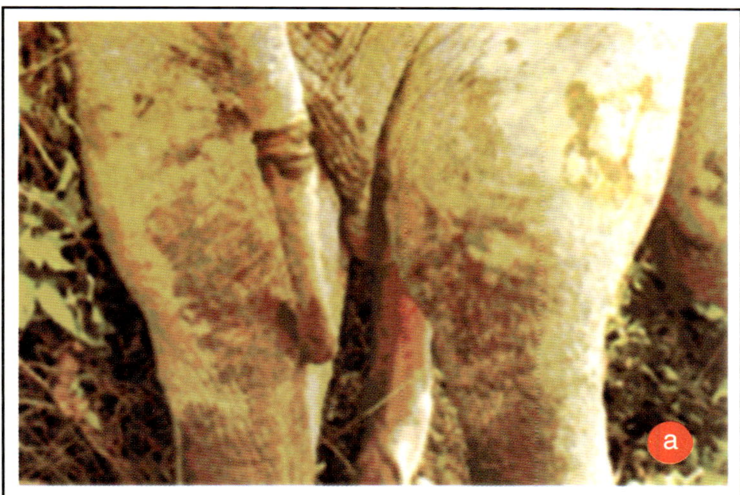

Figure 766: (a) Elephant (*E. maximus*) tail with deep cut up to caudal vertebra due to unattended forgotten band tied 20 years ago (b) Moist gangrene tail in rescued wild elephant calf (Courtesy: Sarma, K.K).

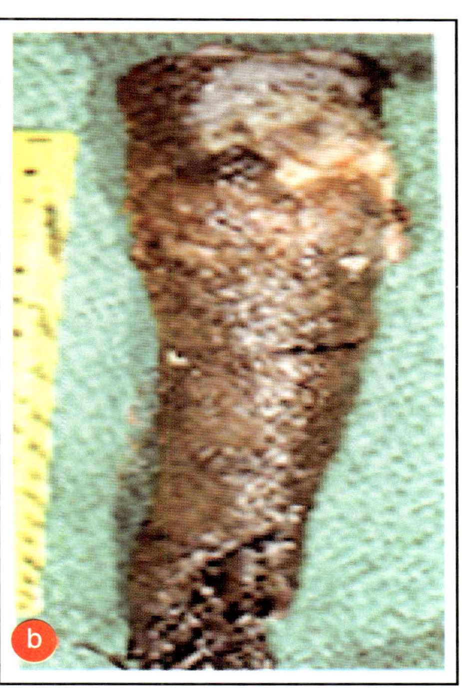

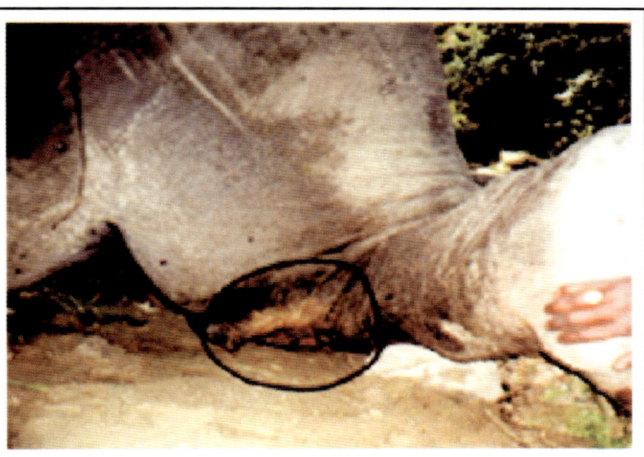

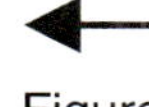

Figure 767: A large deep wound on the antero-lateral aspect of hind limb observed in carcass of an adult male wild elephant belonging to Rajaji National Park (Uttarakhand).

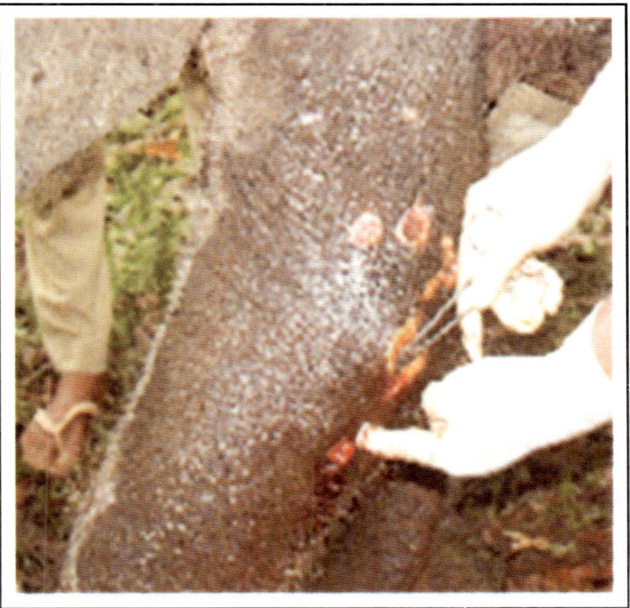

Figure 768: Photograph of wounded trunk of elephant calf at Forest Camp, alleged to tiger (*P. tigris*) attack. It was rescued and treated (Courtesy: Sarma, K.K.).

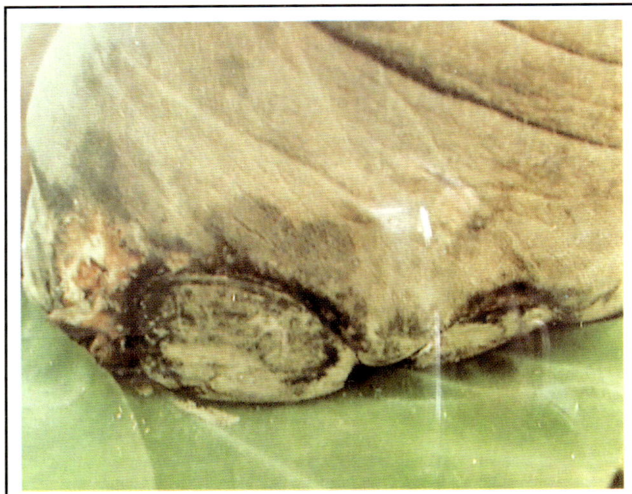

Figure 775: FMD lesion involving nail of elephant (*E. maximus*). The case is already refferred under respiratory and digestive system (Courtesy : Sharma D.K.).

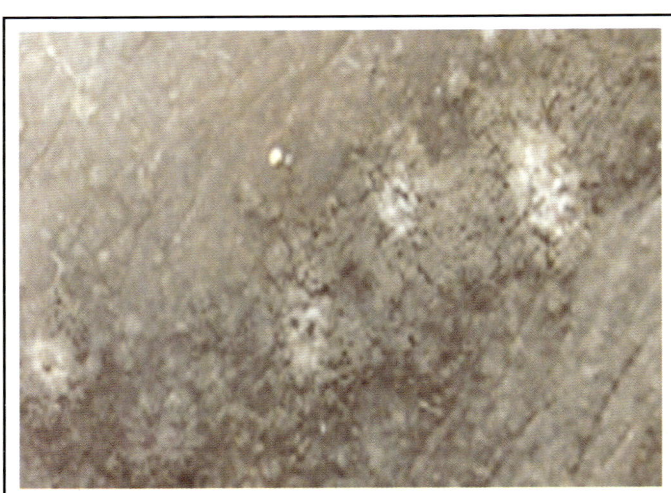

Figure 776: Photograph showing mycotic dermatitis in the abdominal region of elephant (*E. maximus*) caused by *Trichophyton sp.*

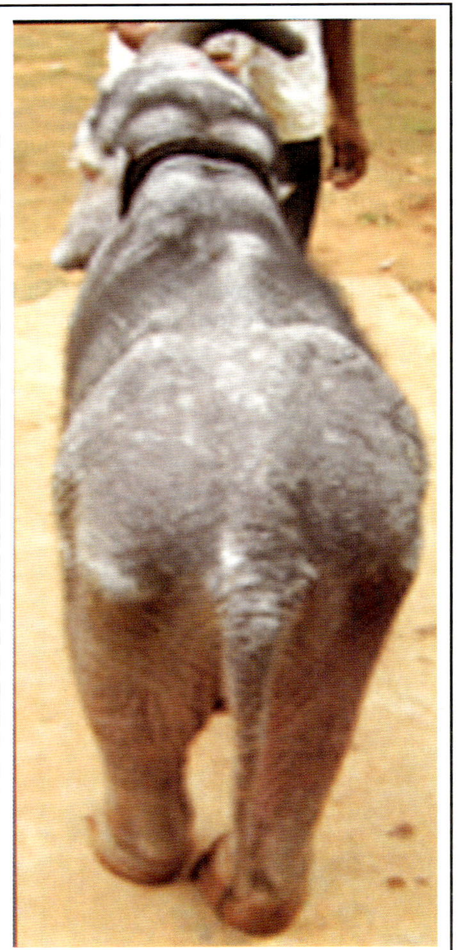

Figure 777: Scaling and dryness of skin noted in 7-8 weeks old elephant calf rescued from wild at Zoological Garden, Mysore (Karanataka).

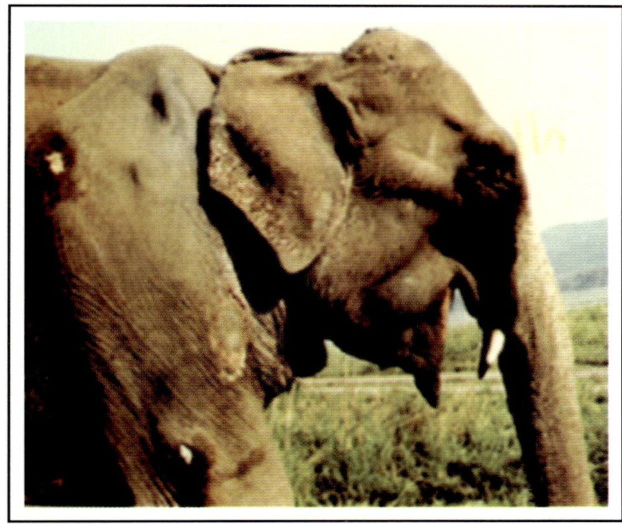

Figure 778: An adult elephant (*E. maximus*) at Corbett National Park, Ramnagar (Uttarakhand) showing several abscesses all over its body.

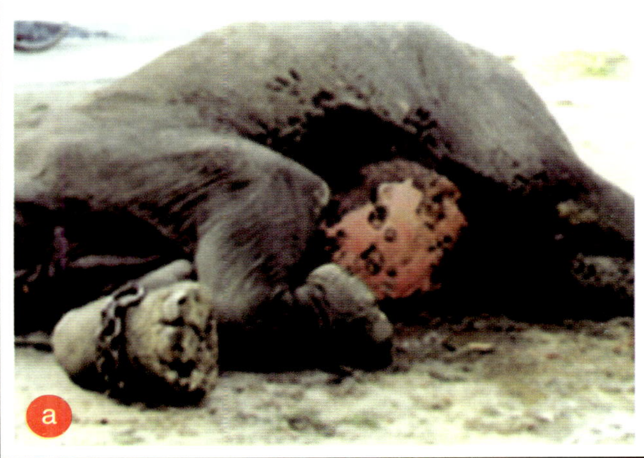

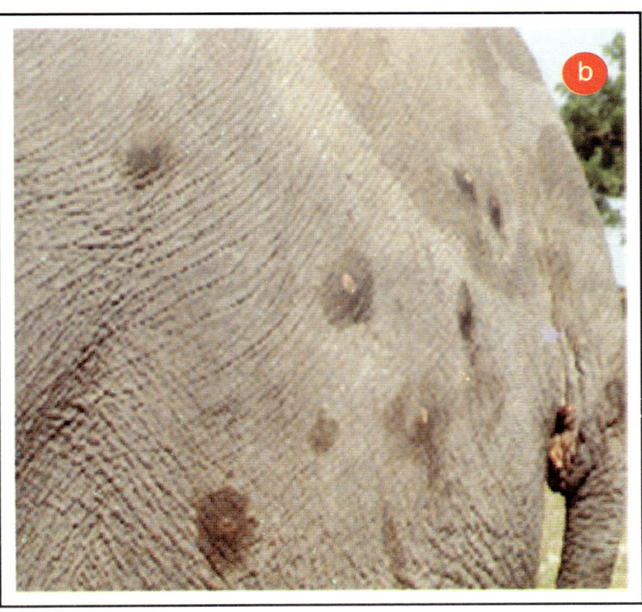

Figure 779: (a) Mycotic dermatitis in the belly region of captive elephant (*E. maximus*). (Courtsey: Choudhury, B.).(b) Photograph showing dermatitis in an adult elephant (*E. maximus*) due to filarial infection (Courtesy: Sarma, K.K.).

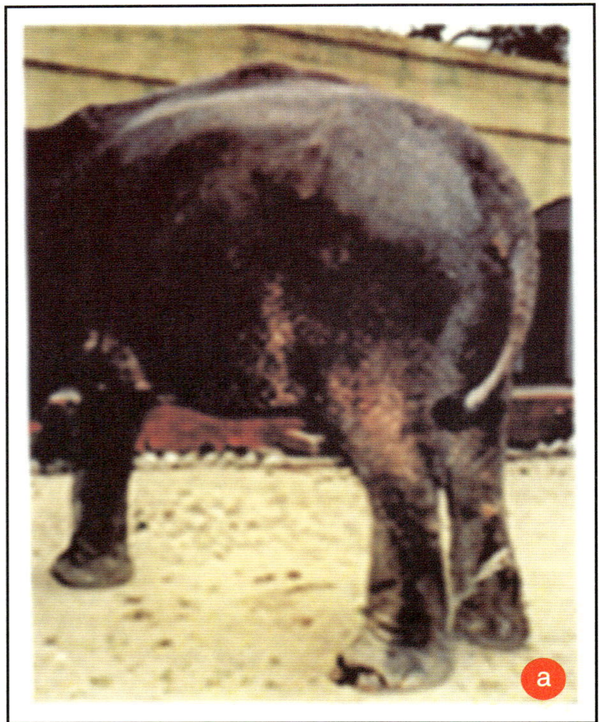

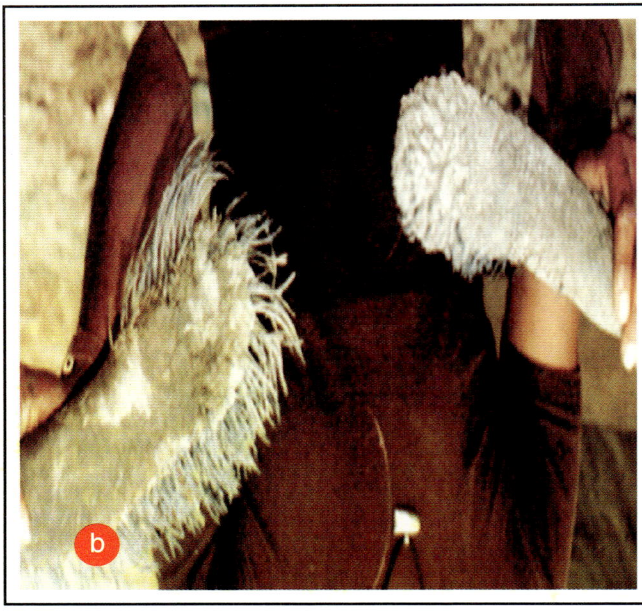

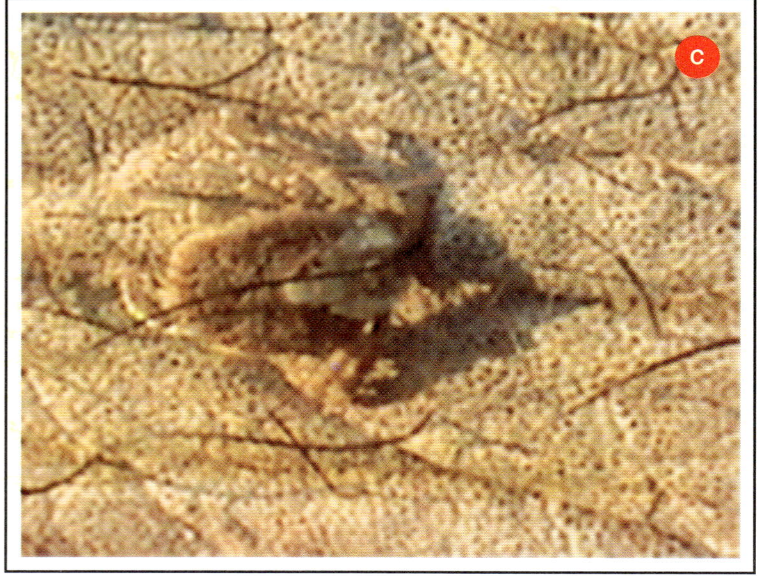

Figure 780: (a) An adult captive elephant (*E. maximus*) infested with *Haematomyzus elephantis* causing dryness and roughness of the skin. (b) *Haematomyzus elephantis* affecting tail in an elephant (*E. maximus*). (c) *Haematomyzus elephantis*.

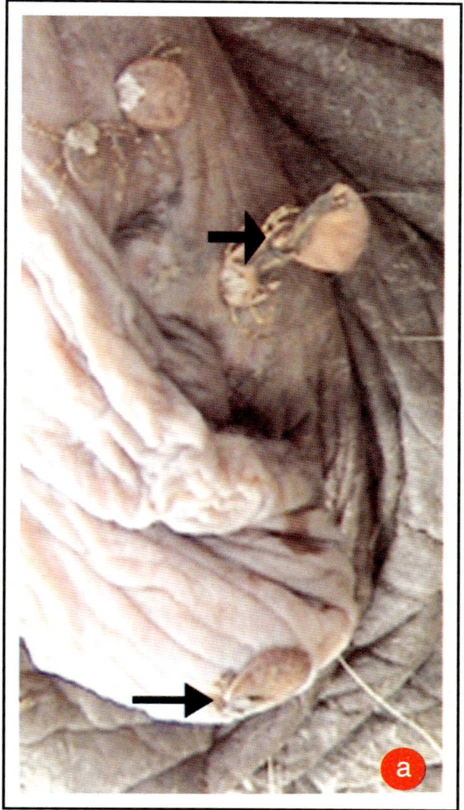

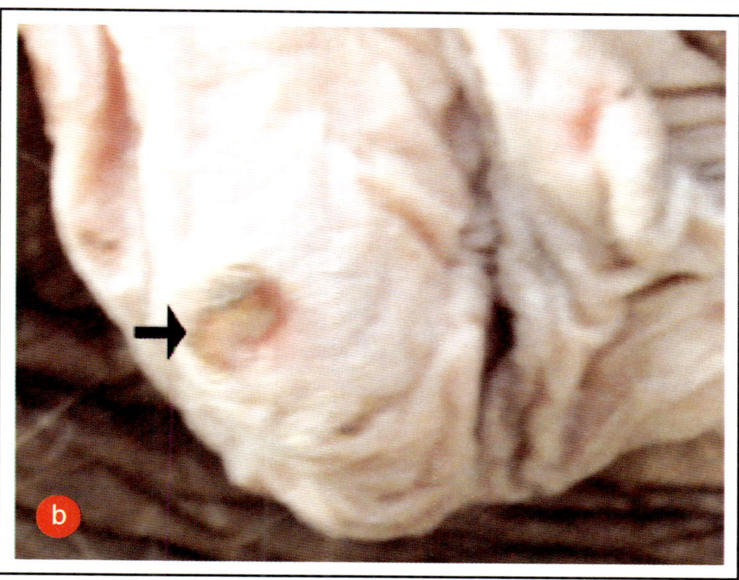

Figure 781: Tick attached to skin and rectal mucosal folds in an adult elephant (*E.maximus*). (b) Scar on skin and rectal mucosal fold due to sticking of tick (Courtesy: Sharmistha Chakaraborty).

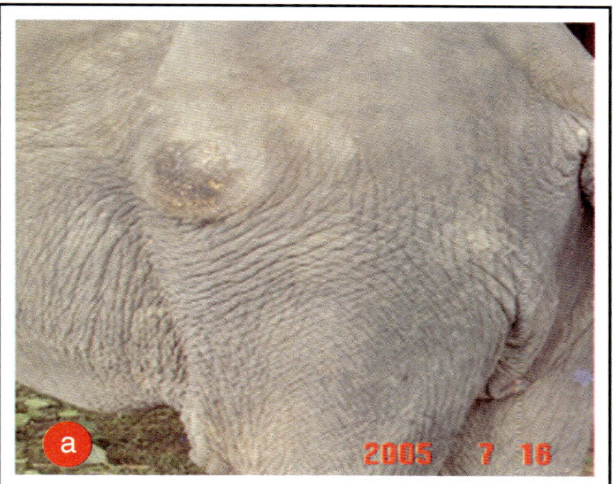

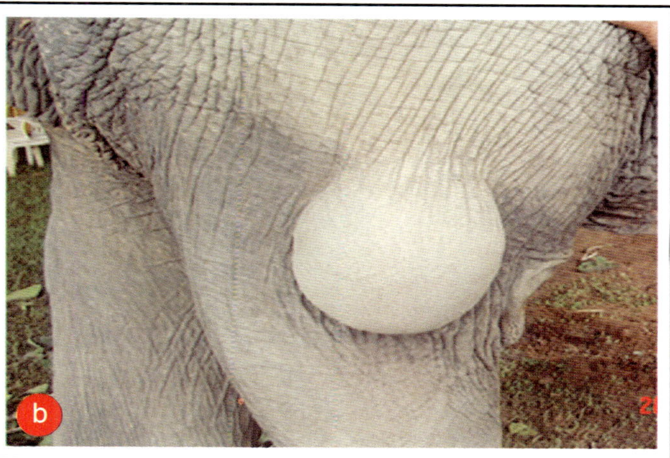

Figure 782: (a)Hard growth over the left stiffle joint of captive elephant (*E. maximus*) clinically diagnosed as fibroma. (b) Hard growth on lateral aspect of left fore limb in an adult elephant (*E. maximus*) belonging to a circus, clinically diagnosed as tumour.

Figure 783: Papillomatous growths on the trunk of an adult captive elephant (*E. maximus*). (Courtesy: Talukdar.A.).

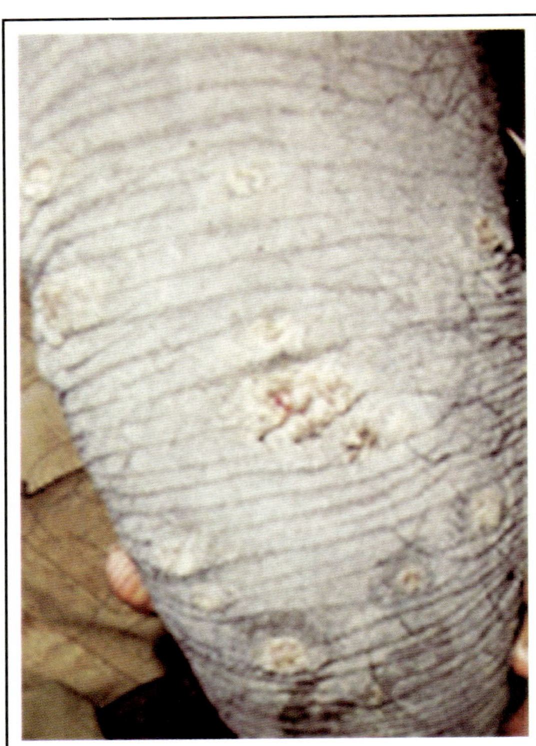

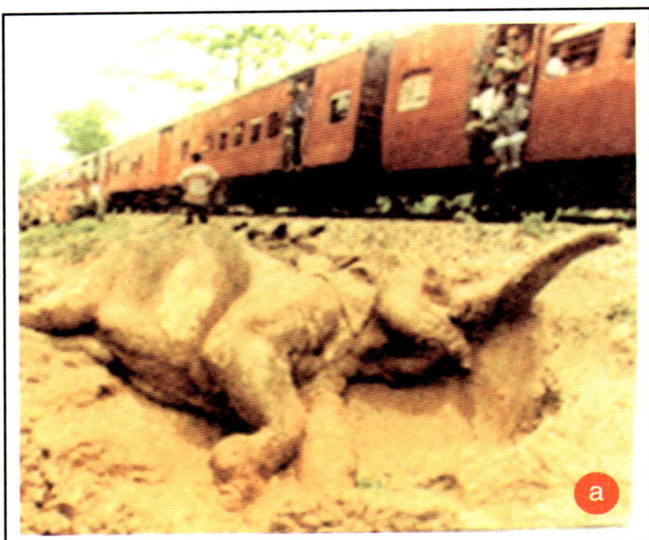

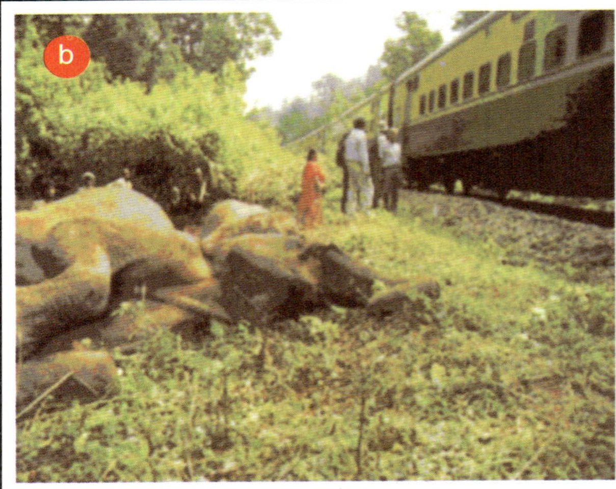

Figure 784: Elephants (*E. maximus*) died after head-on collision with trains. (a) Photo from a National Daily News Paper. (b) Photograph Courtesy: Nigam, P.

Musculo-Skeleton System

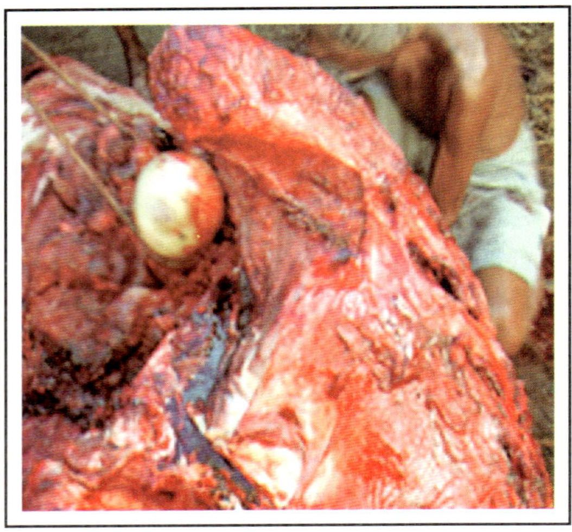

Figure 785: Photograph showing multiple fractures and haemorrhages in an elephant (*E. maximus*) that had died following collision with automobile (Courtesy: Nair, N.D.).

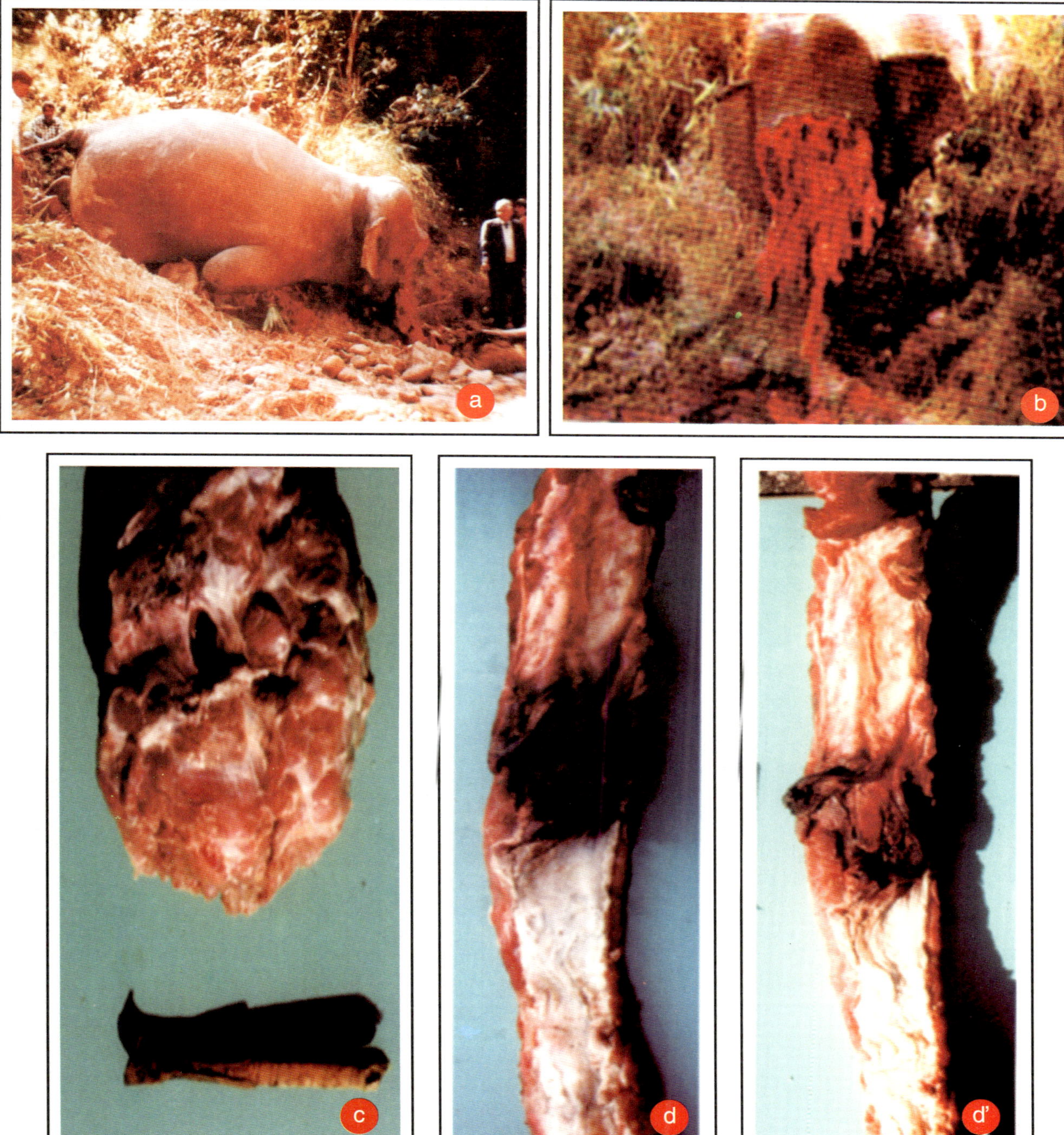

Figure 786: Photographs showing:(a) Side and front(b) views of the carcass of tusker (*E. maximus*) having forehead and trunk chopped off and tusks removed.(c) Lump of muscles showing hole through which dart deeply struck into the body and also showing the spatula shaped iron dart fitted with wooden bar (d,d') Fracture of rib caused as a result of striking of dart.

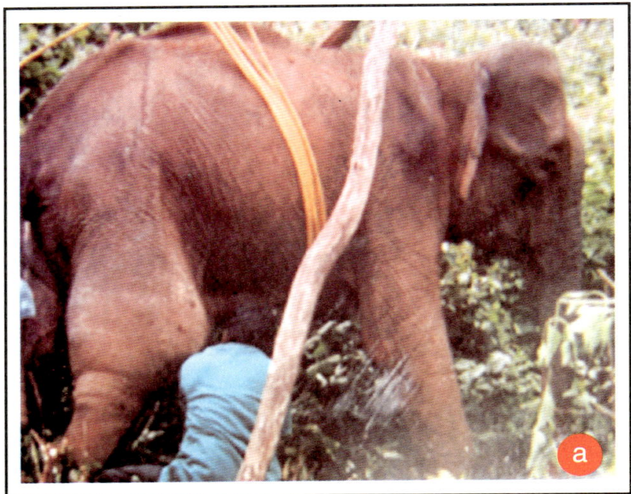

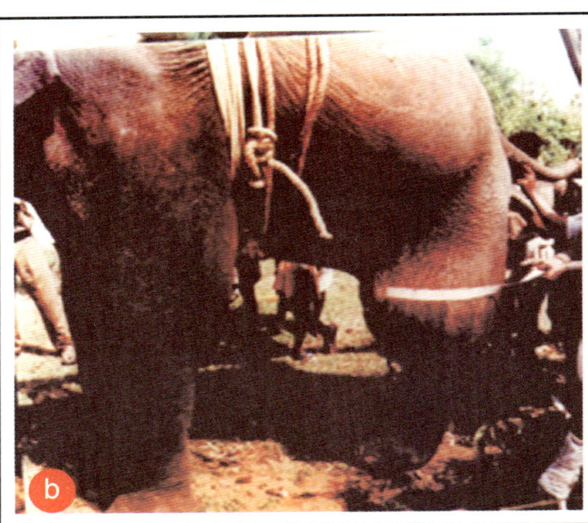

Figure 787: (a)An adult rescued wild elephant (*E. maximus*) cow on sling for surgical management of swelling of her right stifle joint. (b) Wild male adult tusker having a large swelling at its left Stifle joint (Nath *et al.*, 2005).

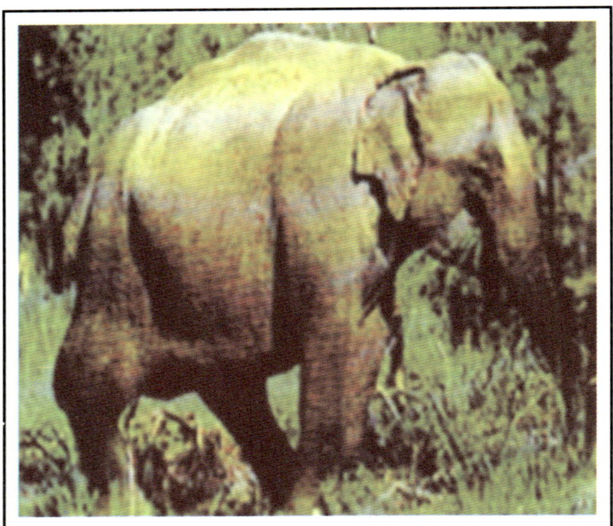

Figure 788: Fracture in right stifle joint of cow elephant in Corbett National Park, Ramnagar (Uttarakhand). (Adopted from Indian Wildlife, with permission from Bedi and Bedi, 1984).

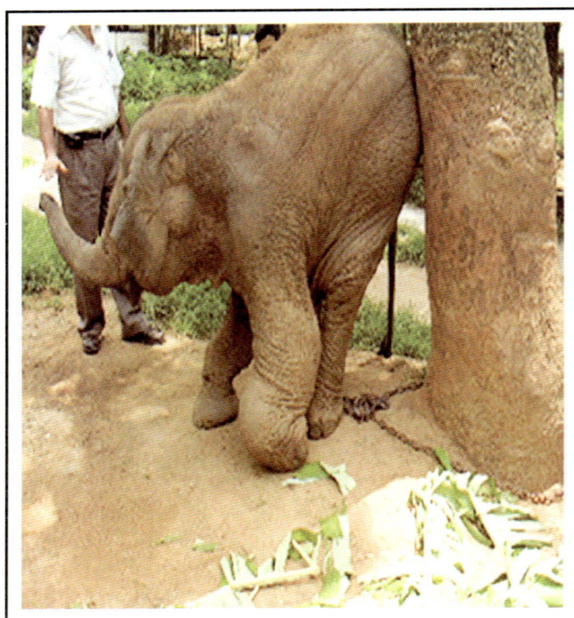

Figure 789: Photograph showing radial paralysis in a calf (*E. maximus*) following fracture of bilateral radial bones (Courtesy: Sarma, K.K.).

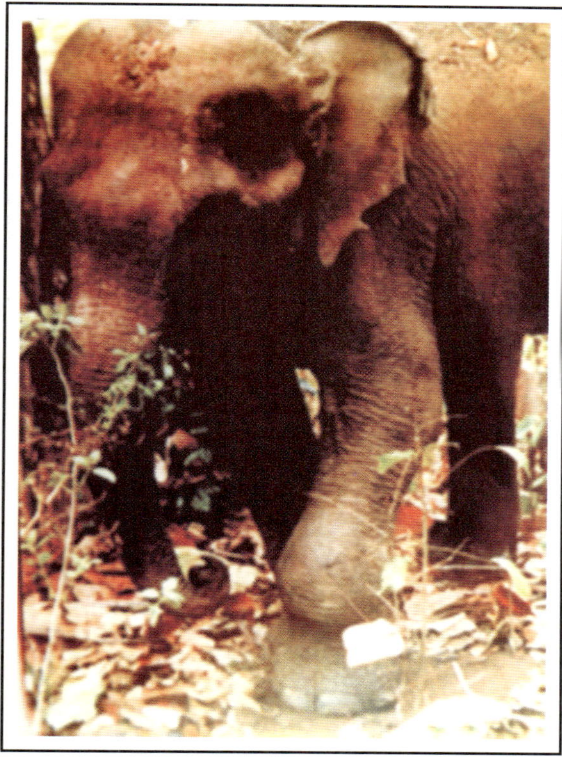

Figure 790: Photograph showing left radio-ulnar carpal joints swollen in an adult cow elephant (*E. maximus*).

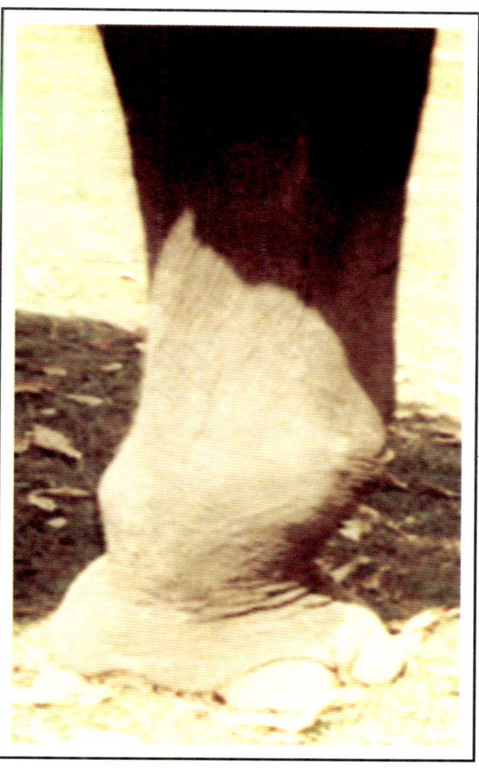

Figure 791: Photograph showing healed fracture of radio-ulnar carpal joints in an adult cow elephant.

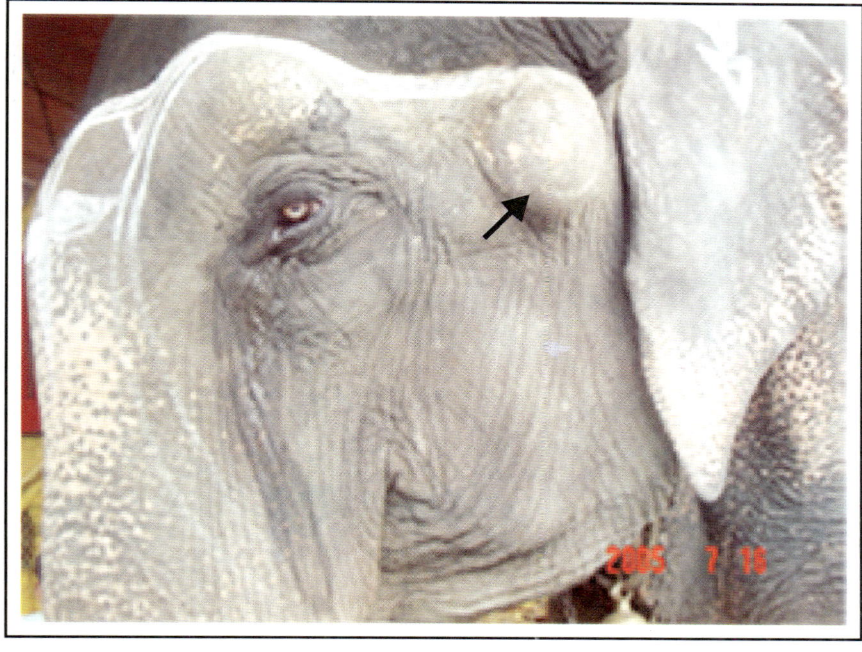

Figure 792 Photograph showing swelling of temporal bone in an adult captive elephant (*E. maximus*), which could be the result of frequentl use of driven spear/hook by Mahout.

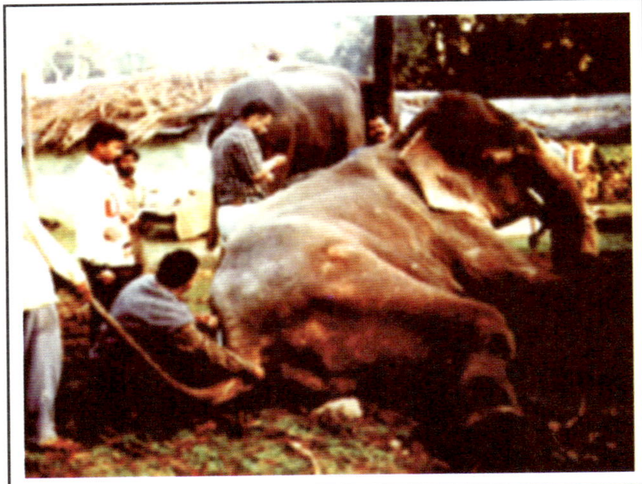

Figure 793: Debiliated elephant (*E. maximus*) cow under treatment at Dudwa National Park(U.P.). Note bed sores on her body.

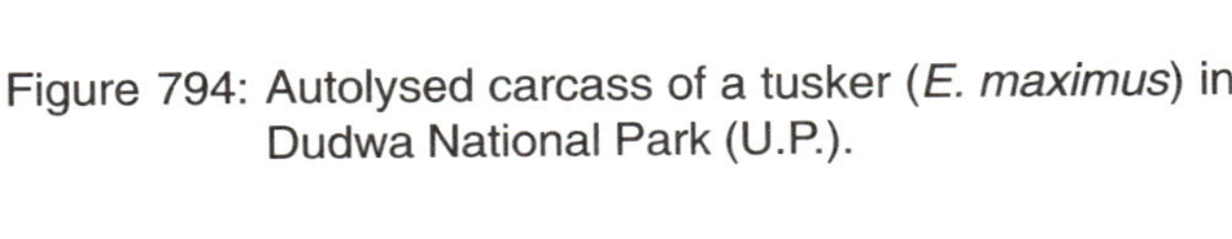

Figure 794: Autolysed carcass of a tusker (*E. maximus*) in Dudwa National Park (U.P.).

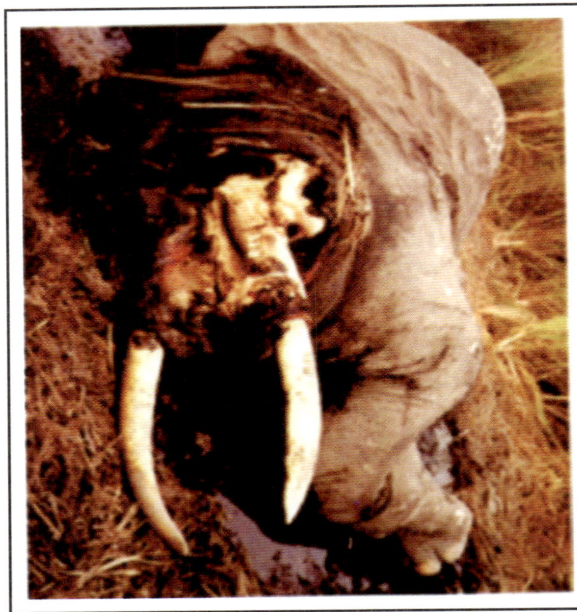

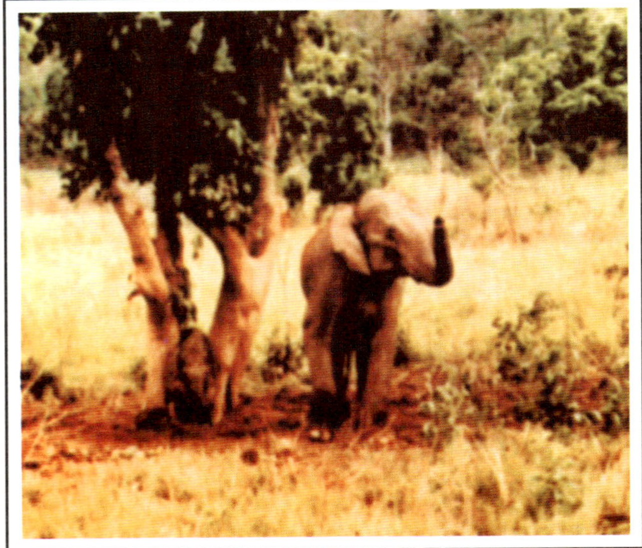

Figure 795: Elephant calf stranded between forked stem of a tree in Corbett National Park (Uttarakhand) and helpless mother standing nearby.

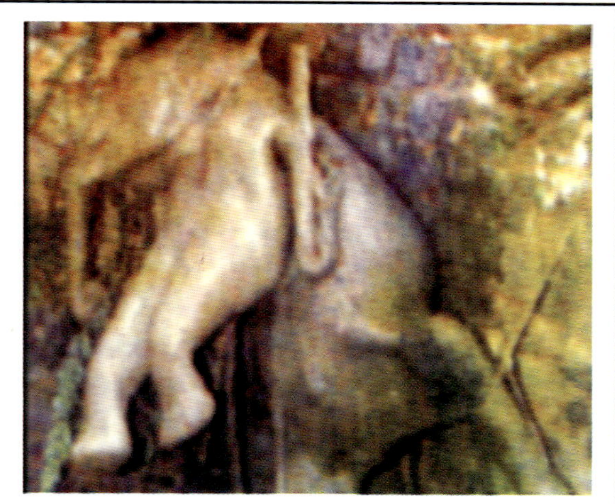

Figure 796: Wild elephant calf being rescued from a well.

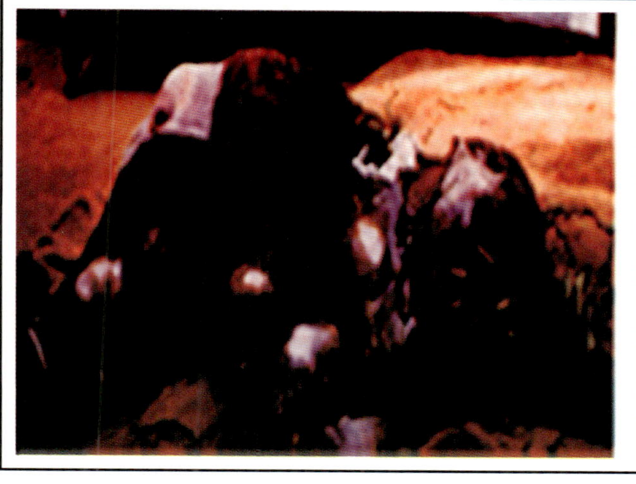

Figure 797: Elephant calf destined for Zoological Park, New Delhi from Zoological Garden, Guwahati fell sick during transportation by road and was downloaded at Zoological Garden, Lucknow (U.P.) for treatment but had died. Stress of transportation by road and cold was attributed for its death.

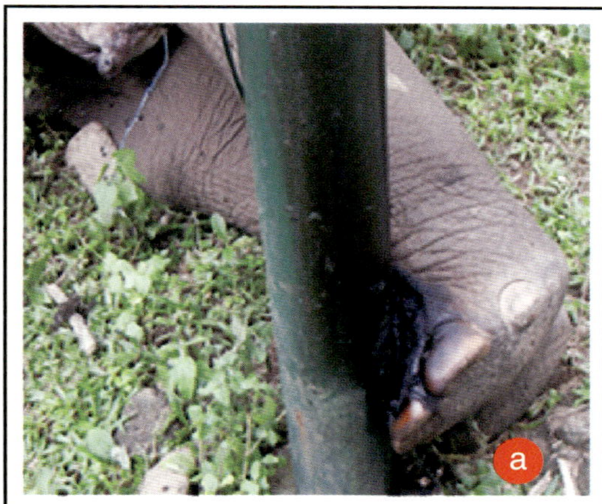

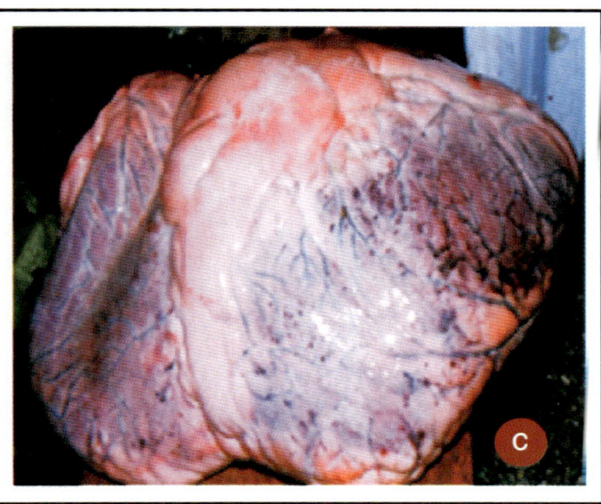

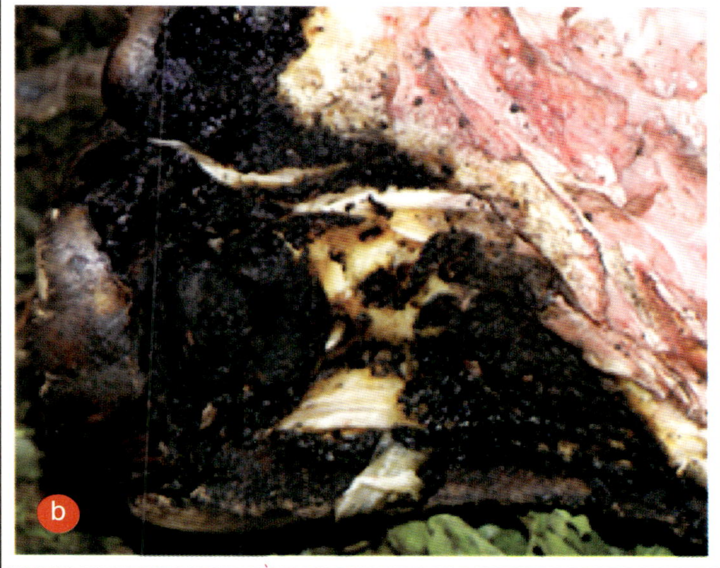

Figure 798: Elephant (*E.maximus*) died of electrocution.(a) Leg of elephant touching an electric post.(b) Electrocuted leg showing burn area. (c) Heart showing massive haemorrhages (Courtesy : Anupam Raskhit).

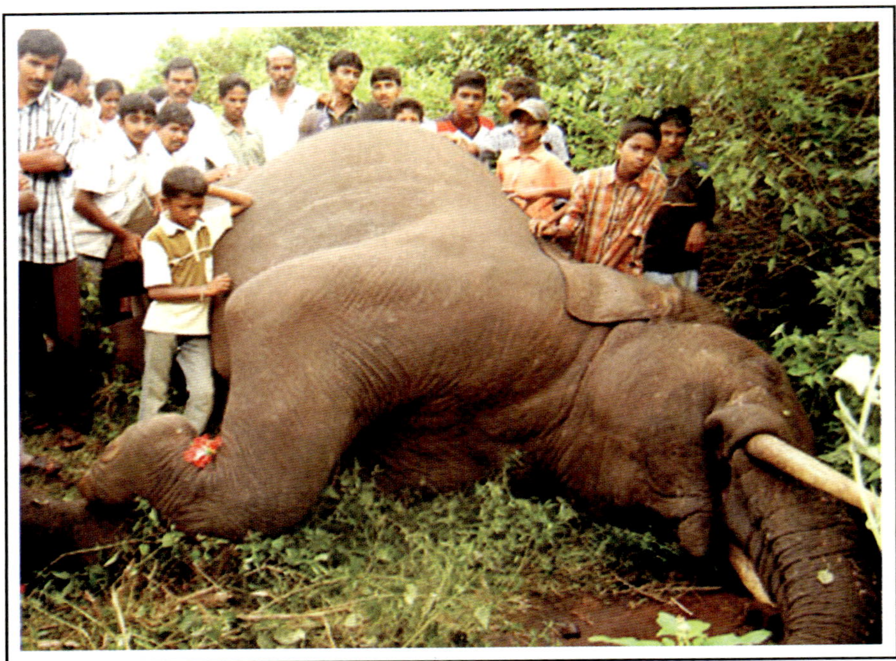

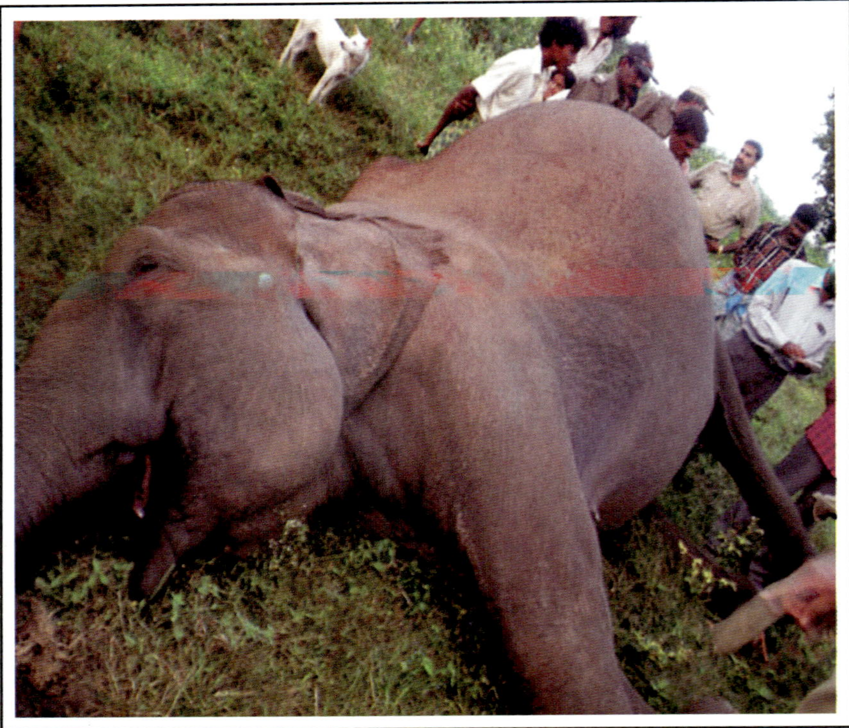

Fig. 799. Photographs of a electrocuted tusker and a cow elephant in Bandipur Wildlife Sanctuary. (Rajkumar, D. ERN Member, E-mail : 09-2-08.)

References

Ajay, A. Desai (1989) In : Proceedings "The Asian Elephant" By Silas, E.G., Nair, M.K. & Nirmalan, G. Pub. Kerala Agricultural University, Trichur.

Arora, B.M. (2003). Indian wildlife diseases and disorders. 1st Edition, Published by Association of Indian Zoo & Wildlife Veterinarians.

Bedi, R. and Bedi, R. (1984). *Indian Wildlife.* Pub. Brijbasi Printers Pvt. Ltd; E-46/11Okhala (Phase II), NewDelhi-110020

Chakraborty. T. and Majumdar, B.K. (1990). Foot and mouth disease in an Indian elephant. In Calcutta Zoological Garden: A case Report. *Indian Vet. Med. J.* 14:213-14.

Chandrasekharan, K. (1989). In : Proceedings "The Asian Elephant" By Silas, E.G., Nair, M.K. & Nirmalan, G. Pub. Kerala Agricultural University, Trichur.

Evans, G.H. (1910).Elephants and their diseases-a treatise on elephant, Rangoon

Islam Saidul *et al.* (1996). Pathology of nephropathies in two elephants. Zoos' Print, 11:5-7.

Manhoran, B.M. *et al.* (2004). Pododermatitis in elephant *Indian Vet J* 81:107.

Nath, K.L. *et al* (2005). Elephant tranquilization and treatment- A report of six cases. In: Souvenir National symposium on Wildlife Health and Husbandry Constraints, Pub. AIZ&WV.

Sharma, D.K. *et al.* (1994). Foot and mouth diseases in baby elephant. *Indian J.Vet.Path.*18 (1): 55-56.

Sarma, K.K *et al.* (2005). Dub-mandubular oedema in a cow elephant affected with *Fascioloa jacksoni. Intas Polivet.* 6 (2) 318.

Talukdar, A. and Choudhury, B. (2007). Management of injured trunk of an elephant (*E. maximus*) calf.In:*Rehabilitation in tree living wild animals,Ed.B.M.Arora, 1st Ed.Pub. AIZ&WV, Bareilly.*

Singh, K. P. *et al.* (1994) *Facioloa jacksoni* infection in elephants. *Indian J. of Anim. Sci.* 64(8):802-04.

AVES

Introduction

The Class- Aves of Phylum vertebrate includes 27 Orders **(Table 6)**, which are comprised of 9, 000 species in the world. From behavioural point of view, they are grouped into walking birds and flying birds. In India, among the 12 hundred bird species recognized, all are flying. Presently the most endangered bird species belonged to family *Pheasanidae* and *Felconiformes*. White winged wood duck (*Cairina scutalata*), pink-headed duck (*Rhodonessaca caryophyllacea*), Pink tailed duck either has vanished or has reached at the brink of extinction. The large sized flying birds such as sarus crane, flamingo, pelican, adjutant and painted storks, pied hornbill, bastard, vultures, require special care in captivity. Keeping these birds in small cages brings them not only misery but also adversely affect their health and reproduction. A large number of migratory bird species during winter season visit the country. They may introduce the disease into the country like bird flu. Therefore monitoring and surveillance disease programme needs to be strengthened.

Table 6: Class –Aves, orders and their species

SN	Order	Species Profile	SN	Order	Species Profile
1	Anseriformes	Waterfowl with long beak, webbed feet,e.g ducks, geese, swan	15	Gruiformes	Marsh birds with long, strong legs, e.g.cranes, rails
2	Apodiformes	Short legged long winged, e.g. swifts and humming birds	16	Passeriformes	Singing and perching small to medium sized birds, large number(over 5,000) species in this Order, e.g. weavers, finches, tangers, sunbirds, tots,birds of paradise, crows, magpies, starlings, swallows, fly catchers, thrushes, blackbirds, nightingles, wrens, larks
3	Apterygiformes	Flightless, grey brown hair like feathers,e.g. Kiwis	17	Pelecaniformes	Large swimming birds with webbed feet, e.g. pelicans, cormorants, frigates birds
4	Caprimulgiformes	Nocturnal birds with long wings and small feet, e.g. nightjars	18	Piciformes	Colourful birds with large or long painted bills, eg. woodpecker, toucans
5	Casuariformes	Large flightless birds, long neck and legs, e.g.Cassowaries	19	Podicipediformes	Aquatic birds, living on fresh waters, partially webbed feet, close plumage, e.g. grebs
6	Charadiiformes	Small to medium sized waders with bulky body, short legs, e.g. gulls, suks, avocets, plovers	20	Procellariformes	Long winged sea birds with tubler nostrils, e.g. albatorosses, petrefs
7	Ciconiiformes	Large long necked birds with beak, e.g.herons, storks, flamingoes	21	Psittaciformes	It is commonly known as Parrot family, root of bill with nostrils is covered by naked skin, very strong beak, e.g. parrots, macaws, cockatoos
8	Coliiformes	Mouse like small birds with long tails, e.g.mouse birds	22	Rheiformes	Latge flightless birds, long neckand legs, e.g. rheas
9	Columbiformes	Medium sized birds with bulky body , short legs, e.g. pigeons , doves	23	Sphonisciformes	Flighless marine birds, flippers instead of wings, body covered with feathers, e.g.penguins.
10	Coraciiformes	Birds with brilliant plumage, usually large bill, long tail and head crested, e.g. king fishers, hornbills, bee eaters	24	Strigiformes	Nocturnal birds of prey, big head, soft plumage, large eyes surrounded by facial disc, strongly hoocked claws, e.g. owls
11	Cuculiformes	Small to medium sized long tail and curved beak, e.g.cuckoos	25	Struthioniformes	Largest living birds, run instead of flying, e.g. ostrich
12	Falconiformes	Birds of prey , have powerfull hooked beak, strong claws, e.g. eagles, felcons, vultures	26	Tinamiformes	Medium sized partridge- like birds, e.g tinamous
13	Galliformes	They are known as game birds, have robust build and powerful, e.g pheasants, partridges, turkeys, quils	27	Trogoniformes	Brightly coloured birds with short broad bills, e.g. tragons
14	Gaviifomes	Duck like birds,with pointed bill,e.g.loons, divers			

Developmental anomalies: Like mammals melanism for white or black form of avian individuals is mutant and as such they are results of presence of identical genes controlling biochemical mechanism inhibiting incorporation of melanoblasts- precursors of normal pigment producing cells melanocytes into the growing hair at the embryonic stage. White specimens such of crow, peafowl, dove **(Figure 65-66)**, jungle babbler, common myna, jungle bush quail are often seen in Zoological collections. No specific congenital organ anomaly in respect of cardio-vascular, digestive, respiratory and urinary systems could be portrayed photographically as no case was found. A small cyst like structure connected with persistent urachus **(Figure 59)** found in a black swan (*Cygnus atratusi, an* exotic sp.). A solitary case of double head brahaminy duck (*Tadorna ferruginea*) chick hatched in captivity is illustrated **(Figure 76)**.

Eco-husbandry associated health hazards: (a) Poisoning: Specific etiology for rapid decline in populations of three species *of* vulture namely, white-backed vulture (*Gyps bengalensis)*, long billed vulture (*Gyps indicus*) and slender billed vulture (*Gyps tenuirostris*) throughout South Asia is alleged to drug toxicity caused by eating carcasses of domestic animals that were treated with diclofenac- non steroidal anti-inflammatory drug (NASID). Some believe that a viral disease may be responsible for enmasse killing of vultures. Thus, results of mortality investigations are at variance. Occasionally malicious poisoning is alleged for mortality of serpentine eagles **(Figure 83)** and vultures **(Figure 19)**. In peafowl mortality with pesticides (organophosphates) particularly during crop sowing seasons has been reported (Arora, 2003)

Alfatoxicosis is related to eating of aspergillus-infected food. Workers have documented lesions of degeneration and necrosis of hepatic cells **(Figure 26)** in parrots and in addition to that extensive bile duct hyperplasia **(Figure 27)** in tuffed pochard ducks (*Aytha fuligatta*)

(b) Physical injuries: Infighting and cannibalism injuries in certain bird species are occasionally registered. Ingestion of foreign matter in the zoo birds are often found during necropsy examination **(Figures 17 to 18).** Predation related mortalities in captive birds are due to vermin **(Figure 85).** Traumatic shock in caged birds often occurs either in capture or transportation operations **(Figure 86)** or owing to presence of some threats in and around their cages causing terrible commotion and distress to them. Transportation of bird is not risk free particularly during summer season. Overcrowding and underfeeding of birds in confinement is misery **(Figure 87)**. During typhoons/storms long bone fractures in growing adjutant and painted stork chicks has been encountered due to felling from the tree nests **(Figures 80- 81)**. Repair of leg fractures in these birds provide a unique challenge, as leg bones possess large medullary cavity and thin cortices. Fracture of beak in one or two cases on a mass capturing of young painted stork and pelican cannot be ruled out. There is high incidence of lacerated wing injuries in large bodied birds of prey caused due to string of flying kites **(Figure 67).** Electrocution losses due to striking against electric transmission lines in free flying birds are not uncommon. During early morning hours certain birds such as parrots, crows, common mynas, and doves are seen picking the food particles on the high ways and when a speedy vehicle approaches, they start flying one by one and in this course one or two birds (particularly parrots) get collided against the speedy vehicles and are either died or get seriously injured.

Nutritional deficiency & Metabolic disorders: Birds in captivity are liable to suffer from deficiency of various vitamins and minerals and certain metabolic disorders, which have not been systematically studied. Deficiencies of vitamins B_1 and A, are experienced in captive birds **(Figures 15, 61)**. Non-supply of water resulted in heavy mortality in small birds **(Figure 89)**. Metabolic disorder like visceral gout in birds is not uncommon. Necropsy examinations have recorded uric acid deposits in visceral organs - over kidneys, liver and heart in vultures-Gyps species **(Figures 50 to 54)** and other birds (Arora, 2003). One case of uric acid deposition in visceral organs in woolly neck storks (*Ciconia episcopus*) died in wild was recorded **(Figure 1a,b).**

Diseases. (A) Infectious & Parasitic: These are poorly studied in wild birds. Certain illustrations produced in the chapter are recounted hereunder.

(a) Cardiovascular system: Avian malaria (*Plasmodium* sp.) infection has been documented in jungle fowl **(Figure 4)**, pea- fowls, partridges and paddy birds. Some workers alleged *Plasmodium gallinaceum* to be one of the causes of declining vulture population in India. Besides the lesions of Zygomycosis in the respiratory and digestive systems of Bengal florican (*Houbaropsis bengalensis*) that died in wild, a large sized raised nodular growth on the heart, and small nodules on the pericardium were marked. Microscopically the lesions showed hyphae of Zygomycetes in fibrinous mass **(Figure 2)**.

(b) Respiratory system: Nocardiosis is an important bacterial disease encountered in Hill myna (G*racula religiosa*). The lesions include nodular caseated or granulomatous lesions with epithelioid and langhans' giant cells in the lungs **(Figure7)** similar to that of tuberculosis. Pulmonary tuberculosis **(Figure 8)** is recorded in chir pheasants (*Catreus wallichi*). Disease was recorded in demoiselle cranes (*Anthropoids virgo),* macaw (*Ara severa*) Muscovy (*Caririna moschata*) and brahminy (*Tadorna ferrugina)* ducks. The lung lesions in these described formation of tubercles embedded in the parenchyma, some coalesced forming irregular masses and others as discrete foci.

Pulmonary mycotic infection caused by *Aspergillus* sp. was found in oriental pied hornbill (*Anthracoceros malabaricus*) died in the wild **(Figure 9-11)** and in red jungle fowl (*G. gallus*) and Millitary Macow (*Ara militaris*, an exotic sp.) in captivity. The gross lesions were whitish nodules in the air sacs **(Figures 10-11).** Zygomycosis was diagnosed in a rescued five months old Bengal florican (*Houbaropsis bengalensis*). The gross lesions included circumscribed raised necrotic nodules (about 2- 4 cm) in the lung and microscopic lesions were multi-focal necrotic foci surrounded by inflammatory cells. Broad, basophilic, aseptated fungal hyphae indistinguishable from those of Zygomycetes could be seen within necrotic lesions **(Figure 12)**.

(c) Digestive system: Ulcerative colitis is said to be of complex etiology. It is recorded in open billed stork (*Anastomus oscitans*). Microscopic lesions included small necrotic foci in the mucosa of intestine, ulcers penetrating into the muscular layer with mononuclear cell and lymphocytic infiltration and oedema in muscular layer. Hepatic cell degeneration and vacuolations with small necrotic foci infiltrated by mononuclear cells **(Figure 20)** are also found**).**

Colibacillosis causing hepatic micro-granulomas was diagnosed in a swan (*Sygnus atratus,* exotic sp.) chick **(Figure21)**. Tuberculous lesions in liver and spleen **(Figure 23-24)** of demoiselle cranes (*Anthropoides virgo*) were of varying in size from miliary granulomas to large coalescing caseo-necrotic types. Special stained sections showed small daughter tubercles without central necrotic zone around a large tubercle with macrophages and giant cells showing acid- fast bacilli.

Workers have described *Cryptococcus neoformans* in intestinal and hepatic granulomatous lesions **(Figures 28-29** in pheasants died in captivity**).** *Candidia* sp. infection causing lesions in the stomach of peafowls and ulcerative lesions in the crop **(Figure 30)** of red jungle fowl (G*allus gallus*). *Candida albicans* and *C. Tropicalis* besides some other *candida* species were isolated from the free ranging wild birds. Mucour infection in proventriculus of chir pheasant (*C. wallichi*) has also been demonstrated in captivity **(Figure 31).** Gross lesions of creamy coloured nodules attached to serosa of intestine near duodenal loop, enlargement of spleen and liver encountered in peafowl (*P. cristatus*) were related to Marek's disease **(Figure 32).**

A case of hepatic histomoniasis in pea- fowls (*Pavo cristatus*) was marked with microscopic lesions of distension of sinusoids, multiple coagulative necrosis in the parenchyma and infiltrated predominantly with lymphocytes and macrophages. Ovoid bodies of protozoa, *H. meleagridis* were either free or within giant cells in the sinusoids **(Figure 33).**

Necropsy of two lesser adjutant storks (*Leptoptilos javanicus*) died in wild showed presence of nodular growths on the intestinal serosa, which were related to an unidentified trematode **(Figure 34)**. Cross section of *Ophistorchis brahmini* and eggs **(Figure 35)** were seen in bile duct of brahminy duck (*Tadorna ferruginea*). Histopathological section of a growth from Adjutant stork (*Leptoptilos dubius*) showed trematode infection in the musculature of gizzard surrounded by caseonecrotic reaction **(Figure 36)**. Intestinal nodular lesions were encountered in open bill stork *(Anastomus oscitans)* casused by tapeworm sp. **(Figure 37).**

Plugging of intestine **(Figure 38)** by *Ascaridia galli* was also encountered in a spotted pelican (*Pelecanus philipensis*). Severe enteritis due to *Capillaria* sp. infection **(Figure 40)**. was recorded in chir pheasant chicks An adult migratory white pelican (*Pelecanus onocrotalus*) had fallen from its flock during flight and died on 5th day due to heavy load of round worms-*Contracaecum spiculegerum* **(Figure 41).**

(d) Urinary system: In Hill myna (*G. religiosa*) lesions of nocardiosis in kidney **(Figure 55)** in addition to the disease lesions in respiratory and digestive system (discussed above) were found**.** Similarly Marek's disease lesions were also observed histopathologically in kidney of pheasants **(Figure 56)** in addition to the lesions in other organs.

(e) Integumentary system: Wild birds are susceptible to pox. Lesions on the head and beak in addition to involvement of mucosal lesions in common myna died in the wild were recorded **(Figure 73).** Ecto parasitism in wild birds is poorly studied.

(B) Neoplasms: Recorded neoplasms in birds include: aortic body tumour **(Figure 6)** from brahminy duck (*Tadorna ferruginea*), lymphomatosis **(Figures 44-45)** in peahen (*P. cristatus*) and pied myna (*Sturnus contra*), hepatic fibrosarcoma **(Figure 46)** in adjutant stork (*Leptoptilos dubius*), heptocellular carcinoma in copper pheasant (*Syrmaticus soemmerringi*, an exotic sp.) and in flamingo (*Phoenicopterus* sp.) died in captivity **(Figures 47,48**) and hepatic lipoma **(Figure 49)** in wild peacock (*Pavo cristatus*).Nephroblastoma **(Figure 58)** was recorded in Copper pheasant (*Syrmaticus soemmerringi*, an exotic sp.). Melanosarcomatous growth **(Figure 74)** on the beak and in lung of white winged wood duck (*Cairina scutulata*), is worth mentioning, as this bird species under WPA is listed as critically endangered. A growth weighing 1.2 kg extirpated from left wing of a captive Adjutant stork (*Leptoptilos dubius*) was diagnosed to be fibrosarcoma **(Figure 75).** The recorded cases allude to that incidence of liver neoplasm in wild birds appears to be high than that of any other organs.

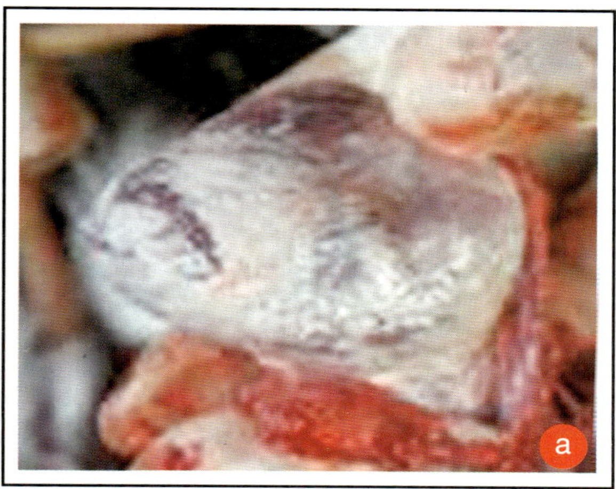

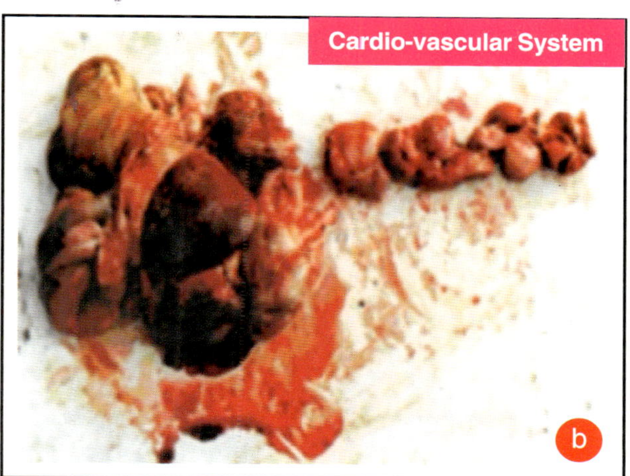

Figure 1: (a) Photographs showing: (a) Urates deposition on the heart of woolly neck stork (*Ciconia episcopus*) died in wild. The case is also referred under digestive system (Courtesy: Talukdar, A.). (b) Urate crystals found on pericardium and visceral surface of liver in vulture (Courtesy: Panda, S.K.and Nath, I.).

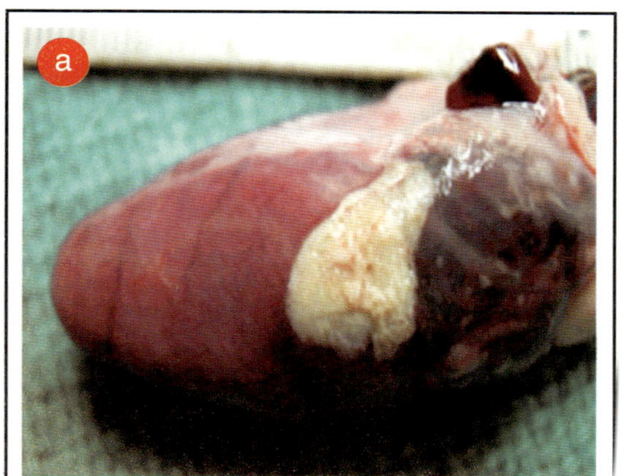

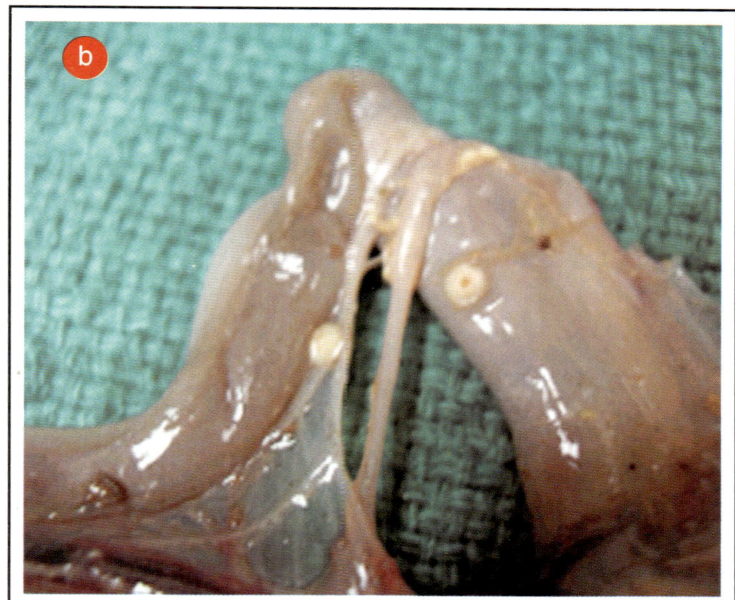

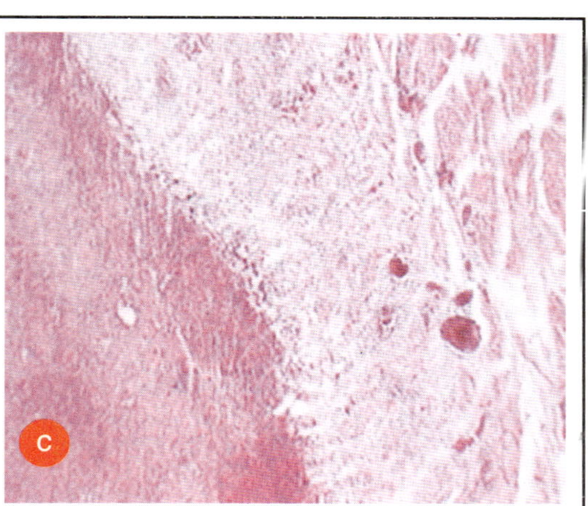

Figure 2: Zygomycosis in Bengal florican (*Houbaropsis bengalensis*). Photograph showing (a) large sized raised nodules on heart and small nodules on the peritoneum and (b) serosal surface of intestine. (c) Photomicrograph of epicardial lesion showing hyphae of Zygomycetes in fibrinous exudates. H & E, x 100. Case is also referred under digestive system. (Das *et al.*, 2007).

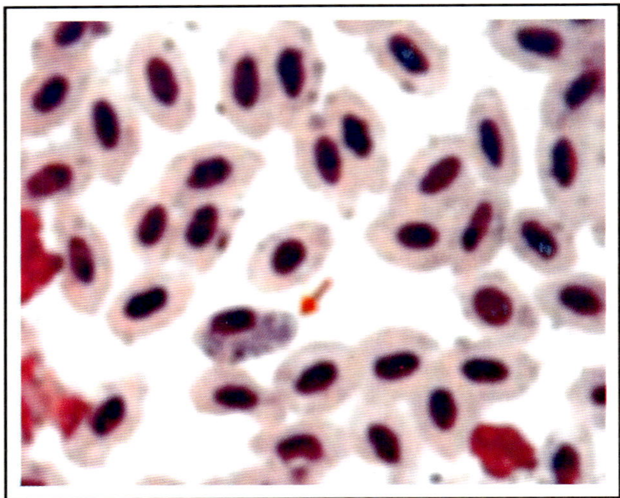

Figure 3: Photomicrograph of blood smears showing *Haemoproteus columbae* in psittacine bird. Note Gamonts in RBCs as crescent or bean shaped bodies which partially encircle the nucleus of the cell in the form of halter. Giemsa stain x 1000.

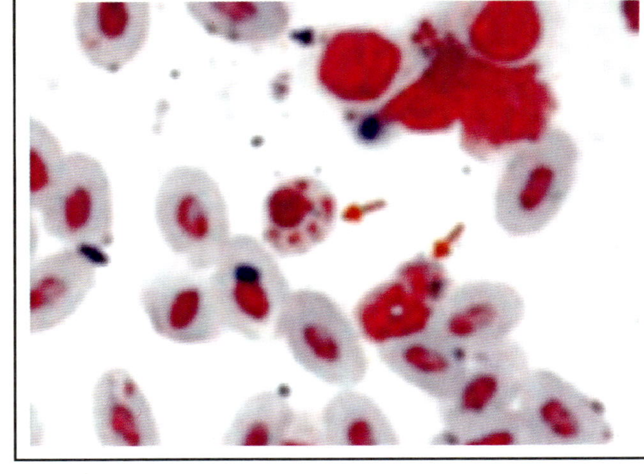

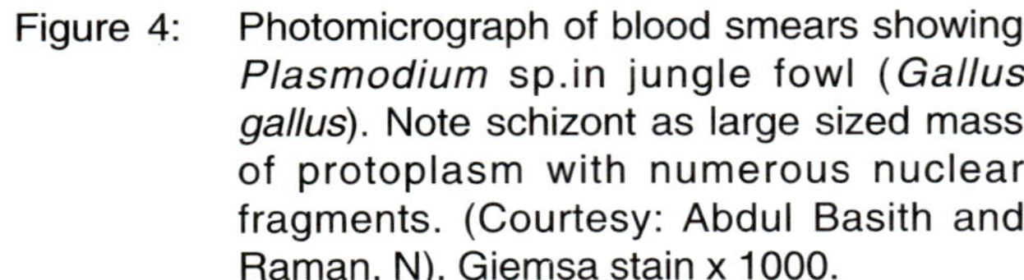

Figure 4: Photomicrograph of blood smears showing *Plasmodium* sp.in jungle fowl (*Gallus gallus*). Note schizont as large sized mass of protoplasm with numerous nuclear fragments. (Courtesy: Abdul Basith and Raman, N). Giemsa stain x 1000.

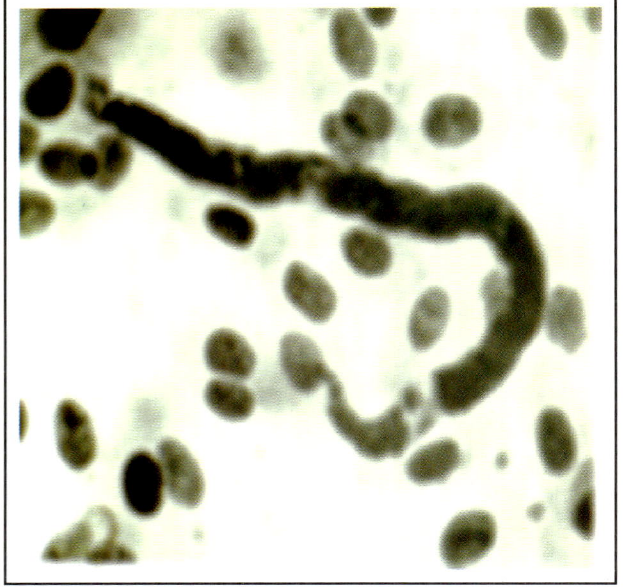

Figure 5: Photomicrograph of blood smear of green magpie (*Cissa chinensis*) showing a mirofilaria. The species is carrier of filarial worms. Wright's stain x 1000.

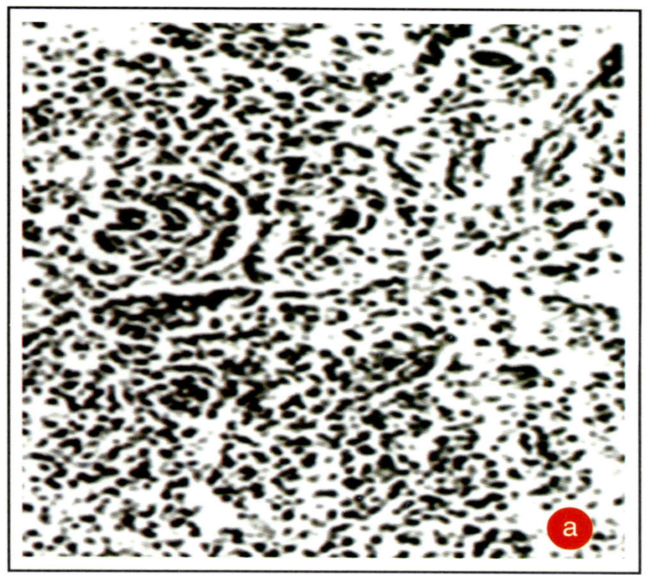

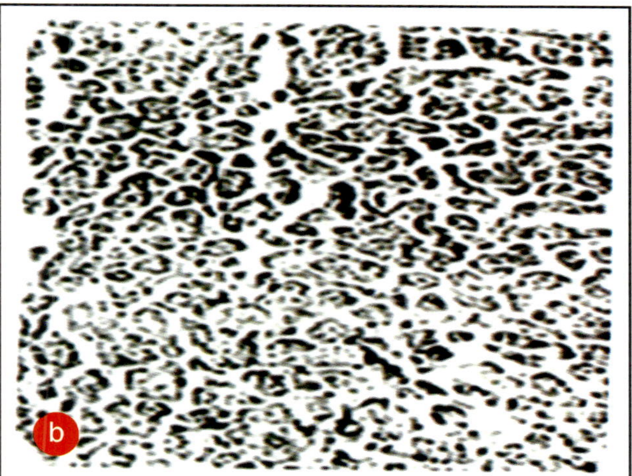

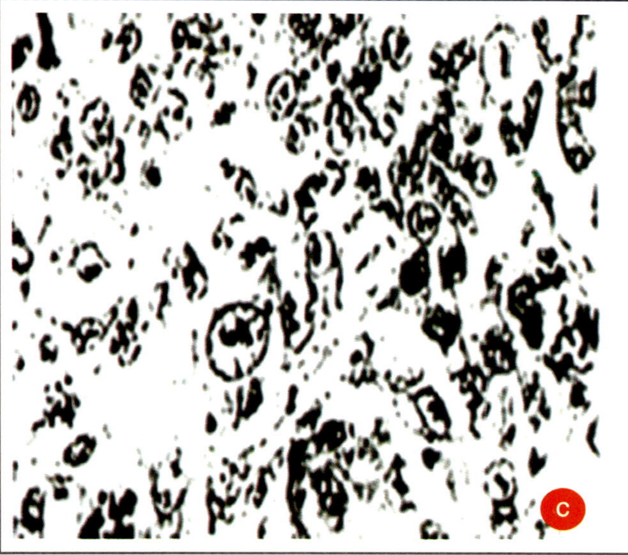

Figure 6: Photomicrographs of aortic body tumour from Brahminy duck (*Tadorna ferraginea*) showing: (a) Tumour cells arranged in sheets .Peritheliomatous arrangement and trabeculae are also seen.H&E, x110. (b) Tumour cells arranged in the form of palisades around capillaries. H&E,x110 (c) Some bizarre cells with vacuolated cytoplasm and large nucleus and nucleolus under higher magnification. H&E,x450 (Sah *et al.*, 1974).

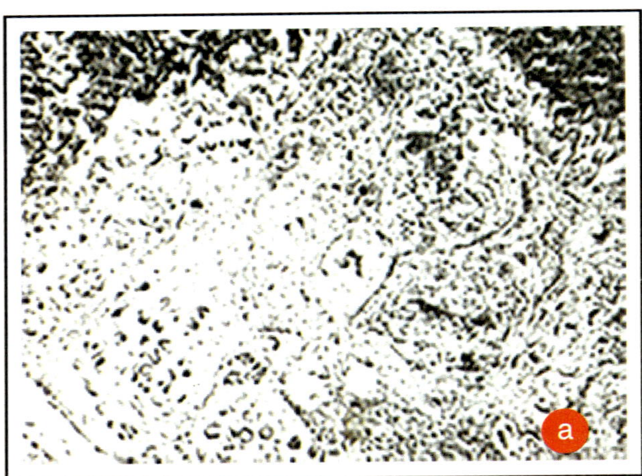

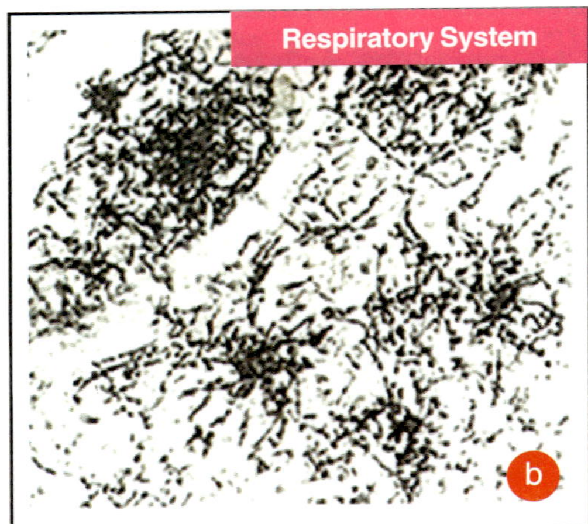

Figure 7: Nocardiosis in Hill Myna (*Gracula religiosa*). (a) Granulomatous lesion in lung containing epithelioid and Langhan's giant cells. PAS & Haemotoxylin,x 65. (b) Gram positive organisms. x 650. The case is also referred under digestive system. (Iyer *et al.*, 1972).

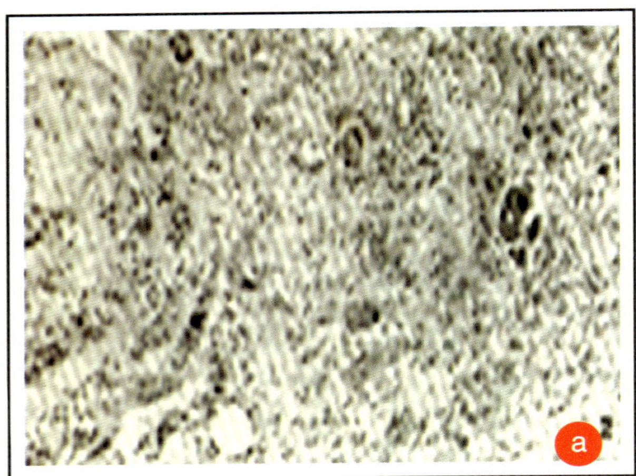

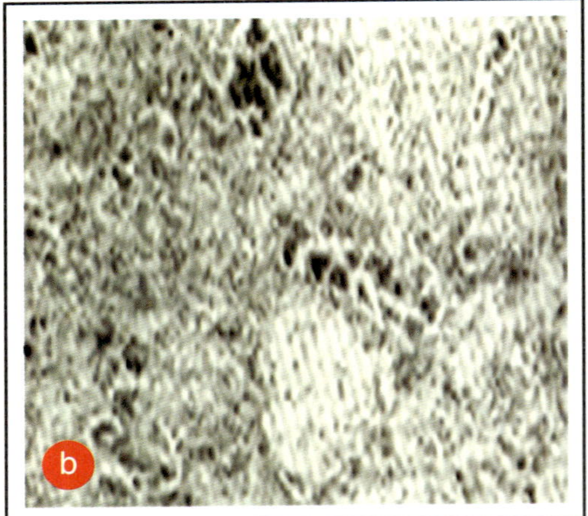

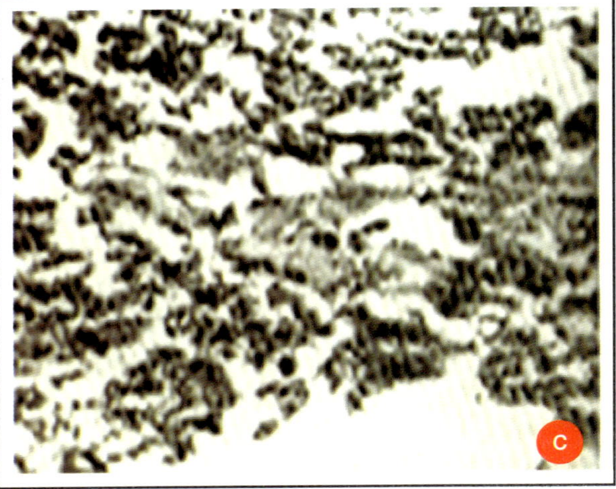

Figure 8: Pulmonary tuberculosis encountered in cheer pheasant (*Catreus wallichi*) died in captivity. Photomicrographs (a, b) showing characteristic changes of caseation and mononuclear cell and giant cell infiltration in nodules. H&E, x 125. (c) Note dust-like particles (Anthracosis) in lung parenchyma H&E,x 125 (Somvanshi *et al.*, 1992). Note: Original photos were not available. Hence black and white prints (a-c) portyed.

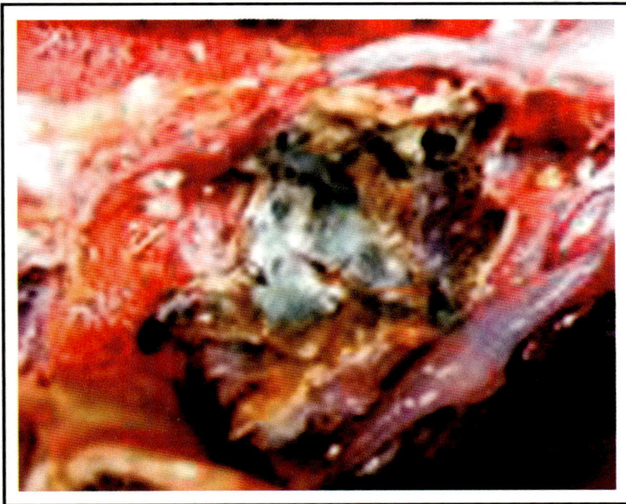

Figure 9: Photograph showing pulmonary mycotic infection in oriental pied horn bill (*Anthracoceros malabaricus*) found dead in Kaziranga National Park, Assam (Courtesy: Talukdar, A.).

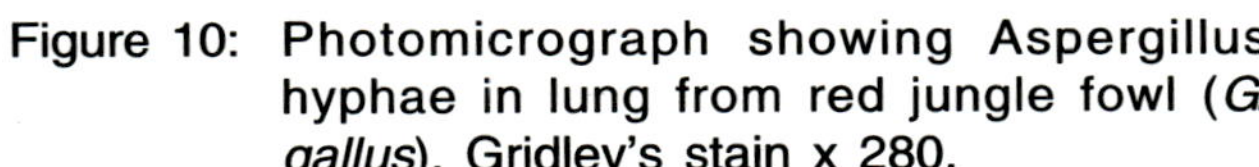

Figure 10: Photomicrograph showing Aspergillus hyphae in lung from red jungle fowl (*G. gallus*). Gridley's stain x 280.

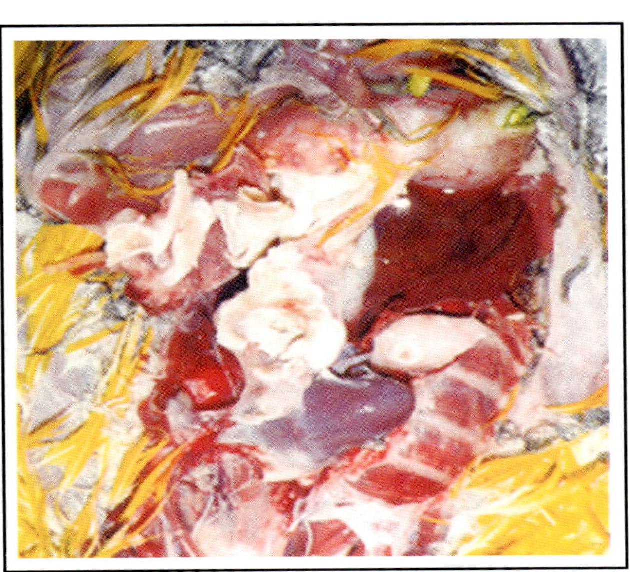

Figure 11: Aspergillus infection encountered in Millitary Macow (*Ara militaris*, an exotic sp.) died in Zoological Garden, Mumbai.Photograph showing white nodules with depressed centre and raised borders in air sacs. (Courtesy: Suryawanshi, D.S.).

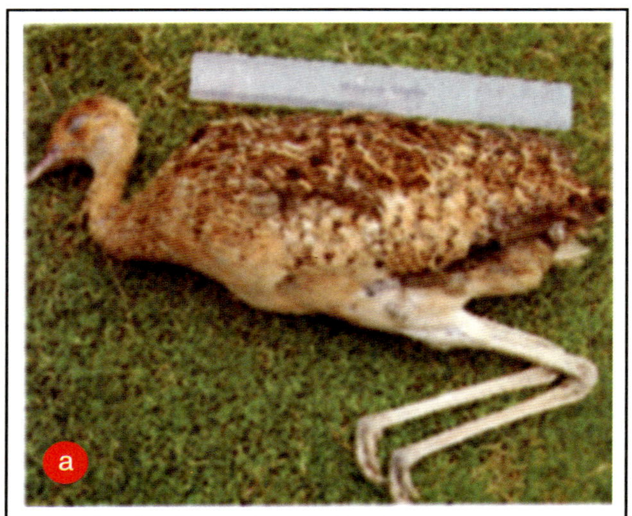

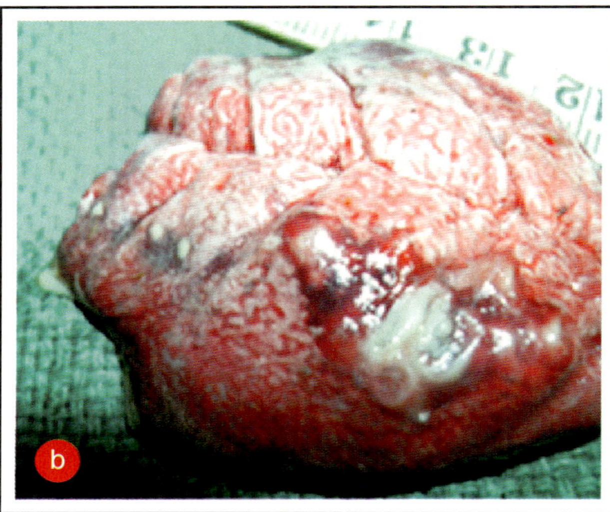

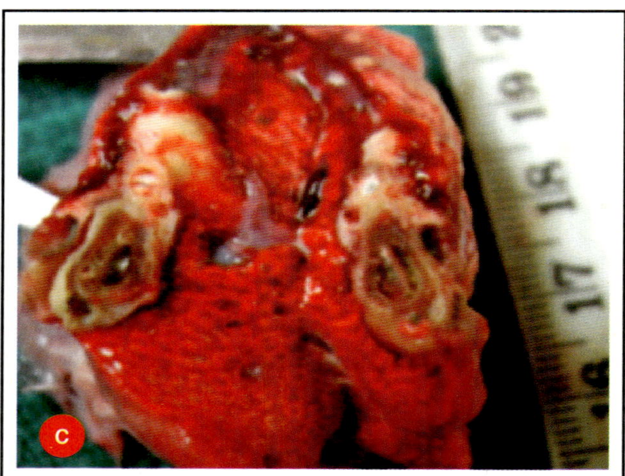

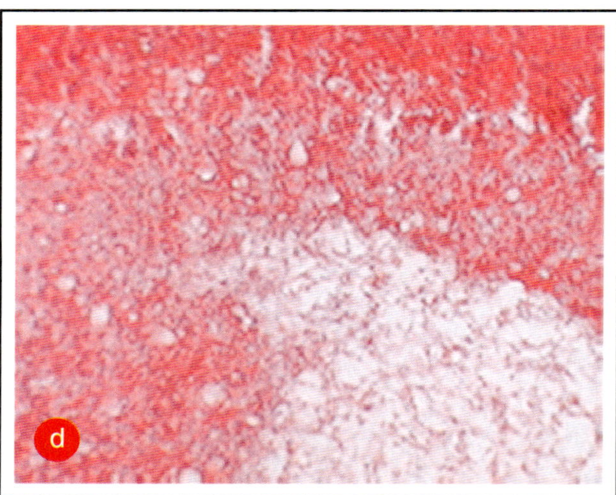

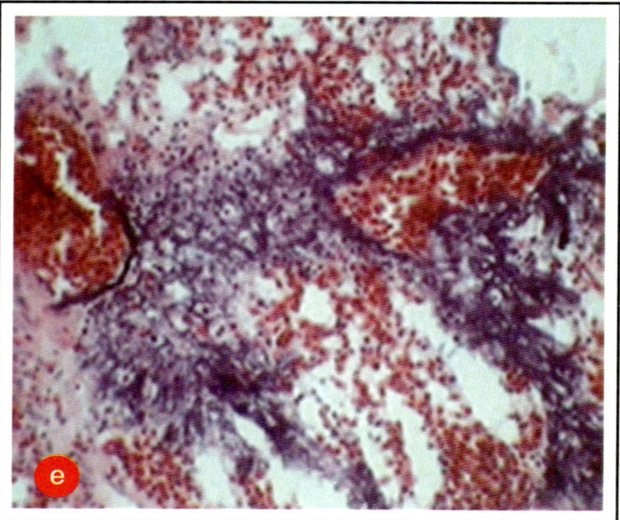

Figure 12: (a) Zygomycosis in a five months old Bengal florican (*Houbaropsis bengalensis*) rescued from Manas National Park (Assam),which later on died in captivity. (b) Photographs showing circumscribed raised necrotic nodules (about 2 cm in dia.) and nodules (3-4 mm dia) in the left diaphragmatic lobe. (c) cut section of (b) showing lesion. Photomicrographs of (b) showing: (d) Multifocal necrotic foci surrounded by inflammatory cells. H & E, x 100 (e) Broad, basophilic, aseptated fungal hyphae indistinguishable from those of Zygomycetes within necrotic lesions. H & E, x 400 (Das *et al.*, 2007).

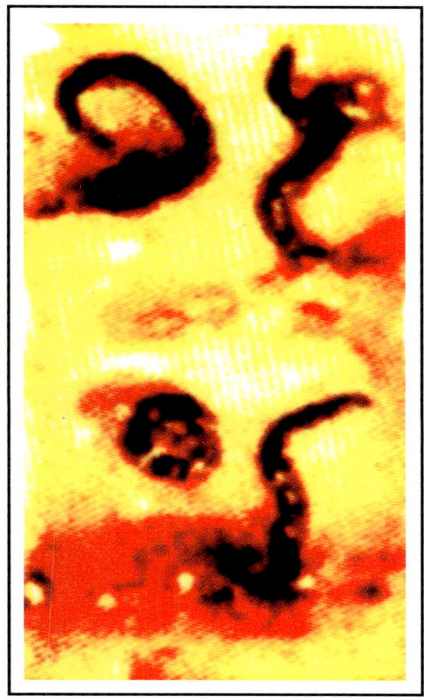

Figure 13: Photograph showing (a) *Syngamus trachea* in the trachea of an adult peafowl (*P.cristatus*). (Courtesy: Subramanian, K.S.).

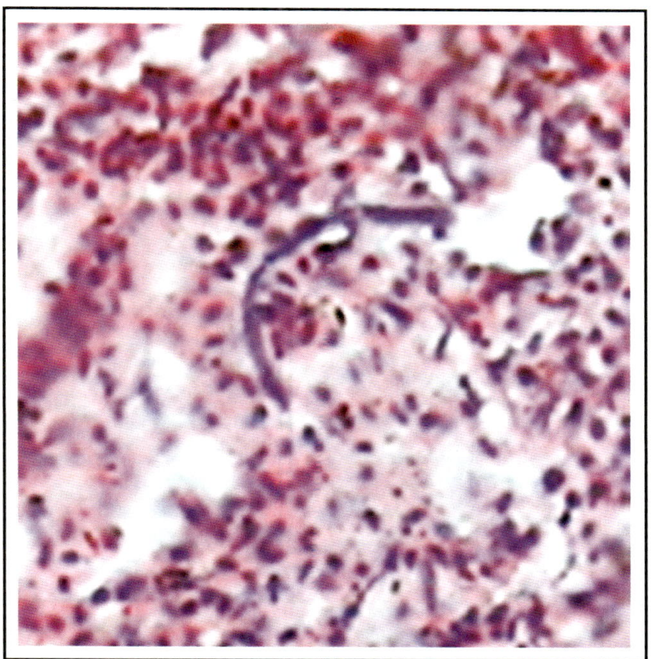

Figure 14: Photomicrograph showing microfilaria in the lung of green pigeon (*Ducula* sp.). Note haemorrhage and polymorpho nuclear cells infiltration. H&E, x400.

Digestive System

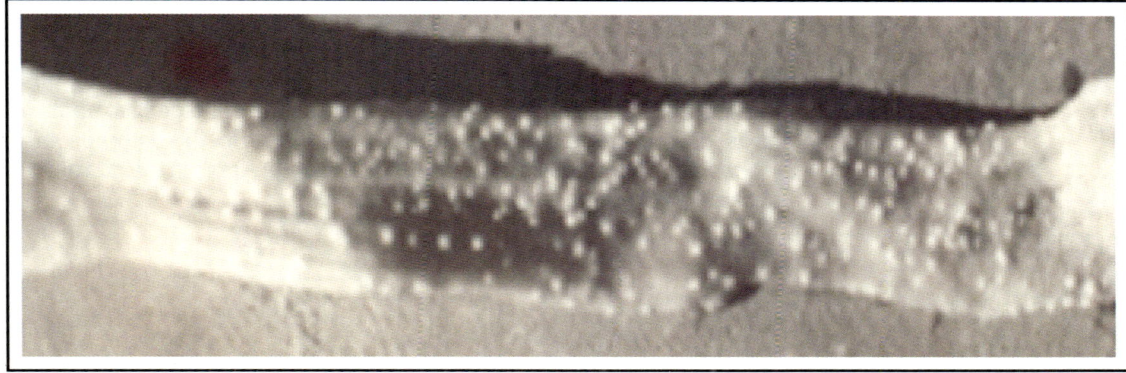

Figure 15: Oesophagus of peacock (*P. cristatus*) cut opened showing pastules due to deficiency of vitamin 'A'.

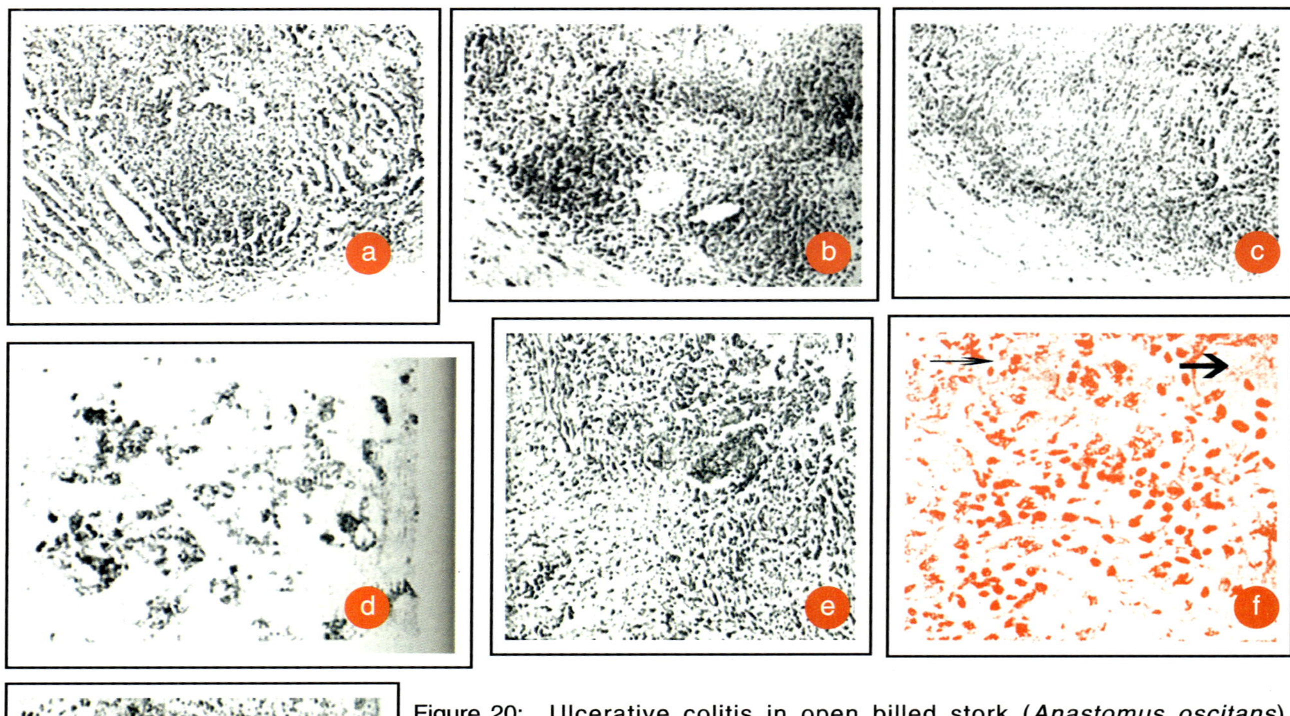

Figure 20: Ulcerative colitis in open billed stork (*Anastomus oscitans*). Photomicrographs showing: (a) Small necrotic foci in the mucosa of intestine and mild infiltration of mononuclear cells in adjoining areas. H&E,x100. (b) Ulcers penetrating into the muscular layer with mononuclear cell infiltration. H&E,x100. (c) Lymphocytic infiltration and oedema in muscular layer. H&E,x100 (d) Gram positive rods,MacCallum Goodpasture stain, x100. (e)Intestinal congestion, focal area of necrosis and infiltration of lymphocytes. H&E,x100 (f) Hepatic cell degeneration and vacuolations with small necrotic foci infiltrated by mononuclear cells,H&E,x400 (g) Coalescing foci of necrosis with degenerated cellular debris in spleen. H&E,x100 (Sah *et al.*,1972).

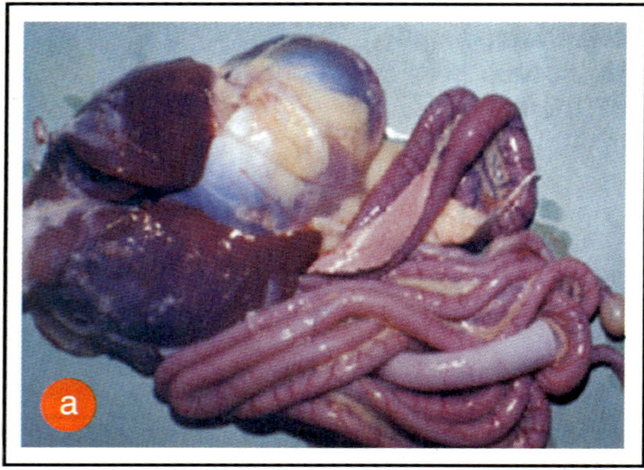

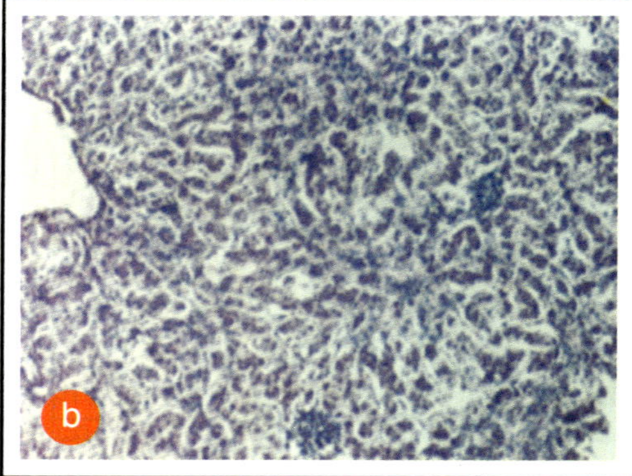

Figure 21: Collibacillosis in 2-day-old black swan (*Cygnus atratrus,* an exotic sp.) chick. (a) Photograph showing severe congestion of serosal capillaries and fibrinous deposits over the surface of liver due to enterotoxic effect of *E. coli.* (b) Photomicrograph of liver of (a) showing small microgranulomas and necrosis of hepatocytes associated with *E.coli* infection. H& E, x100 (Courtesy: Suryawanshi, D.S.).

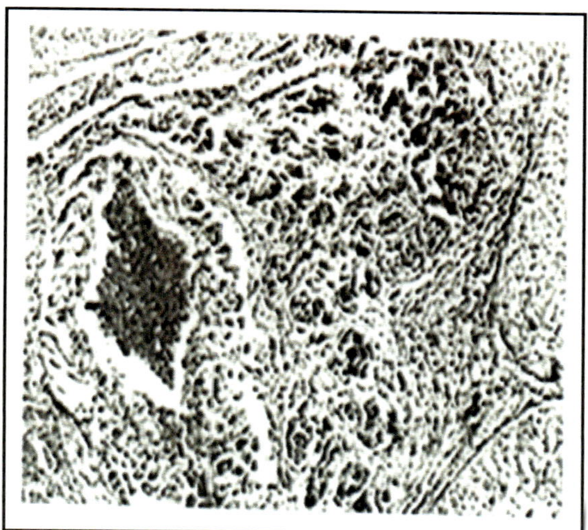

Figure 22: Nocardiosis in Hill Myna (*Gracula religiosa*). Photomicrograph of proventriculus showing granulomatous lesions. Surrounding the caseo-necrotic area of a distinct zone of epithelioid and Langhan's giant cells, which merged with granulation tissue on the outside. H&E,x65. The case is also referred under urinary system and sense organs (Iyer *et al.*, 1972).

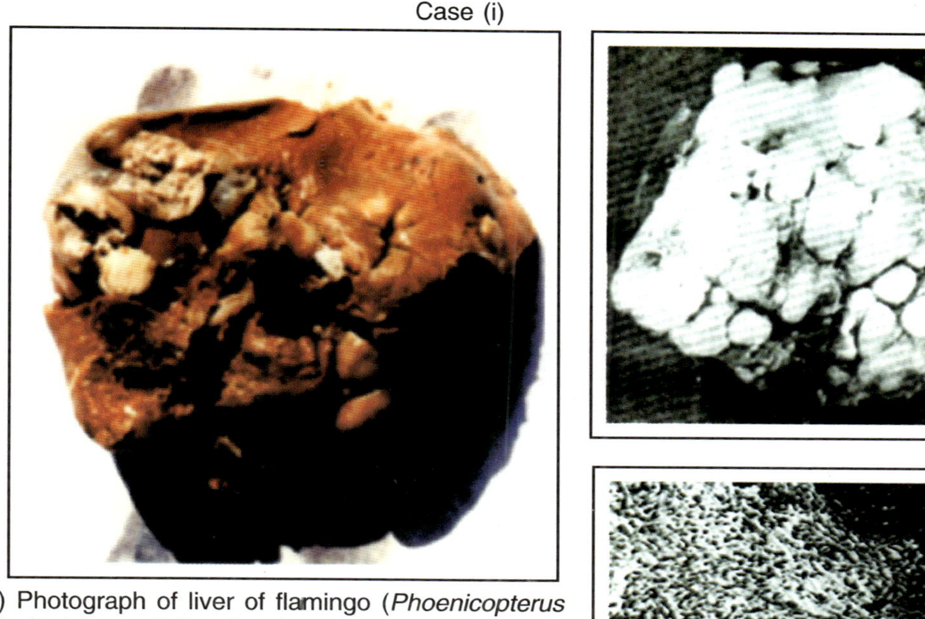

Figure 23: Case (i) Photograph of liver of flamingo (*Phoenicopterus roseus*) died in captivity showing whitish-grey multiple tuberculous nodules.Case (ii-a) Photograph of liver from demoiselle crane (*Anthropoides virgo*) showing multiple greyish white nodular lesions. Case (ii-b) Photomicrograph of (-a) showing granulomatous lesions with caseonecrotic zone,cellular infiltration and connective tissue capsule. H&E, x128 (Sashoo *et al.*,1992).

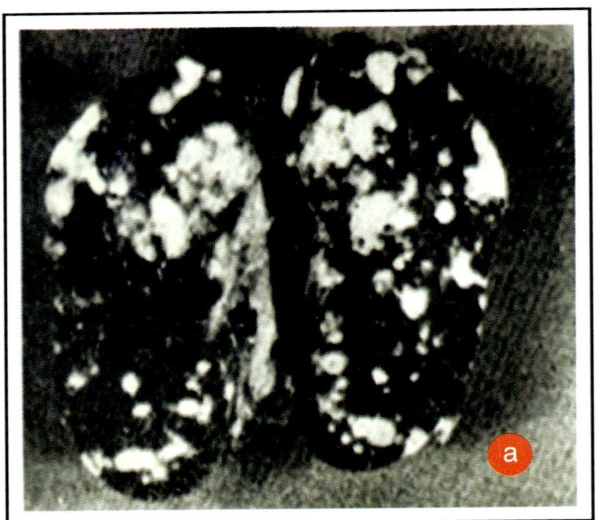

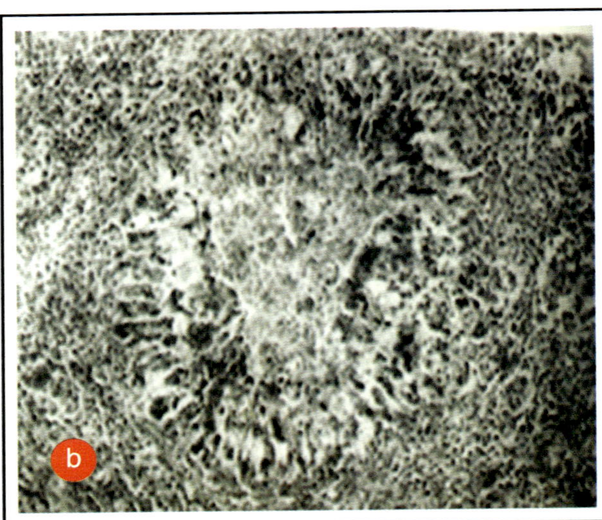

Figure 24: (a) Photograph of spleen from demoiselle crane (*Anthropoides virgo*) showing caseous tuberculous nodules on its cut surfaces. (b) Photomicrograph of (a) showing a granuloma associated with inflammatory cells.H&E,x120 (Sah *et al.*, 1985).

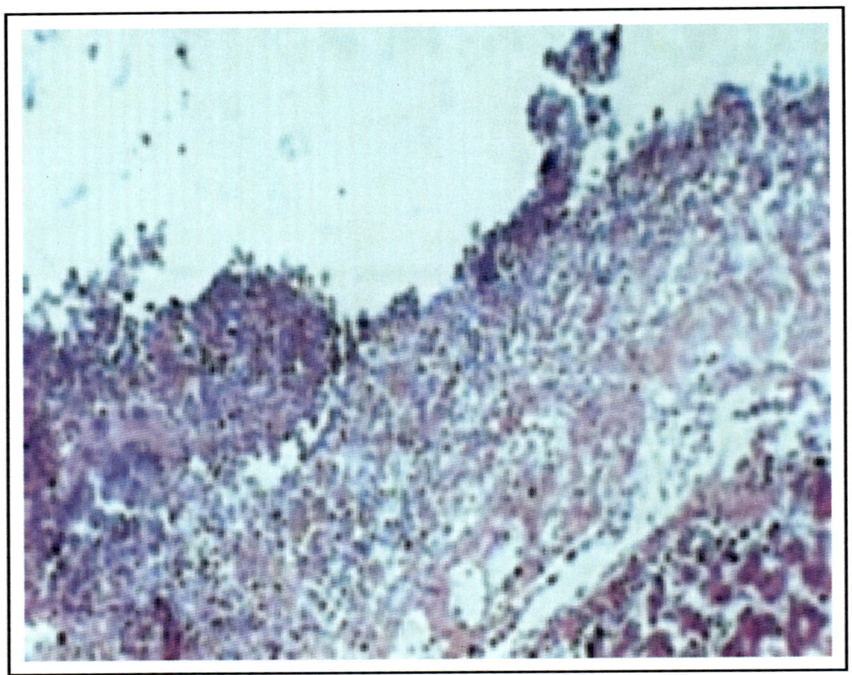

Figure 25: Zygomycetes infection in Bengal florican (*Houbaropsis bengalensis*). Photomicrograph showing intestinal nodular lesion with necrosis and infiltration of inflammatory cells. H & E, x 100. (Das *et al.*, 2007). The case is also referred under respiratory system.

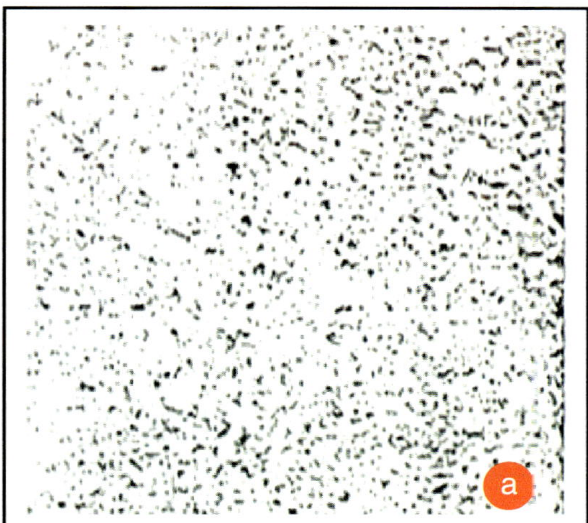

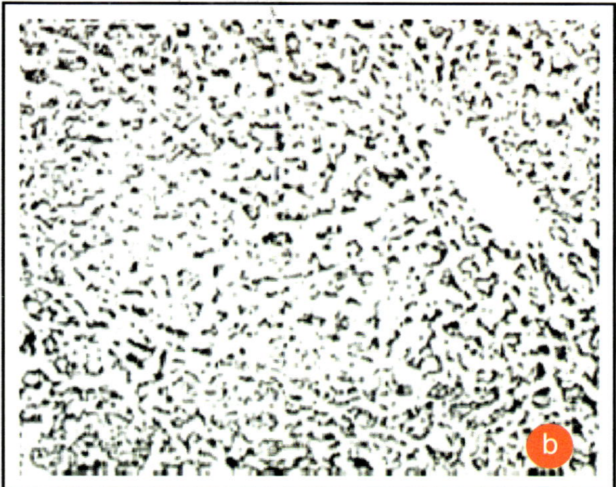

Figure 26: Alfatoxicosis in parrots. Photomicrographs (a,b) of liver showing congestion, haemorrhages,degeneration and necrosis of hepatic cells. H&E,x 100 (Chakraborty *et al.*, 1988).

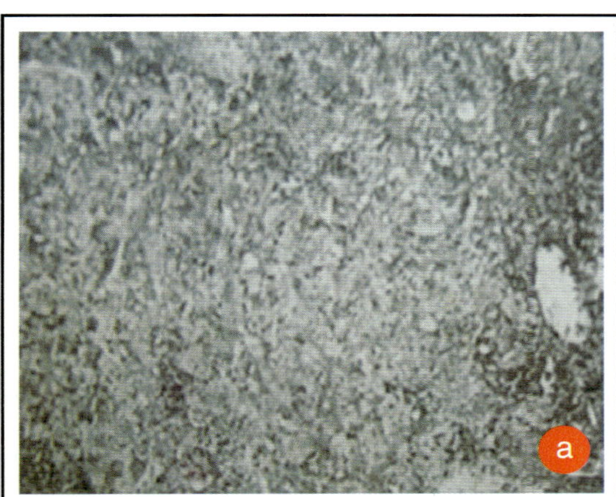

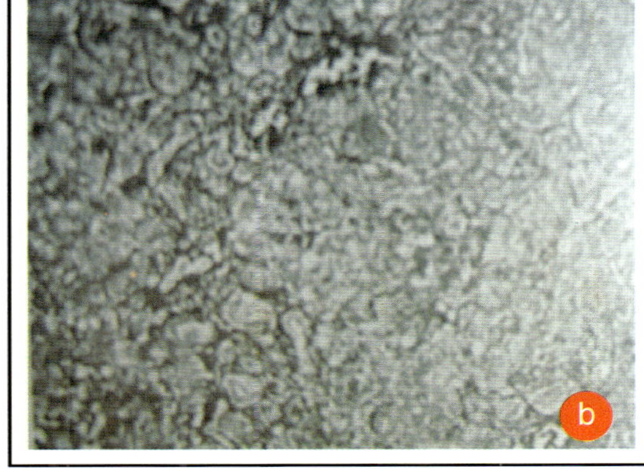

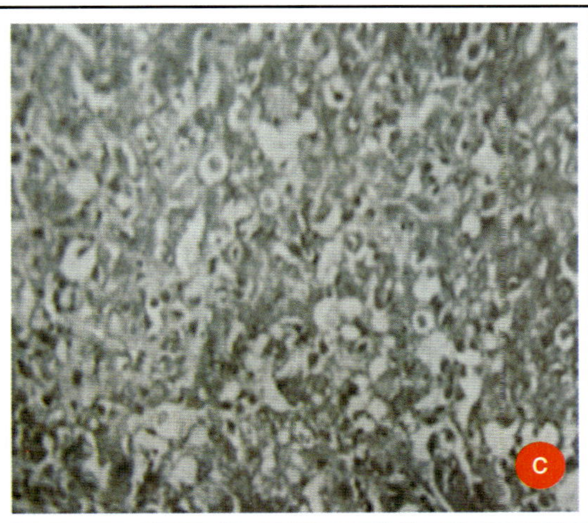

Figure 27: Aflatoxicosis in tuffed pochard ducks (*Aytha fuligatta*).Photomicrographs of liver showing : (a) Severe hepatic cell necrosis involving the peripheral zone with extensive bile duct hyperplasia. (b)Reticular fibers dividing the hepatic lobule altering the liver structure. Gomori reticulum stain, x100. (c) Eosinophilic hyaline bodies in the degenerating hepatocytes. H&E,x250 (Sheikh Meera Mohiuddin *et al.*, 1977).

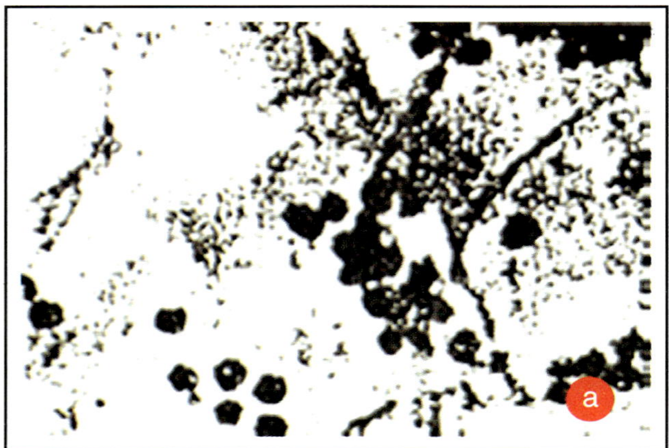

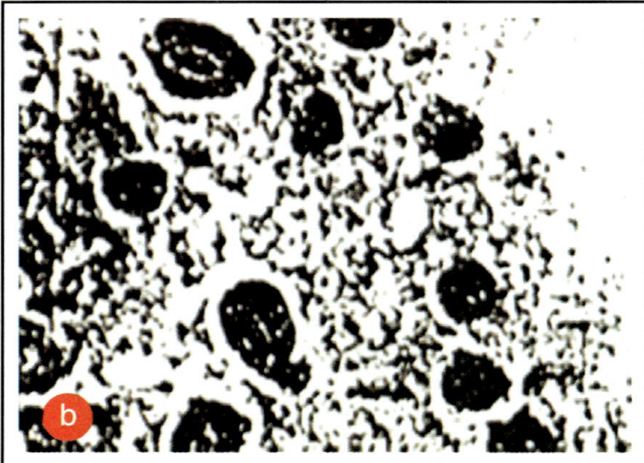

Figure 28: Cryptococcosis (*Cryptococcus neoformans*) in Golden pheasant (*Chrysolophus pictus*).Photomicrographs of smears from (a)intestine and (b) liver demonstrated clusters of encapsulated light-stained spherical bodies of 4μ and 15μ of diameters, respectively. Note capsules were stained dark while the encircled bodies were reddish. Leishman's stain x 800 No connecting filaments observed (Nayak *et al.*,1985).

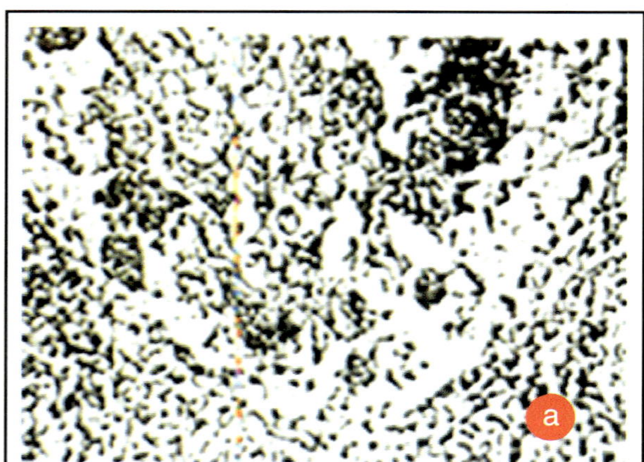

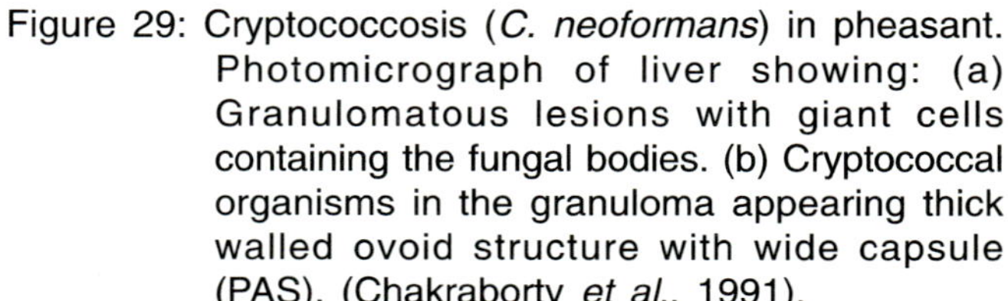

Figure 29: Cryptococcosis (*C. neoformans*) in pheasant. Photomicrograph of liver showing: (a) Granulomatous lesions with giant cells containing the fungal bodies. (b) Cryptococcal organisms in the granuloma appearing thick walled ovoid structure with wide capsule (PAS). (Chakraborty *et al.*, 1991).

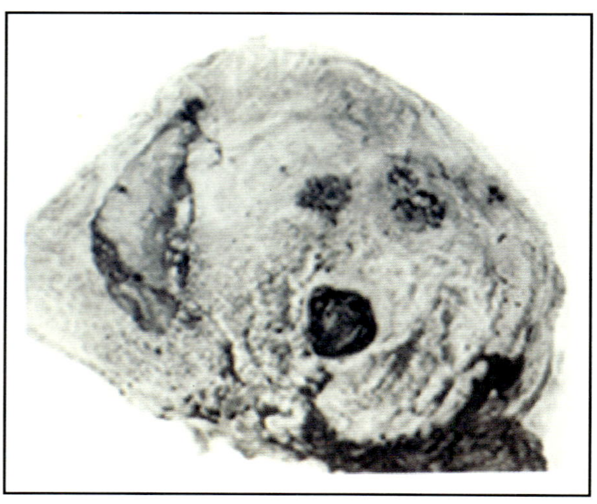

Figure 30: Photograph showing ulcerative lesions in crop due to *Candida albicans* sp. infection in red jungle fowl (*Gallus gallus*).

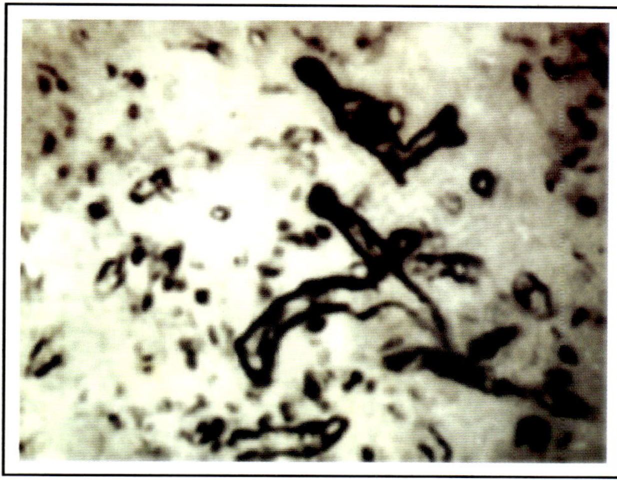

Figure 31: Mucour infection in proventriculus of chir pheasant (*C. wallichi*) died in captivity.

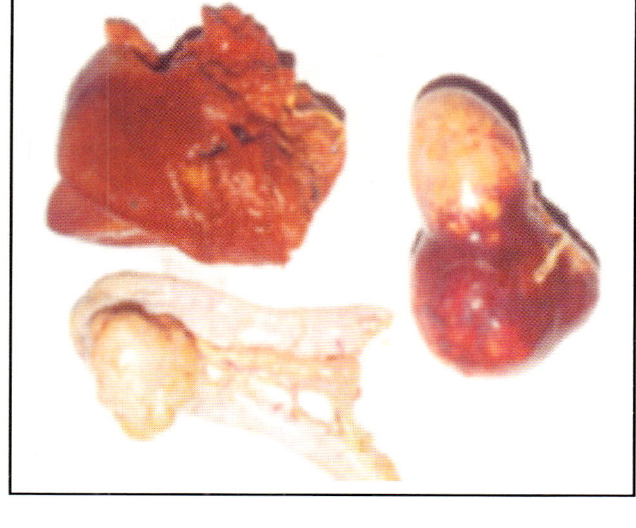

Figure 32: Marek's disease lesions in peafowl (*P. cristatus*). Photograph showing creamy coloured nodules attached to serosa of intestine near duodenal loop. Note also enlargment of spleen and liver (Courtesy: Suryawanshi, D.S.).

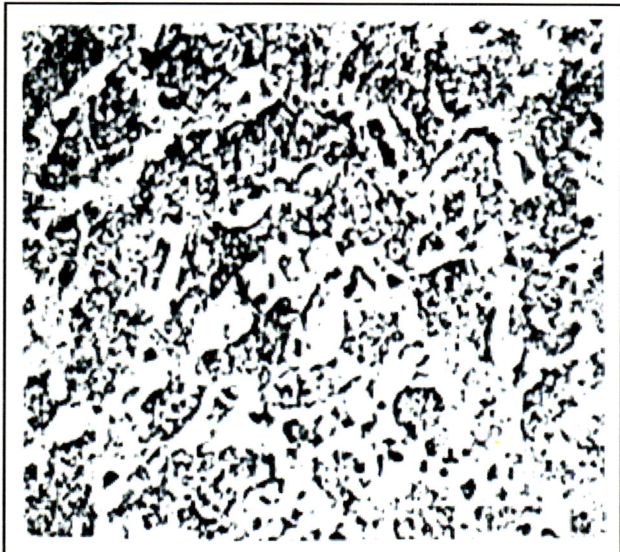

Figure 33: Histomoniasis in a peafowl (*P. cristatus*). Photomicrograph of liver showing hyperaemic with distersion of sinusoids, multiple coagulation necrosis in the parenchyma and necrotic areas infiltrated predominantly with lymphocytes and macrophages. Ovoid bodies of protozoa, *H. meleagridis* were either free or within giant cells in the sinusoids . They were stained light pink with H&E and appeared to be surrounded by a clear space. (Damodaran & Vishwanathan, 1978).

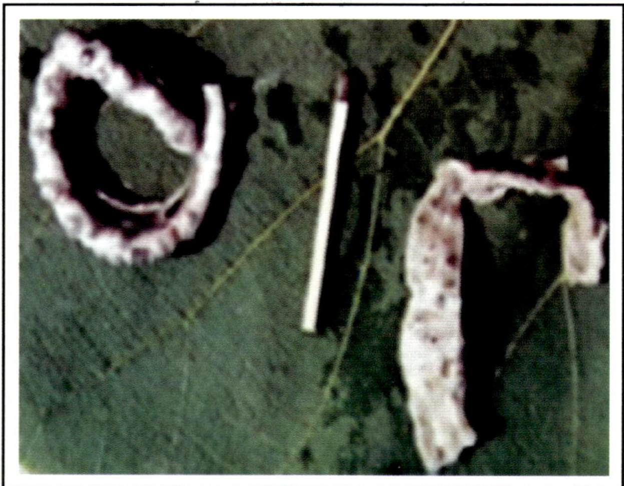

Figure 37: Intestine from open billed stork (*Anastomus oscitans*) showing nodular lesions caused by tapeworm sp. (Courtesy: Talukdar, A.).

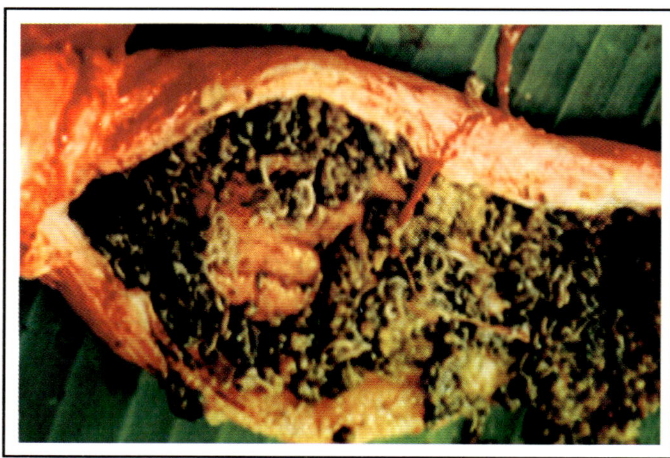

Figure 38: Photograph showing *Ascaridia galli* in the intestine of spotted pelican (*Pelecanus philipensis*) found dead in wild (Courtesy : Choudhury, B).

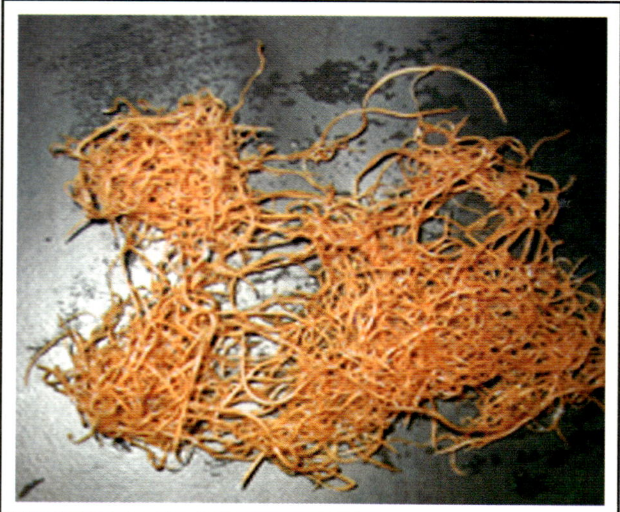

Figure 39: Photograph showing *Ascaridia columbae* collected from intestine of common pigeon (*Columba livia*) died in captivity.

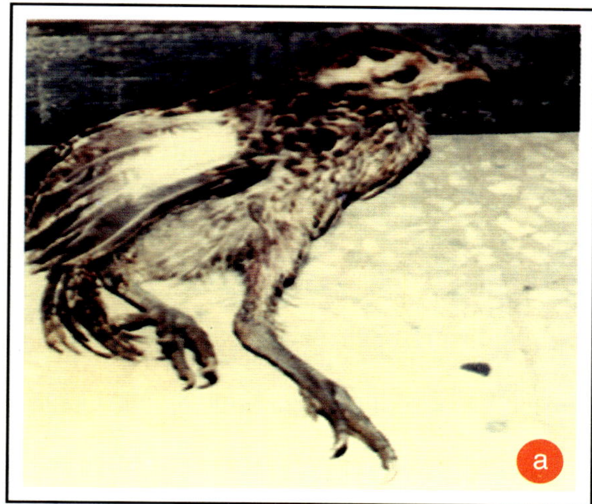

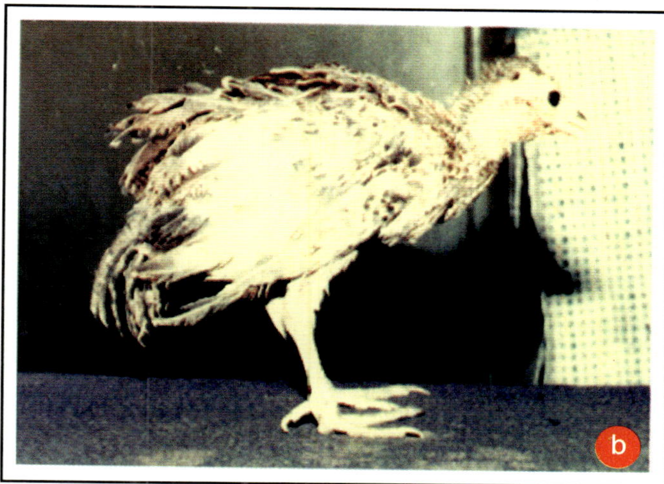

Figure 40: (a,b) Sick chir pheasant (*Catreus wallichi*) chicks suffering from capillariasis at IVRI Pheasantry.

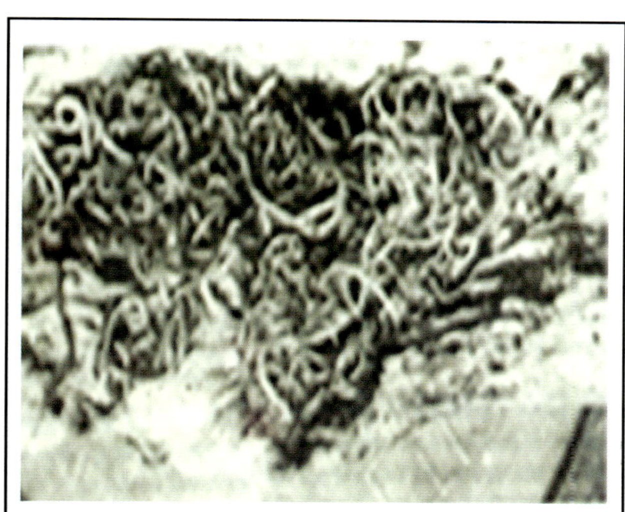

Figure 41: Photograph showing intestine of a migratory white pelican (*Pelecanus onocrotalus*) (Band No Moskowa KK3439)packed with round worms- (*Contracaecum spiculegerum*). Pelican had fallen from its flock during flight. It was unable to stand and eat,and had died on 5th day. (Maradia, 1994).

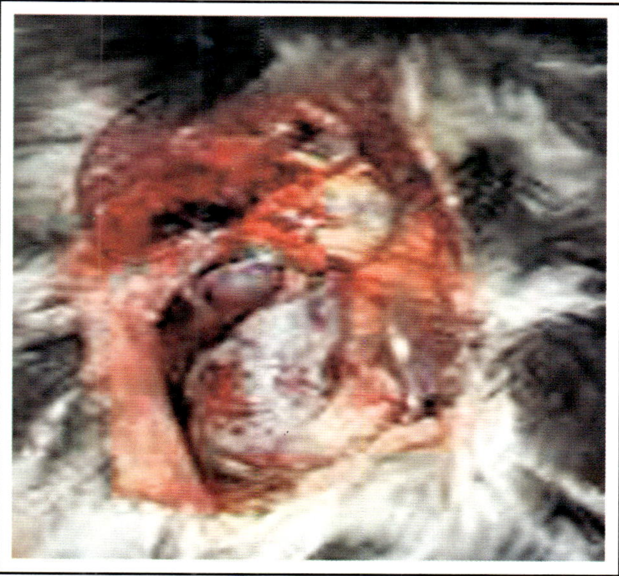

Figure 42 : Photograph showing urates deposition on the liver of woolly neck stork (*Ciconia episcopus*) found dead in wild. The case is also referred under cardiovascular system (Courtesy: Talukdar, A.).

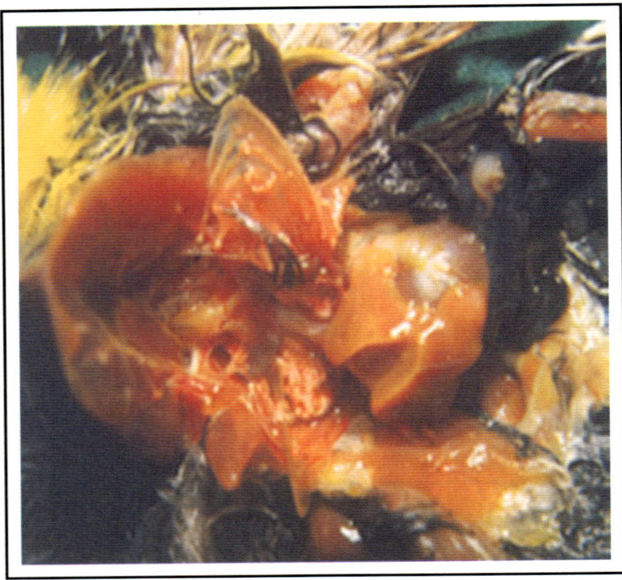

Figure 43 : Photograph showing yellowish discolouration of the visceral organs due to jaundice in love bird (*Agapornis sp.*) died in captivity (Courtesy: Suryawanshi, D.S.).

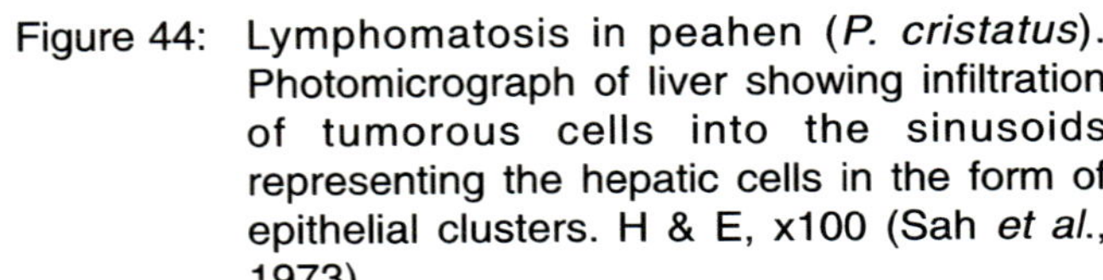

Figure 44: Lymphomatosis in peahen (*P. cristatus*). Photomicrograph of liver showing infiltration of tumorous cells into the sinusoids representing the hepatic cells in the form of epithelial clusters. H & E, x100 (Sah *et al.*, 1973).

Figure 45: Lymphamatosis in pied myna (*Sturnus contra*). Photomicrograph of spleen showing diffuse infiltration of tumorous cells into the sinuses and red pulp. H&E.x100. The case is also referred in urinary system (Sah *et al.*, 1973).

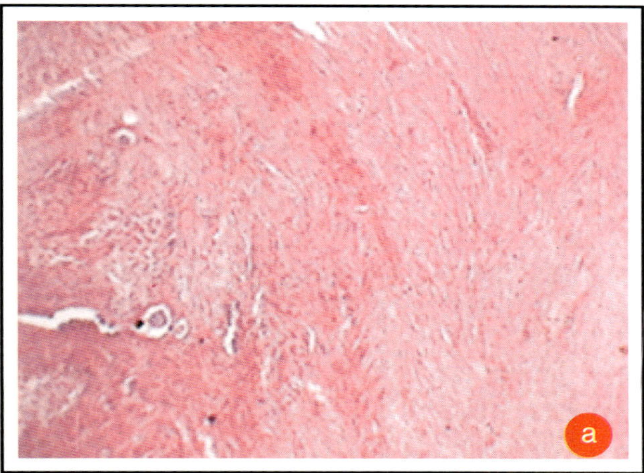

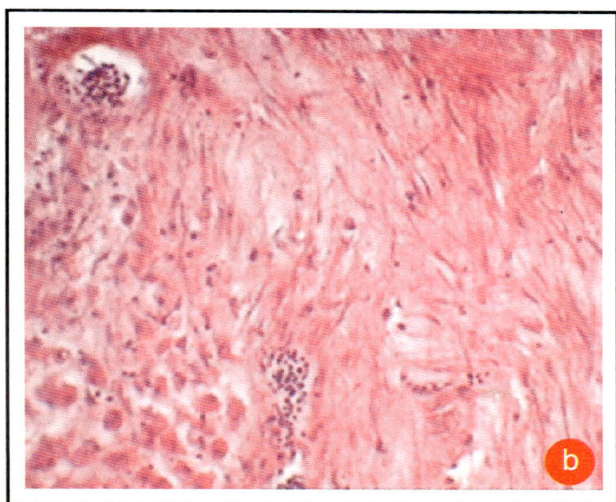

Figure 46: Photomicrgraphs of liver from Adjutant stork (*Leptoptilos dubius*) showing: (a) Metastatic fibrous connective tissue replacing the liver parenchyma characteristics of fibrosarcoma. Proliferation of new blood vessels were also observed. H&E,x100 (b) Fibrous connective tissue with few entrapped hepatic cells and new blood vessels. H&E,x 400.

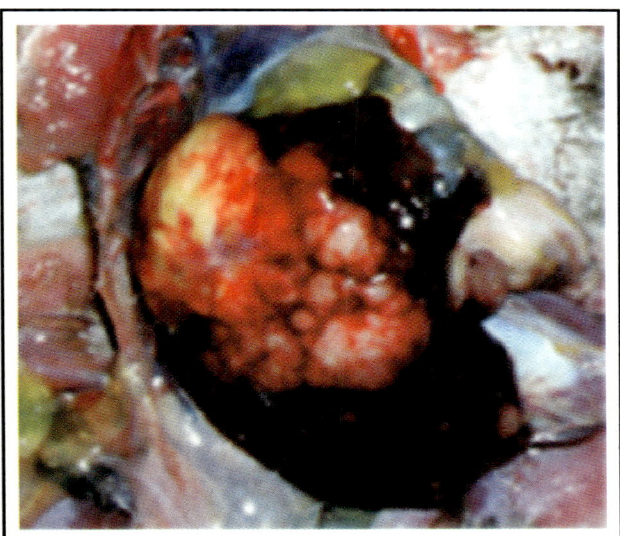

Figure 47: Photograph showing hepatocellular carcinoma in an adult Copper pheasant (*Syrmaticus soemmerringi*, an exotic sp) died in captivity. (Courtesy: Singh,S.D.).

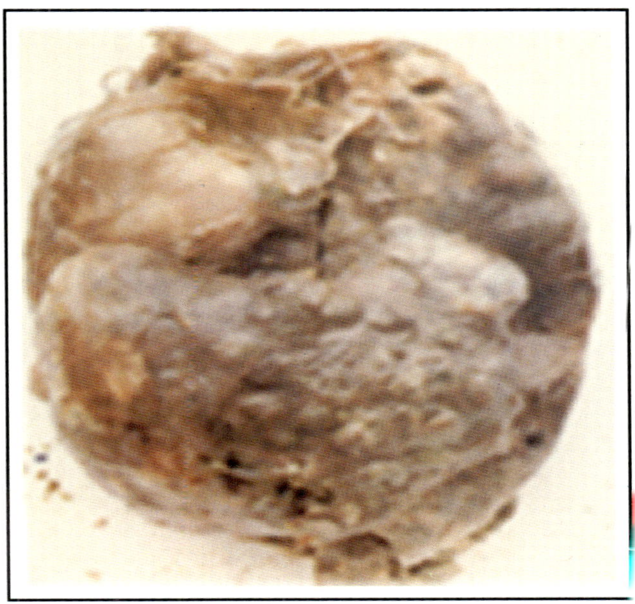

Figure 48: Photograph showing hepato cellular carcinoma encountered in a flamingo (*Phoenicopterus* sp.) died in captivity.

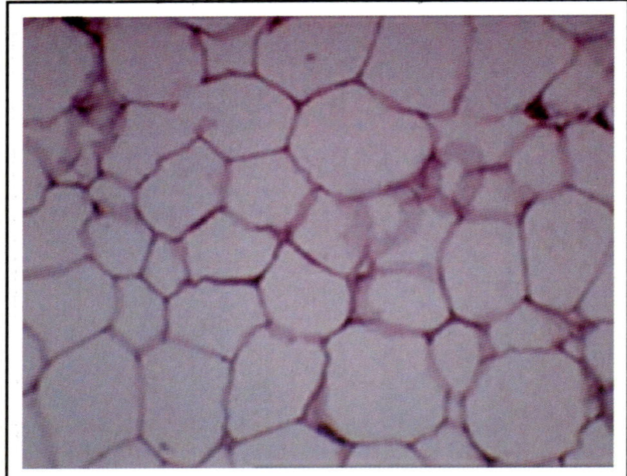

Figure 49: Hepatic lipoma encountered in wild peacock (*Pavo cristatus*). Photomicrograph of liver showing large fat vacuoles replacing the cytoplasm with peripherialization and compression of nuclei. H&E, x 400.

Urinary System

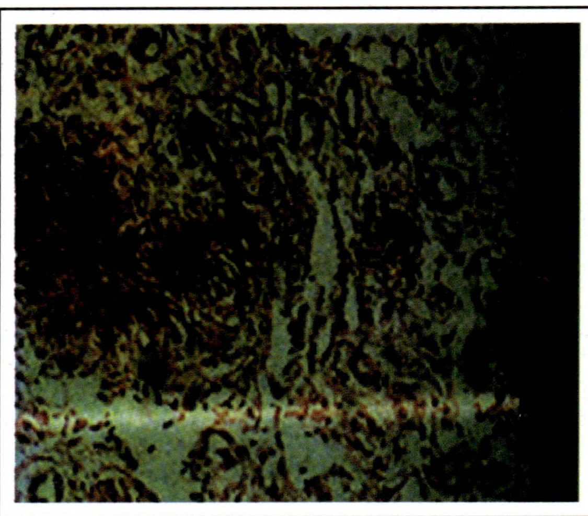

Figure 50: Photomicrograph of kidney of Copper pheasant (*Syrmaticus soemmerringii*, an exotic sp) showing radiating uric acid crystals with mononuclear cell reaction at the periphery. H&E,x200. (Courtesy: Singh,S.D.).

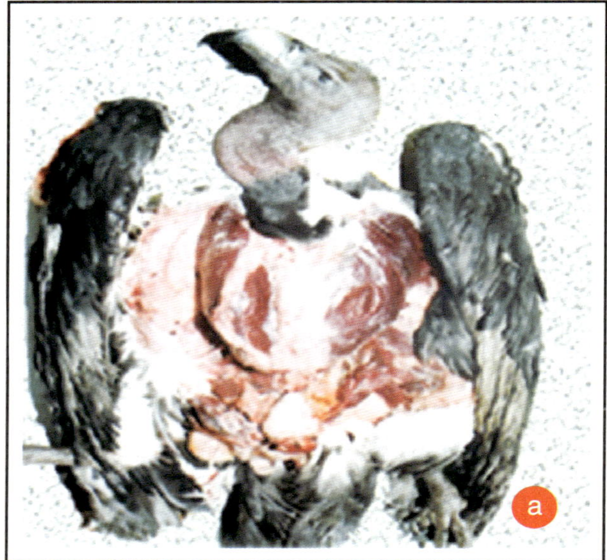

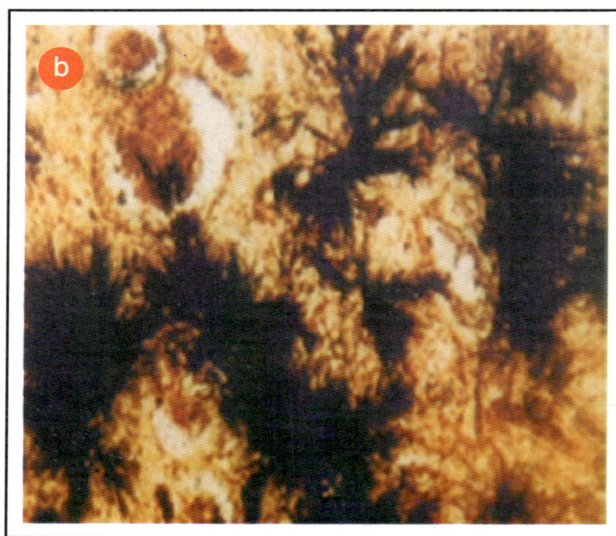

Figure 51 : (a) Dissection of king vulture (*Sarcogyps calvus*) showing visceral gout in the kidneys. Photomicrograph (b) of kidney showing uric acid deposition predominately in the kidney tubules. DeGalanthas stain. (Courtesy : Panda, S.K)

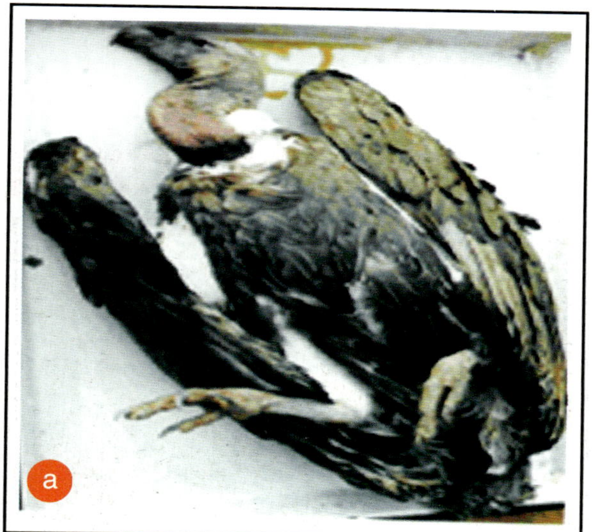

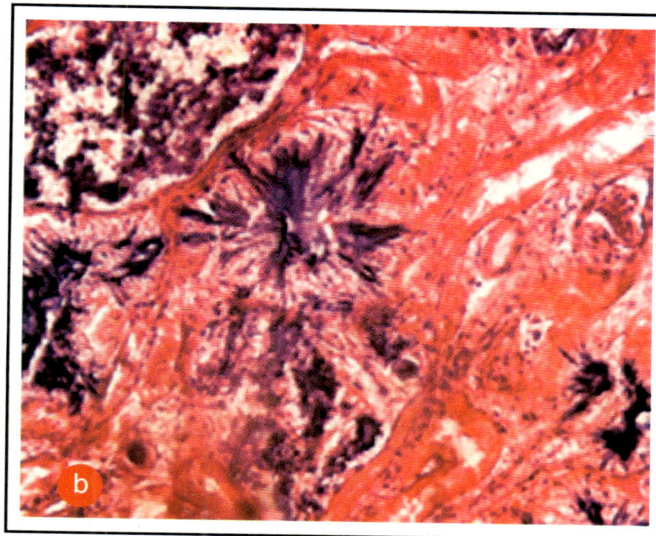

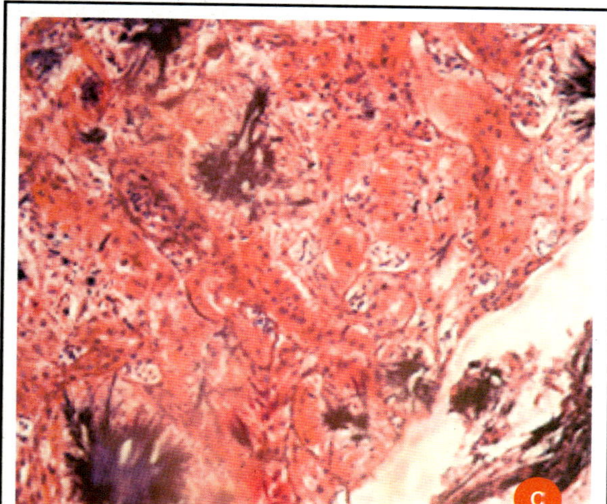

Figure 52 (a):Carcass of white- backed Bengal vulture (*Gyps bengalensis*) died in a captive facility. Photomicrographs showing: (b) Presence of urate tophi with marked congestion. H&E,x128. (c) Urate tophi arranged in radiating pattern. H&E,x240. (Courtesy: Panda, S.K.& Nath, I.).

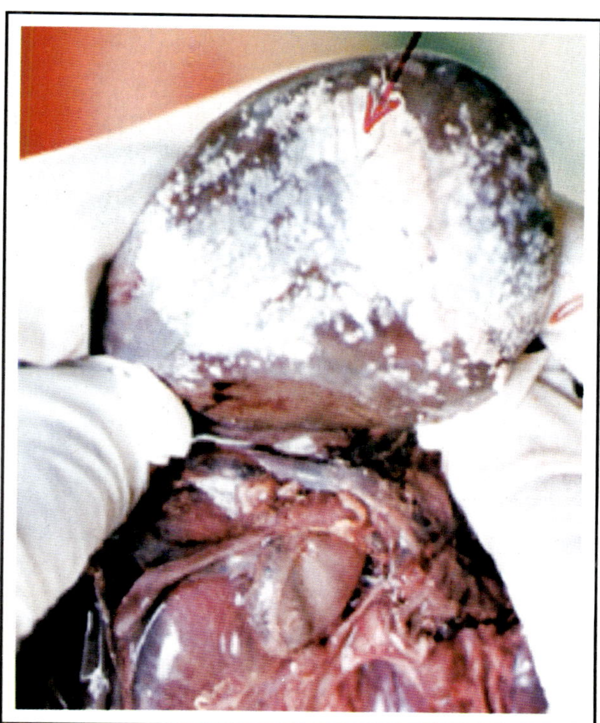

Figure 53: Photograph showing visceral gout, predominately in kidney in vulture.Note deposition of whitish crate or uric acid crystals. (Courtesy: Dept. of Wildlife Science, C.V.Sc,Chennai, T.N).

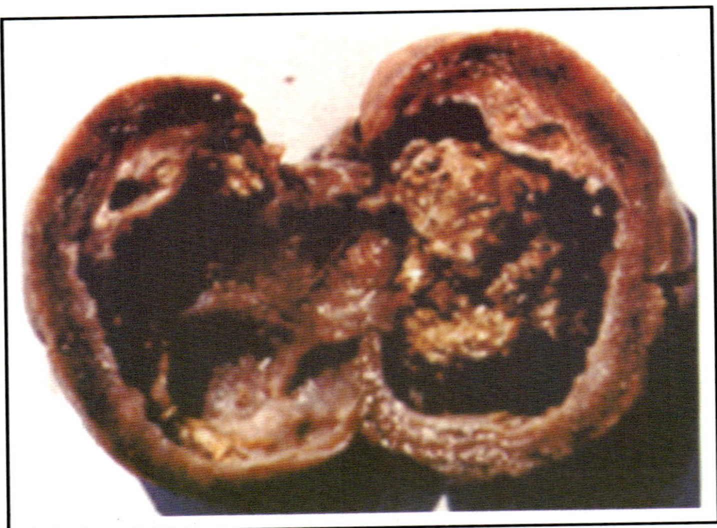

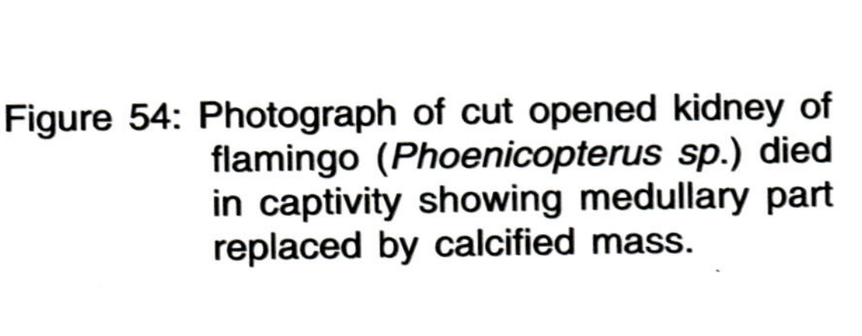

Figure 54: Photograph of cut opened kidney of flamingo (*Phoenicopterus sp.*) died in captivity showing medullary part replaced by calcified mass.

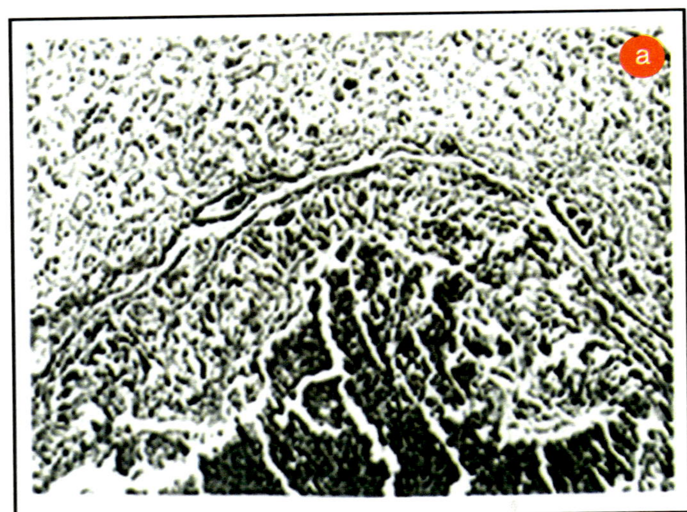

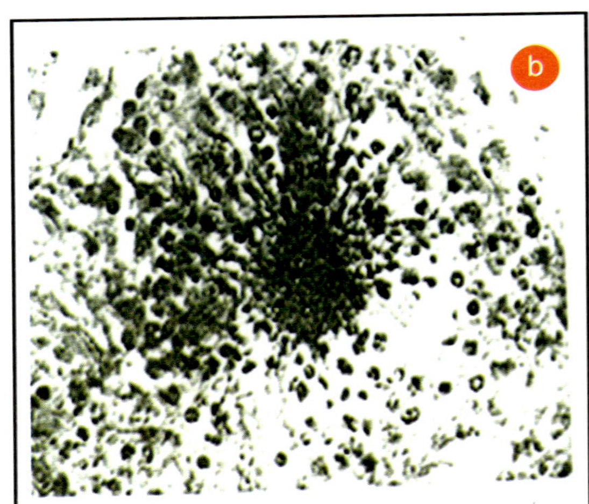

Figure 55: Photomicrographs of kidney of Hill myna (*G. religiosa*) showing (a) Granulomatous lesions of Nocardia infection. H&E, x65. (b) Thin PAS positive filamentous in an area of abscess, PAS & Haematoxylin, x 650 (Iyer *et al.*, 1972).

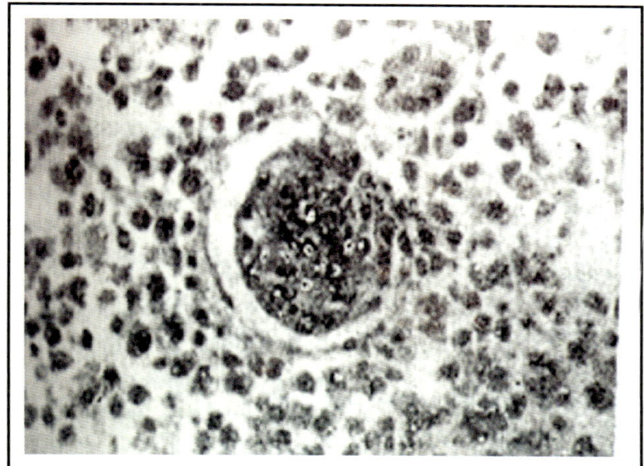

Figure 56: Marek's disease in captive pheasants (*Chir, Kalij, Mikado*).Photomicrograph of kidney showing diffuse infiltration of pleomorphic lymphoid cells around glomerulus.The case is also referred under Nervous system. H&E,x520. (Sah *et al.*,1982).

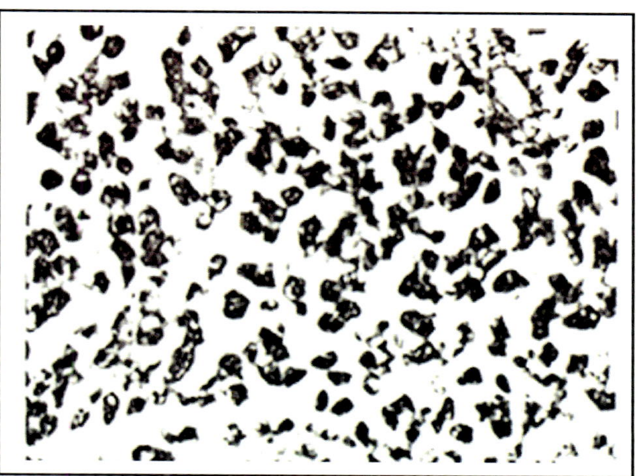

Figure 57: Lymphomatosis in a peafowl (*Pavo cristatus*). Photomicrograph of kidney showing diffuse tumorous cell infiltration in the intertublar spaces. H&E,x400 (Sah *et al.*, 1973).

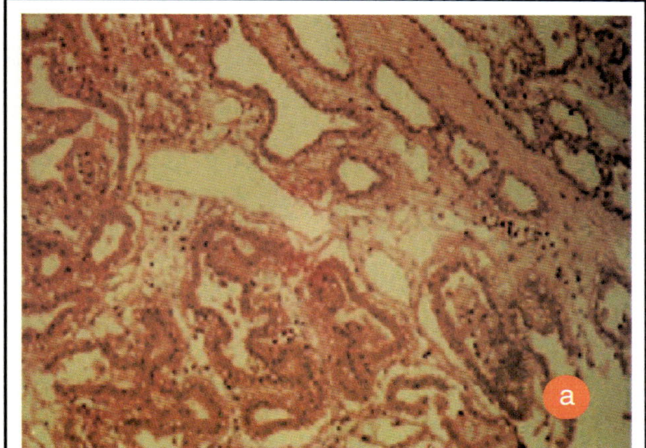

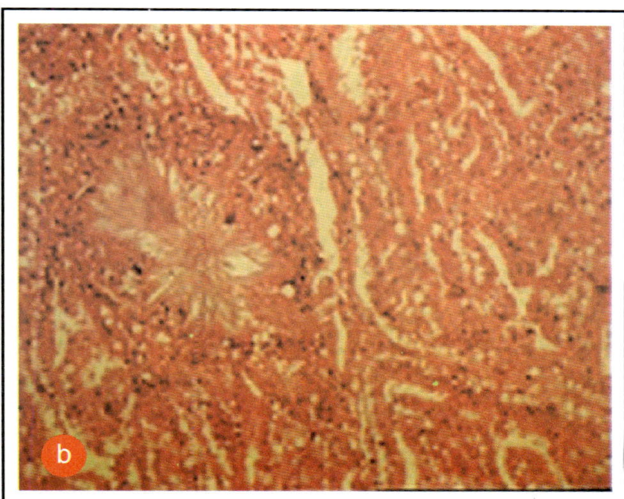

Figure 58: Nephroblastoma in Copper pheasant (*S.semmerringii*, an exotic sp.)died in captivity.Photomicrograph of kidney showing: (a)Bizarre shaped hyper chromatic tubuli in a fairly cellular connective tissue stroma.H&E,x200 (b) Presence of radiating hyphae of uric acid crystals and granulomatous reaction at the periphery. H&E,x200 (Courtesy: Singh, S.D.).

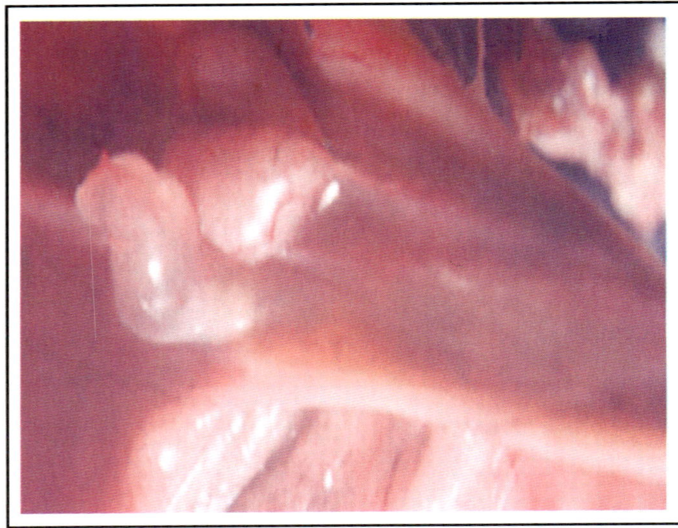

Figure 59: Photograph showing persistant urachus in black swan (*Cygnus atratus*,an exotic sp.).Note small elongated cyst like structure filled with fluid connected to bladder (Courtesy: Suryawanshi, D.S.).

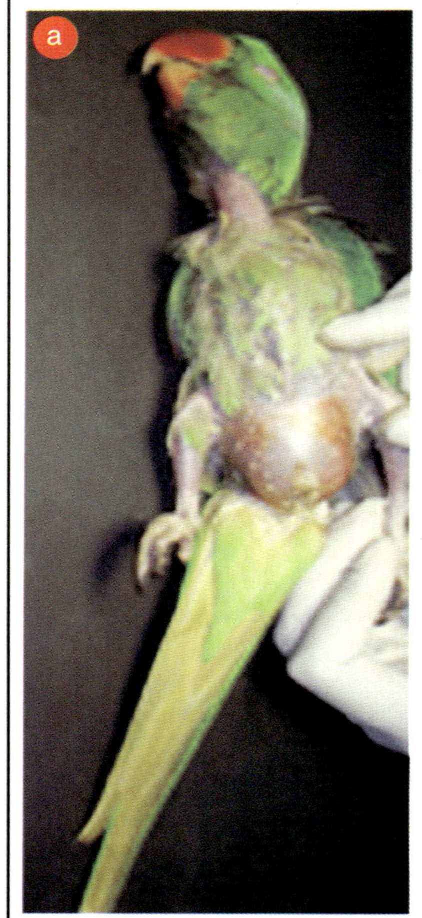

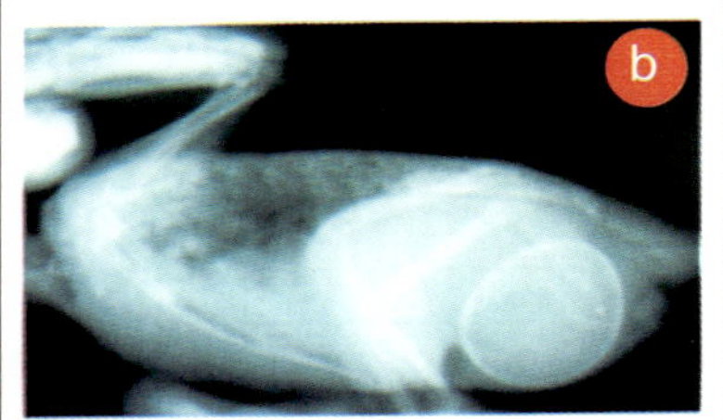

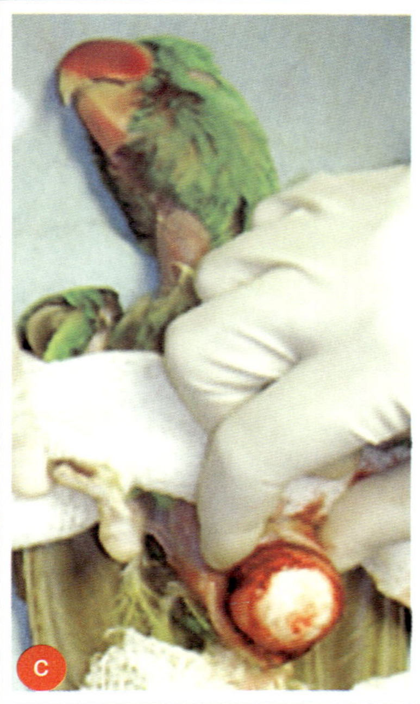

Figure 60: (a) Rosy parrot, having bulging ventral region. (b) Lateral radiograph of (a) showing retained egg in the posterior of abdomen. (c) Surgical management (laparotomy) to extricate the retained egg (Courtsey: Kanwar, M.S.).

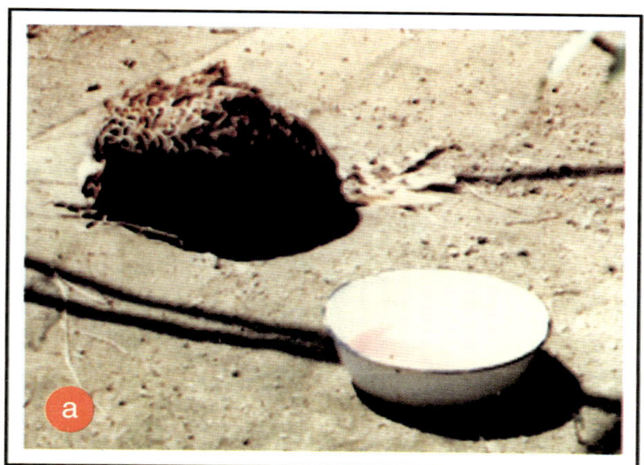

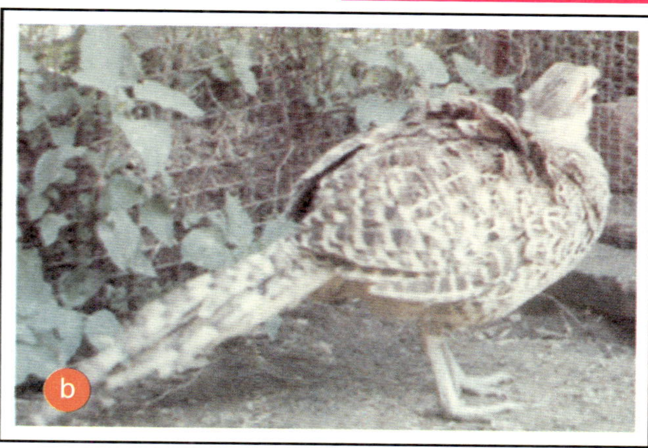

Figure 61: (a) Completely paralysed Chir pheasant (*Catreus wallichi*). (b) The same is recovered after treatment with Berin (Vit. B_1).

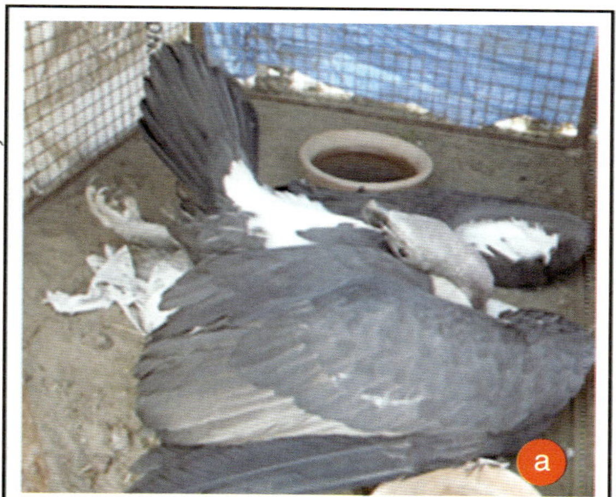

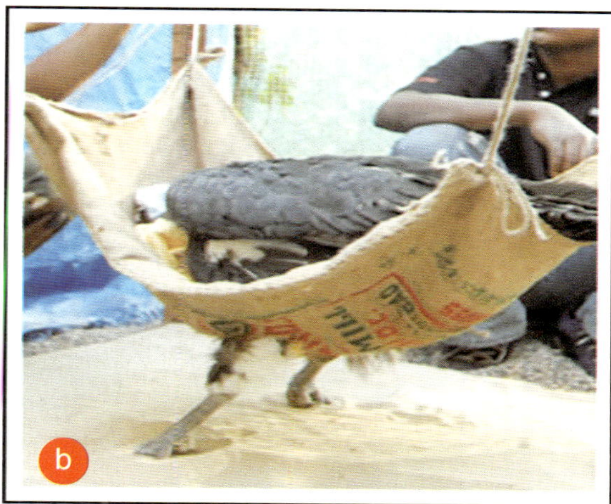

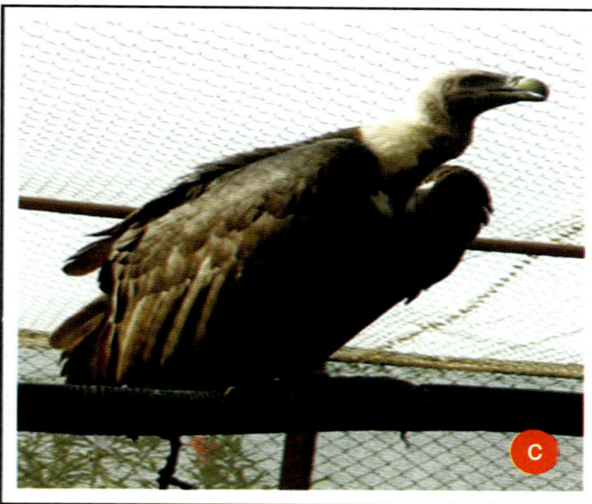

Figure 62: (a) White backed vulture (*Gyps bengalensis*) lying flat on the ground with extended legs and retracted head was unable to regain normal posture. (b) Vulture (a) on sling under treatment. (c) Completely recovered (a). (Disale *et al.*, 2007).

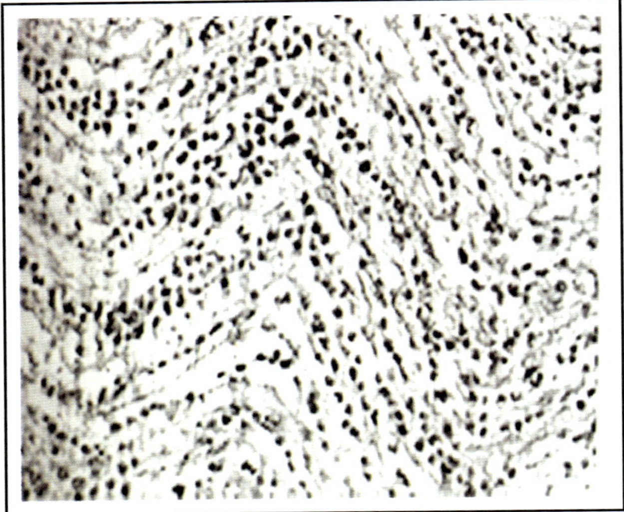

Figure 63: Marek's Disease in captive chir, Kalij, Mikado (an exotic sp.)pheasants. Photomicrograph showing Sciatic nerve having pleomorphic lymhoid cell infiltration and oedema. H&E, x 250. The case is also referred under urinary system. (Sah *et al.*,1982).

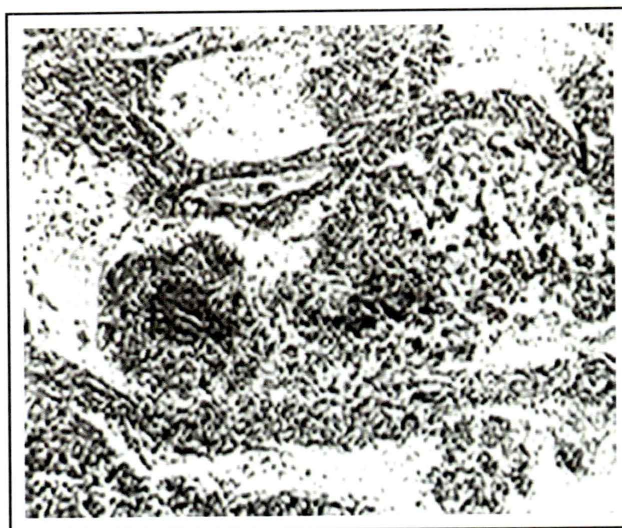

Figure 64: Photomicrograph of affected eyes of Hill myna (*G religiosa*) showing caseo- necrotic lesion in Ciliary body. H&E x65. The case is also referred under respiratory, digestive and urinary systems. (Iyer *et al.*, 1972).

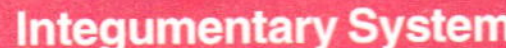

Integumentary System

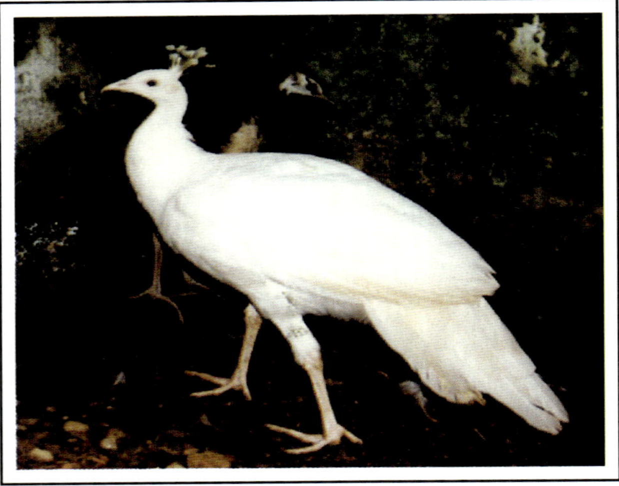

Figure 65: White peafowl (*Pavo cristatus*) often seen in captive facilities.

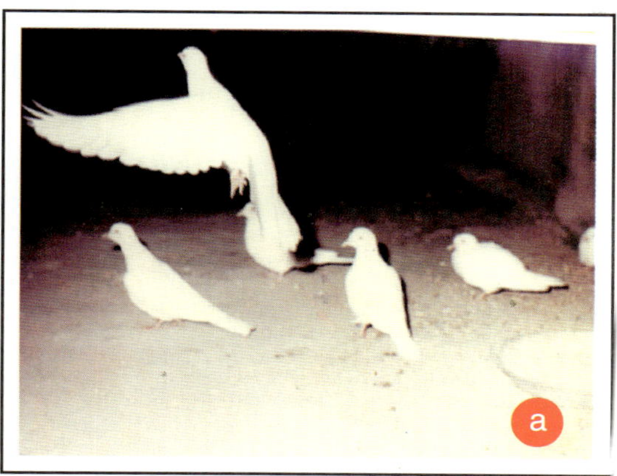

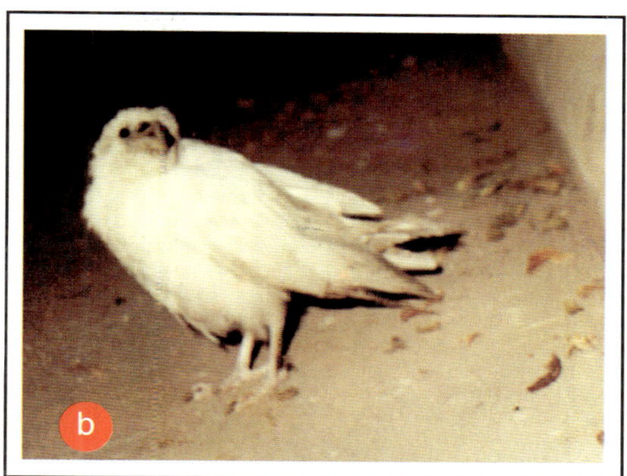

Figure 66: (a) White dove (*Streptopelia sp.*) and (b) white crow (*Corvus sp.*) in Zoological Park, Chhatbir (Chandigarh).

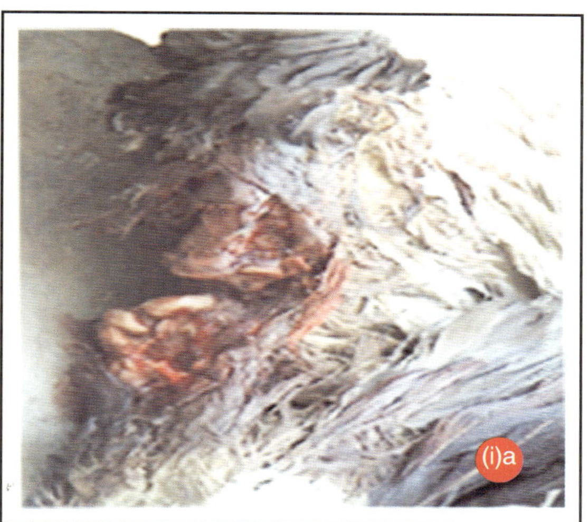

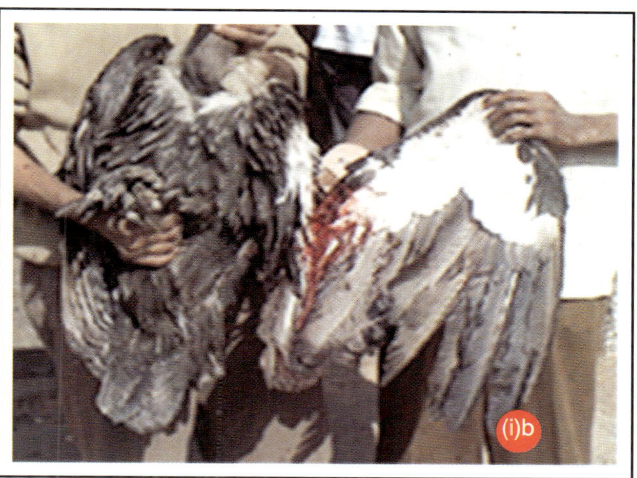

Figure 67: Photographs showing lacerated deep wounds caused by flying kite thread in (i) white backed vultures (*Gyps bengalensis*). (a) In the leg muscles. (b) Under left wing (Courtesy B.K.Gupta). (ii): Common eagle under treatment for wound under the left wing caused by flying kite string.

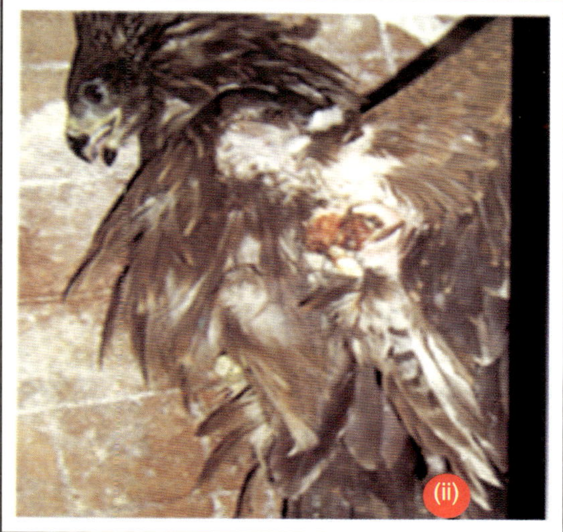

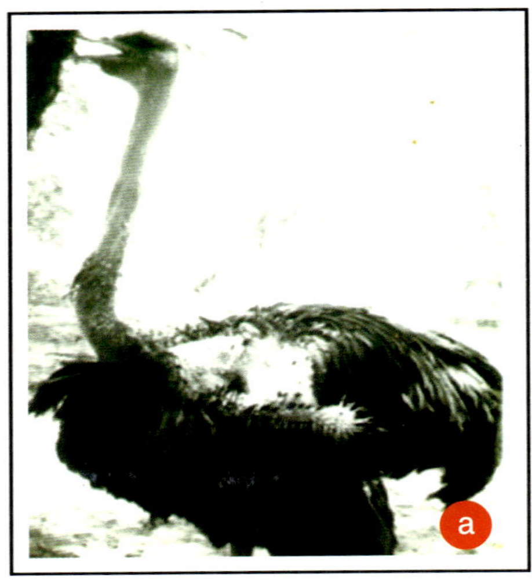

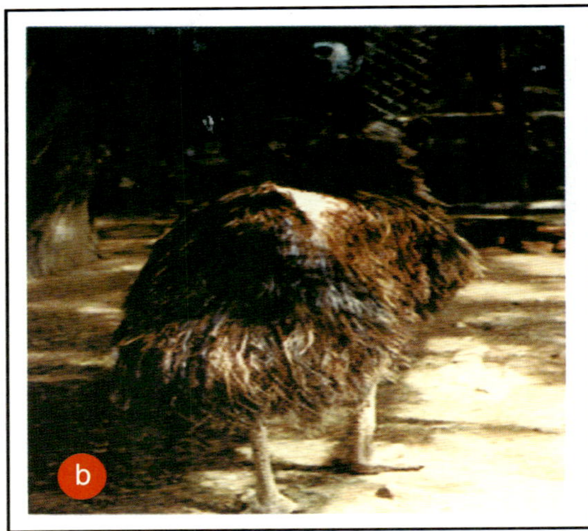

Figure 68: Photograph showing burnt feathers due to lighted cigarette thrown on the body of ostrich (*S. camelus*, an exotic land bird) by a visitor in National Zoological Park, New Delhi. (b) Another -land bird-rhea (an exoitic land bird) also has similar fate.

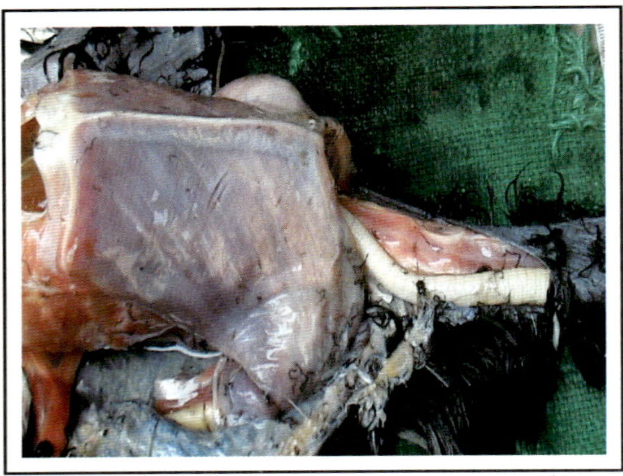

Figure 69: Photograph showing breast muscle dystrophy due to Vit. E deficiency encountered in a young horn bill (*Buceros bicornis*) died in Zoological Garden, Guwahati, Assam.

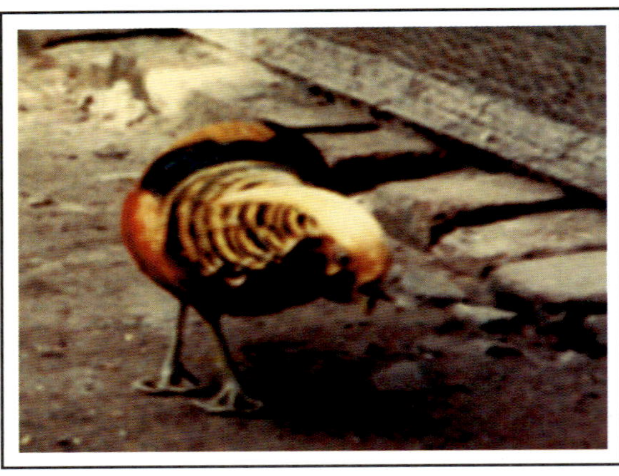

Figure 70: Golden pheasant (*Chrysolophus pictus*, an exotic sp.) having developed curling of toes.

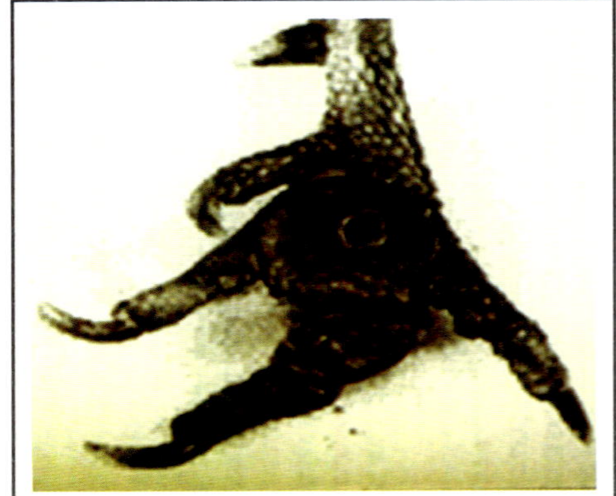

Figure 71: Photograph showing bumble foot in chir pheasant (*C. wallichi*) caused by *Staphylococcus aureus* (Courtesy: Somvanshi, R.).

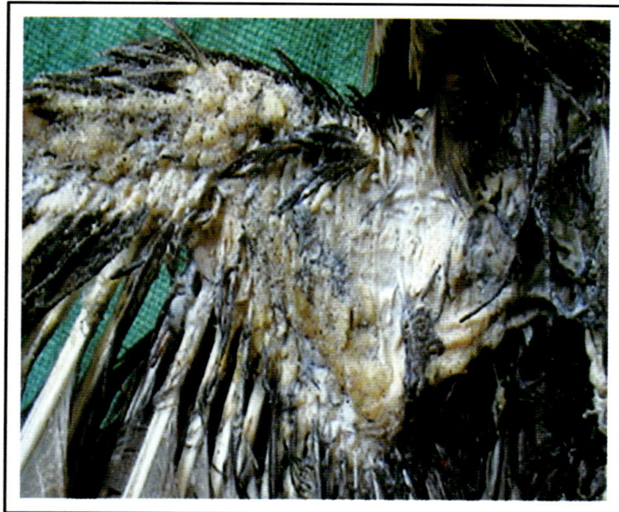

Figure 72: Silver pheasant (*Laphura nycthemera*, an exotic sp.) suffering with mycotic dermatitis of its wings in Zoological Garden, Guwahati Assam.

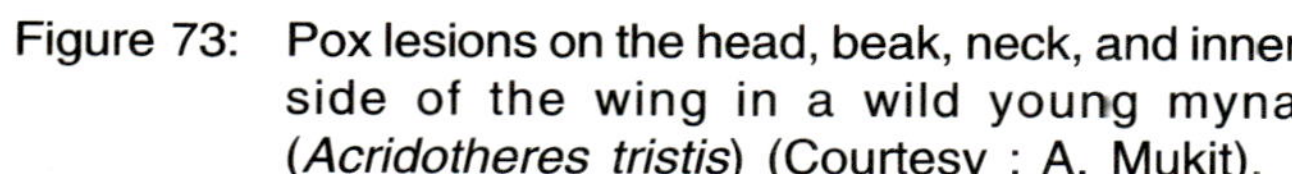

Figure 73: Pox lesions on the head, beak, neck, and inner side of the wing in a wild young myna (*Acridotheres tristis*) (Courtesy : A. Mukit).

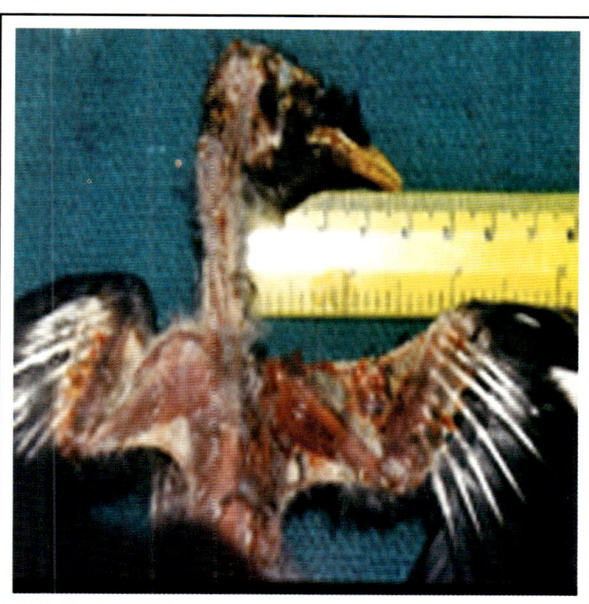

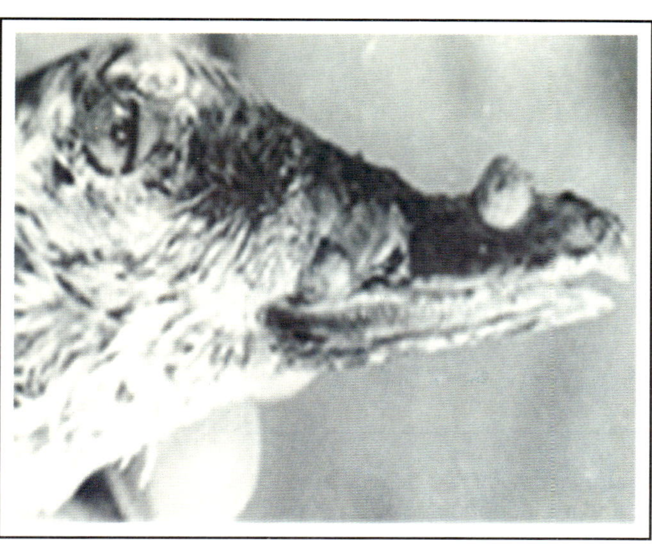

Figure 74: Growth of sarcoma melanoma on the beak of white winged wood duck (*Cairina scutulata*) of Maio aviary (Arunachal Pradesh).

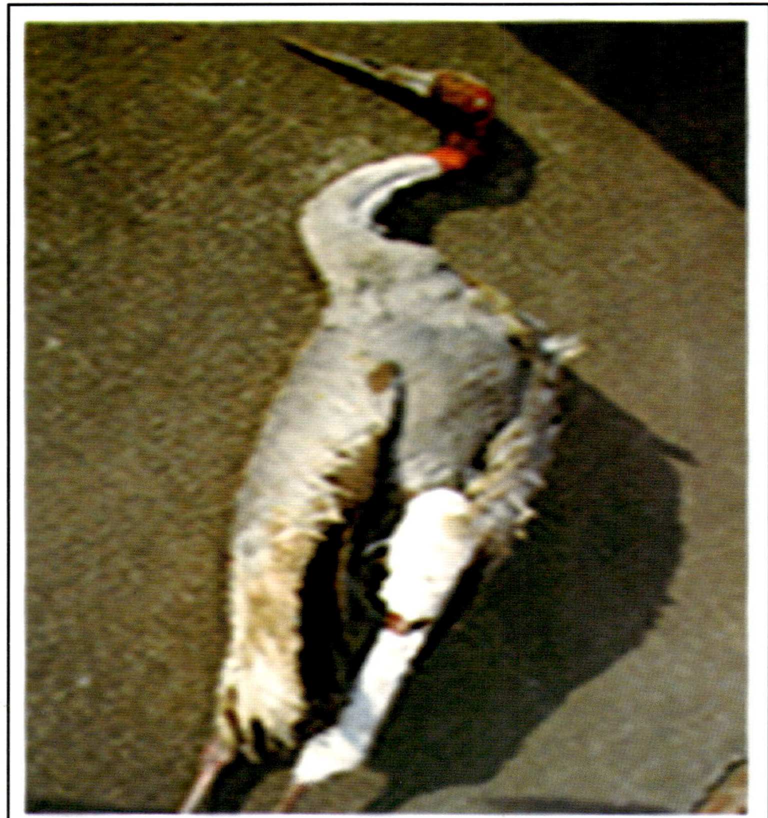

Figure 78: Siberian crane (*Gurus antigone*) with leftlimb fractured under surgical management.

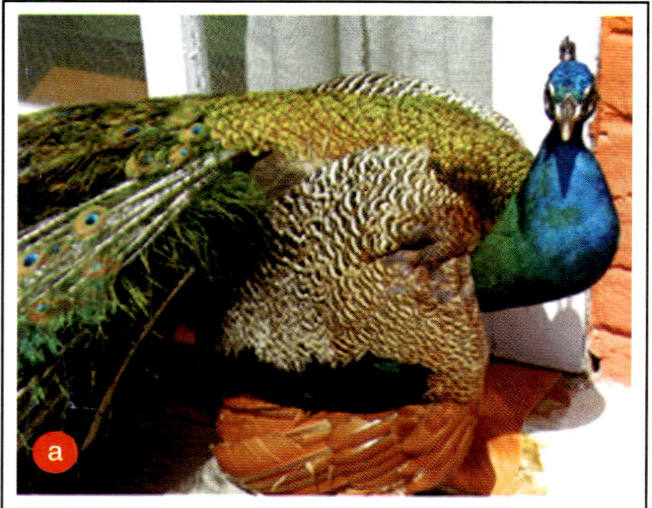

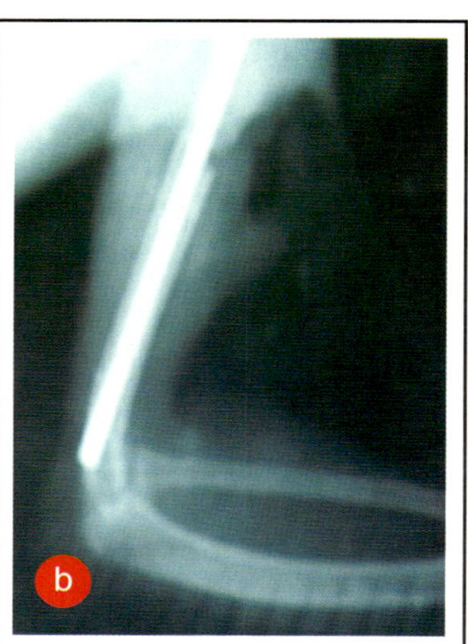

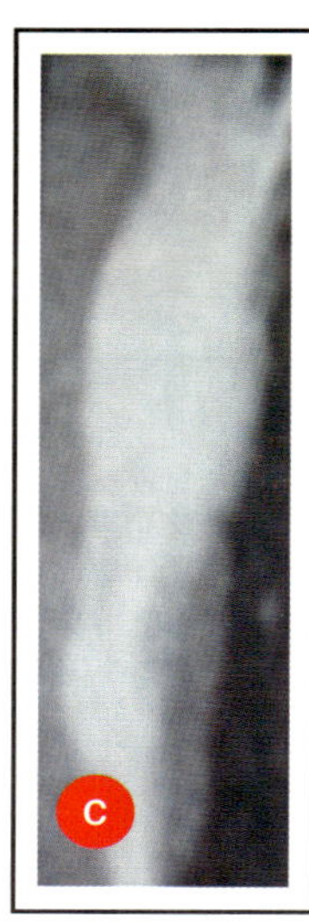

Figure 79: (a) Left tibia shaft fractured in peacock (*Pavo cristatus*). (b,c) Using medullary pin the same was managed. (Courtesy: Kanwar,M.S.).

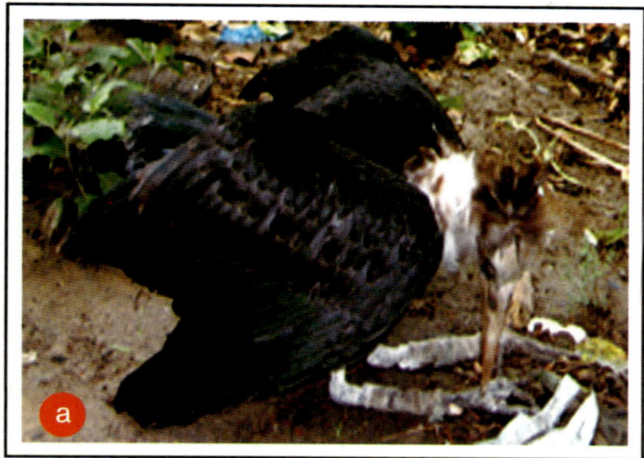

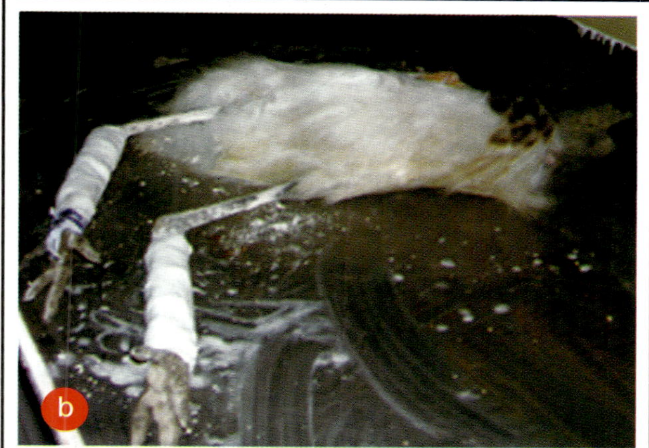

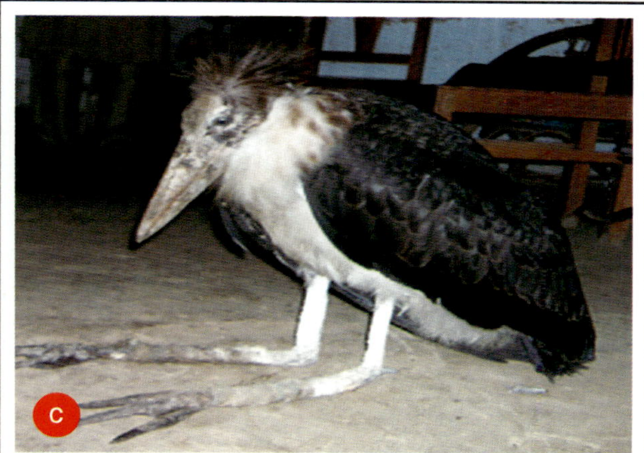

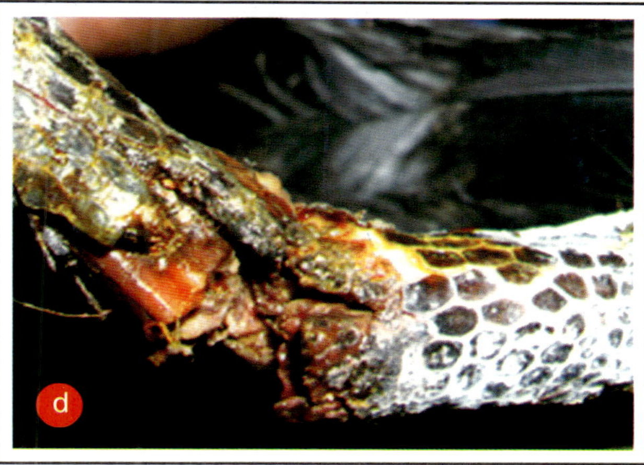

Figure 80: Fractures encountered in growing lesser adjutant storks (*Leptoptilos javanicus*). (a) Bird unable to sit in normal posture due to fracture in its tarsal bones. (b) Surgical management of fracture of tarsal bone in both legs using bamboo splint and plaster to set fracture. (c) the fracture was cured and the stork was able to bear weight on its legs in due course. (d) Another case of tarsal bone fracture. (Courtesy: Das, B.J.).

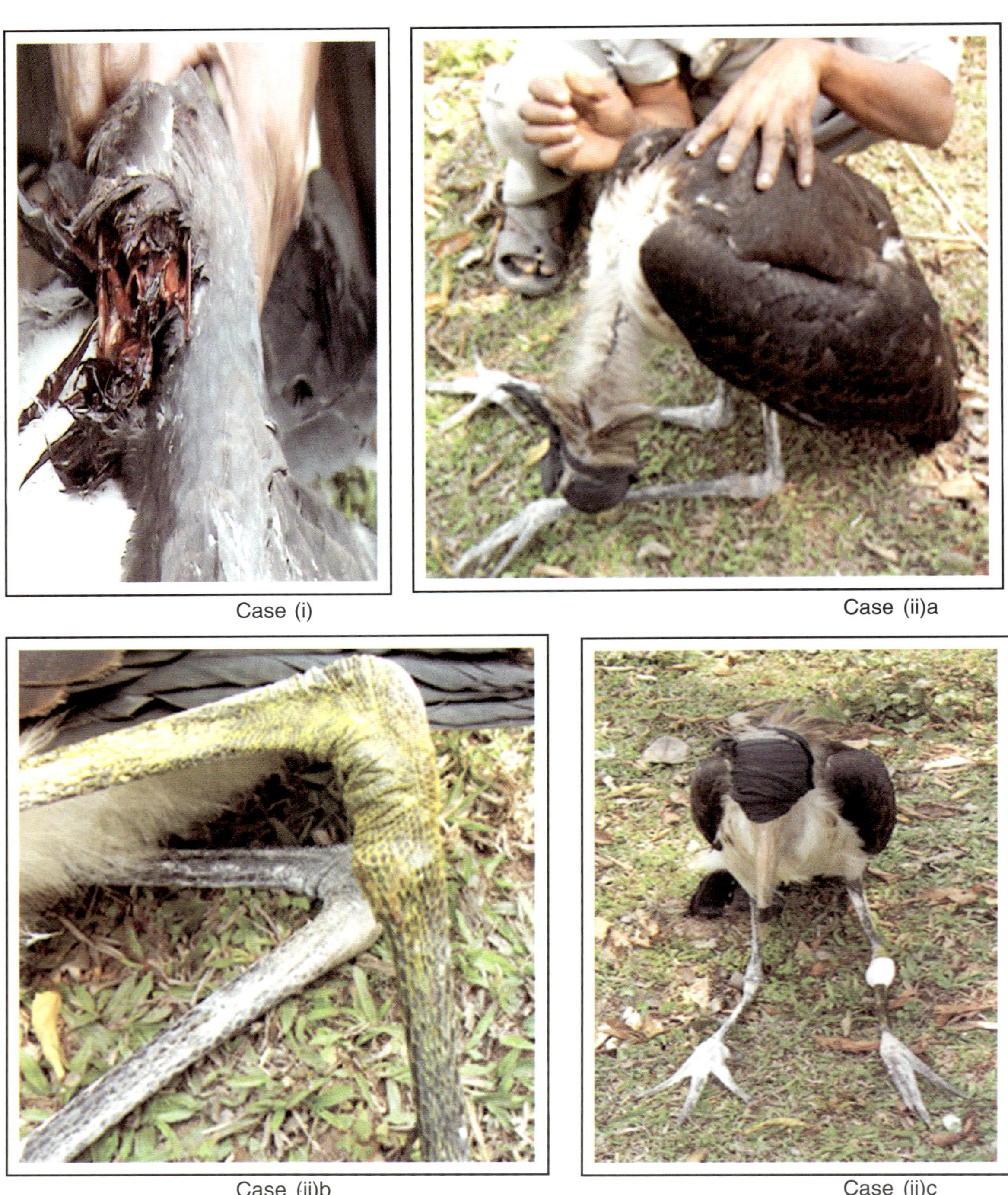

Figure 81: Photographs showing fractures in growing greater adjutant stork (*Leptoptilos dubius*) which had fallen from tree during storm: Case (i) Fractured right wing. Case (ii-a) Stork unable to sit in normal posture due to fracture in its left tarsal bone Case (ii) b,c. Management of fracture undertaken. (Case-ii, Courtesy : Das, B.J.).

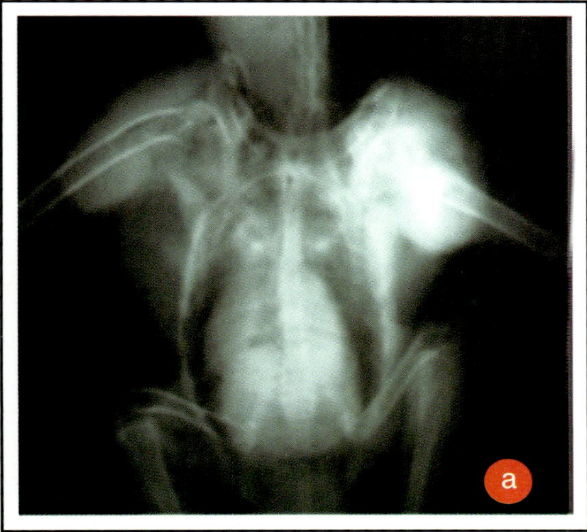

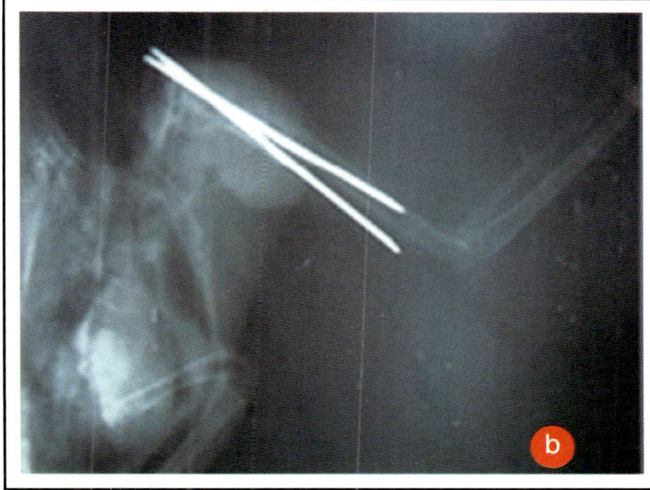

Figure 82: (a) Radiograph showing fracture of humerus in a black kite (*Milvus nigrans*). (b) insertion of intra-medulary pin intramedulary pins in position. (Disale *et al.*, 2007)

Miscellaneous

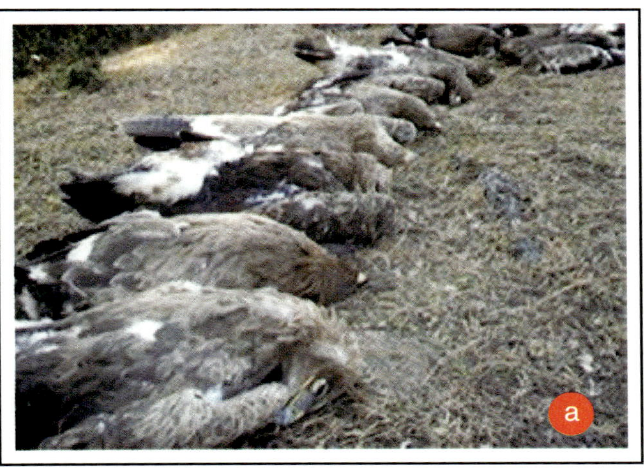

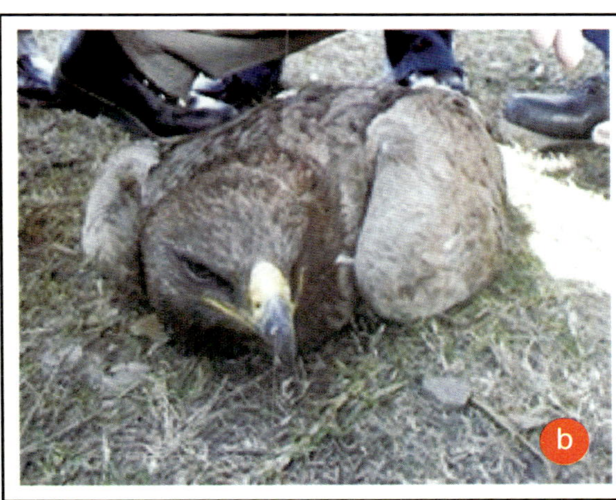

Figure 83: (a) En-mass demise of Steppe eagle (*Aquila nipalensis*) related to Organo-phosphate poisoning encountered during 2005 near Ranikhet in Uttarakhand. (b) A sick Steppe eagle sitting on strenum due to spastic paralysis of legs, and marked for salivation and gasping respiration (Courtesy: Choudhury, B.).

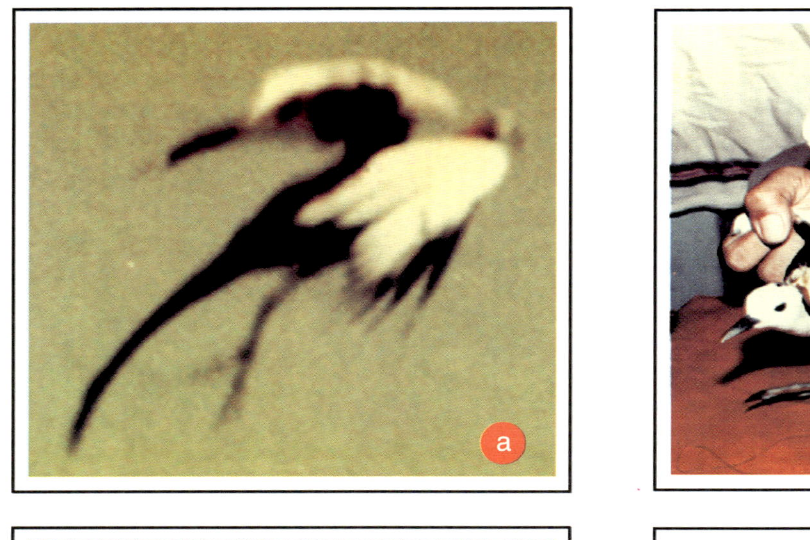

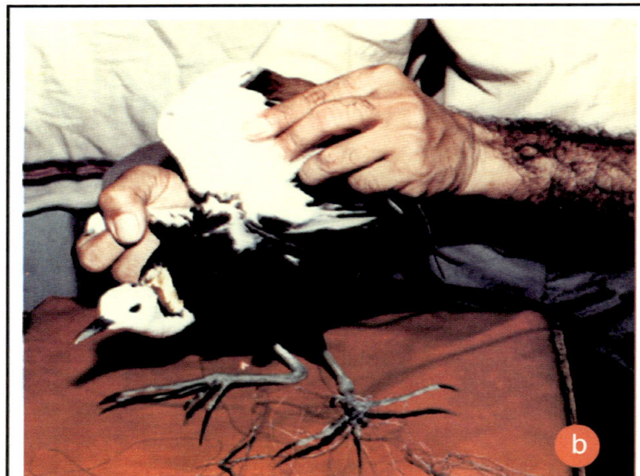

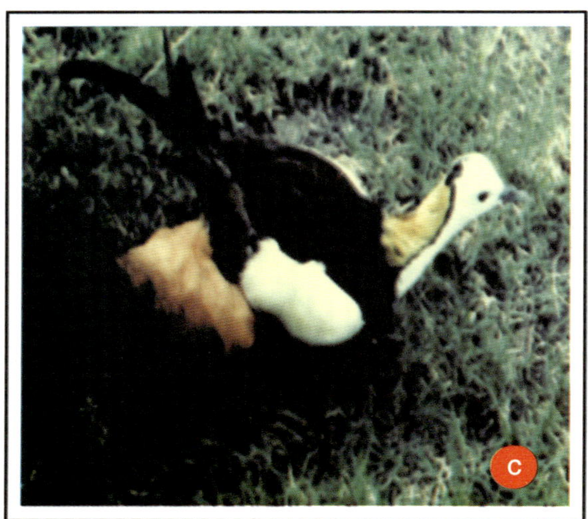

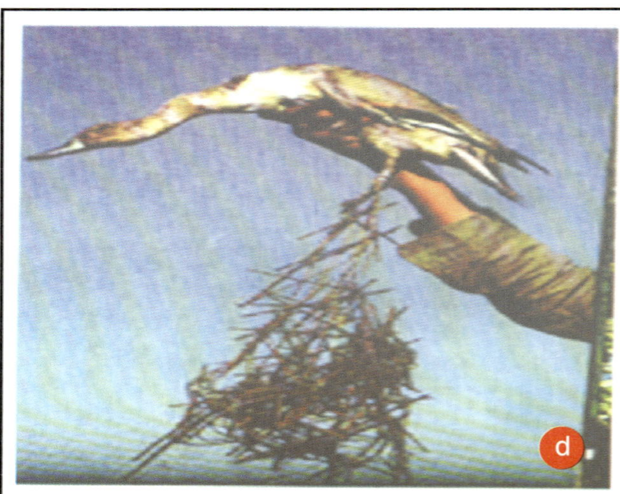

Figure 84: (a) Pheasant tailed Jacana (*Hydrophasianus chirurgus*) legs entangled with kite string hanged in air. (b) Kite string being removed. (c) After thread removed the bird being released back to wild. (d) A pintail trapped in a net (Photo from Indian Wildlife, Bedi & Bedi, 1984)

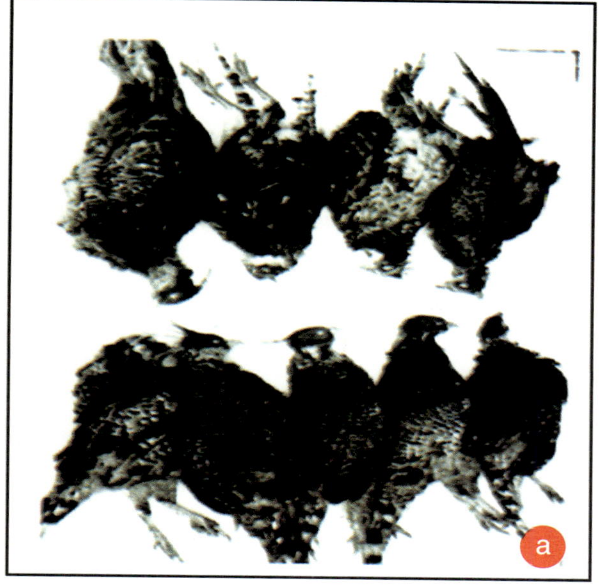
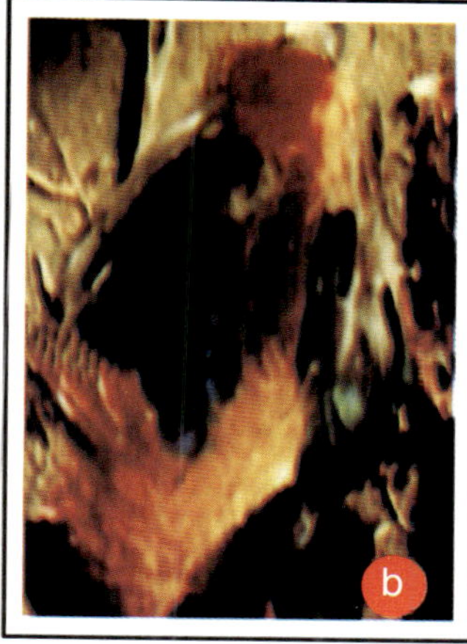
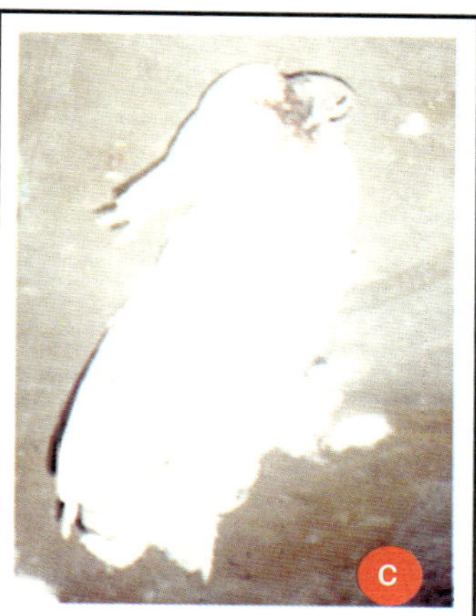
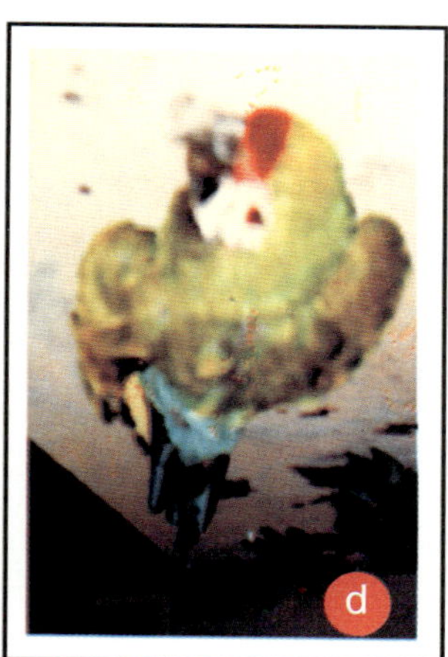
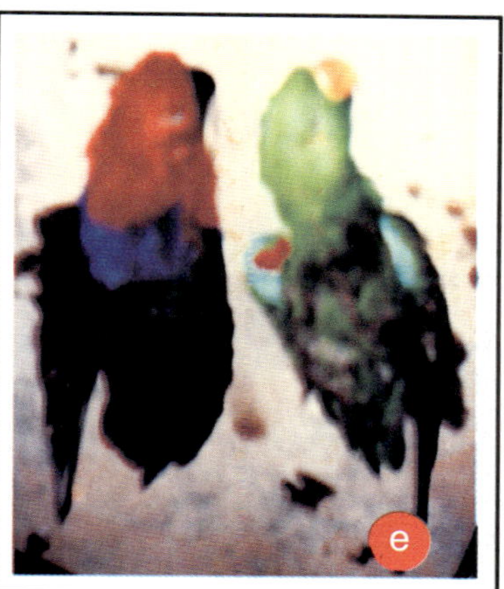
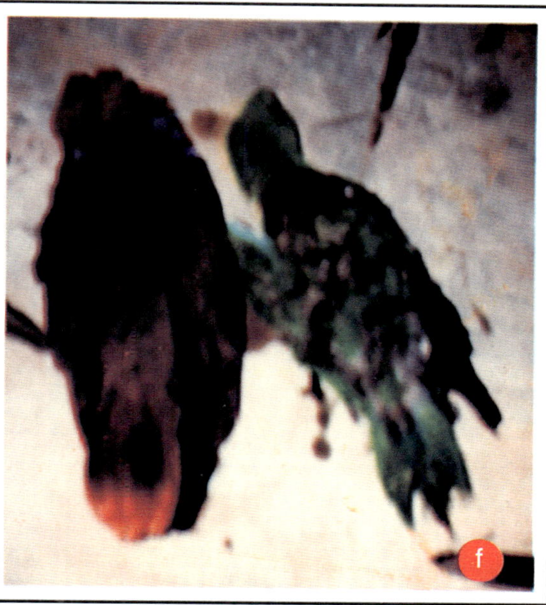

Figure 85: Birds in captivity killed by vermin. Carcasses of: (a) Chir pheasants (*C.wallichi*) and exotic bird species- (b) Golden pheasant (*Chrysolophus pictus*), (c) White cockatoo (*Kakatoe sp*), (d-f) Lorikeet (*Loriculus vernalis*).

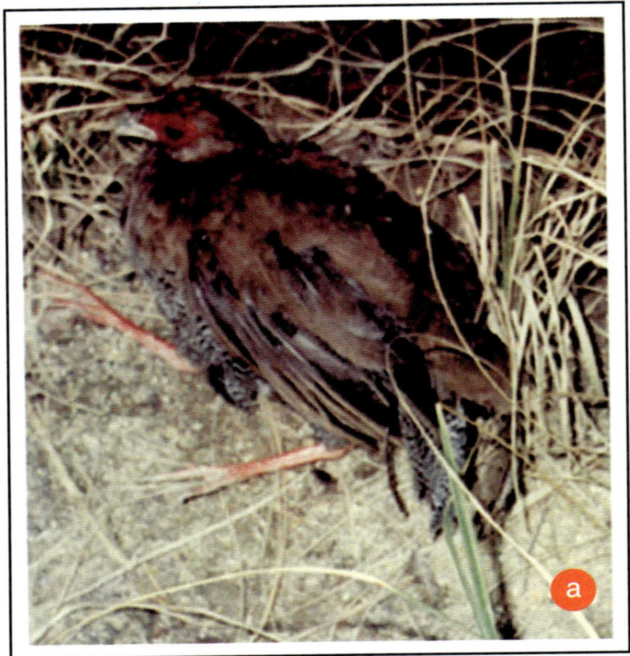

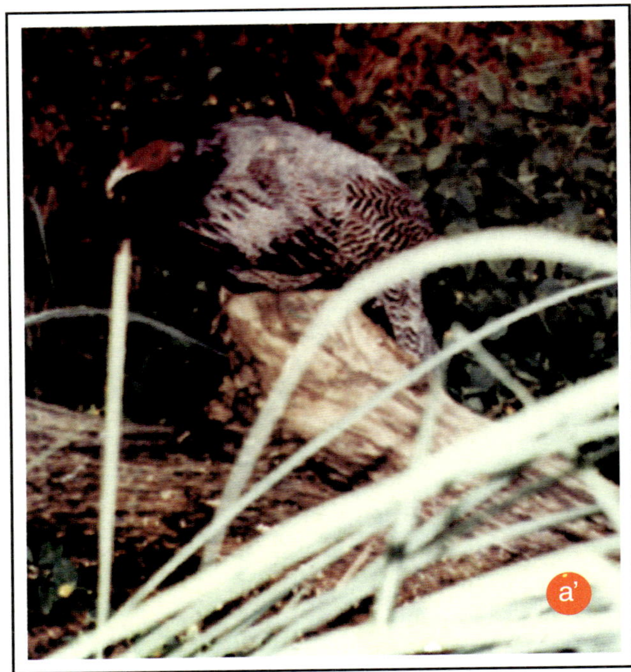

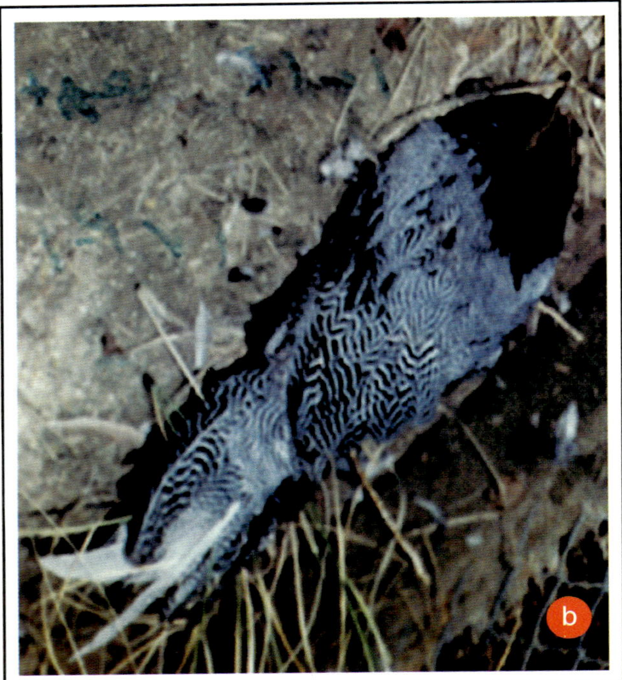

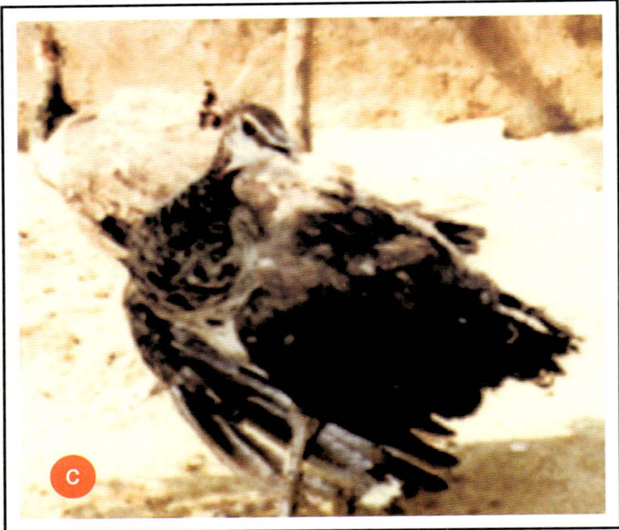

Figure 86: Photographs showing impact of stress and shock due to long distance tansportation by vehicle of: (a, a') Two female and (b) a male Kalij pheasants (*Lophura leucomelanoa*). (c) Pea fowl (*Pavo cristatus*).

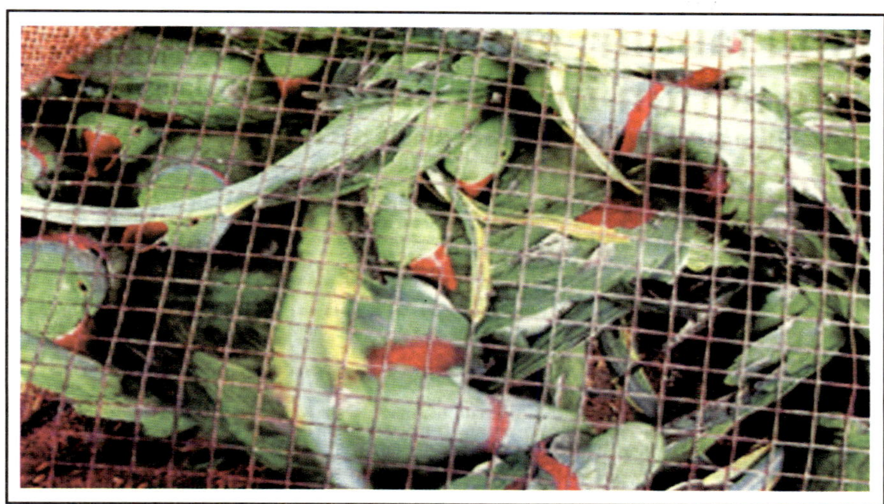

Figure 87: Alexandrian parakeets, popularly known as Gaggrani tota in Rajasthan were seized during the raid in Jaipur. Birds were found squeezed into 2.5x 2 feet wooden cages. Later on, they were kept in Jaipur zoo (Hindu Oct 10, 2006).

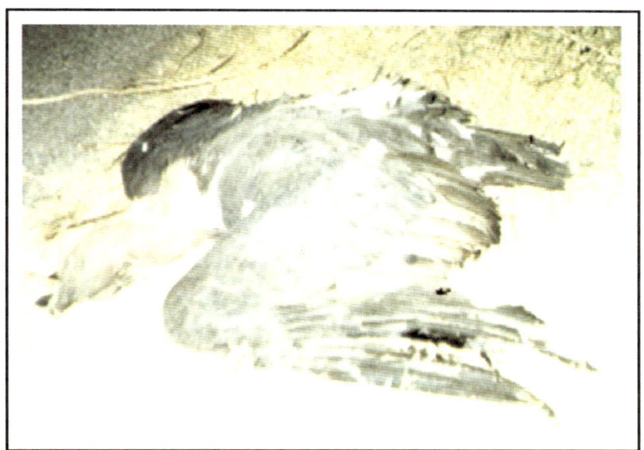

Figure 88: Carcass of White backed vulture,lying crushed on a metalic road, due to over run by some motor vehicle. Remnants of mutilated small animal carcass was also noticed nearby.

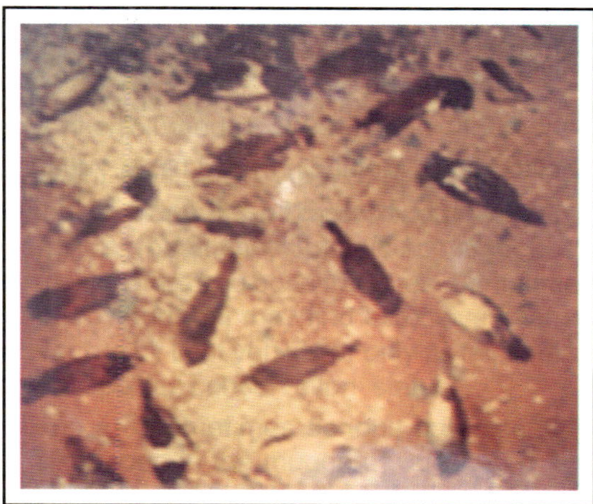

Figure 89: Death of a large number of munia (*Lonchura* sp.) due to water deprivation in their cage-in Zoological Garden, Mysore (Courtesy: Naga Raju , S.).

Figure 1: A large blood clot in pericardium of crocodile died in captivity.

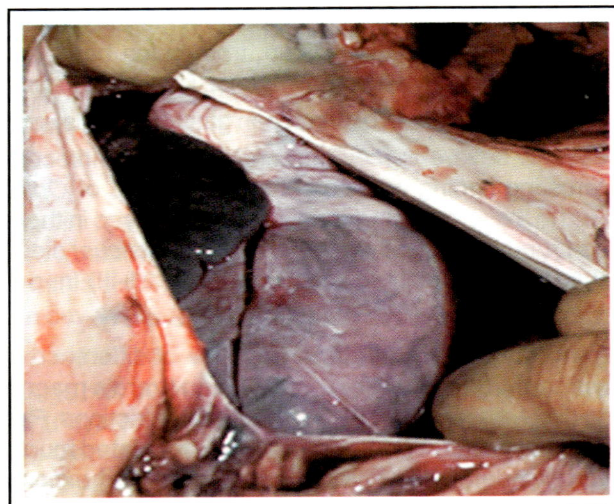

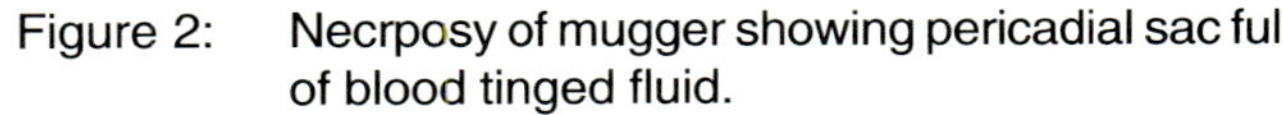

Figure 2: Necrposy of mugger showing pericadial sac full of blood tinged fluid.

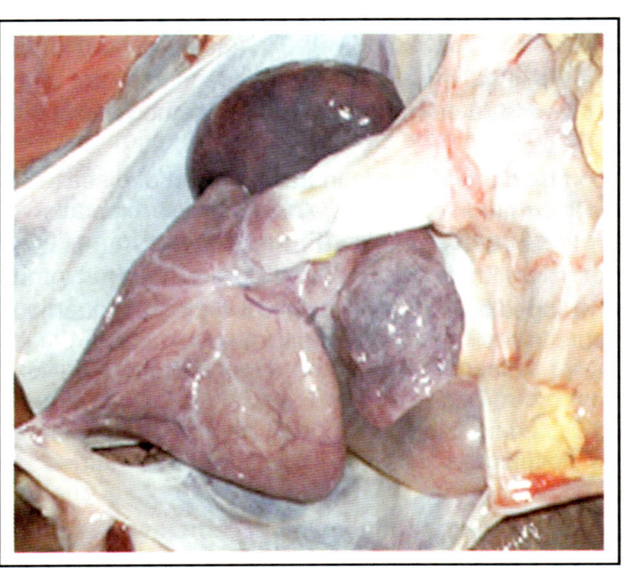

Figure 3: Photograph showing hydropericardium and dilated auricles in tortoise died in captivity (Photos 1 to 3 Courtesy: Suryawanshi,D.S.).

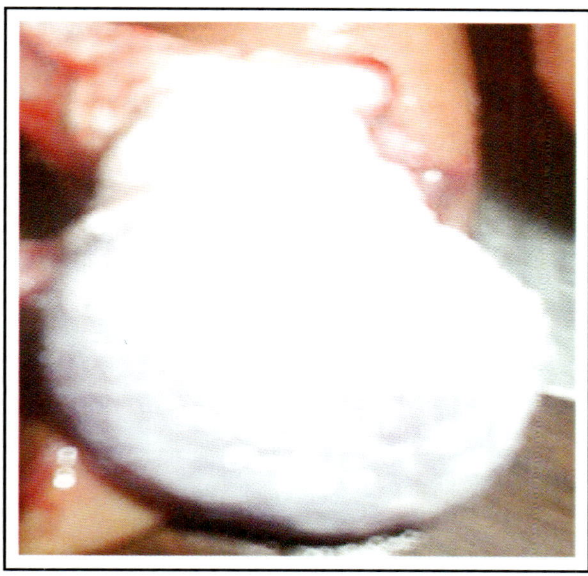

Figure 4 : Photograph showing chalky white material (visceral gout) on the pericardium of monitor lizard. (Courtesy: Suryawanshi,D.S.).

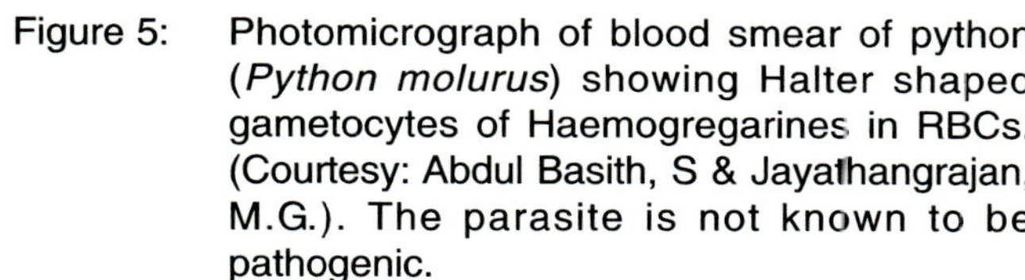

Figure 5: Photomicrograph of blood smear of python (*Python molurus*) showing Halter shaped gametocytes of Haemogregarines in RBCs. (Courtesy: Abdul Basith, S & Jayathangrajan, M.G.). The parasite is not known to be pathogenic.

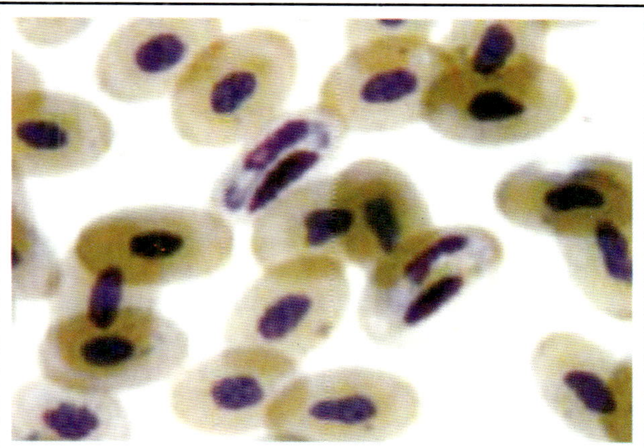

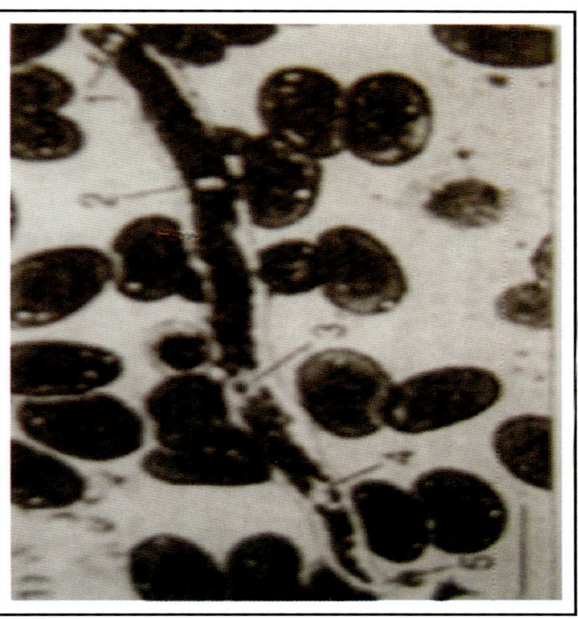

Figure 6: Photomicrograph of blood smear of toad (*Bufo melanostictus*) showing microfilaria (Roy & Sarkar,1999).

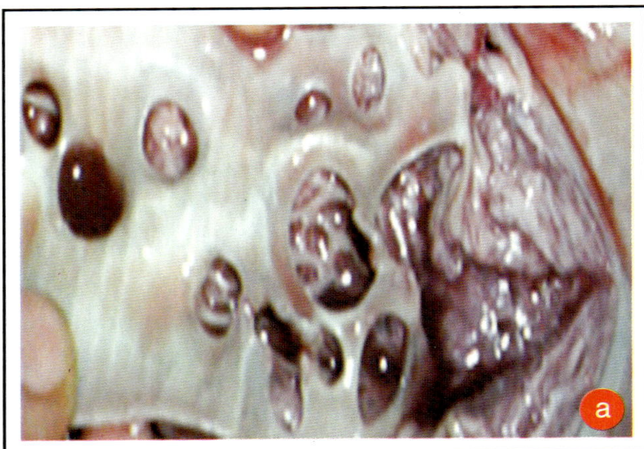

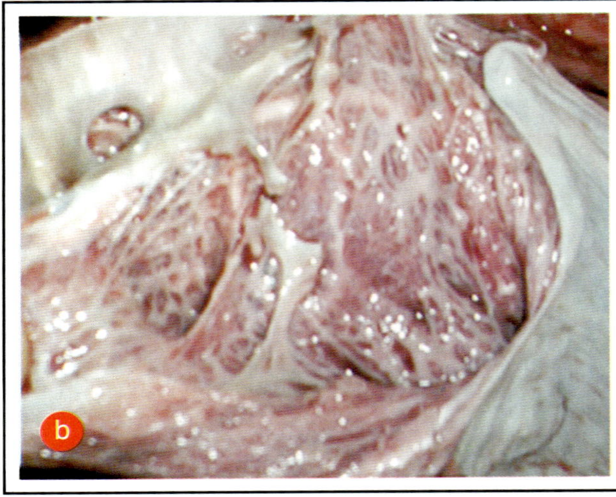

Figure 7: Photographs showing: (a) Ulcers in the trachea and (b)oedema of lung. Bronchi contained reddish fluid in a mugger died in captivity (Courtesy: Suryawanshi, D.S.)

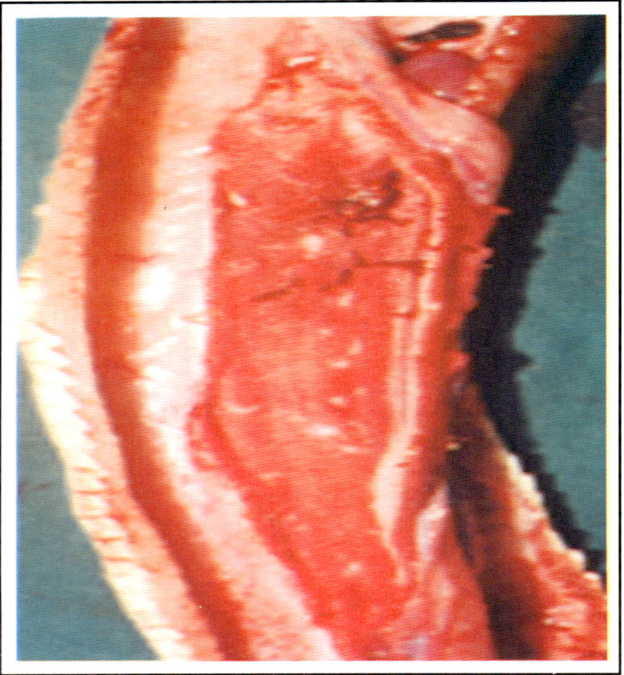

Figure 8: Photograph showing congestion and oedema of lung in a snake died in captivity.

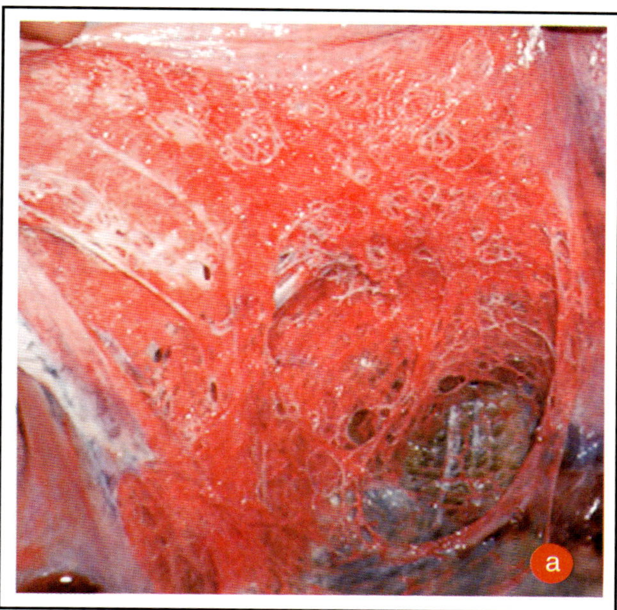

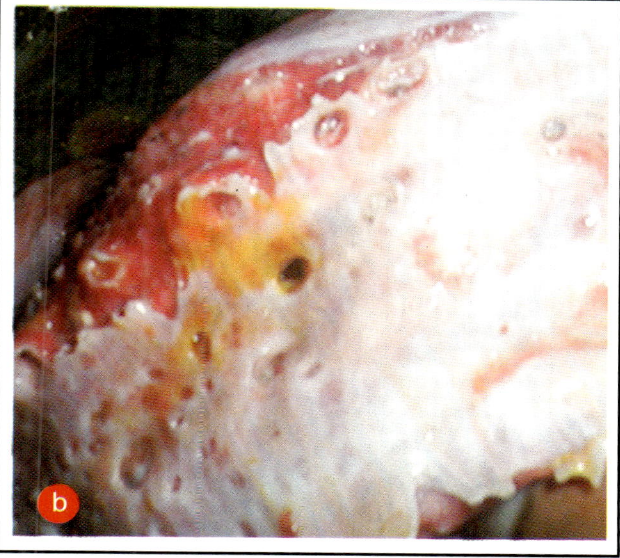

Figure 9: Photographs (a,b) showing congestion and oedma of lung encontered in tortoise died in captivity. (Courtesy: Suryawanshi,D.S).

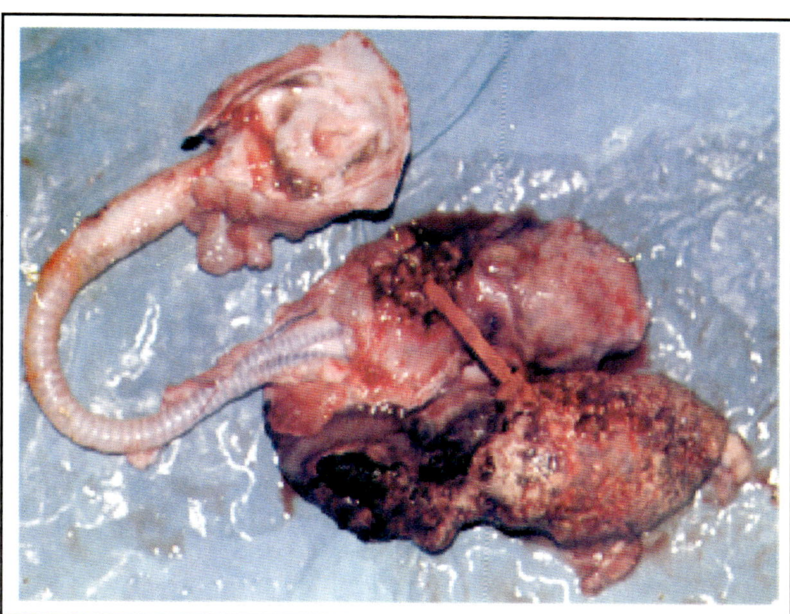

Figure 10: Photograph of lung, heart and liver showing creamy colored, thickened nodules of Pseudo tuberculosis (*Corynebacterium* sp. infection) in caiman crocodile (Courtesy: Harish, B R).

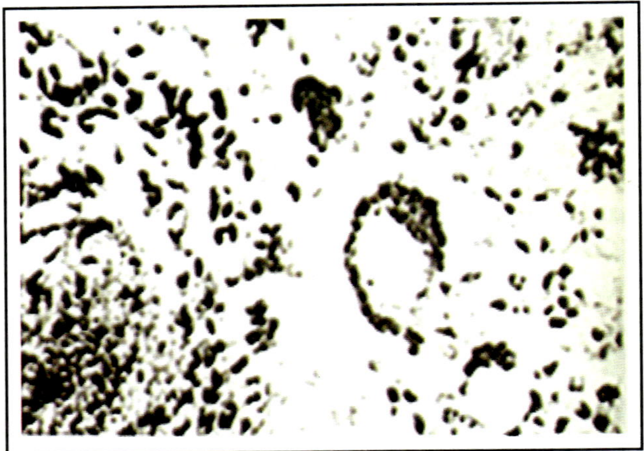

Figure 11: Photomicrograph of lung of crocodile showing serofibrinous exudate,mononuclear cells and giant cells related to *Proteus sp.* infection. H&E, x 450. (Chakraborty *et al.*, 1988).

Digestive System

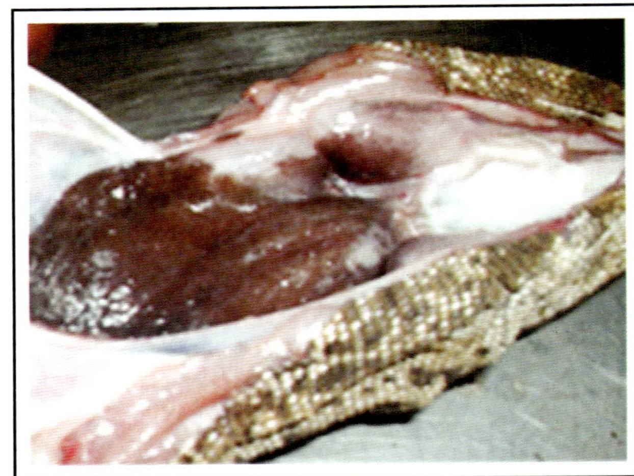

Figure 12: Photograph showing haemorrhages in the pharynx in lizard (Courtesy: Suryawanshi, D.S.).

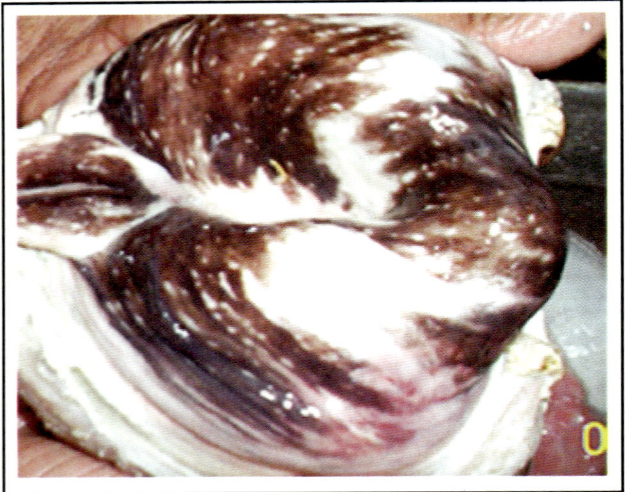

Figure 13: Photograph showing haemorrhages in the pharyngeal mucosa in crocodile (Courtesy: Suryawanshi, D.S.).

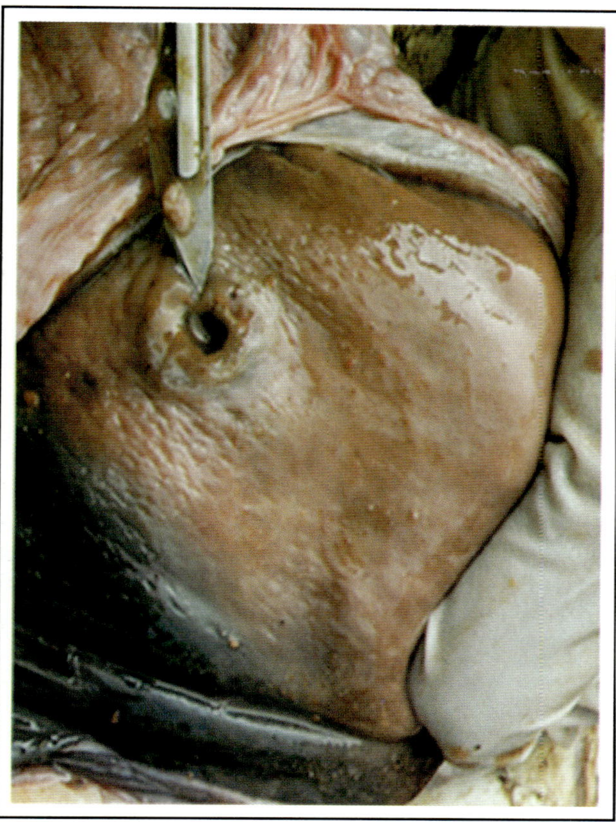

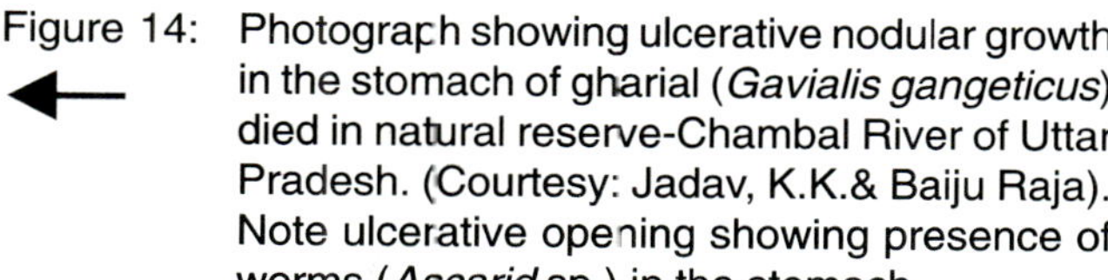

Figure 14: Photograph showing ulcerative nodular growth in the stomach of gharial (*Gavialis gangeticus*) died in natural reserve-Chambal River of Uttar Pradesh. (Courtesy: Jadav, K.K.& Baiju Raja). Note ulcerative opening showing presence of worms (*Ascarid* sp.) in the stomach.

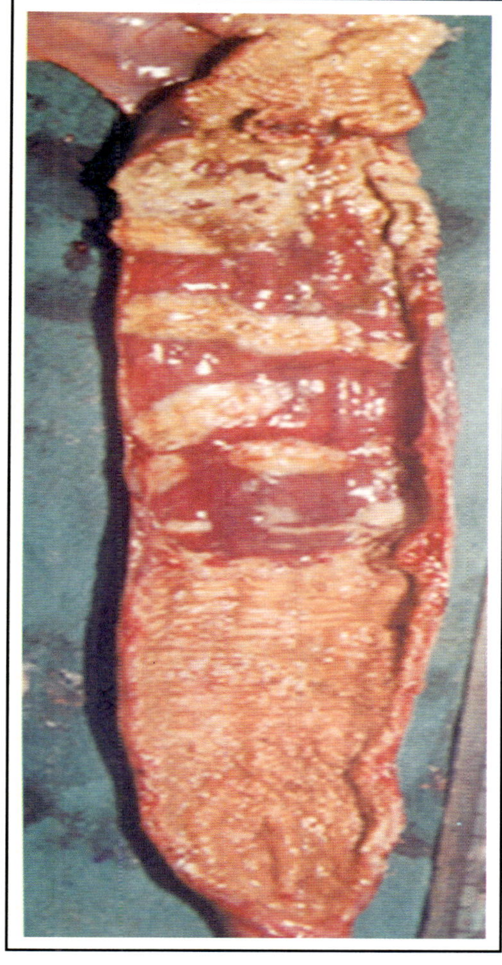

Figure 15 : Photograph showing diphtheritic colitis due to Salmonella infection in snake (Courtesy: Suryawanshi, D.S.).

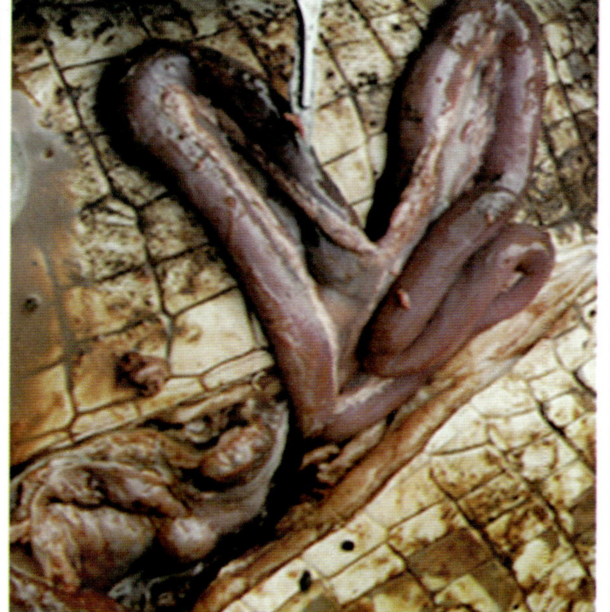

Figure 16: Haemorrhagic enteritis in a gharial (*Gavialis gangeticus*) died in natural reserve-chambal river. Note severely congested serosal surface of intestine. Dissection of intestine showed presence of blood tinged intestinal contents. (Courtesy: Jadav, K.K.& Baiju Raja).

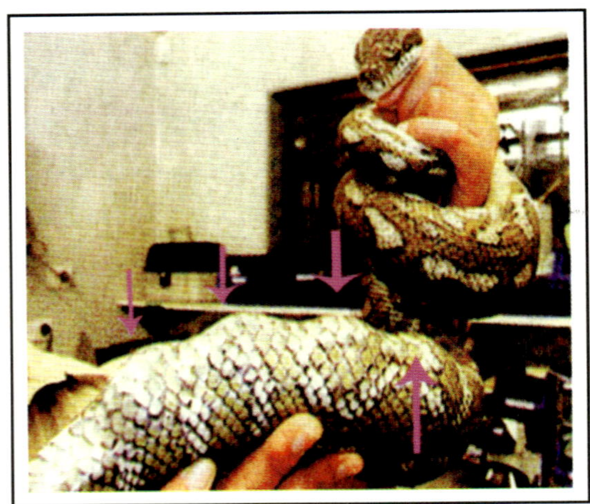

Case (ia)

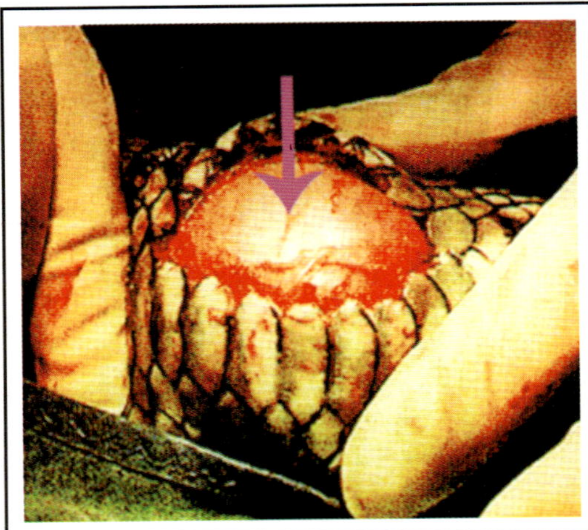

Case (ib)

Figure 17: Case (i) A keeper holding a carpet python (an exotic sp) that swallowed four golf balls, mistaking them for chicken eggs, at currumbin on Australia's Gold Coast. (b) A veterinarian operating (a) to remove the balls from its intestine. Source: News paper - Times of India, page 18 dated 5th January, 2008. Case (ii) Python (*P. molurus*) had swallowed a man (E. mail Photo: Ajinder Singh Chawla, Member ERN, WTI).

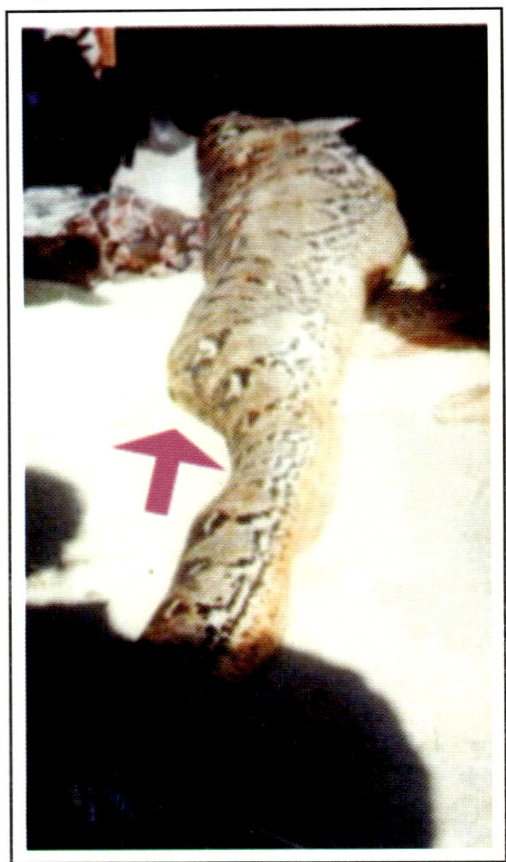

Case (ii)

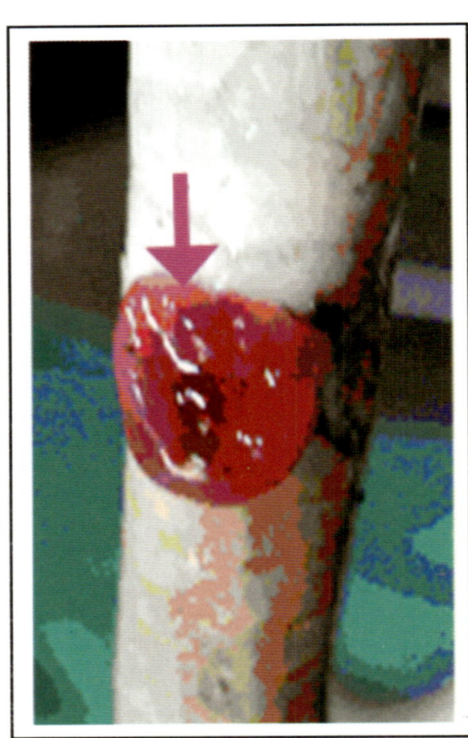

Figure 18: Prolapse of rectum in cobra (*Naja naja*) rescued from wild (Courtesy: Nath, I)

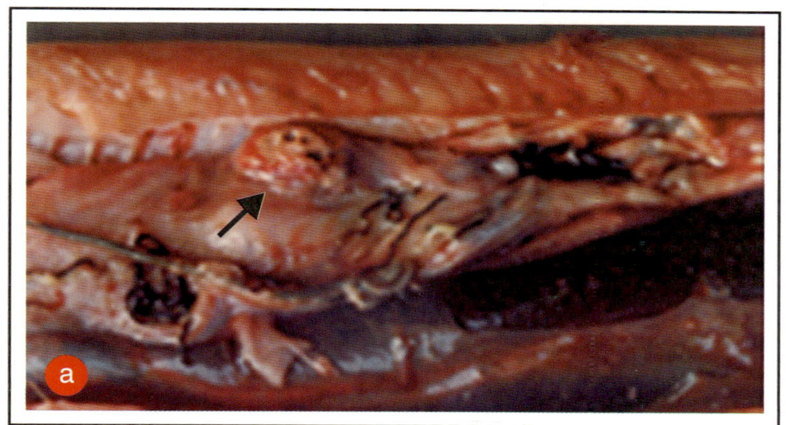

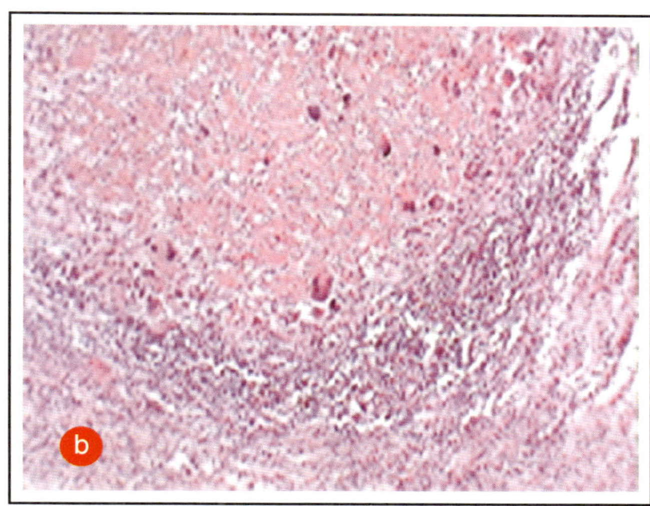

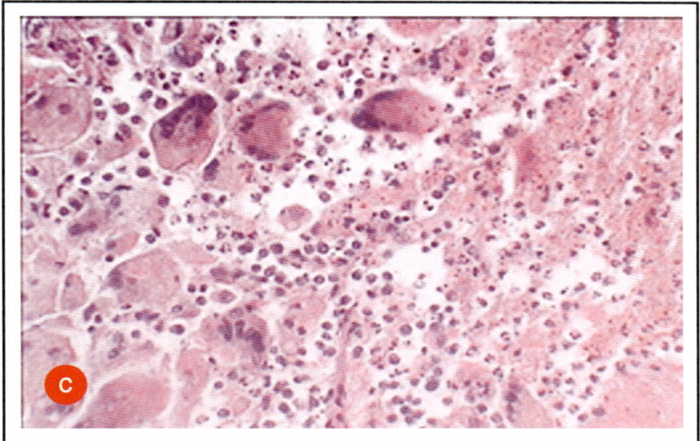

Figure 19: (a)Tuberculous nodule (arrow) in the intestine of python (*M.molurus*). Also note *Ophidascaris ajgaris* (b) Photomicrographs of (a) showing typical granuloma with large number of giant cells around necrotic area H&E,x10. (c) A well developed tubercle with numerous Langhan's giant and epithelioid cells.H&E,x 400.

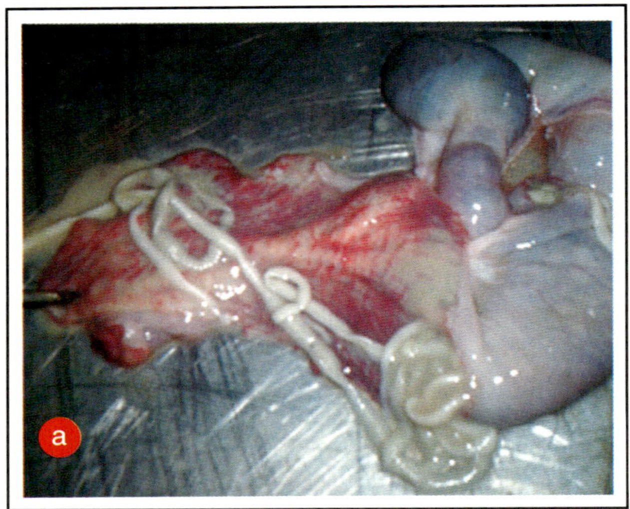

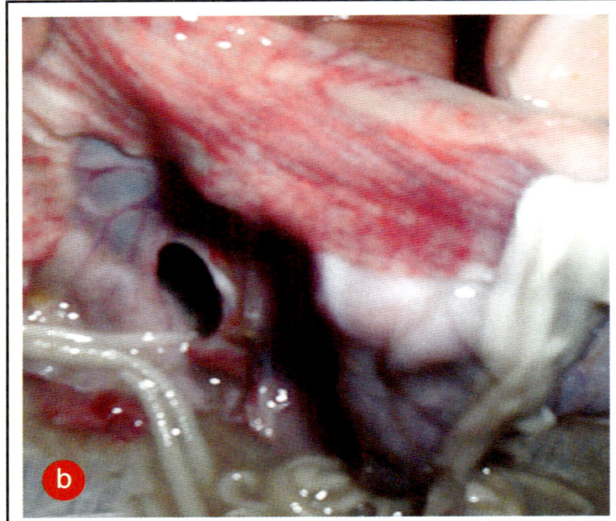

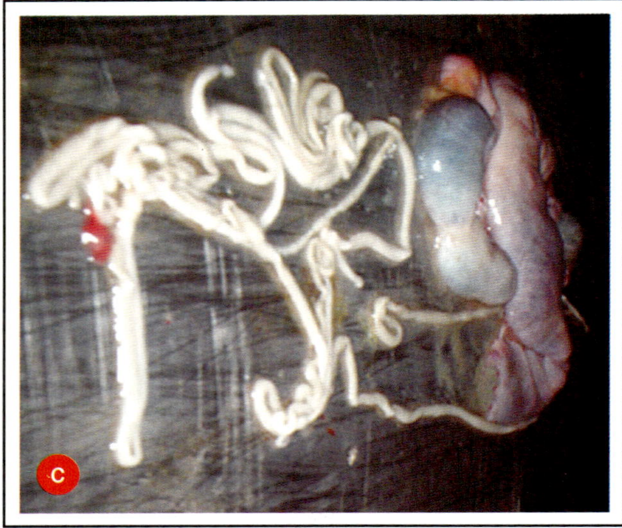

Figure 20: Photographs showing: (a,b) Congestion of intestine infected with tape worms encountered in monitor lizard. (c) Tape worms (Courtesy: Suryawanshi, D.S.).

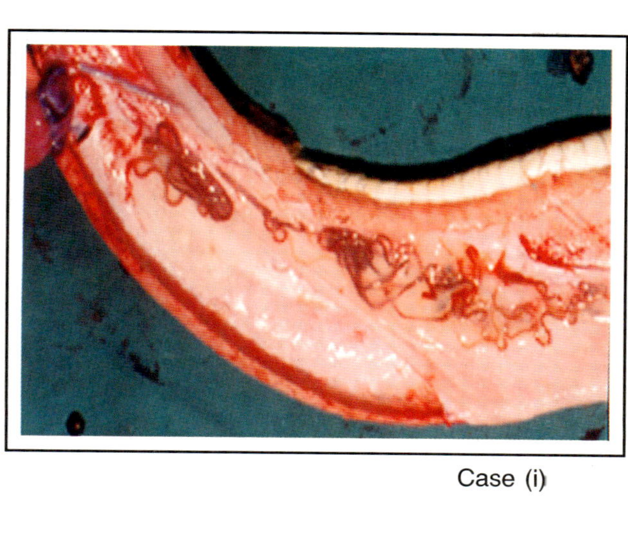

Case (i)

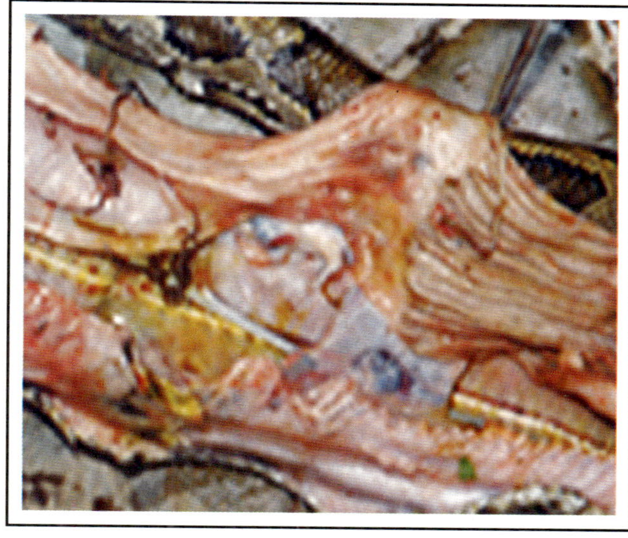

Case (ii)

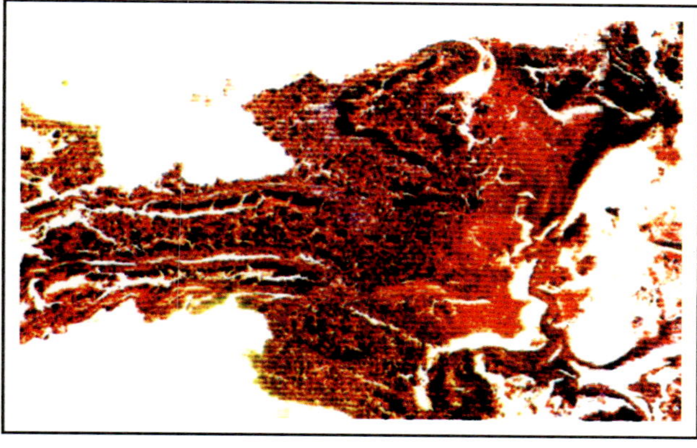

Case (iii)a

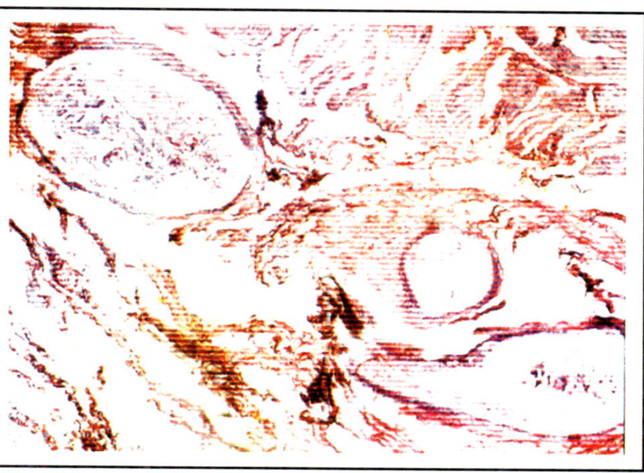

Case (iii)b

Figure 21 Case (i) : Masses of round worms- *Ophidascaris ajgaris* in the stomach of snake (Courtesy: Suryawanshi, D.S). Case (ii). *Ophidascaris ajgaris* deeply embedded in the lining and ulcers formation in the intestinal tract of python (*P. molurus*) died in captivity. Case (iii) Photomicrographs (a & b) of intestine showing degeneration and desquamation of the epithelium and marked cellular infiltration into lamina propria of python (*P. molurus*) (b) Cross section of parasite. (Courtesy: Mohapatra, H.K.).

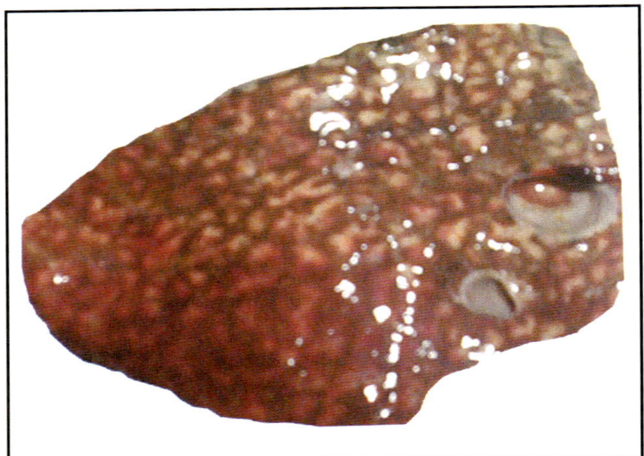

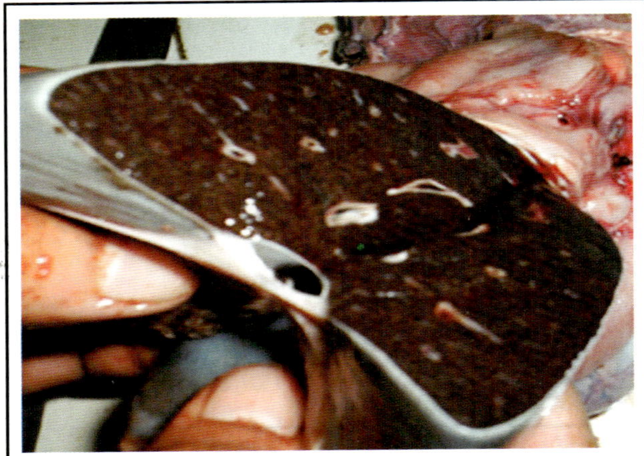

Figure 25 : Photographs (a,b) showing nutmeg appearance of liver encountered in tortoise and crocodile. (Courtesy: Suryawanshi, D.S.).

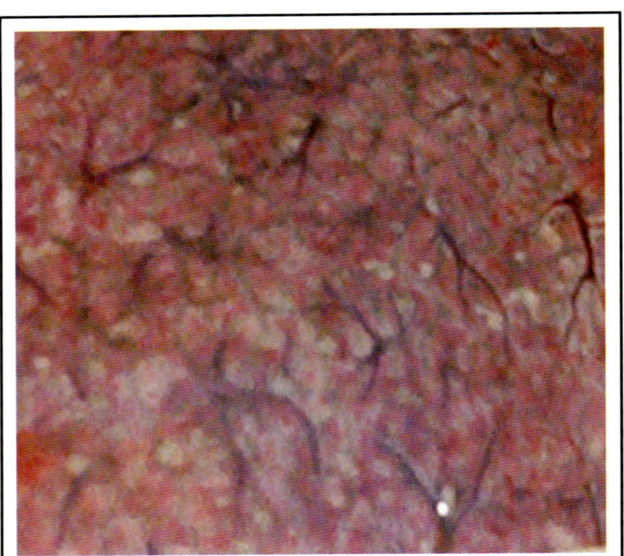

Figure 26 : Photograph showing necrotic foci in liver of tortoise (Courtesy: Suryawanshi, D.S.).

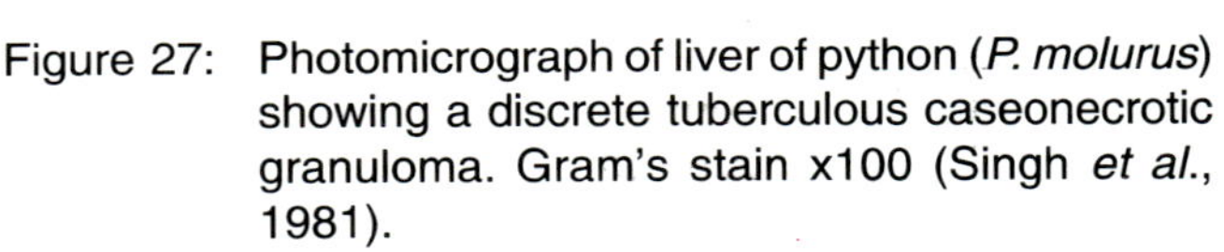

Figure 27: Photomicrograph of liver of python (*P. molurus*) showing a discrete tuberculous caseonecrotic granuloma. Gram's stain x100 (Singh *et al.*, 1981).

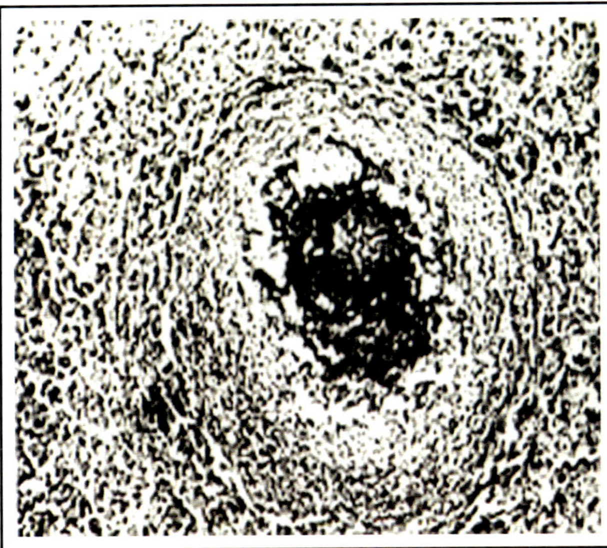

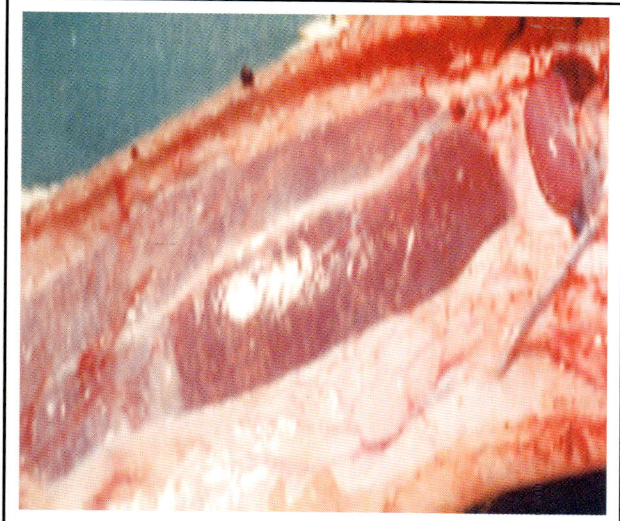

Figure 28: Photograph showing necrotic splenitis in snake related to *Salmonella* infection (Courtesy: Suryawanshi, D.S.).

Urinary System

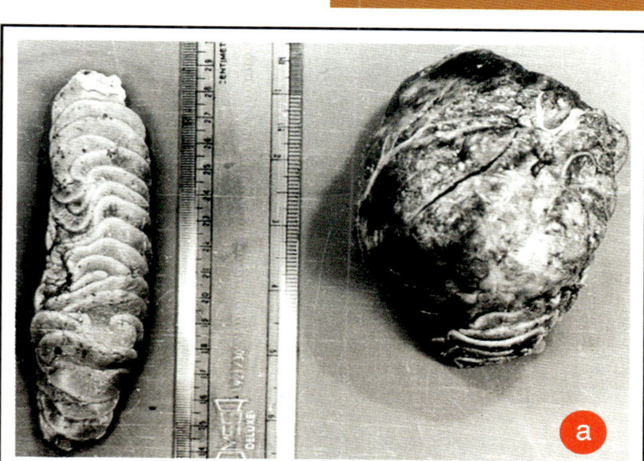

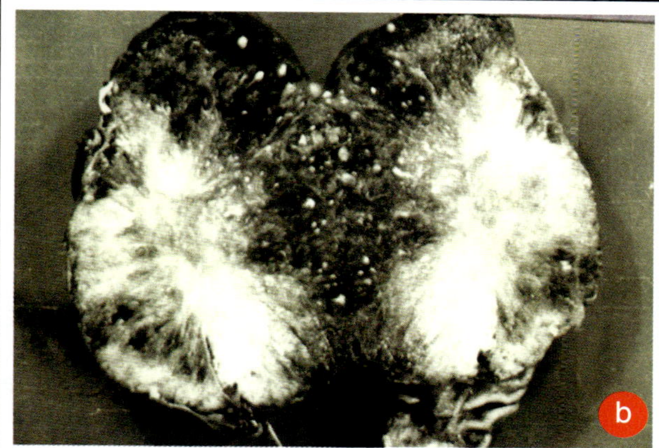

Figure 29: (a) Photograph showing right normal kidney and left kidney enveloped by tumourous growth in Python. (b) Section of abnormal growth of left kidney (c) Photomicrograph of renal tissue and cancerous growth in alveolar connective tissue of (b).H & E. x 52. (d) Formation of cell nest- Typical squamous cell carcinoma. H.& E, x 155.

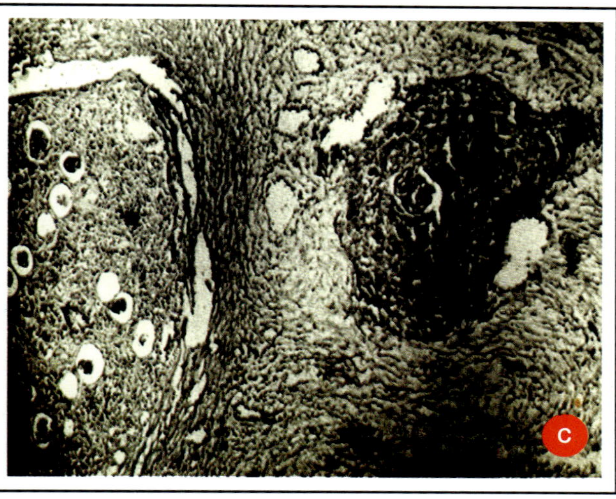

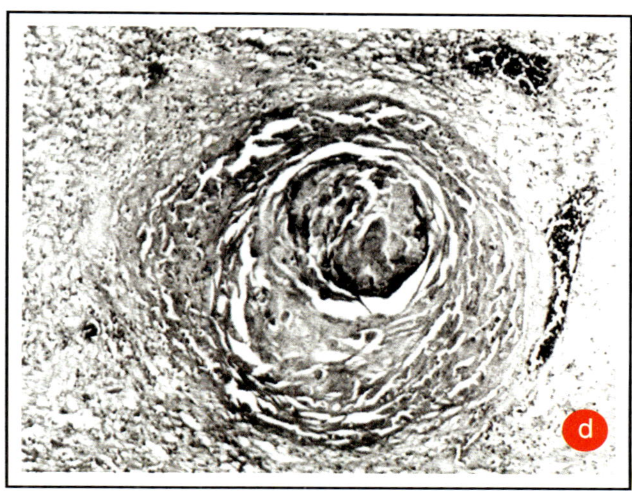

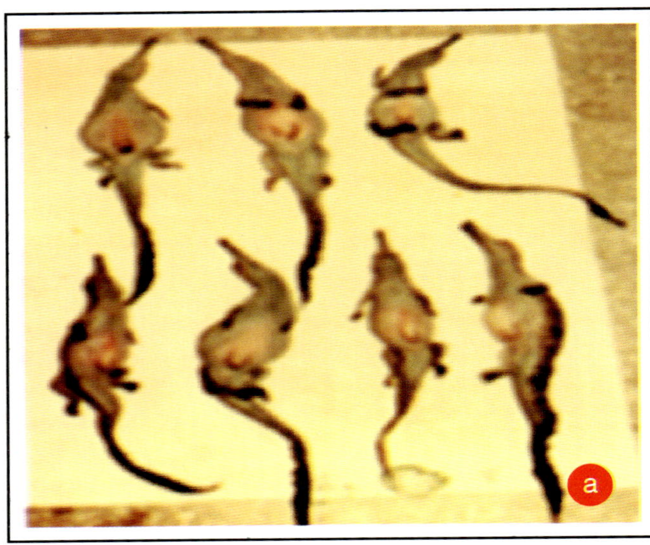

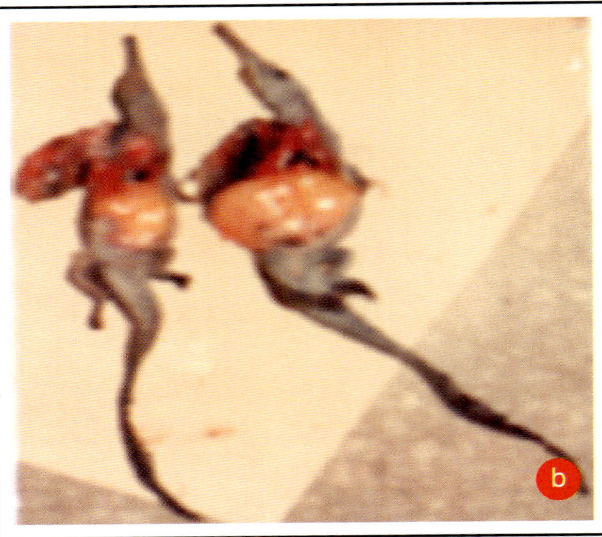

Figure 30: Photographs (a, b) showing unabsorbed yolk in the die offs of gharial (*Gavialis gangeticus*) hatchlings. Condition could be incubation under unfavourable environmental situations.

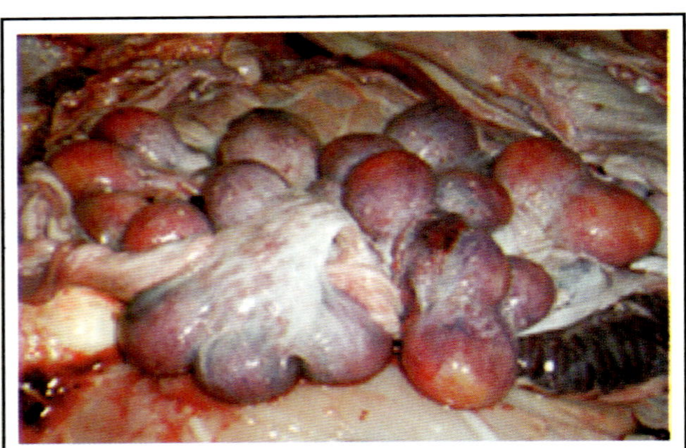

Figure 31: Photograph showing oophoritis in tortoise (Courtesy: Suryawanshi, D.S.)

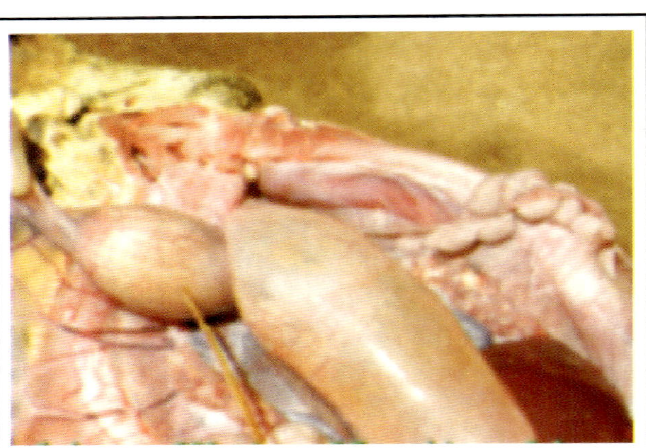

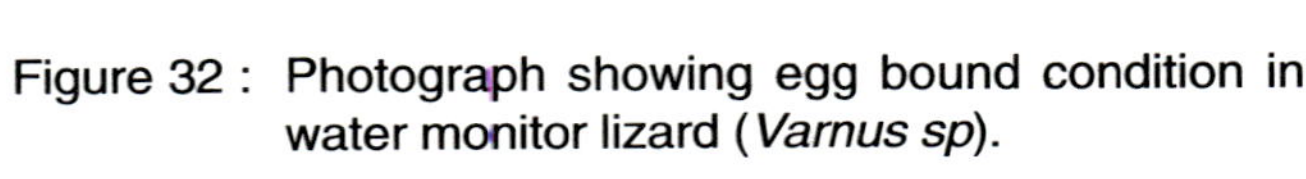

Figure 32 : Photograph showing egg bound condition in water monitor lizard (*Varnus sp*).

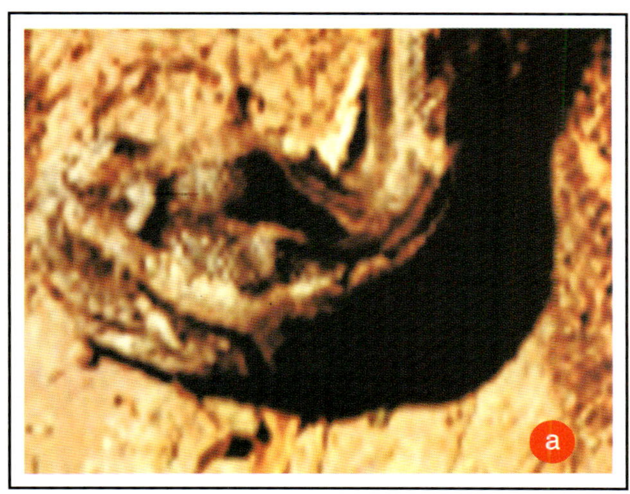

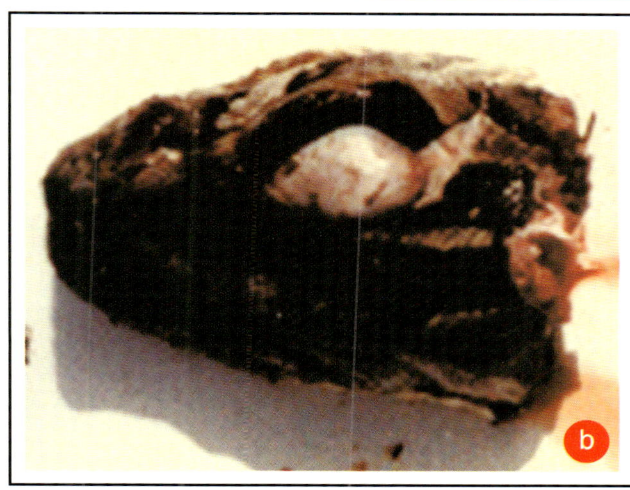

Figure 33: (a)During necropsy of an adult python (*P. molurus*) died in captivity a protuberance at its dorsal of the head was observed. (b) Dissection of the same showed a large elliptical white stone like mass weighing about 7 g partially embedded in the brain substance.

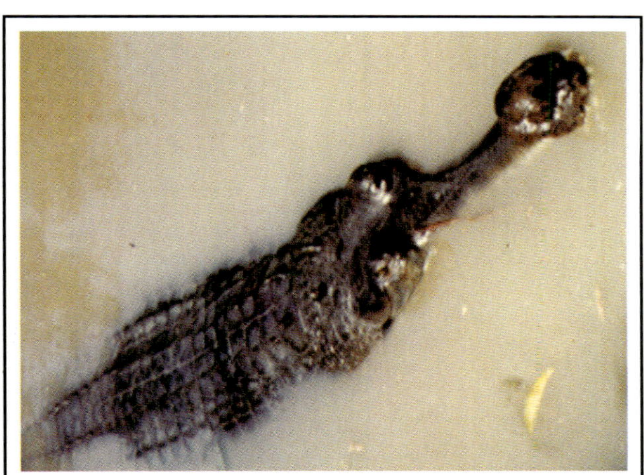

Figure 34: Photograph showing a congenitally blind gharial (*Gavialis gangeticus*) swimming in water pond at Crocodile Breeding Centre, Kukrail, Lucknow (U.P).

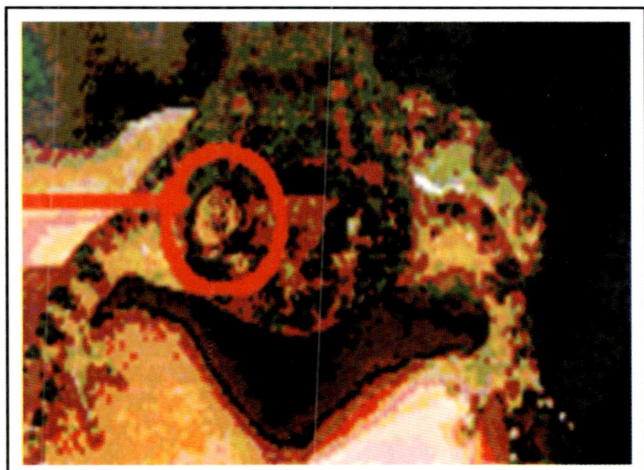

Figure 35: Photograph showing deformed eye in sacred pond night frog (*Nyctibatrachus sanctipalustris*). Photo credit Kudremukh Wildlife Division (Karthikeyan Vasudevan *et al.*, 2007).

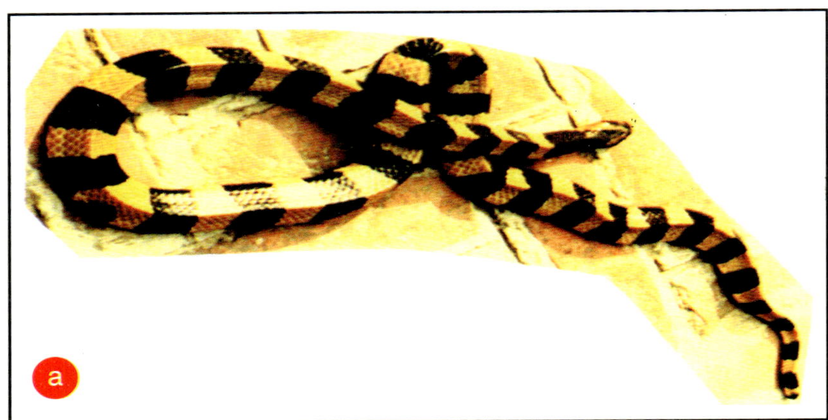

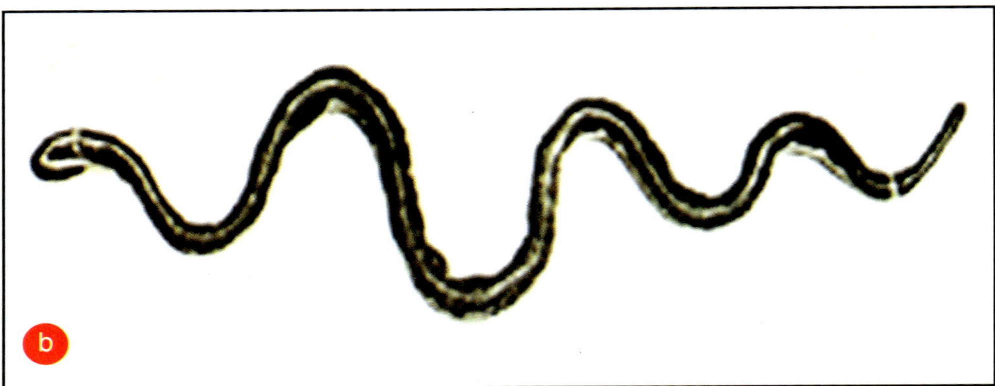

Figure 36: Photographs of Banded Krait (*B. fasciatus*) of: (a) Normal coloration (b) Aberrant coloration- juvenile specimen. (Whitaker, 1968).

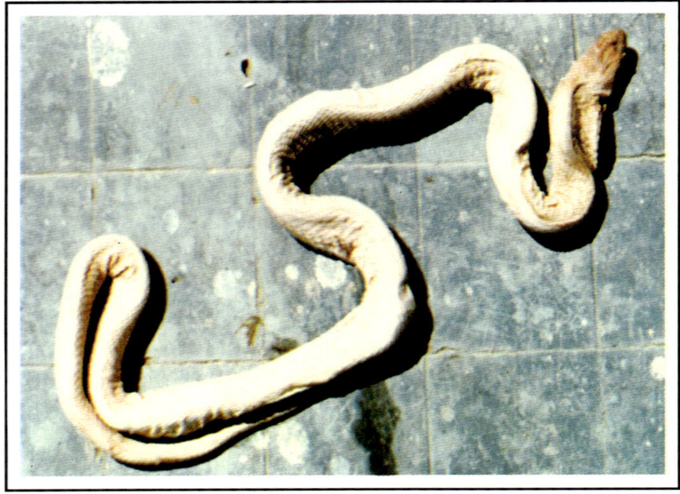

Figure 37: Photograph of carcass of white colour (eye colour pinkish) cobra (*Naja naja*) at Z.G., Lucknow,Uttar Pradesh. (Courtesy: Late Dr Das, R.K., Zoo Deputy Director).

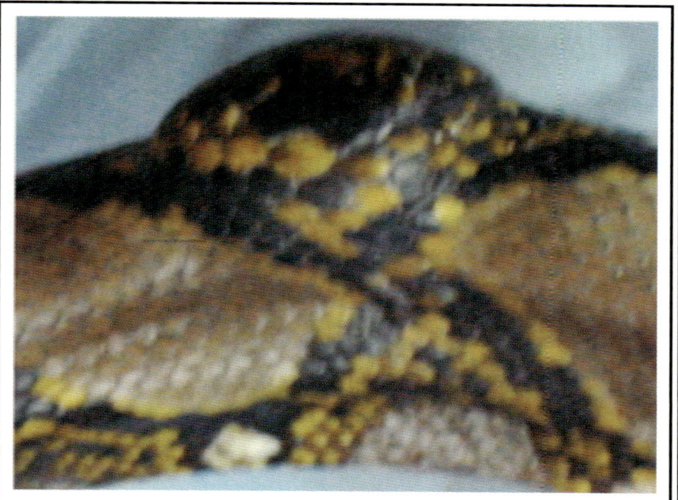
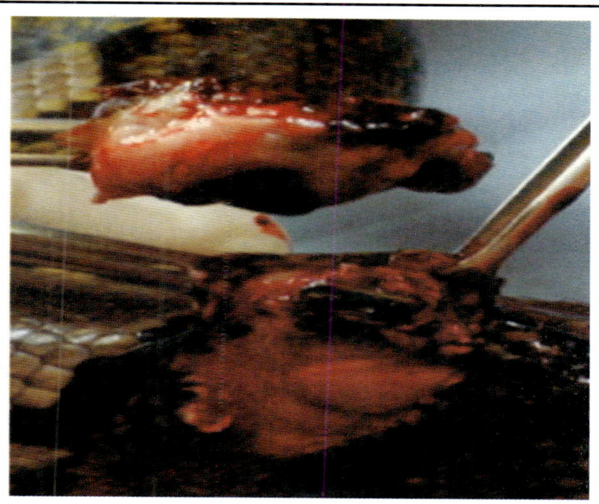

Figure 38: Cutaneous abscesses in reticulated python (*Python reticulatus*) being surgically operated at Zoological Park, Chennai (Pathan Nasrulla Khan *et al.*, 2005).

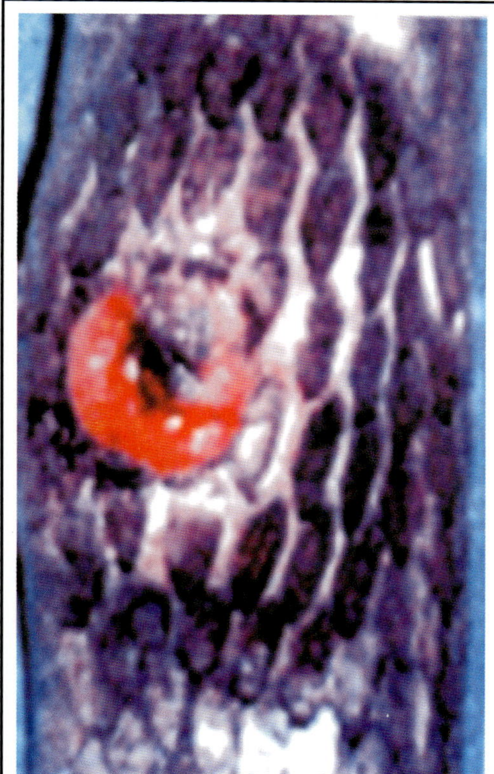

Figure 39: Photograph showing a large deep ulcer in the body musculature in king cobra (*Ophiophagus hannah*) in captivity. (Courtesy: Aiyasami, S.S).

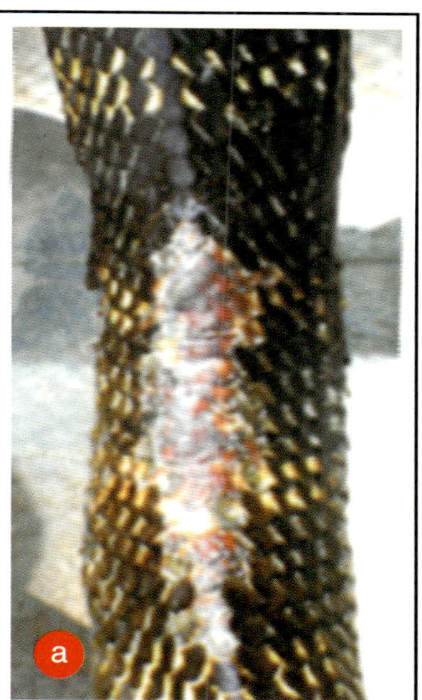

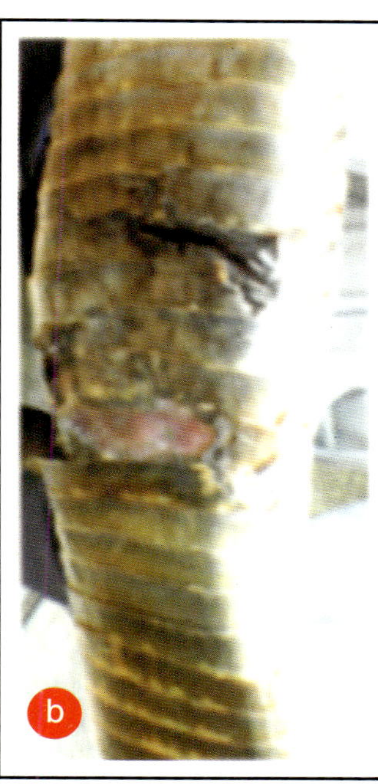

Figure 40: Photographs showing traumatized king cobras (*Ophiophagus hannah*) under treatment in captivity (a,b): Wounds on dorsal and ventral aspects of the body of the snake belonging to Z.G,Mysore,Karnataka.

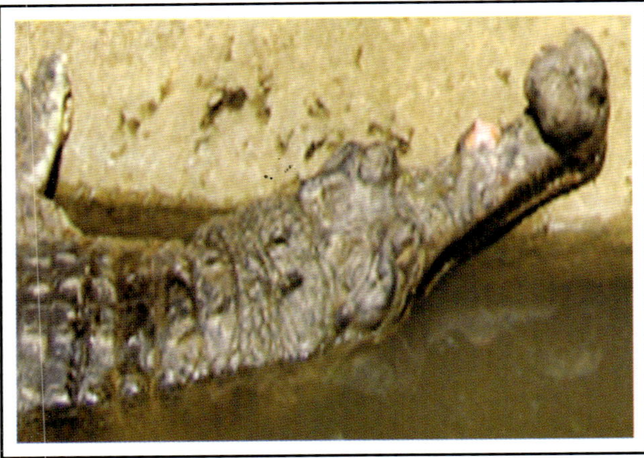

Figure 41: Photograph showing an abscess nearly middle of the upper jaw in young gharial (*Gavialis gangeticus*) in Zoological Park, Patna (Bihar).

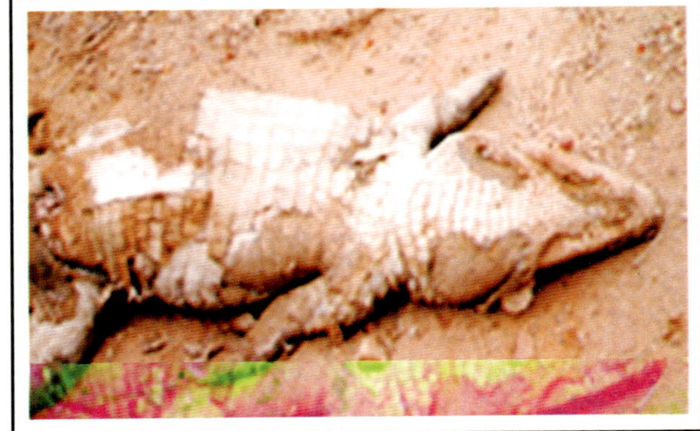

Figure 42: Photograph showing sloughing of the skin in muggar (*Crocodylus palustris*) suspected for bacterial infection (Courtesy: Dept. of Wildlife Science, C.V.Sc, Chennai. T.N.).

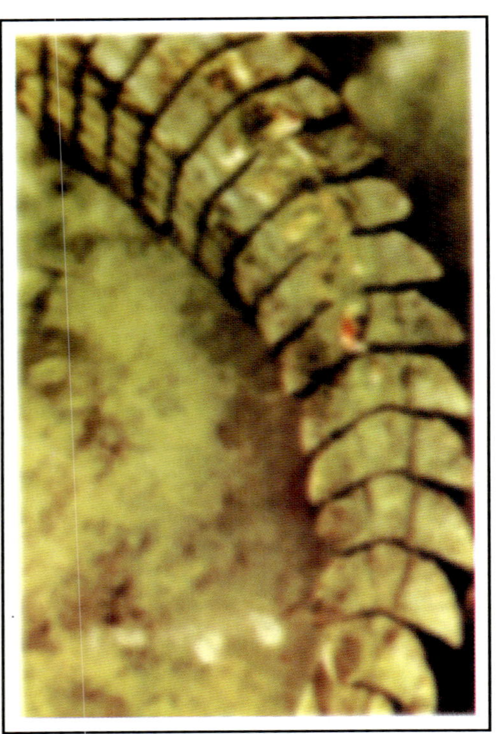

Figure 43: *Aeromonas hydrophila* dermatitis in an adult gharial (*G gangeticus*).

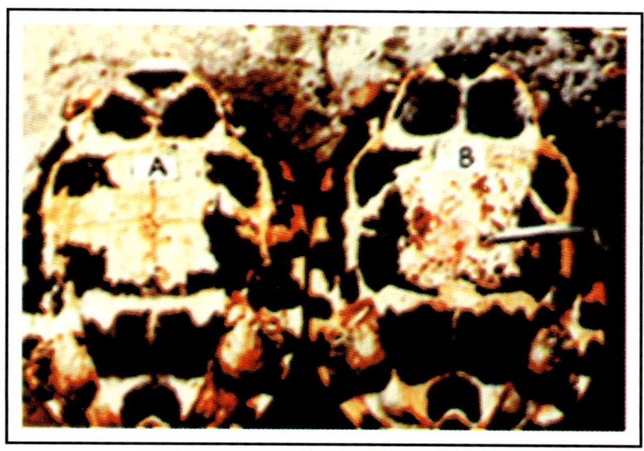

Case (i)

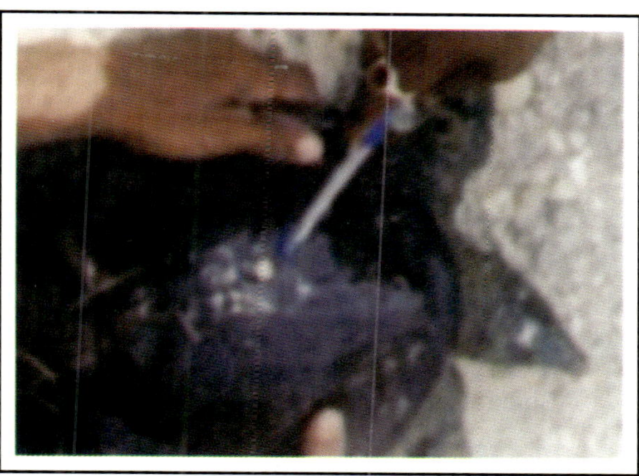

Case (ii)

Figure 44: Case (i) Spotted black terrapin (*Eochemys hamilton*) from wild: (a) Normal (b) Showing excoriation of plastron associated with *Proteus* sp. infection. Case (ii) Necrotic lesions in carapace of wild tortoise related to *Klebsiella* sp. (Courtesy: Pralay Mandal).

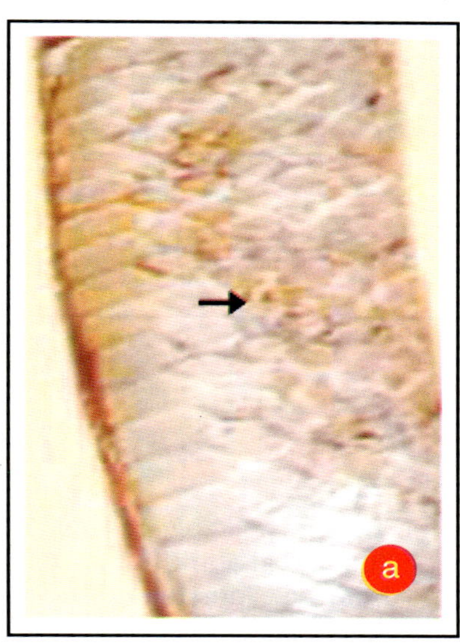

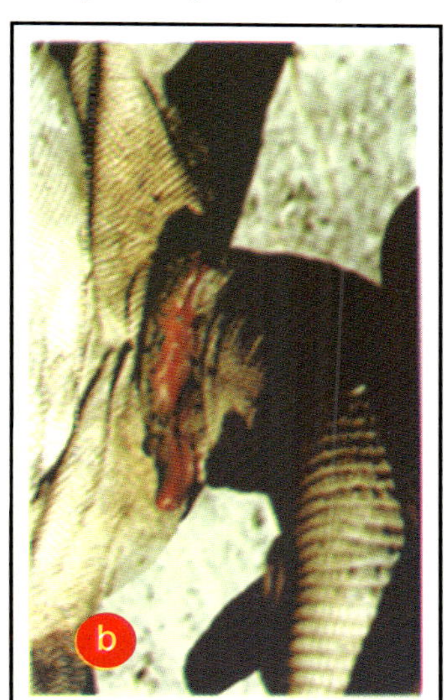

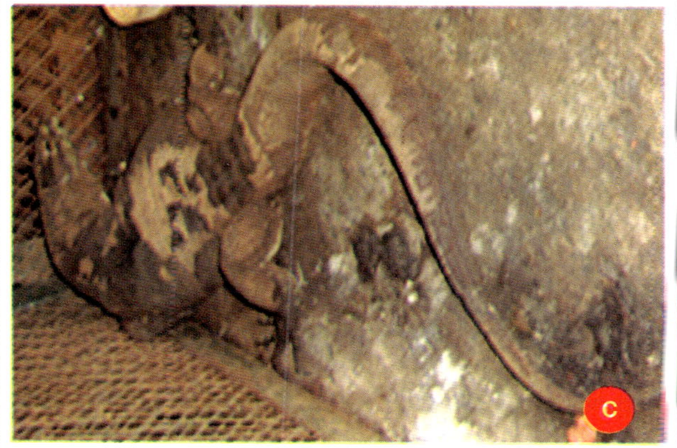

Figure 45: (a) Photograph showing skin infection in python (*Python molurus*) with *Aponomma gerviasi* ticks. (Courtesy: Abdul Basith, S.). (b) Skin lesions in monitor lizard (*Varnus bengalensis*) infested with tick at clocal region (Courtesy: Gupta, B.K.) (c) Another case of monitor lizard (*V. bengalensis*) showing skin lesion (dermatitis) due to tick infestation.

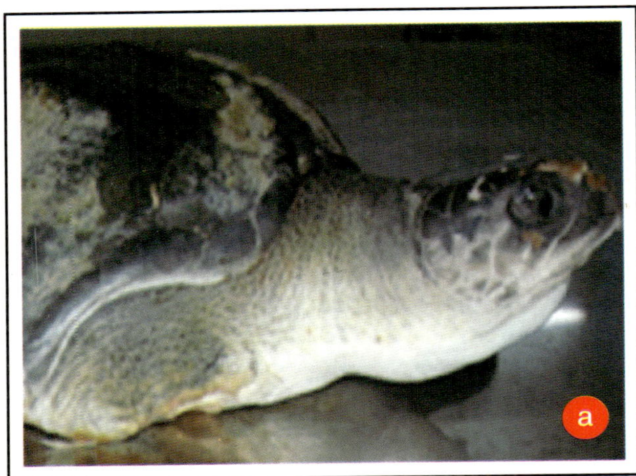

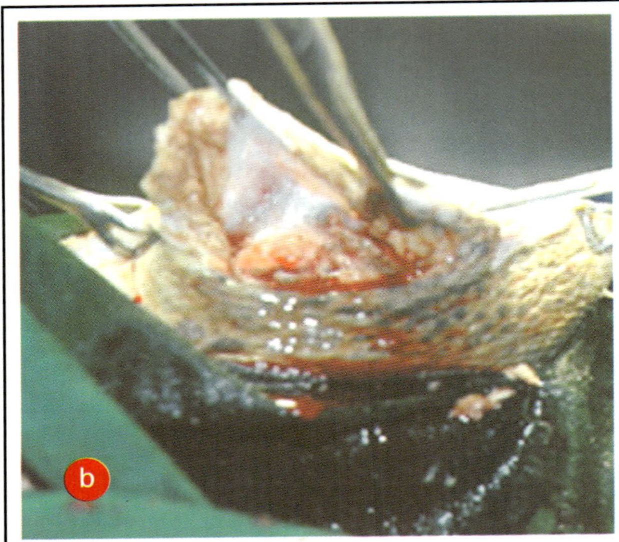

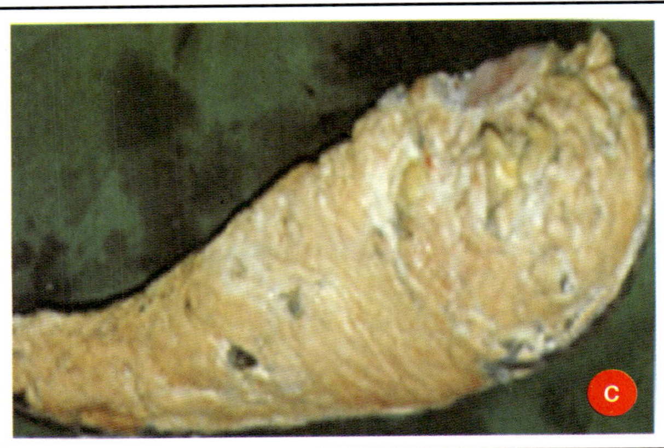

Figure 49: (a) Olive Ridley turtle (*Lepidochelys olivacea*) with its right fore flipper injured. (b, c) Photographs of extirpated flipper. (Source: Pralhad Shankar Chaudhary & Vipin Vinayk Rao, 26-7-2007 with Courtesy of Darshan Desai).

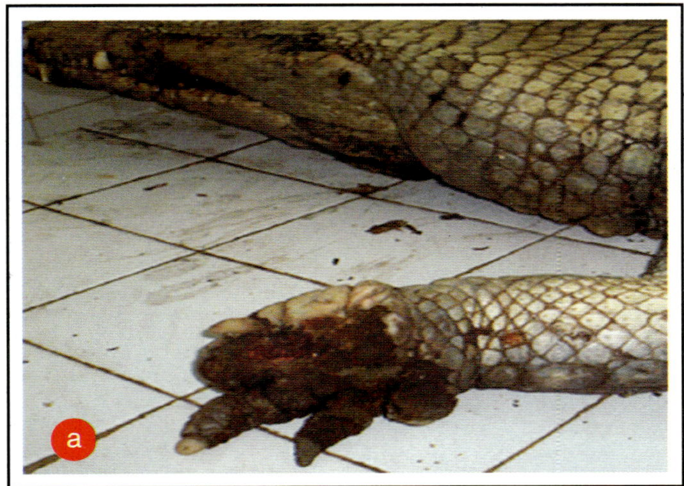

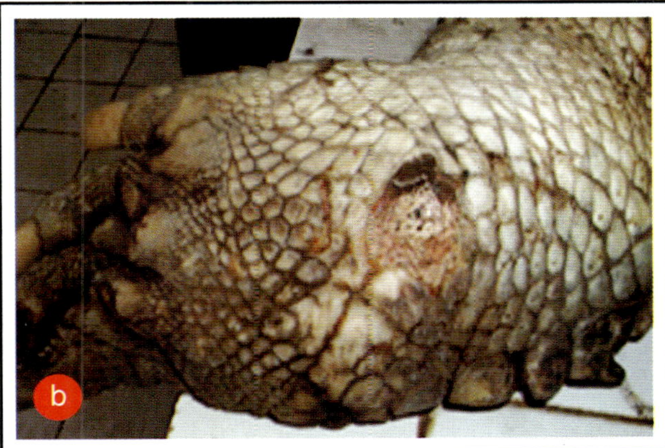

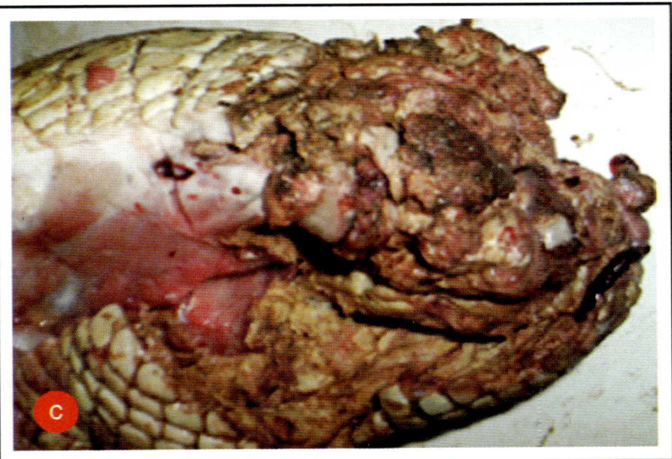

Figure 50: Photograph showing foot pad injury in captive crocodile. (a) Injury to foot pad of the left fore leg. (b) A large suppurative wound in the foot pad. (c)Necrosed claws and foot pad. (Courtesy: Suryawanshi, D.S.).

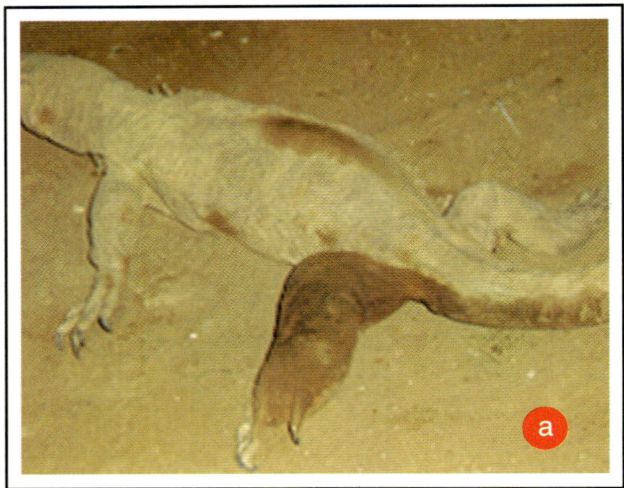

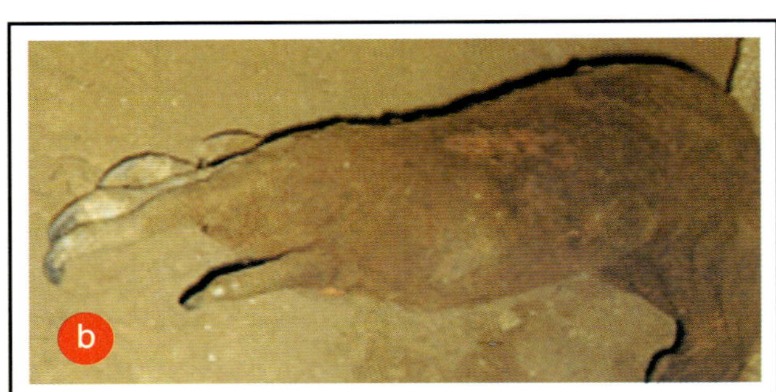

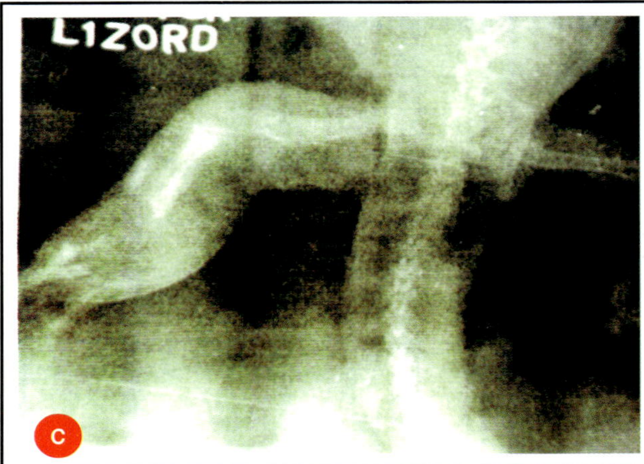

Figure 51: Photographs of monitor lizard (a, b) showing left hind leg swollen due to fracture. (c) Radiograph of (a) showing disjoint femur and tibia at articulation and also fracture in the shaft of tibia.

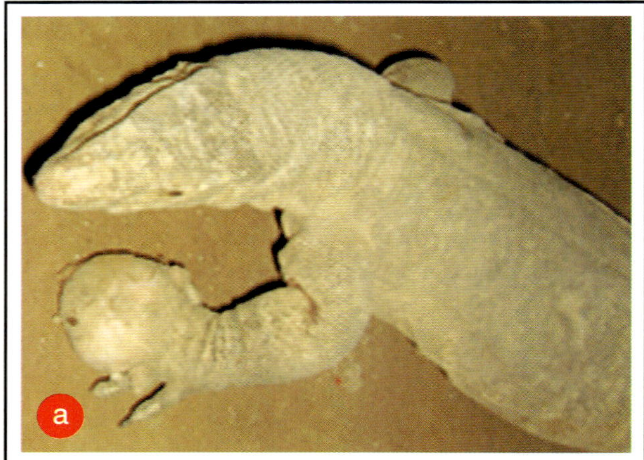

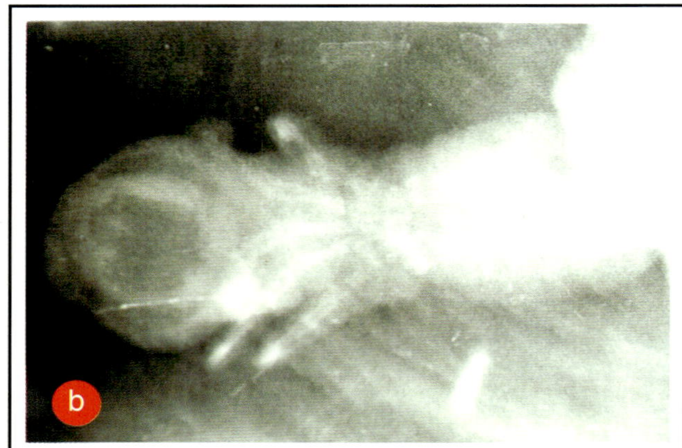

Figure 52: Abscessation in monitor lizards (*V. bengalensis*) belonging to National Zoological Park. Photograph showing tenis ball size abscess in left fore paw (b) Radiograph of (a) showing suppurative lesions involving digits-palmar view.

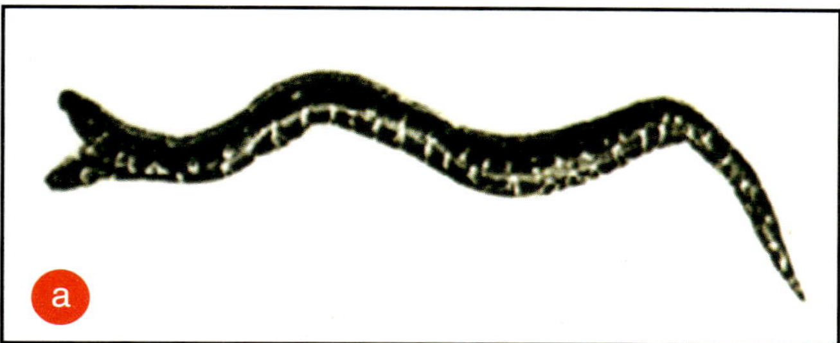

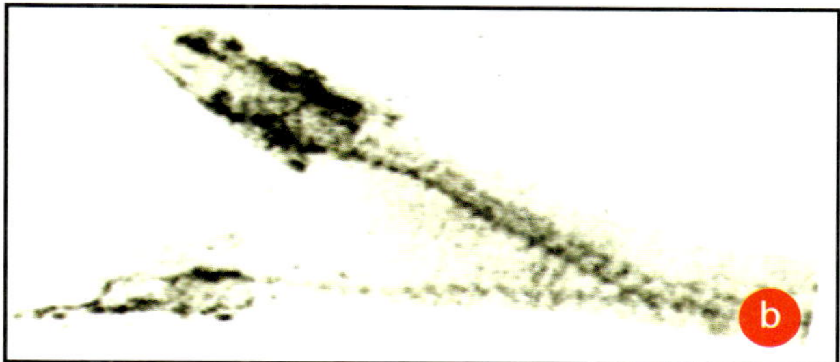

Figure 53: (a) Photograph showing two headed earth snake (*Eryx conicus*). (b) Radiograph of the anterior portion of (a)showing two separate skulls and portions of the vertebral column (Desai,1983).

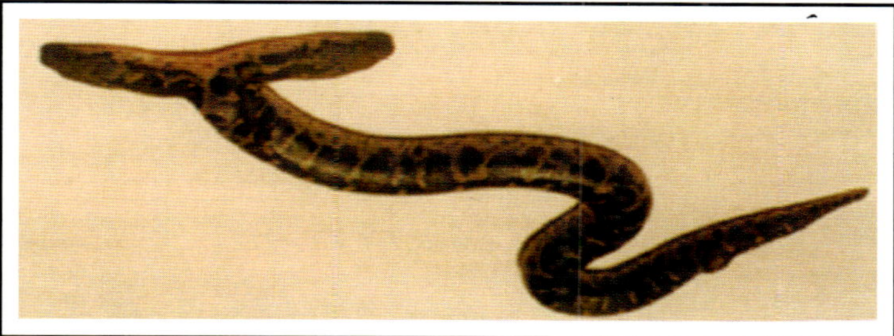

Figure 54: Photograph showing two headed sand boa (*Eryx johnii*). Courtesy: Pune Snake Park.

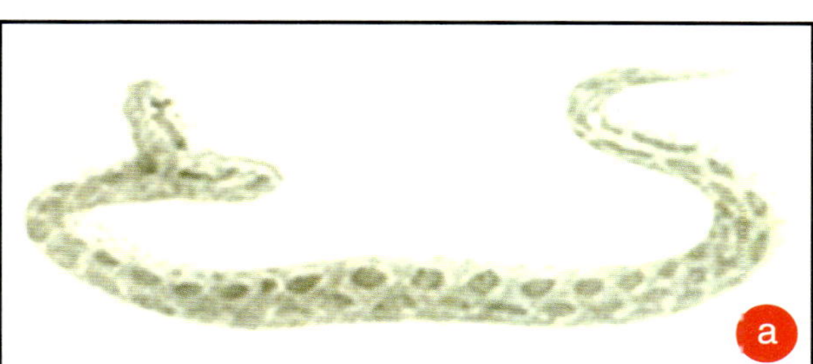

Figure 55: Double headed Russell's viper (*Viper ruselli*). (a) Mitra (1994) . (b) Courtesy Mishra,K.K.

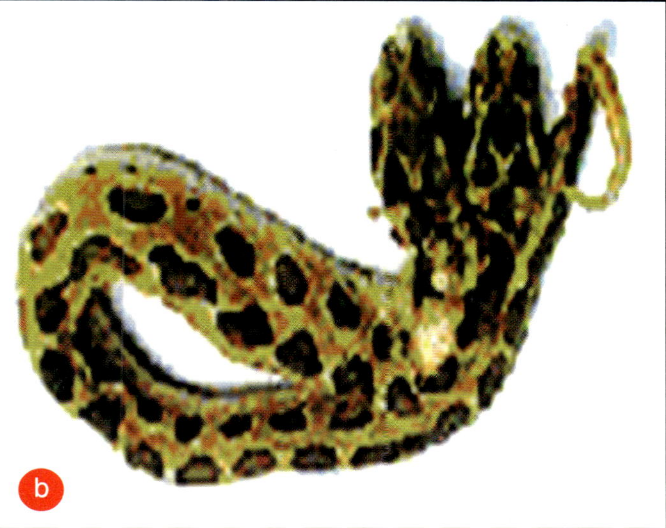

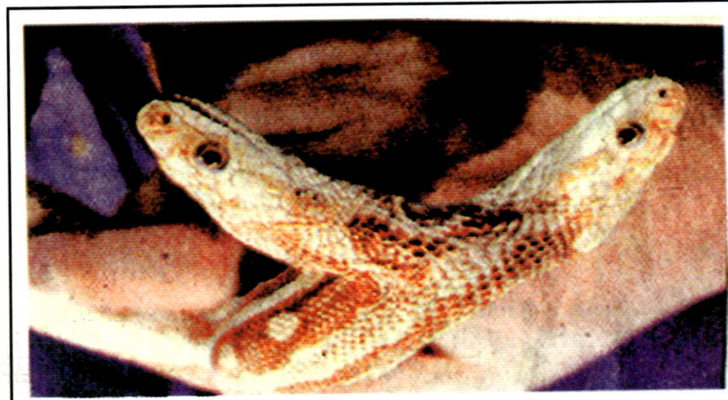

Figure 56: Double headed snake an exotic sp. AmarUjala News paper (Bareilly ed.) dated 4.1.06

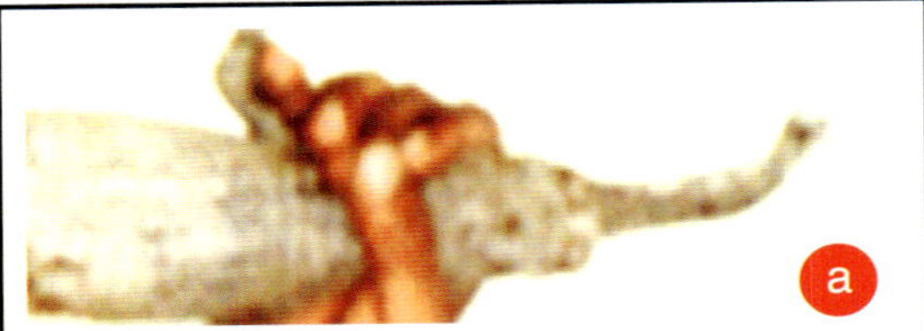

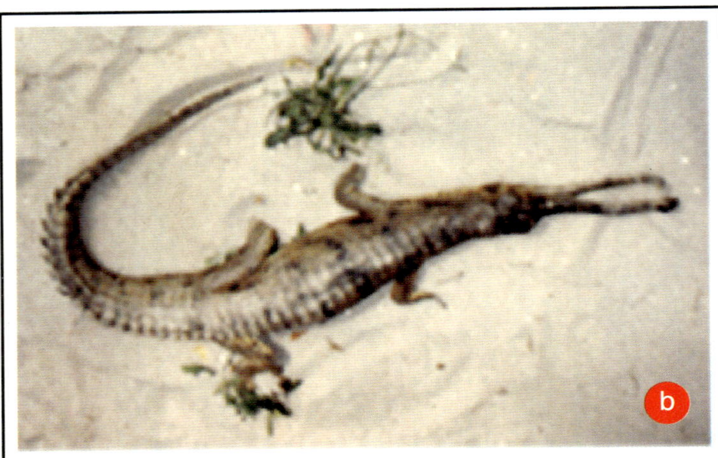

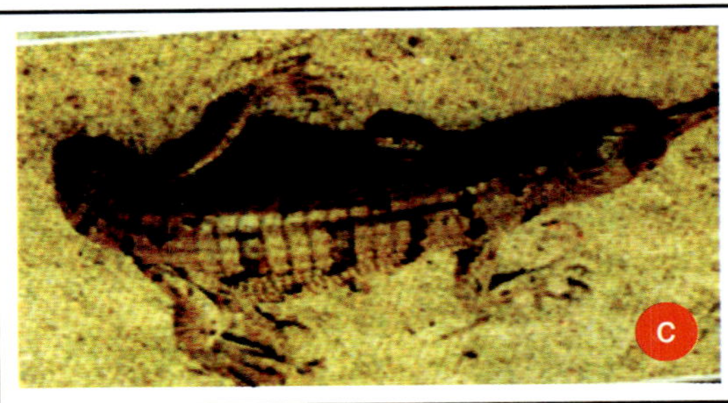

Figure 57: Photographs showing congenitally deformities in gharial hatchlings (*G. gangeticus*) at Crocodile Breeding Centre,Kukrail, Lucknow (U.P). (a,b) upper and lower jaws bent (c) Stump tailed

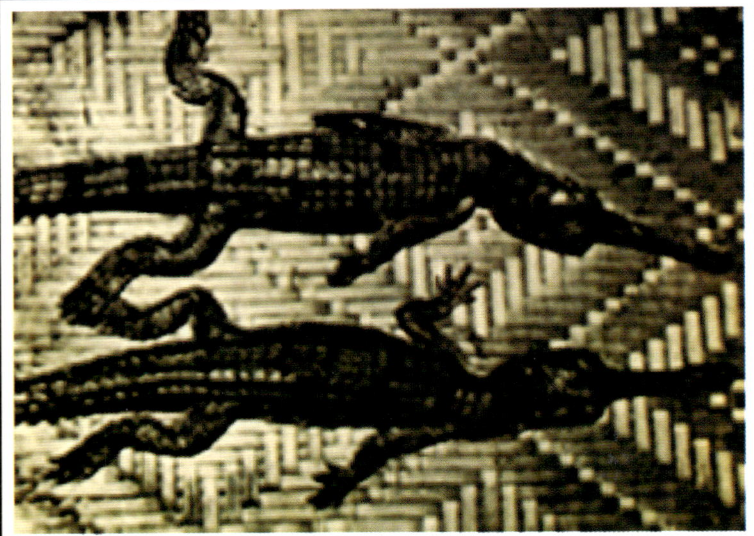

Figure 58: Bent neck condition in young gharial hatchlings (Adopted from: Elliot Jacobson Field Document No 11 FAO/India74/046)

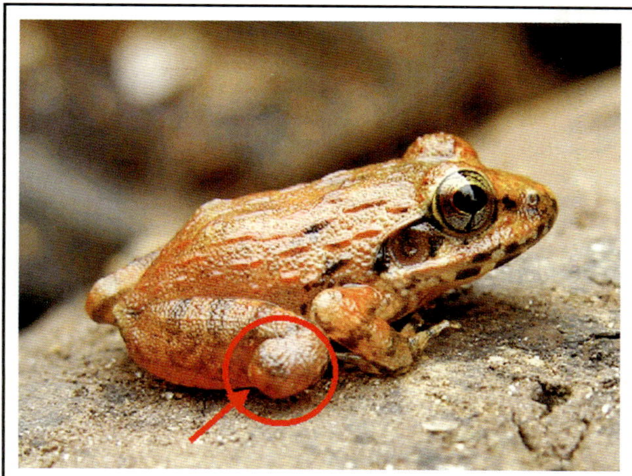

Figure 59: Right hind limb missing (Amelia) in short legged litter frog (*Indirana brachytarsus*). Photo credit Kudremukh Wildlife Division. (Karthikeyan Vasudevan *et al.*, 2007).

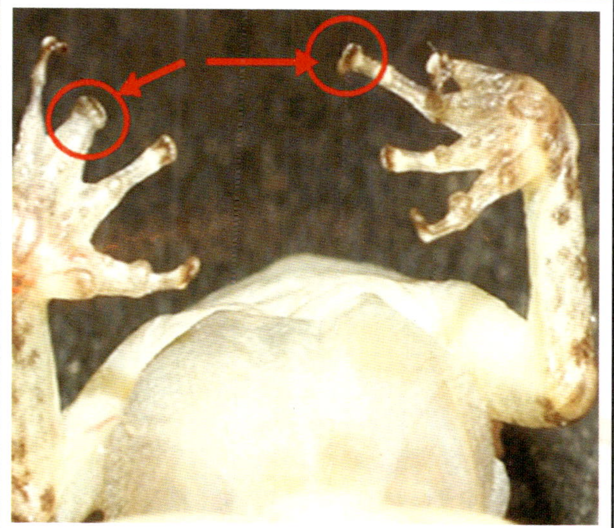

Figure 60: Brachydactyly in short legged litter frog (*Indirana brachytarsus*). Note shortened toes though number of metatarsals bones were normal but number of phalanges was found to be reduced. Photo credit Varun Torsekar. (Karthikeyan Vasudevan *et al.*, 2007).

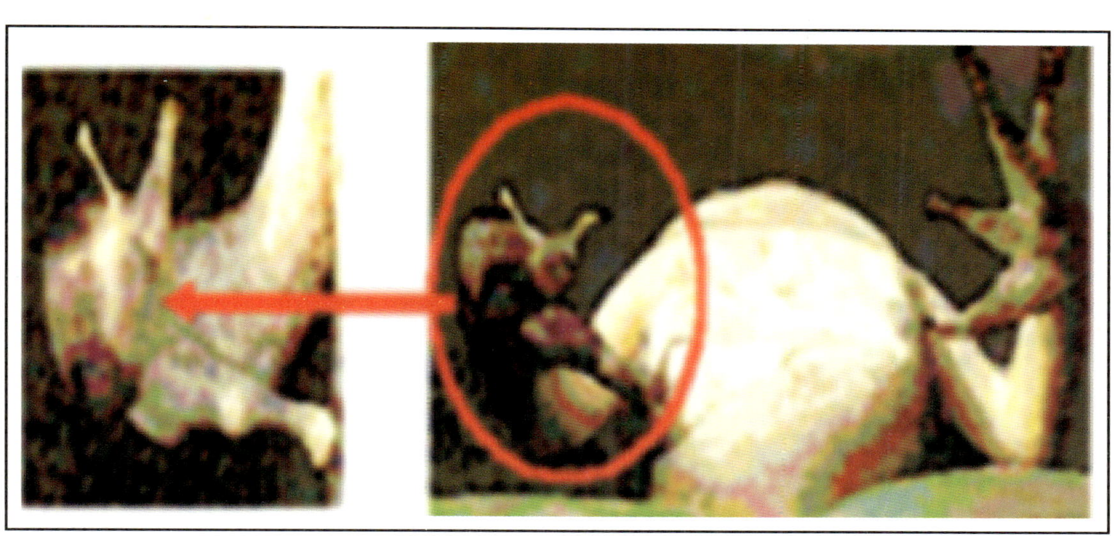

Figure 61: Ectrodactyly (missing of digits including metatarsals) in short legged litter frog (*Indirana brachytarsus*). Photo credit Varun Torsekar. (Karthikeyan Vasudevan *et al.*, 2007).

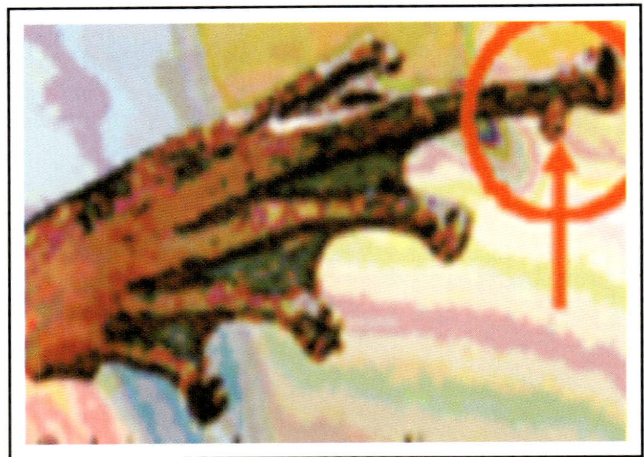

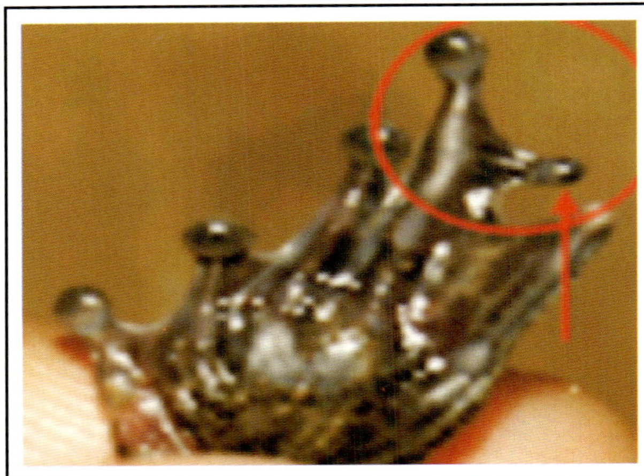

Figure 62: Photograph showing polydactyly in : (a) Bronzed frog (*Sylvirana temporalis*). (b) Karnataka night frog (*Nyctibatrachus hussaini*). Photo credit Kudremukh Divison. (Karthikeyan Vasudevan *et al.*, 2007).

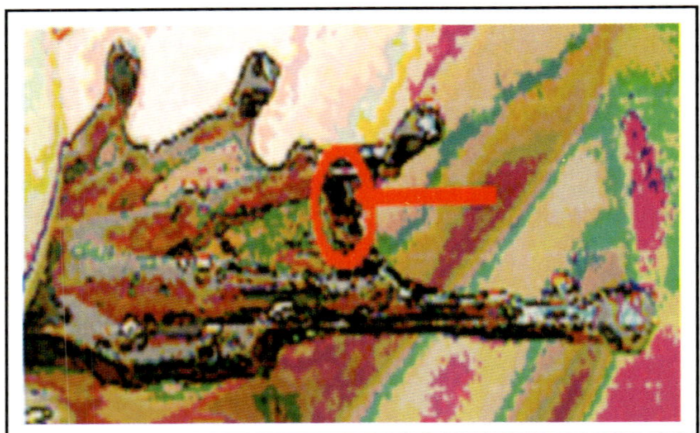

Figure 63: Photograph showing variation in number of phalangeal bones in bronzed frog (*Sylvirana temporalis*) belonged to Kudremukh Wildlife Div. (Karthikeyan Vasudevan *et al.*, 2007).

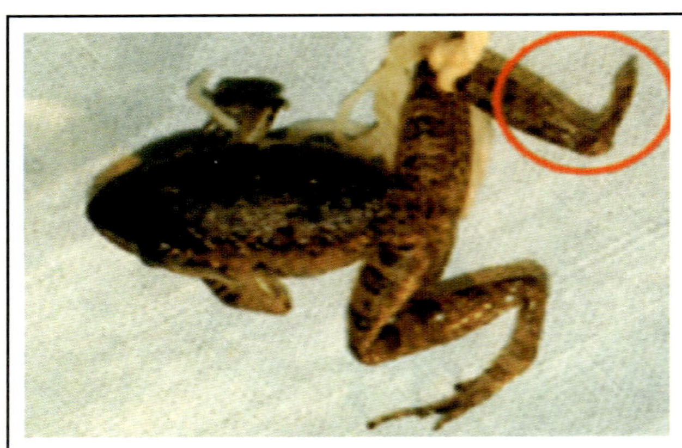

Figure 64: Ectromelia (Missing toes). Distinguished from brachydactyly, refers to a completely missing digit including the metatarsal bone and phalanges in short legged litter frog (*Indirana brachytarsus*). (Karthikeyan Vasudevan *et al.,* 2007).

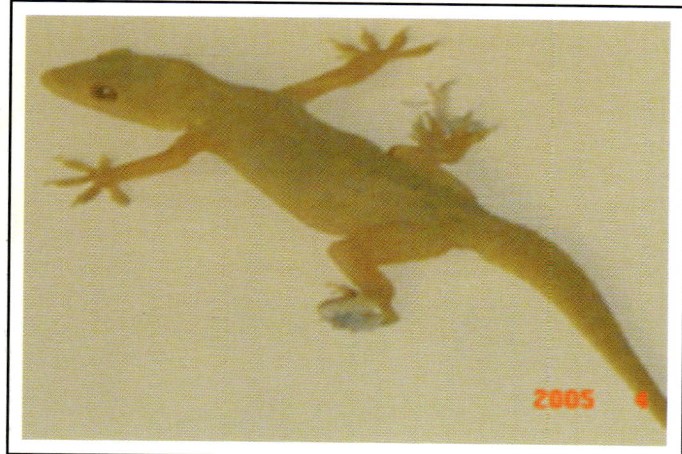

Figure 65: Common house wall lizard having defective digits of both hind limbs.

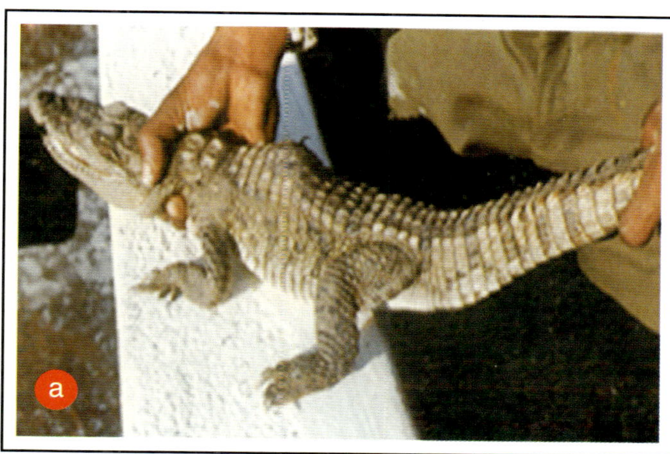

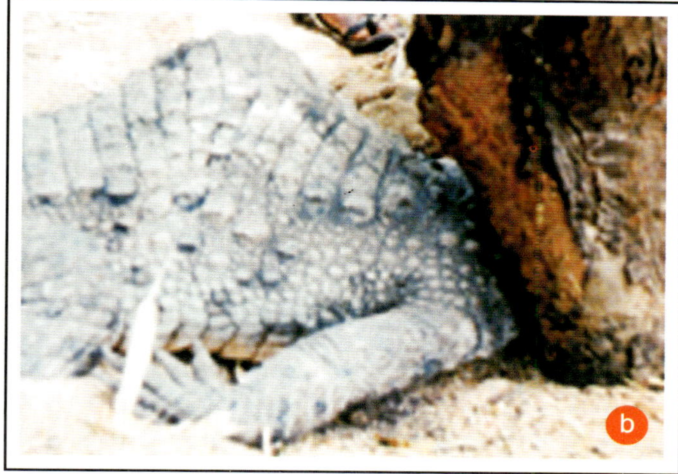

Figure 66: Photographs showing hunchback in muggers (*Crocodylus palustris*). (a) A subadult. (b) Another case. The condition is not uncommon in this species breeding in captivity.

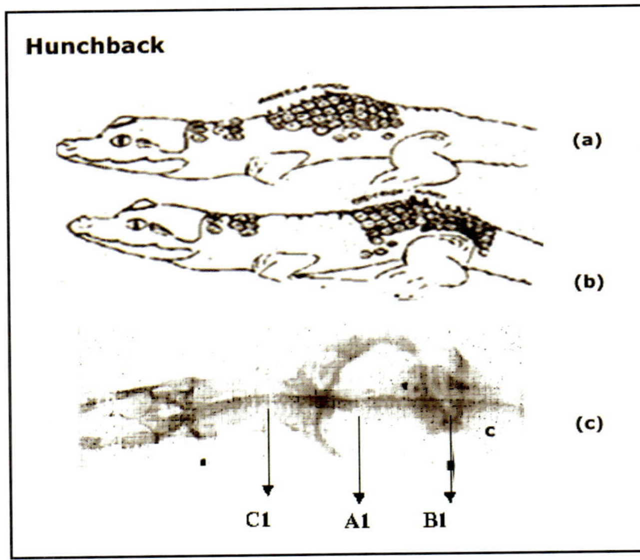

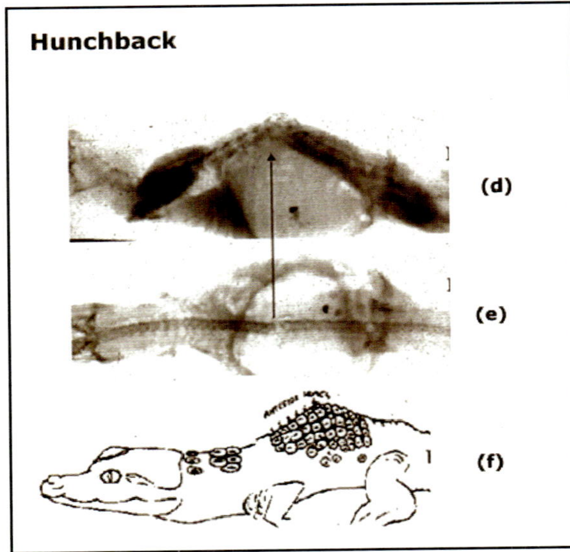

Figure 67: (a,b) Sketches showing the anterior and posterior areas of hunchback condition encountered in muggers. (c) Radiograph showing the potential areas of 8th, 20th and 27th vertebrae , in which de-ossification is marked prominantly. (d, e) Radiographs (lateral and dorsal views) showing vertex of the hunchback formation with de-ossification of vertebrae and their thining in mugger.Sketch (f) presents the thoracic area shown in radiographs. (Singh *et al.*, 2001).The condition is related to inadequate supply of calcium rich diet.

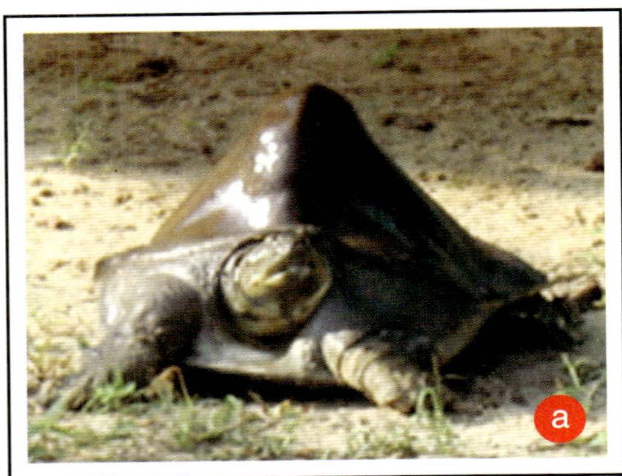

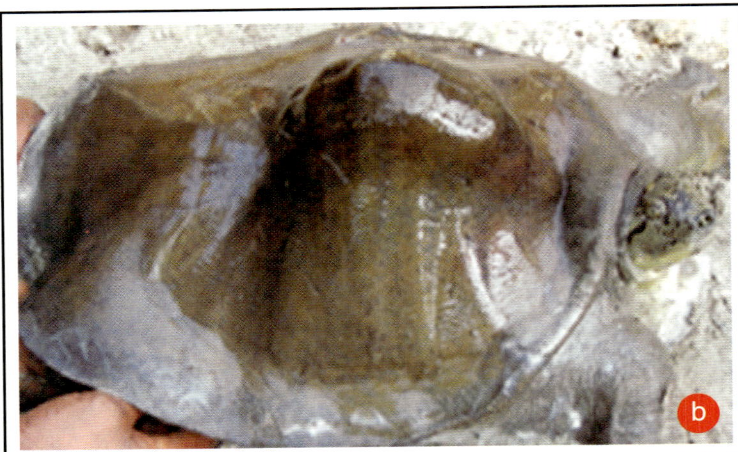

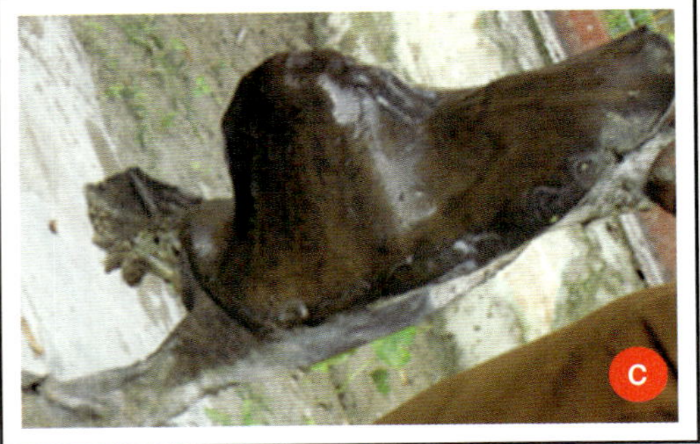

Figure 68 : Photographs (a, b and c from different angles) of adult tortoise (*Aspiderctes gangeticus*) having pyramid shaped hunchback condition due to defect in its vertebral column at Crocodile Rehabilitation Centre, Kukrail, Lucknow (U.P.).

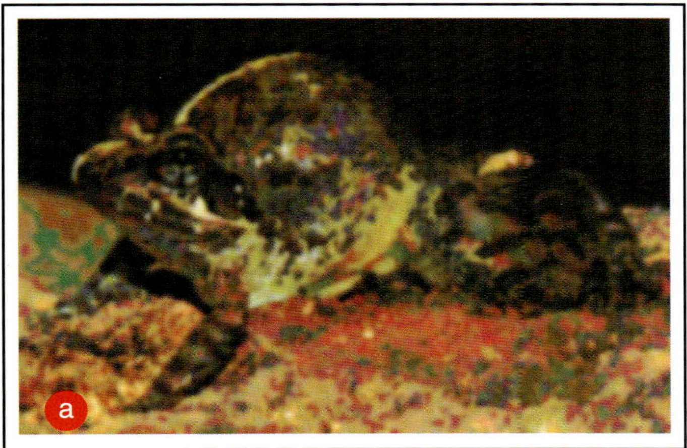

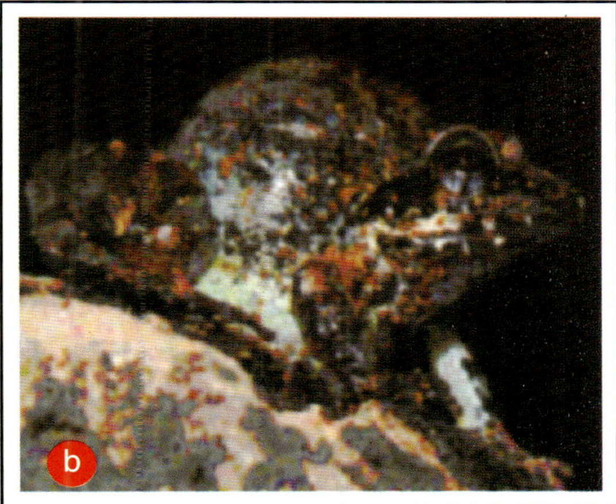

Figure 69 (a,b): Hunch back condition encountered in short legged litter frog (*Indirana brachytarsus*)- Two cases (Karthikeyan Vasudevan *et al*., 2007).

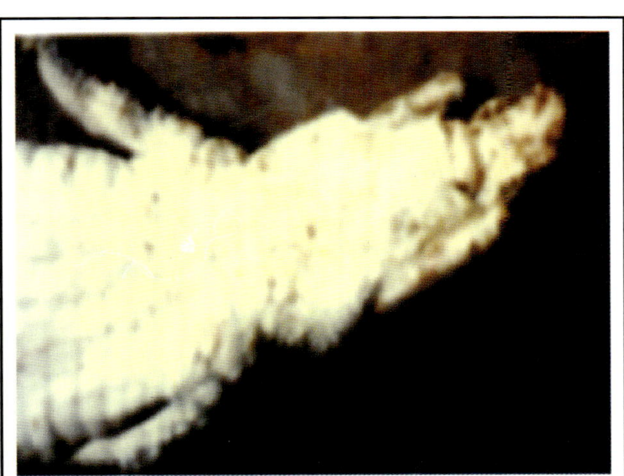

Figure 70: Fracture of the lower jaw of mugger (*Crocodylus palustris*)owing to infighting in captivity.

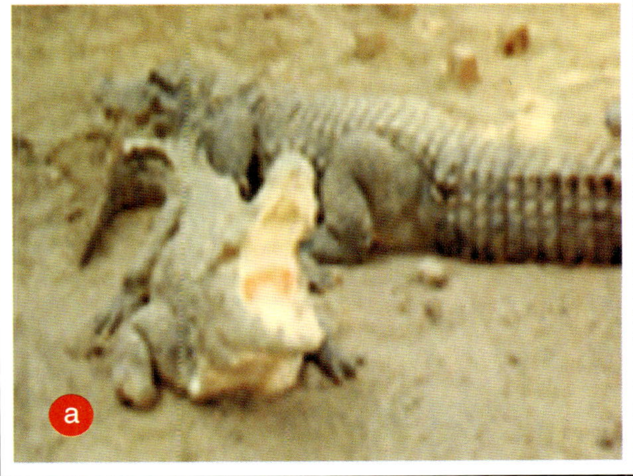

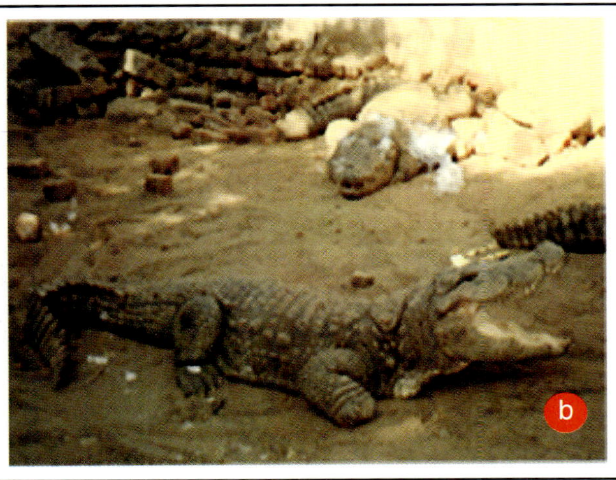

Figure 71: (a,b): Lower portion of the fore legs among muggers (*Crocodylus palustris*) chopped off as a result of infighting or cannibalism.

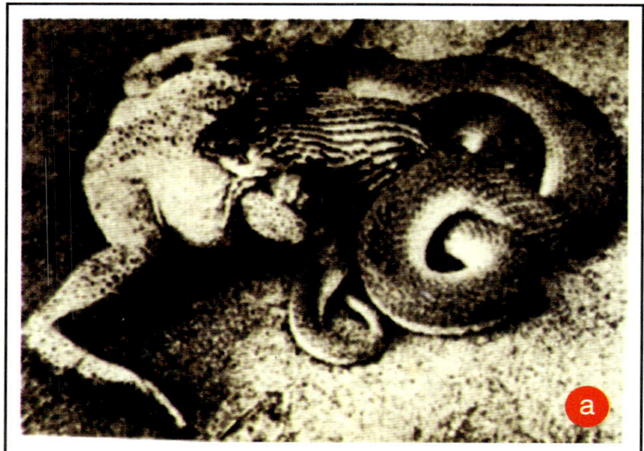

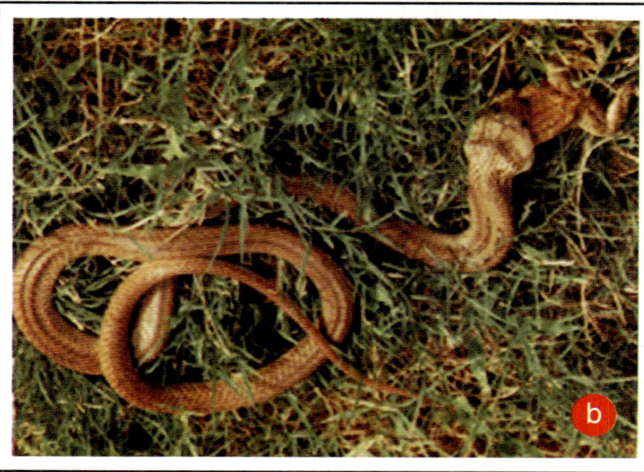

Figure 72: Predation for food in nature.Photographs showing: (a) Cobra swallowing toad in 1940 photo by O.C.Edwards (Pub. in a daily news paper). (b) Courtesy: Pune Snake Park

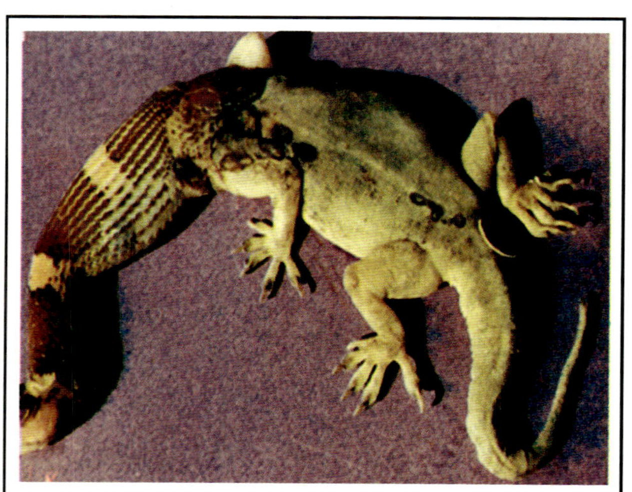

Figure 73: A snake while eating a lizard in an agriculture field was crushed under the tractor wheel.

Figure 74: A sharp object pierced the body of monitor lizard into disbowelling (*V. bengalensis*) resulted with intestines coming out.

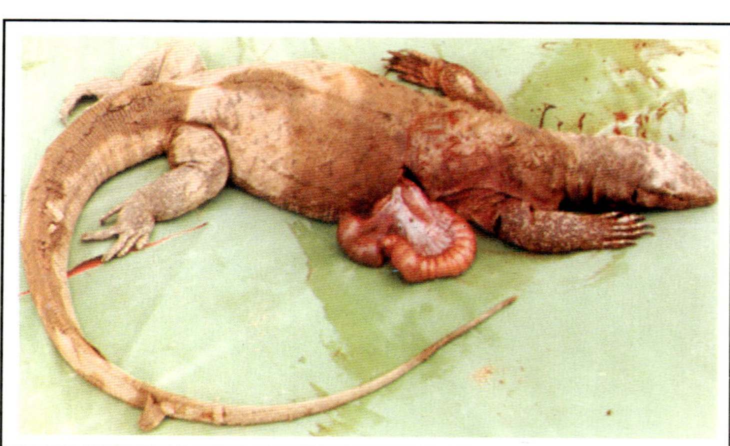

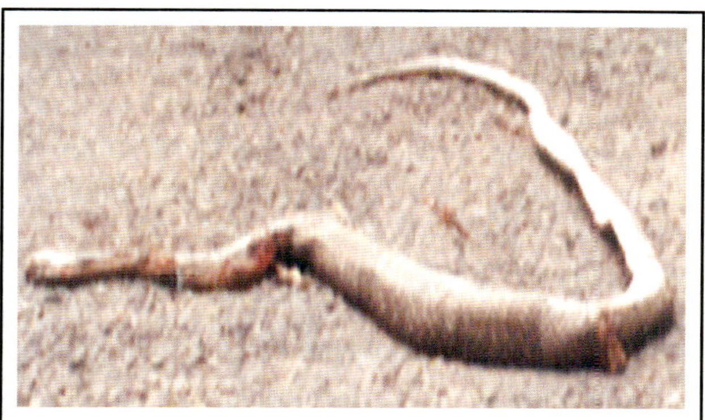

Figure 75: Russell's snake (*Vipera ruselli*) crushed by a speedy vehicle.

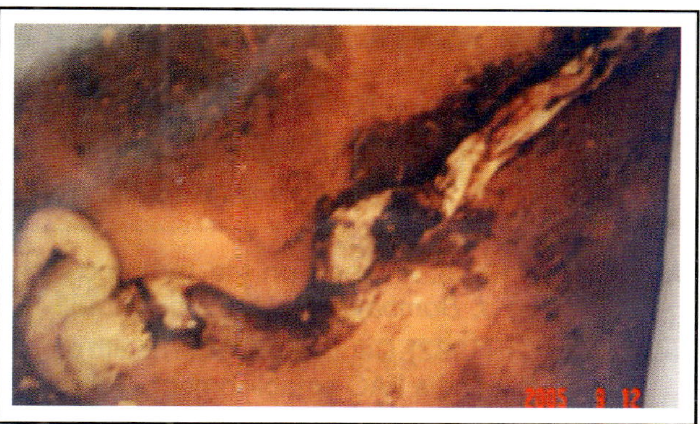

Figure 76: An adult python (*Python molurus*) burnt by miscreants in a captive facility.

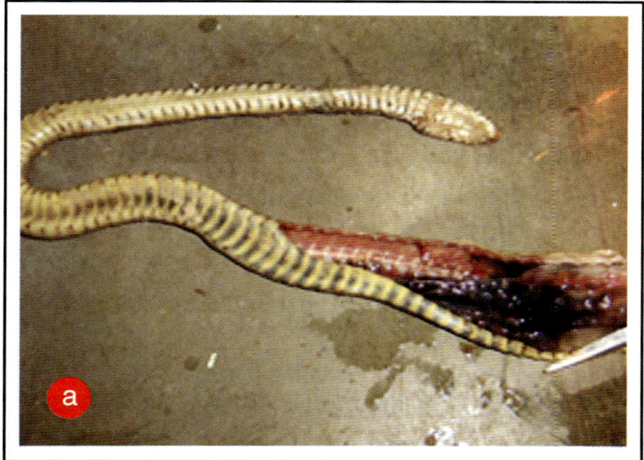

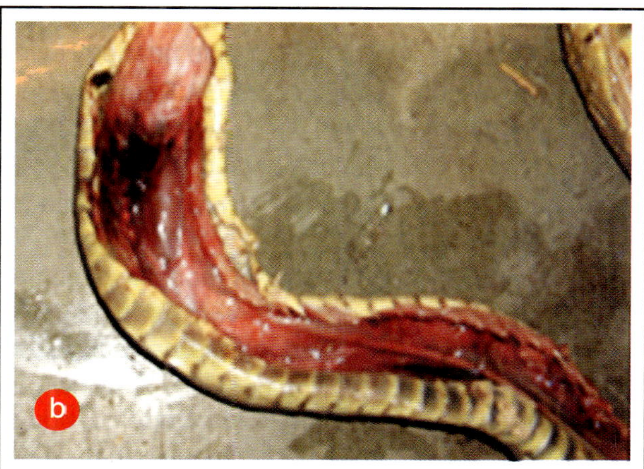

Figure 77: (a,b) Photograph of a dissected dhamin snake (*Ptyas mucosus*) showing haemorrhages throughout its body). It was pulled out forcibly from a pit and then kept in captivity to feed to king cobra (*O. hannah*). However, it had died after two days of its capture.

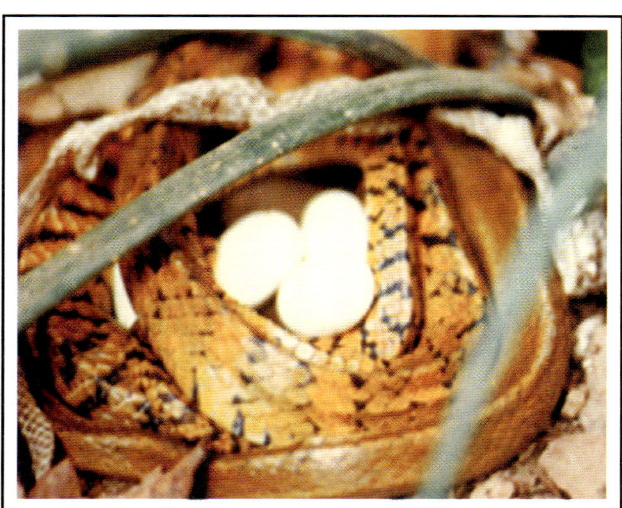

Figure 78: Photograph showing signs of dehydration of a rat snake incubating eggs at Snake Park, Pune (MS).

Name of Contributor	Figure No.
Dr. Garg, U.K. Associate Professor of Pathology, College of Vet. Sci. Mhow (M.P)	Mammals: 331(a); 388
Mr. Gupta, B. K. Scientist C.Z.A., Bikaner House, New Delhi-110011	Aves: 67 Reptiles: 45(b)
Dr. Gupta, M.P. Associate Professor Dept. of Veterinary and A.H. Extension GADVASU, Ludhiana (Pb)	Mammals: 14; 90; 119
Dr. Gupta, V. K. Associate Professor, Dept. of Veterinary Pathology, College of Vet. Sci.& Animal Sciences, Palmpur-176062 (H.P)	Mammals: 303; 350;
Dr. Harish, B. R., Institute of Animal Health & Vet Biologicals, Southern Regional Disease Diagnostic laboratory, (Min. of Agriculture), Banglore, Karnataka	Mammals: 33; 276(b); 318; 322; 333; 369; 386; 511; 557; 686; 726; 727(a); 733;743; 752; Reptiles: 10; 24
Dr. Illayaraja, S. Wildlife Veterinary Officer, Wildlife S.O.S(R) Agra Bear Rescue Centre, Agra (U.P) .	570; 572(a); 587
Dr. Jadav, K.K. Wildlife Veterinary Officer, Wildlife S.O.S(R) Agra Bear Rescue Centre, Agra (U.P)	Mammals: 564; 572(a) Reptiles:14; 16
Dr. Jacob Alexander, ADCP, Clinical Laboratory District Vet. Centre, PMG, Junction, Kerala	Mammals: 13; 191; 192; 736.
Dr. Jani, R. G. Prof. of Medicine, Wildlife Health Centre College of Veterinary Science & A.H., Anand-388001(Gujarat)	Mammals: 277; 286(b); 361; 393; 700;
Dr. Jayathangrajan, M.G. Professor& Head, Dept of Wildlife Science, Madras Vet. College, Chennai-600007 (TN)	Reptiles: 5
Dr Jayakumar, C,.S Vet. Surgeon, Zoological Garden, Trivendrum, Kerala	Mammals: 13; 191; 192.
Mr. Joshi, H. C. Range Officer, Zoological Garden, Nainital (Uttarakhand)	Mammals: 414 (b); 422(a)
Dr. Kallappa, S. Veterinary Officer, Wildlife Division, Shimoga, Karnataka	Mammals: 318; 512(c); 535
Dr. Kanwar, M. S. Dept. of Surgery, College of Vet Sci& A.H, Palmpur (H.P.)	Mammals: 453; Aves: 60; 79.
Dr. Kishore bhai Kotecha, Wildlife Conservation Trust, Rajkot (Gujarat).	Mammals: 286 (a); 420
Dr. Kishtwaria, R.S. Associate Professor& Incharge Vet. Clinical Complex College of Vet. Sci & Animal Sciences, Palmpur -1760062	Mammals: 181; 207; 239; 313; 401 ;404; 421; 422(b); 585; 591 Aves : 16;
Dr. Lal Kishan, Assistant Director General (AS) ICAR, New Delhi	Mammals: 350

Name of Contributor	Figure No.
Mr. Mishra, K.K. Wildlife Conservationist & Nature photographer77 Kanal Road Shiv Colony, Lakhimpur Kheri (UP)	Reptiles: 55(b)
Dr. Mohapatra, H.K. Ex- Professor of Pathology , College of Veterinary Science, Bhubneshwar, Orissa	Reptiles: 21 (c)
Dr. Mukhopadhayay, S.K. Head, Dept. of Pathology, Faculty of Vet. & Animal Sciences, WBUAFS, Kolkatta-700037(WB)	Mammals: 100; 125
Dr. Mukit, A Veterinary Officer, Dept. of A.H., West Bengal	Aves: 73
Dr. Murthy, S. Vet. Officer Bannerghatta Zoological Park, Banglore (Karnataka)	Mammals: 325
Dr. Naga Raju, S. Former Assistant Director, Zoological garden, Mysore. Director of Extension, KVAFSU, Banglore	Mammals: 26 Aves: 89
Dr. Nair, N.D. Dept. of Pathology, College of Vet Sc., Thrissur, Kerala	Mammals: 785
Dr. Nanjappa, K.A. Deputy Director, Zoological Garden, Mysore (Karnataka)	Mammals: 85, 135, 356; 535; 650;666;
Dr. Nath, I. Associate Professor , Dept. of Surgery, College of Veterinary Science, Bhubneshwar (Orissa)	Mammals : 279(a); 365; 417; 434; 483; 705; Aves- 1(b) ;52 Reptiles:18
Dr. Nigam, P. WII, Chandrabani, Dehra Dun-248001 Uttrakhand	Mammals: 196; 483; 784(b)
Dr. Panda, S.K. Associate Professor of Pathology. Orissa College of Veterinary Science, Bhubneshwar (Orissa)	Mammals: 279(a); 365; 483; 705 Aves: 1(b) ; 51; 52
Mr. Pandey, R.K DFO Katarniaghat (UP)	Mammals: 450
Dr.Parihar,N.S. Ex-Head,Div.of Pathology,IVRI,Izatnagar (UP)	Mammals:556
Drs. Prald Shankar Choudhury & Vipin Vinayk Rao Deshmukh Nandini Hospital, Surat - Gujarat	Reptiles: 49
Dr. Pralay Mandal Forest Veterinary Officer Jaldapara WLS, West Bengal	Mammals: 95 Reptiles: 44 (b)
Dr. Ramman, N. Dept. of Parasitology, CVSc, Chennai (TN)	Aves: 3 to4

Name of Contributor	Figure No.
Dr. Ranukaprasad, C Institute of Animal Health& Vet Biologicals, Southern Regional Disease Diagnostic laboratory, (Min. of Agriculture), Banglore, Karnataka	Mammals: 92; 187; 557; 752;
Dr Sarma, K.K Associate Professor, Dept. of Surgery College of Vet. Sci, Guwahati-781022 (Assam).	Mammals: 735(b); 759; 766; 768 ;779; 789
Dr. Shanker, K.S.M. Deputy Director, Zoo& Wildlife Himalyan Zoological Park, Gangtok, Dikkim-737103	Mammals: 165; 394;
Dr. Sharma Deepak Padamaja Nadu Himalyan Zoological Park,Darjeeling-734101(WB).	Mammals: 574
Dr. Sharma, D.K. College of Vet. Sc, Guwahati, Assam	Mammals: 775
Dr. Shamistha Chakaraborty Dept of Pathology, C.V.Sc, Guwahati-781022 (Assam)	Mammals: 676; 781;
Dr. Sharma, A.K Principal Scientist Division of pathology, IVRI, Izatnagar (U.P).	Mammals: 347c; 576; 758
Dr. Shivashankar IAH&B, Bangalore (Karnataka)	Mammals: 33; 511
Dr. Singh, K.P., Senior Scientist, CADRAD, IVRI, Izatnagar-243122 (UP)	Mammals: 10; 49; 127
Mr. Singh, K. K. DFO, North Kheri, Lakhimput kheri (U.P)	Mammals: 549
Dr. Singh, R. Principal Scientist, CADRAD, IVRI, Izatnagar-243122 (UP)	Mammals: 302; 572 (b)
Dr. Singh, S. D. Principal Scientist, Div. of Pathology, IVRI, Izatnagar- 243122 (UP)	Aves: 47; 50; 58
Dr. Somesh Singh Assistant Professor (Wildlife Science), College of Forestry, A.A.I. - D.U, Allahabad-211007	Mammals: 32;116;129
Dr. Somvanshi, R. Principal Scientist& Head, Div. of Pathology, IVRI, Izatnagar-243122 (U.P)	Aves: 71
Dr. Srivastava , A.B. Professor, Dept. of Pathology, College of Vet. Sci.& A.H., Jabalpur-482001 (M.P)	Mammals: 15(b); 324; 331(b); 419; 609. Aves: 17(a)
Dr. Sudhan, N. A. Dean, College of Veterinary Science, SKUAST- Jammu (J&K)	Mammals 166, 189,
Dr. Subramanian, K.S. Assistant Professor Dept of Wildlife Science, Madras Vet. College, Chennai-600007 (TN)	Aves: 13

Name of Contributor	Figure No.
Dr. Suryawanshi, D.S. Assistant Professor, Dept of Pathology Bombay Veterinary College, Mumbai-400012 (MS)	Mammals: 9, 38; 87; 115; 118; 122; 136; 288b; 295; 326; 328; 344; 367; 377; 396. Aves: 11; 21; 32; 43; 59. Reptiles & Amphi: 1 to 4; 7; 9; 12; 13; 15: 20;21(i); 22; 25; 26; 28; 31; 48(a); 50
Dr. Talukdar, A. Wildlife Vet. Officer , Centre for Wildlife Rehabilitation & Conservation,, WTI, Kaziranga NP (Assam)	Mammals: 205; 484 ; 713; 647; 741; 761; Aves: 1(a); 9; 37; 42
Dr. Thirumurugan, R. Arignar Anna Zoological Park, Chennai	Mammals: 84; 289(c); 296; 354(a); 641; 670. Reptiles: 23;48(c)
Dr. Vishwanath, G.K. Vet. Officer, Bannerghatta, National Park, Banglore (Karnataka).	Mammals: 134,

List of Contributors: (B) Veterinary Institutes

Name organization	Figure No.
Dept of Pathology, College of Veterinary Science,Anand(Gujarat)	Mammals:351(a);429
Dept. of Wildlife Science, College of Veterinary Science, Bangalore, Karnataka	Mammals: 348
Dept. of Wildlife Science, College of Veterinary Science, Chennai (TN)	Mammals: 31; 36; 81(b); 189(b); 291; 354; 375; 520; 523; 525; 527. Aves: 53.
Dept of Pathology, College of Veterinary Science, Nagpur (MS).	Mammals: 15(a); 47;139 ; 288c; 282; 290(b); 338; 355; 373; 398;510; 531.
Dept of Pathology, College of Veterinary Science, Tirupati (AP)	Mammals: 91; 284; 360
Dept. of Preventive Medicine& Epidemiology, College of Veterinary Science, Mumbai(MS)	Mammals: 197
Indian Veterinary Research Institute, Izatnagar & Campus, Kolkata(WB)	Mammals: 12; 280(b); 515;723
ERN-Members, Wildlife Trust of India (WTI), NEW DELHI-110065	Mammals:269;799 Reptiles:49

ARTIODACTYLIDS : 1-119

AVES : 393-434

CARNIVORES : 121-285

NON-HUMAN PRIMATES : 287-320

PERISSODACTYLIDS : 327-347

PROBOSCIDS : 349-387

REPTILES & AMPHIBIANS : 435-472

RODENTS & PANGOLINS : 322-326